THE ASIAN SKIN

THE ASIAN SKIN
A REFERENCE COLOR ATLAS OF DERMATOLOGY

Edited by

GOH Chee Leok
MD, MBBS, M.Med (Int. Med), FRCP (Edin), FAMS
Senior Consultant Dermatologist
National Skin Center, Singapore

CHUA Sze Hon
MBBS, FRCP (Edin), FAMS
Senior Consultant Dermatologist
National Skin Center, Singapore

NG See Ket
MBBS, M.Med (Int. Med)
Senior Consultant Dermatologist
National Skin Center, Singapore

Mc Graw Hill

Singapore • Boston • Burr Ridge, IL • Dubuque, IA • Madison, WI • New York • San Francisco
St. Louis • Bangkok • Bogotá • Caracas • Kuala Lumpur • Lisbon • London • Madrid
Mexico City • Milan • Montreal • New Delhi • Santiago • Seoul • Sydney • Taipei • Toronto

The Asian Skin
A Reference Color Atlas of Dermatology

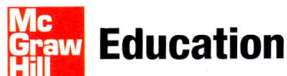

McGraw Hill Education

1 2 3 4 5 6 7 8 9 10 MPM 09 08 07 06 05

When ordering this title, use ISBN 007-124119-1

Printed in Singapore

Contributors

ANG Por
MBBS, MRCP (UK), FAMS
Consultant Dermatologist
National Skin Center, Singapore

CHAN Roy Kum Wah
MBBS, FRCP (Lond),
Dip. Derm (Lond), Dip. Ven (Lond), FAMS
Senior Consultant Dermatologist
National Skin Center, Singapore

CHAN Yuin Chew
MBBS, MRCP (UK)
Associate Consultant Dermatologist
National Skin Center, Singapore

CHIO Martin Tze-Wei
MBChB, MRCP (UK)
Registrar
National Skin Center, Singapore

CHONG Wei Sheng
MBBS, MRCP (UK), M.Med (Int. Med)
Registrar
National Skin Center, Singapore

CHUA Sze Hon
MBBS, FRCP (Edin), FAMS
Senior Consultant Dermatologist
National Skin Center, Singapore

EE Melvin Hock Leong
MBChB, MRCP (UK)
Registrar
National Skin Center, Singapore

FOO Christopher Csian Ian
MBBS, MRCP (UK)
Registrar
National Skin Center, Singapore

GIAM Yoke Chin
MBBS, M.Med (Paed), FAMS
Senior Consultant Dermatologist
National Skin Center, Singapore

GOH Boon Kee
MBChB, MRCP (UK)
Registrar
National Skin Center, Singapore

GOH Chee Leok
MD, MBBS, M.Med (Int. Med),
FRCP (Edin), FAMS
Senior Consultant Dermatologist
National Skin Center, Singapore

GOON Anthony Teik Jin
MBBS, MRCP (UK), FAMS
Consultant Dermatologist
National Skin Center, Singapore

KHOO Lawrence Shih Wee
MBBS, MRCP (UK), FAMS
Senior Consultant Dermatologist
National Skin Center, Singapore

KWAH Raymond Yung Chien
MBBS, MRCP (UK)
Registrar
National Skin Center, Singapore

LEE Joyce Siong See
MBBS, MRCP (UK), M.Med (Int. Med)
Associate Consultant Dermatologist
National Skin Center, Singapore

LEOW Yung Hian
MBBS, M.Med (Int. Med), FAMS
Senior Consultant Dermatologist
National Skin Center, Singapore

LOH Henry Teck Hong
MBBS, MRCP (UK)
Associate Consultant Dermatologist
National Skin Center, Singapore

NG Patricia Pei Lin
MBBS, MRCP (UK), FAMS
Consultant Dermatologist
National Skin Center, Singapore

OOI Colin Gek Ghee
MBBS (Adelaide)
Assistant Registrar
National Skin Center, Singapore

Prasad KUMARASINGHE
MBBS, MD
Senior Consultant Dermatologist
National Skin Center, Singapore

Priya SEN
MBBS, MRCP (UK)
Associate Consultant Dermatologist
National Skin Center, Singapore

SEOW Chew Swee
MBBS, M.Med (Int. Med)
Senior Consultant Dermatologist
National Skin Center, Singapore

TAN Hiok Hee
MBBS, MRCP (UK), FAMS
Consultant Dermatologist
National Skin Center, Singapore

TAN Suat Hoon
MBBS, M.Med (Int. Med),
Dip. RC Path (DMT), FAMS
Senior Consultant Dermatologist
National Skin Center, Singapore

TAN Audrey Wei Hsia
MBBS, MRCP (UK), M.Med (Int. Med)
Associate Consultant Dermatologist
National Skin Center, Singapore

TANG Mark Boon Yang
MBBS, MRCP (UK), M.Med (Int. Med)
Associate Consultant Dermatologist
National Skin Center, Singapore

THENG Colin Thiam Seng
MBBS, MRCP (UK), M.Med (Fam. Med)
Registrar
National Skin Center, Singapore

WONG Siew Ngoh
MBBS, MRCP (UK), Dip. Derm (Lond)
Senior Consultant Dermatologist
National Skin Center, Singapore

WONG Su-Ni
MBBS, MRCP (UK), M.Med (Int. Med),
FAMS
Associate Consultant Dermatologist
National Skin Center, Singapore

Contents

Foreword I

Although the cellular and molecular elements of skin of all races are basically the same, some quantitative and qualitative differences exist. These differences account for the different hues that are seen in the skin of various individuals and for a small number of the variations that are seen in the clinical presentations of various diseases in individuals of varied racial and ethnic backgrounds. Clinical experience and literature reviews indicate that certain skin diseases are indeed more common in some racial and ethnic groups and that some commonly occurring diseases may have widely varying clinical presentations. Psoriasis, atopic dermatitis, lichen simplex chronicus, melanoma and many other diseases have varied clinical presentations amongst individuals of Caucasian, Asian and African backgrounds. Environmental and behavioral differences as well as local customs may also contribute to the varied clinical diseases and presentations seen in these individuals. Making a correct diagnosis often depends on knowledge of these differences.

The Asian Skin: A Reference Color Atlas of Dermatology is a comprehensive pictorial illustration of a spectrum of skin diseases seen in Asian individuals. Virtually all of the clinical photos come from Singapore's National Skin Center, an internationally renowned clinical, research and teaching center. The extensive clinical experience of the Center is captured in the Atlas.

The Atlas will serve the many general physicians and dermatology specialists throughout Asia because it focuses directly on the presentation of skin diseases in people indigenous to this part of the world. It will also serve physicians in other parts of the world because Asians comprise a considerable percentage of the population in many major metropolitan areas throughout the world.

Congratulations to Professor C.L. Goh and Doctors S.H. Chua and S.K. Ng and their many colleagues at the National Skin Center for compiling this impressive atlas and for providing the succinct commentaries that accompany the illustrations.

STEPHEN I. KATZ, MD, PHD
Director, National Institute of Arthritis and
Musculoskeletal and Skin Diseases
National Institutes of Health
Department of Health and Human Services
Bethesda, Maryland

Foreword II

Almost 30 years ago, I left Melbourne to undertake further postgraduate study at St John's Hospital for Diseases of the Skin in London. At that time, there was a large population of people with colored skin who were presenting, along with other English people, for treatment of common skin diseases at St John's Hospital. The first patient I saw with dark skin had an itchy skin eruption that I was unable to diagnose. I asked my senior consultant, Professor Malcolm Greaves, what was this condition. He replied "Eczema. You are obviously not used to looking at skin conditions in people with colored skin!" It became very clear to me then that there is a difference in appearance of the same skin condition in people with different skin types. There is also a predisposition for different skin conditions in people from different parts of the world, unrelated to skin color.

This Atlas fulfills the criteria of illustrating a wide range of skin conditions in Asian people. It gives a clear demonstration of the clinical appearance of many common and not so common skin conditions in people with Asian skin. It also presents examples of skin conditions that tend to be more common amongst or are peculiar to Asian people, either because of their cultural practices or because of their genetic constitution.

The world is becoming a smaller place for many reasons, not the least of which is the ease of movement of individuals and populations from one region to another. Asian people have always migrated, not only within their own region, but also to many other parts of the world. There are substantial populations of Asian people now living in many countries throughout the world. Classic examples include the United Kingdom, the United States, Canada and Australia. But there are many more. Thus, an Atlas like this will have value in not only the traditional regions of the Asian countries, but also in many more countries to which large numbers of Asian people have migrated and now live.

Twenty-first century dermatologists, and other medical practitioners providing care for people with cutaneous disease, all need to be aware of the variations that occur in the clinical appearance of these diseases when they occur in people with different skin types. This Atlas attempts to fill a gap. I am sure it will enhance the medical practitioner's ability to reach the correct diagnosis. This, in turn, will permit the correct therapy to be selected, where appropriate, for these people both in the Asian region and in the many other countries throughout the world in which they are living.

ROBIN MARKS, MBBS, MPH, FRACP, FACD
Professor of Dermatology
University of Melbourne
Department of Medicine (Dermatology)
St Vincent's Hospital
Melbourne, Australia

Preface

Several excellent color atlases of dermatology already exist but most depict dermatoses affecting Caucasian skin, whilst very few devote themselves to Asian skin. Dermatologists in Asia have long noticed that certain dermatoses affecting the Asians have different clinical appearances from those affecting Caucasians. This is due to the inherent differences in skin color in the different races. The different pigmentary responses following skin inflammation and injury also contribute to the characteristic clinical presentation of dermatoses in Asians. In addition, inherent genetic differences and unique Asian cultural practices may also influence the characteristic presentation of various dermatoses in Asians.

This dermatologic atlas on Asian skin was motivated by the ever-growing need for a reference color atlas that depicts the characteristics of dermatoses that are uniquely seen in Asians. It also includes dermatoses that primarily affect Asians. Most of the color pictures in this atlas comes from the medical photograph archives of the National Skin Center, Singapore, a tertiary skin referral skin center which attends to a predominant Asian population of multi-racial and multi-cultural origins.

The authors believe that this color atlas will complement existing dermatologic atlases. The contents will be particularly informative to dermatologists in Asia. With widespread global travel and emigration, Asians are present in sizeable communities in most major cities of the world. Hence, this atlas will also be a useful reference guide for dermatologists in other countries outside Asia.

This atlas is divided into 18 chapters that cover a comprehensive range of dermatologic conditions. The division of chapters is based on either morphologic presentation of the dermatoses, e.g. acneiform disorders, papulosquamous disorders; by etiology of the dermatoses, e.g. infections and infestations; or by dermatologic subspecialty, e.g. photodermatology, immunodermatology. The last two chapters are devoted to dermato-venereology. A degree of repetition and overlap may occur in some chapters but this is kept minimal. Each chapter begins with an introduction which gives the reader a general overview of the topic and the captions of each color plate contain succinct and up-to-date information about the dermatoses depicted.

The authors hope that this atlas will serve as a useful pictorial reference and a valuable companion to the dermatology textbook for all dermatologists in Asia and other parts of the world.

Acneiform Disorders

Chong W.S. and Wong S.N.

Acneiform disorders are conditions which are characterized by the presence of non-inflammatory comedones and/or inflammatory papules or pustules centered around the pilosebaceous units. Acne vulgaris is one of the most common dermatological problems affecting adolescents and young adults. Mimics of acne vulgaris, presenting with acne-like lesions, are not uncommon. A careful history (with particular attention to the occupation, drug ingestion, medicament application and contactant exposure) together with clinical examination (with particular attention to the site of involvement and special morphological features) allows differential diagnoses to be made in most cases. In more difficult cases, a skin biopsy for histology may be helpful.

ACNE VULGARIS (Figures 1–1 to 1–9)

Acne vulgaris, the archetype of the acneiform disorders, is a common chronic inflammatory disease of the pilosebaceous unit. It is characterized by the formation of non-inflammatory comedones and inflammatory papules, pustules, nodules, and cysts. Acne is extremely common, affecting about four in five (80%) of adolescents and young adults aged 11 to 30 years. Although acne usually starts during the teenage years, it can start for the first time in their 20s or 30s.

The lesions usually involve the face, back, and chest, with associated seborrhea of varying severity. A combination of non-inflammatory comedones and inflammatory lesions is often present. Severe inflammation may result in the formation of fluctuant cysts and sinus tracts. Inflammatory lesions may heal with scarring with the risk greatest in nodulocystic variants of acne vulgaris. Acne scars include ice-pick, boxcar, rolling, hypertrophic and keloidal scars. Hyperpigmentation often accompanies acne scars, especially in darker-skinned Asians, as a result of inflammation or from treatment with minocycline.

Although acne vulgaris may not lead to serious medical complications, its psycho-social impact can be tremendous. Adolescents and young adults affected by severe acne often have a poorer quality of life due to diminished self-image and negative perception by peers. Permanent scars left by acne may cause negative psycho-social effects years after the acne has subsided.

OCCUPATIONAL ACNE

Jobs that involve contact with certain chemicals may result in worsening of acne or may cause acne. These chemicals include insoluble cutting oils (in the engineering and manufacturing industries), crude petroleum (in the oil refinery industry), diesel oil (in motor mechanics), and halogenated aromatic hydrocarbons (in industries manufacturing conductors/insulators and insecticides/fungicides/herbicides).

DRUG-INDUCED ACNE

Certain drugs are well-documented to aggravate or even cause acne. These include corticosteroids given either orally or systemically, lithium which is used to treat manic-depressive illness, testosterone pills or injections which may be used by professional athletes and bodybuilders to increase muscle mass, and danazol, which is given to women for endometriosis. Other acnegenic drugs include isoniazid and phenytoin. Cushing's syndrome resulting from endogenous cortisol excess may present with steroid acne in addition to other clinical features such as moon facies, buffalo hump, supraclavicular fat pads, centripetal obesity, and abdominal striae.

COSMETIC ACNE

Most people using cosmetic products do not experience any acne problem, but a small group of cosmetic users do develop cosmetic acne. This presents as multiple small comedones over the face where the cosmetic has been applied. Since cosmetic acne usually appears gradually after several months of repeated use of a comedogenic product, many do not connect their outbreaks with the given product. The woman with cosmetic acne suffers a vicious cycle: the more acne she has, the more make-up she uses to cover it up and this only leads to a worsening of the acne. Ingredients in cosmetics that may aggravate acne include lanolin, analogs of isopropyl myristate, algae extract, cocoa butter, laureth-4, lauric acid, octyl palmitate, coconut oil, and D&C red pigments.

ACNE EXCORIÉE

This is a form of neurotic excoriation where the underlying primary psychiatric disorder is often an obsessive-compulsive disorder. Scarring and pigmentary changes can result. Behavioral and psychotherapeutic intervention in combination with medication such as fluoxetine and paroxetine are often needed to decrease the compulsive urge to pick at the acne.

ROSACEA

Rosacea is less commonly seen in Asians as compared to Caucasians. In rosacea, the centro-facial area is predominantly affected with papules, papulopustules, erythema, telangiectasia and flushing episodes. Comedones are notably absent. In severe cases, papules are numerous enough to be confluent. Rosacea patients are predisposed to blushing and flushing. Sunlight and heat are aggravating factors. Useful therapy includes topical metronidazole gel and systemic tetracyclines. A relapsing course is common.

INFECTIVE ACNEIFORM LESIONS

Infections resulting in acneiform lesions may mimic acne vulgaris. Gram-negative folliculitis is a complication of long-term treatment of acne vulgaris with oral antibiotics. It is a gram-negative bacterial infection and presents as inflammatory papules and pustules. Pityrosporum folliculitis is caused by the organism *Malassezia furfur*. It usually presents as a sudden eruption of monomorphic papules and pustules over the shoulders and upper trunk of healthy young adults, especially those working in hot, humid environments.

ACNE AGMINATA

Acne agminata, formerly known as *lupus miliaris disseminatus faciei*, is an uncommon condition which presents with brownish or red, closely packed acneiform papules on the face. It is now generally accepted that acne agminata is a variant of rosacea and is not related to tuberculosis. The cause remains unknown. Possible inciting antigens suggested by different authors include disintegrating hair follicles, degenerating elastic fibers, and *Demodex folliculorum* mites. However, evidence to prove the direct pathogenetic role of these agents remains elusive.

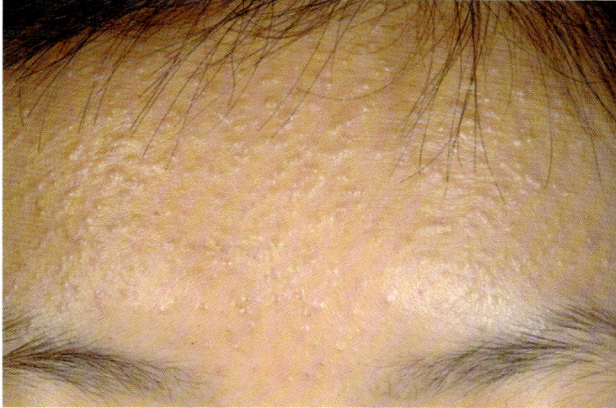

Figure 1–1 □ Acne vulgaris – closed comedones. Acne vulgaris makes its debut with the non-inflammatory lesions or comedones which can be classified as closed or open. Closed comedones are also known as whiteheads. They are small, whitish keratin-filled papules found on the face, chest, and back. This young lady has multiple closed comedones located on the forehead.

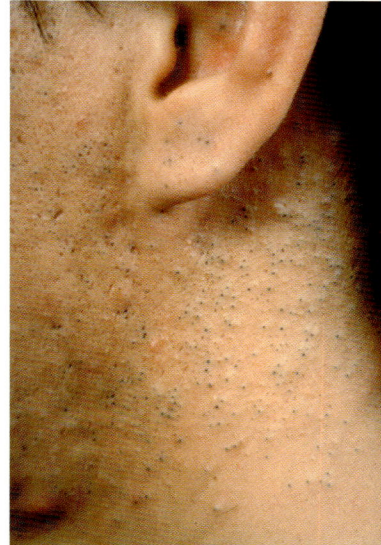

Figure 1–2 □ Acne vulgaris – open comedones. These non-inflammatory acne lesions are also known as blackheads. The black color is due to melanin. They may progress to inflammatory papules and pustules. This young man has multiple open comedones involving the left cheek and left side of his neck. Comedones may be treated with comedolytic agents such as the topical retinoids. Persistent lesions may be removed by physical methods such as comedone extraction and light electrocautery.

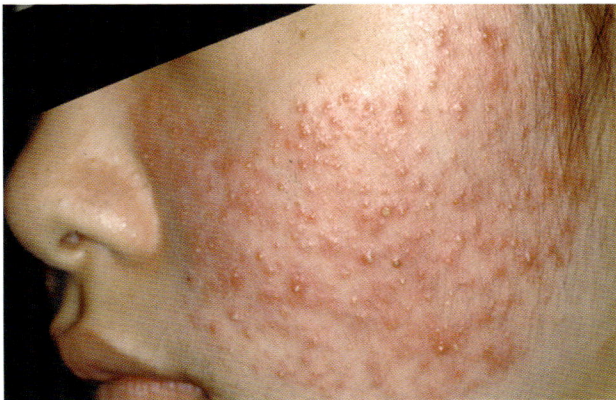

Figure 1–3 □ Acne vulgaris – papulo-pustular lesions. Comedones can secondarily develop into inflammatory papules and pustules. These papules and pustules may progress to inflammatory nodules and cysts, with subsequent scarring. This lady has multiple inflammatory papules and pustules on her cheeks.

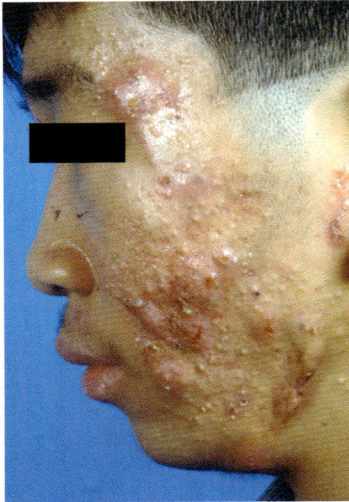

Figure 1–4 □ Nodulocystic acne. The inflammatory lesions consist of deep-seated nodules and cysts. Acne cysts are not true cysts as they are not lined by an epithelium. Such lesions can be very painful. These inflammatory nodules and cysts can result in extensive scarring. This man has multiple inflamed nodules and cysts involving his temples, cheeks, and sides of his face.

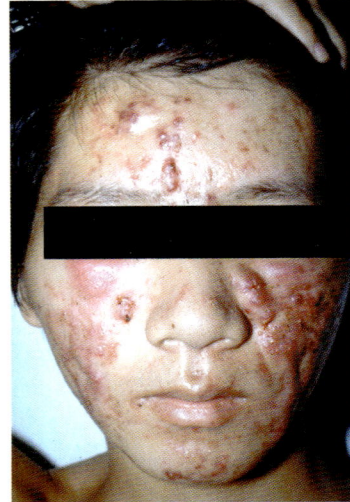

Figure 1–5 □ Acne conglobata. This is the most uncommon but severe form of acne, with lesions occurring on the face, trunk, and upper limbs. Nodules are characteristic, fusing to form multiple draining sinuses. Extensive scarring often results. Early and aggressive treatment, often with the use of systemic isotretinoin, is needed to minimize the risk of scarring in this severe variant of acne vulgaris.

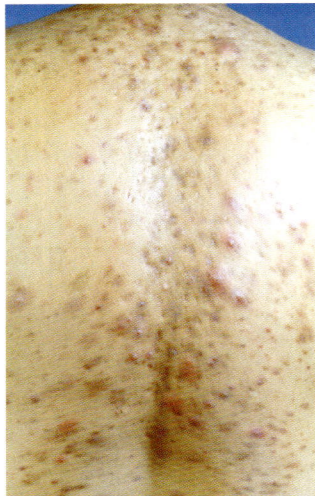

Figure 1–6 □ Truncal acne. This condition presents as inflamed papules, pustules, and small nodules located on the upper chest and back. Truncal acne is often quite persistent, often lasting months and years with a fluctuating course. Response to conventional acne therapy is generally slower compared to facial acne.

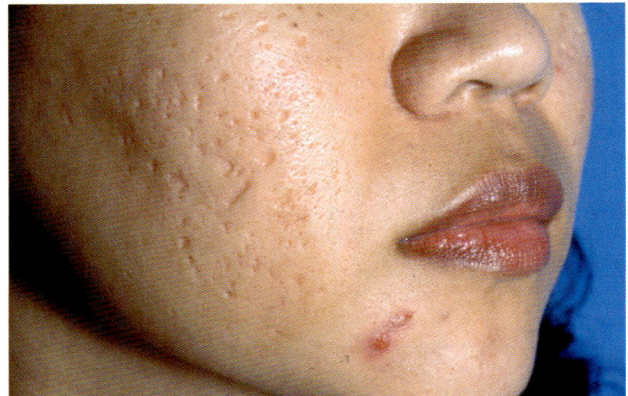

Figure 1–7 □ Acne scars – box-car, ice-pick. Depressed acne scars are the most common type of acne scars. They vary in their appearance and depth. Dermatologists classify them as ice-pick scars (narrow, deep-pitted scars), box-car type scars (round and oval depressions with sharply demarcated vertical edges), and rolling scars (scars with an undulating appearance of the overlying skin) to fine-tune their techniques to improve them. In most patients, a combination of the above types of acne scars is often present.

This young lady has multiple box-car and ice-pick acne scars on her cheeks.

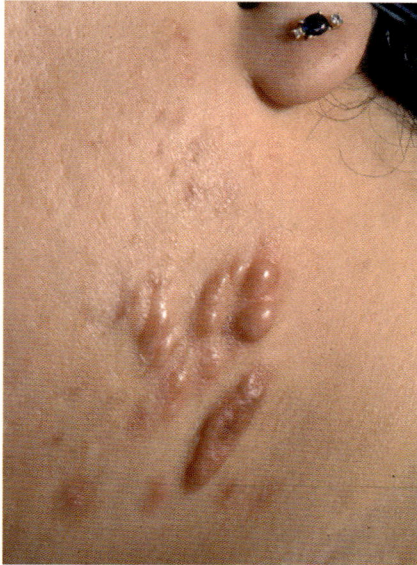

Figure 1–8 □ Acne scars – keloidal. These are thickened and cord-like scars resulting from excessive scar tissue. Such scars are more frequently seen in individuals with a past history of keloid formation. Keloidal acne scars are more common over the jaw line, anterior chest, and shoulder region. This lady has multiple flesh- to red-colored keloidal acne scars along the jaw line.

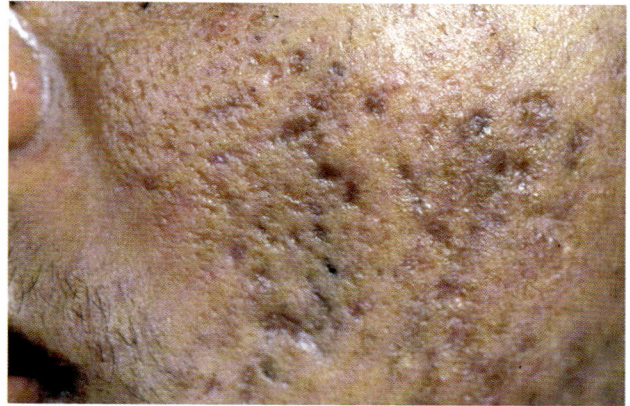

Figure 1–9 □ Acne scars – minocycline-induced hyper-pigmentation. Pigmentation is sometimes seen with minocycline which is commonly used in the treatment of acne vulgaris. One presentation is bluish-black discoloration seen in and around acne scars. The pigmentation is due to the interaction of minocycline with iron in the dermis, basal hypermelanosis, and quinone-like derivative formed by oxidation of minocycline. Cessation of minocycline often leads to gradual clearance of the pigmentation over weeks.

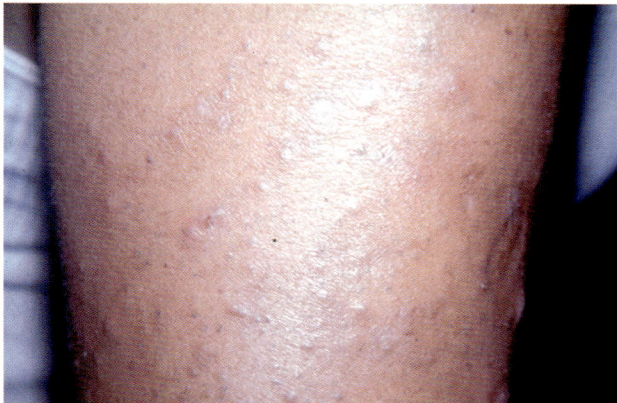

Figure 1–10 □ Occupational acne due to oils and tars. This is an uncommon acneiform eruption occurring in areas in contact with oils and tars. It affects workers in the oilfield, refinery and engineering industries. Comedones are prominent with occasional inflammatory papules and pustules. The thighs and lower arms are especially affected although any site may be involved. This oil refinery worker with occupational acne presents with multiple comedones with few inflammatory papules over his lower arms.

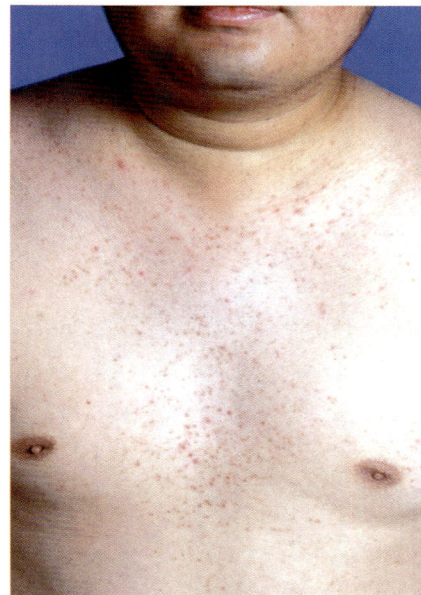

Figure 1–11 □ Steroid acne. Corticosteroids may provoke an acneiform eruption whether they are given orally, topically, or intramuscularly. They induce cornification in the upper part of the pilosebaceous duct. Comedones, inflamed papules, and pustules may be present on the face, back, and chest. The inflammatory lesions are more monomorphic than those seen in acne vulgaris. This man who was started recently on oral prednisolone therapy for his nephrotic syndrome has developed steroid acne over his chest.

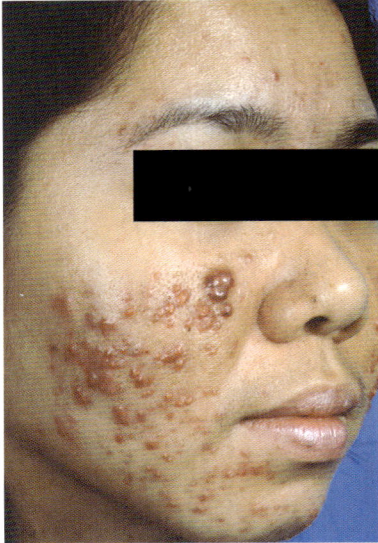

Figure 1–12 □ Drug-induced acne – isoniazid. Acne can be precipitated or aggravated by certain orally administered or topically applied agents. Anti-tuberculous drugs (isoniazid), anti-epileptics (phenytoin), and anti-psychotics (lithium) are some of the common drugs that can induce acne. This lady who received anti-tuberculous drugs including isoniazid for pulmonary tuberculosis subsequently developed acneiform lesions on her face four months after initiation of therapy.

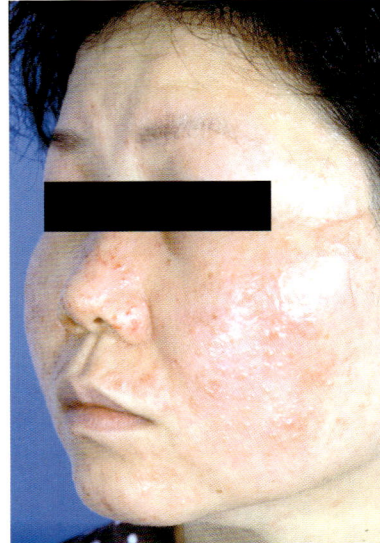

Figure 1–13 □ Cosmetic acne. This is associated with the use of comedogenic cosmetics. Most patients are young to middle-aged females who have been enthusiastic users of cosmetics. The acneiform lesions usually occur over the cheeks and perioral area after the comedogenic cosmetics have been used for several months. A list of comedogenic ingredients is available and patients must be taught to read the cosmetic labels carefully to avoid these ingredients.

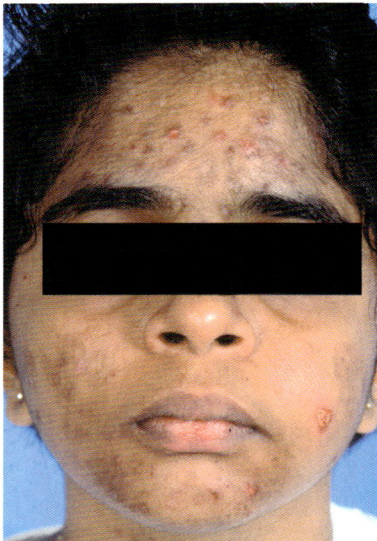

Figure 1–14 □ Acne excoriée. This variant of acne occurs primarily in females who have mild acne but excoriate even the smallest of lesions. There is often an underlying personality or psychiatric problem such as obsessive-compulsive disorder. Such patients may require a combination of oral antibiotics and anti-psychotic therapy. This Indian lady, who has underlying obsessive-compulsive disorder, has multiple self-inflicted excoriations on her forehead, cheeks, and chin with prominent post-inflammatory hyper-pigmentation typical in darker-skinned Asians.

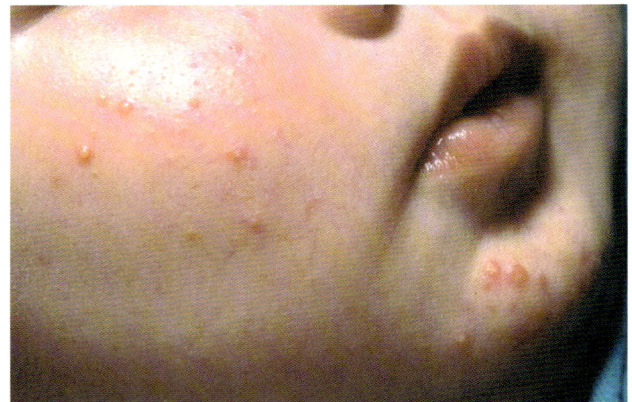

Figure 1–15 □ Infantile acne. This mainly occurs in a child between the ages of 3 to 24 months. Comedones, papules and pustules, are present, usually on the cheeks and chin. This condition is probably due to maternal androgenic hormonal influence. It is usually not associated with an underlying hyperandrogenic state. This three-month-old baby has multiple comedones, papules, and pustules on the cheeks and chin.

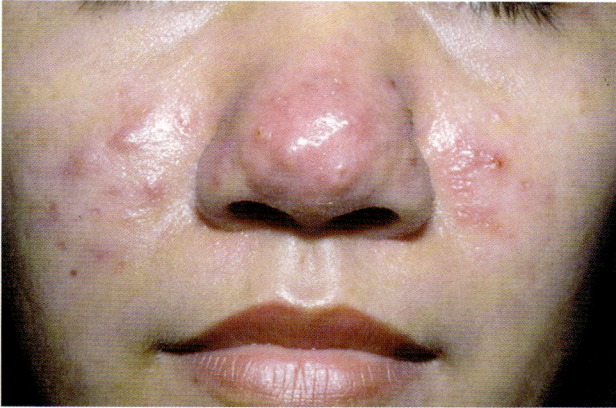

Figure 1–16 □ **Rosacea.** The lesions of rosacea which initially occur in the central convex areas of the face, consist of inflamed papules and pustules against a background of erythema, telangiectasia, edema, and eventual permanent induration and thickening of affected skin. It may present as gross enlargement and deformity of the nose (rhinophyma) in its most extreme form (see Figure 1–17). This lady has multiple inflammatory papules and pustules on a background of erythema and telangiectasia located on her cheeks and nose.

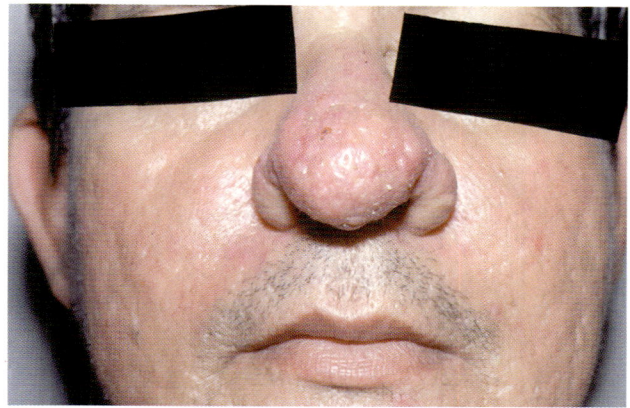

Figure 1–17 □ **Rhinophyma.** This man has rhinophyma, presenting with gross enlargement of the nose with telangiectasia and erythema.

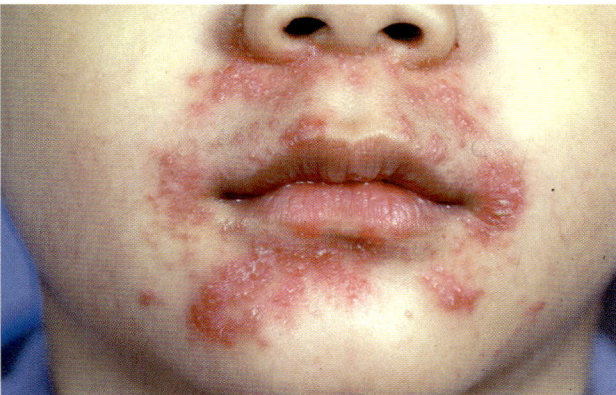

Figure 1–18 □ **Perioral dermatitis.** This is a persistent erythematous eruption consisting of tiny monomorphic papules and pustules with a distribution primarily around the perioral region. It is often a consequence of prolonged topical steroid application. This man developed multiple erythematous papules and pustules around his mouth after applying moderately potent topical steroid cream for his perioral eczema. Treatment with systemic tetracyclines and stopping further application of topical steroids to the affected areas are usually effective.

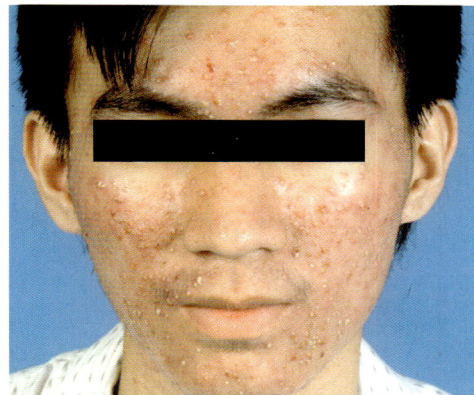

Figure 1–19 □ **Gram-negative folliculitis – face.** This is a complication of long-term treatment of acne with oral antibiotics. It presents with a sudden eruption of multiple small follicular pustules. Microbiological culture from the lesions usually reveals gram-negative organisms, such as *Escherichia coli*, *Klebsiella*, *Pseudomonas* or *Proteus species*. This young man presents with multiple inflamed pustules on his forehead, cheeks, chin, and neck three months after he was started on oral tetracycline for his acne vulgaris.

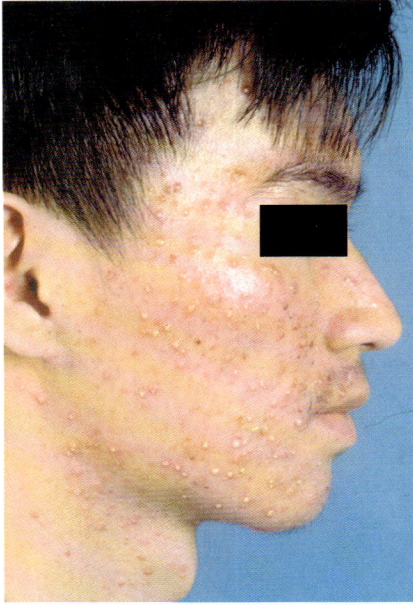

Figure 1–20 □ Gram-negative folliculitis – face. This view shows the same patient with multiple pustules on the side of his face and neck. Microbiological culture from the lesions grew *Escherichia coli,* and his lesions resolved quickly after treatment with systemic cotrimoxazole.

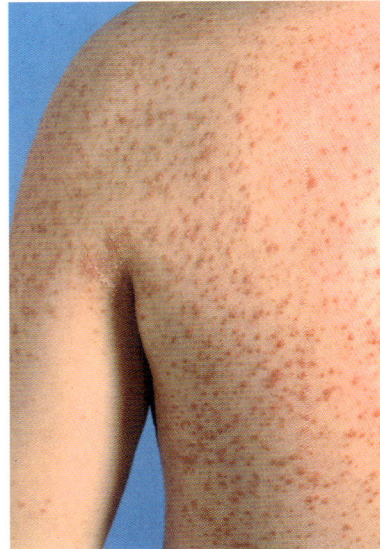

Figure 1–21 □ Pityrosporum folliculitis. This presents as multiple scattered monomorphic papules and pustules without the presence of comedones. This condition results from a host reaction to the normal skin commensal *Malassezia furfur.* In Singapore, this condition is most commonly seen as a sudden eruption of monomorphic acneiform papules and pustules over the shoulders and upper trunk of healthy young adults working in a hot, humid environment or serving their National Service in the army.

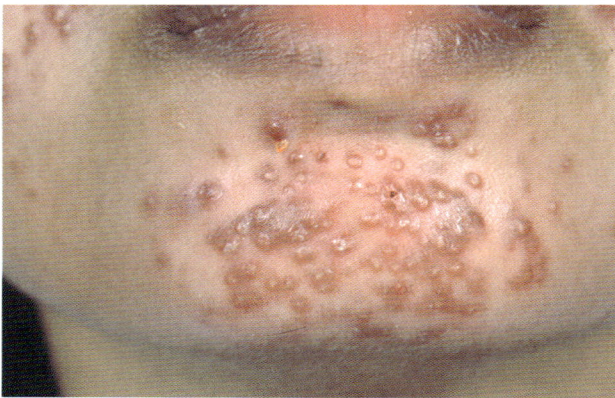

Figure 1–22 □ Acne agminata. This lady presents with multiple small discrete brownish papules over the chin. Acne agminata is a rare centro-facial papular eruption that usually occurs in young adults. Clinically, the condition presents with discrete flesh-colored or erythematous papules and pustules that characteristically involve the periorbital and muzzle area of the face. If left untreated, acne agminata runs a self-limiting course with spontaneous resolution of the lesions over 12 to 24 months, often leaving disfiguring scars. Early treatment is recommended to prevent scarring. Tetracyclines, dapsone, and clofazimine have been reported to be useful.

Eczema

Goh C.L., Goon A.T.J., and Ooi C.G.G.

Eczema or dermatitis is an inflammatory disorder of the skin caused by endogenous and exogenous factors. It is the most common skin disorder seen in most outpatient clinics as well as the most common skin disorder seen in Asians. Many Asian countries are located in the tropics where heat, humidity, and ultimately frequent perspiration tend to trigger or exacerbate eczema.

Eczema is a descriptive sign of superficial skin inflammation and its different phases are classified as acute, subacute, and chronic eczema (see Figures 2–1 to 2–4). Acute eczema presents clinically as erythema, papules, edema, vesiculation, and occasionally bullae. Chronic eczema presents as lichenified, scaly, erythematous patches, occasionally with fissures, excoriations, and pigmentary changes. Subacute eczema presents with mild erythema, edema, and occasional vesiculation. Other less common manifestations of eczema include prurigo and generalized exfoliative dermatitis.

Eczema is classified into endogenous and exogenous eczema. Endogenous eczema refers to a group of eczemas that are constitutional and often have a genetic basis. Exogenous eczema refers to the group of eczemas that is caused by an external agent and includes contact dermatitis and photocontact dermatitis.

ENDOGENOUS ECZEMA

Endogenous eczema can be classified according to its clinical presentation, course of disease, and prognosis. This group classically includes atopic eczema, discoid eczema, seborrheic eczema, stasis eczema, asteatotic eczema, hands and feet eczema, and lichen simplex chronicus. In addition, there remains a group of unclassifiable endogenous eczema whose pattern and clinical presentation do not fit into the above categories and in which no exogenous factors are identified. There is no diagnostic test for endogenous eczema. Diagnosis is based on clinical history, physical examination, and exclusion of exogenous eczema.

Atopic Dermatitis (Figures 2–5 to 2–13)

Atopic eczema is one of the most common endogenous eczemas, occurring in about 20% of the population in most countries, including those in Asia. Environmental and genetic factors contribute to this condition. Often, patients with atopic eczema have a personal or family history of asthma, eczema, or allergic rhinitis.

Eczema appears on the face and trunk during infancy and becomes predominantly flexural in distribution as the child grows older. Occasionally, eczema can be very extensive. Pruritus is often a predominant symptom.

Excoriation and lichenified patches develop quickly on the skin, especially on the flexures. Secondary bacterial infection with *Staphylococcus aureus* is common. The disease tends to run a chronic course to adulthood but childhood atopic eczema tends to improve toward puberty. As for Asian skin, post-inflammatory hyperpigmentation can be particularly prominent in previously affected areas.

Discoid Eczema (Figures 2–14 to 2–17)

Discoid eczema presents as well-circumscribed discoid or nummular eczematous patches on the limbs and occasionally on the trunk. It usually presents around adolescence and tends to persist for many years. The lesions of discoid eczema tend to be wet and oozy, with secondary *Staphylococcus aureus* infection. The lesions are often very pruritic and recalcitrant to treatment.

Seborrheic Eczema (Figures 2–18 to 2–21)

Seborrheic eczema tends to occur on seborrheic areas of the skin. It has a varied clinical presentation, with a yellowish greasy cradle cap on the scalps of infants; erythema with greasy scales on the nasolabial folds or cheeks, eyebrows, scalp, chest and back, axillae and groin areas. In adults, it usually appears in their 50s. Seborrheic eczema is often not pruritic and the eczema tends to persist.

Stasis Eczema (Figures 2–22 and 2–23)

Stasis eczema occurs on the lower legs and ankles. It is always associated with varicosities and tends to occur in the elderly. The medial malleolus is a particularly common presenting site. The clinical picture is characteriztic, appearing as dusky brown to black discoloration on the medial malleolus and lower legs. The pigmentary changes are due to deposition of hemosiderin in the skin. The skin is eczematous – dry, scaly, and edematous. Chronic ulcers may appear on the ankles. Secondary allergic contact dermatitis to topical medicament is common.

Asteatotic Eczema (Figures 2–24 and 2–25)

Asteatotic eczema is often seen in the elderly. The eczema presents as dry, scaly, inflamed, and "cracked" skin. It is also called eczema craquelé. It often occurs on the lower limbs and is often pruritic. Superficial fissuring on the anterior tibial aspect of the legs is the classical presentation, and the affected skin takes on a "cracked porcelain" appearance. Heat, low humidity, and excessive washing aggravate asteatotic eczema.

Hands and Feet Eczema (Figures 2–26 to 2–29)

Endogenous hands and feet eczema often presents as chronic eczema with periodic exacerbation. It is common amongst those exposed to irritants, especially housewives who do domestic chores. Hands and feet eczema is often multifactorial in etiology. Hands and feet eczema presents as dry, scaly, and erythematous patches on the dorsum and palms and soles of the hands and feet respectively. The palms and soles are often affected and painful fissuring on the finger and toe pulps and on the palms and soles may occur. Vesiculation, as a manifestation of eczema on the palms and soles, is referred to as pompholyx.

Lichen Simplex Chronicus (Figures 2–30 and 2–31)

Lichen simplex (neurodermatitis) presents as localized, well-circumscribed lichenified plaques. The plaques of lichen simplex chronicus result from repeated rubbing and scratching. Itch is a prominent symptom and the vicious cycle of scratch and itch results in lichenification. Besides lichenification, the plaques are often scaly with pigmentary changes. Excoriation is prominent. The common sites for lichen simplex chronicus are areas that are accessible to scratching, including the ankles, elbows, hands, neck and genitals (scrotum and vulva) and perineum.

Prurigo Nodularis (Figure 2–32)

Prurigo nodularis refers to firm lichenified nodules that can appear in patients with long-standing endogenous eczema. It is often aggravated by repeated rubbing and picking. The surface of the nodules is often excoriated. The nodules tend to appear on the limbs, but the trunk and face may also be affected.

Unclassifiable Endogenous Eczema

Unclassifiable endogenous eczema refers to a group of endogenous eczema that does not fit into any of those mentioned above. Patients often present with some features of atopic dermatitis with localized or generalized patchy eczema but do not have all the characteriztic features of atopic dermatitis.

Generalized Exfoliative Dermatitis (Figure 2–33)

Generalized exfoliative dermatitis (GED) refers to generalized skin erythema and exfoliation affecting more than 95% of the total body skin surface area. There are several causes of GED, including severe endogenous eczema (e.g. atopic dermatitis, seborrheic eczema), severe contact dermatitis, psoriasis, pityriasis rubra pilaris, drug eruptions, and malignancy (lymphoproliferative diseases). GED is often seen in the elderly and, in most cases, the exact cause cannot be ascertained. Patients with GED may have abnormalities in temperature regulation, hemodynamic problems leading to cardiac failure, fluid and electrolyte imbalance, and anemia.

EXOGENOUS ECZEMA

This refers to the group of eczema that develops after contact with a noxious substance or an allergen. Exogenous eczema includes contact dermatitis (irritant and allergic) and photocontact dermatitis (phototoxic and photo-allergic).

Whilst the majority of contact dermatitis is eczematous, some cases may present with non-eczematous lesions (Figures 2–75 to 2–78). These include erythema multiforme-like reactions (e.g. flavin), purpuric contact dermatitis (e.g. rubber chemicals), granulomatous eruptions (e.g. mercury and gold), and pigmented contact dermatitis (e.g. rubber chemicals).

Contact urticaria, although not eczematous in clinical presentation, is included in this chapter to complete the spectrum of contact skin reactions.

Irritant Contact Dermatitis (Figures 2–34, 2–35, 2–37 to 2–47)

Skin inflammation from direct noxious injury to the skin results in irritant contact dermatitis. Acute irritant dermatitis results from skin contact with strong irritants such as acid and alkali. Strong irritants cause acute irritant contact dermatitis in almost all individuals after only short contact. The clinical presentation progresses through erythema, vesiculation (occasionally absent), exudation, and sometimes erosions, and finally crusting, scaling, residual erythema, and post-inflammatory hyperpigmentation.

Cumulative insult irritant contact dermatitis occurs after multiple episodes of cumulative wear and tear damage due to one or more weak irritants, with the next insult occurring before complete recovery from the damage caused by the previous insult. This is the most common cause of contact dermatitis. Clinically, cumulative irritant contact dermatitis presents as chronic dermatitis with dry, scaly erythematous skin. This pattern of irritant contact dermatitis usually occurs in individuals who have an underlying predisposition, such as in those with atopic dermatitis. The most common irritants include water, detergents (contact from performing domestic chores), topical medicaments (especially counter-irritants and traditional medications), and solvents (contact at the workplace).

There is no diagnostic test for irritant contact dermatitis. Diagnosis is based on history, clinical features and a negative patch test.

Allergic Contact Dermatitis
(Figures 2–36, 2–48 to 2–78)

Allergic contact dermatitis is not due to direct injury, but rather due to an immune response mediated by sensitized T lymphocytes. This is a type IV delayed hypersensitivity reaction. Only individuals who have been exposed and sensitized to the allergen will develop allergic contact dermatitis. The process whereby the individual acquires allergy to a substance is called the *sensitization phase*, which takes at least four days. The *elicitation phase*, when the individual develops allergic contact dermatitis, occurs upon subsequent contact with the same allergen. This reaction peaks between 48 and 72 hours. The clinical spectrum of allergic contact dermatitis ranges from acute vesiculobullous eczema after contact with high doses of a strong allergen to chronic lichenified, fissuring eczema after repeated contact with low concentrations of a weak allergen. The common allergens in Asia include metals (nickel, chromates, cobalt), fragrance, medicaments, and preservatives.

Allergic contact dermatitis can be confirmed by a relevant positive patch test reaction. In patch testing, non-irritant concentrations of allergens are applied on the back for 48 hours and reactions recorded 48

hours after application of the patch and again after 96 hours. A positive reaction will appear as a localized eczematous patch.

Photocontact Dermatitis
(Figures 2–79 to 2–86)

Photocontact dermatitis occurs when a substance causes dermatitis only in the presence of ultraviolet light. There are two subtypes, *viz.* phototoxic contact dermatitis and photo-allergic contact dermatitis.

Phototoxic contact dermatitis may manifest as an exaggerated sunburn reaction (e.g. due to coal tar) or hyperpigmentation (e.g. from plant psoralens). It occurs in most patients exposed to the phototoxic substance.

Photo-allergic contact dermatitis is an immune reaction, presenting as eczematous eruptions like allergic contact dermatitis. Common photocontact allergens include topical anti-inflammatory agents (e.g. indomethacin, ibuprofen, diclofenac gels), sunscreens, antiseptics (e.g. in medicated soaps), topical medicaments (e.g. phenergan, chlorpromazine), plants, and some fragrances.

Photo-allergic contact dermatitis can be confirmed by a positive photopatch test. The photopatch test procedure is similar to the patch test procedure, except that a duplicate set of test allergens is irradiated with UVA at 48 hours.

Contact Urticaria (Figures 2–87 and 2–88)

Contact urticaria is an adverse contact reaction where an urticarial eruption develops at the site of contact with an offending substance. This reaction occurs rapidly (within 20 minutes) and disappears within one to several hours. Repeated contact urticaria can present with eczematous lesions (protein contact dermatitis). Contact urticaria may be immunologically or non-immunologically mediated. The former reaction is usually localized. It is an immediate hypersensitivity (type I hypersensitivity reaction which is IgE-mediated) reaction and may be life-threatening and complicated by anaphylaxis. The common causes of allergic contact urticaria are natural rubber latex proteins, proteinaceous foodstuff (e.g. seafood and meat), and plants (e.g. vegetables). Immunologic contact urticaria can be confirmed by a skin prick test and occasionally a RAST test. Non-immunological contact urticaria is caused by histamine releasers, e.g. drugs such as codeine, and food additives such as lactic acid and sorbic acid.

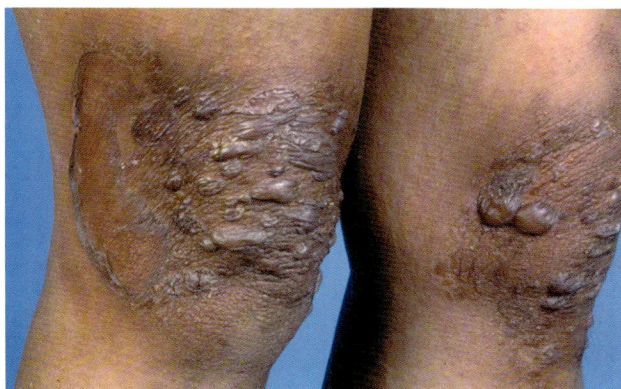

Figure 2–1 □ Acute eczema. This picture illustrates the features of acute dermatitis involving the extensor surface of the knees. There is erythema, edema, weeping, and a vesicobullous reaction. This has occurred in a patient with irritant contact dermatitis due to dithranol. Acute dermatitis may occur as part of endogenous eczema or develop as part of allergic or irritant contact dermatitis reactions.

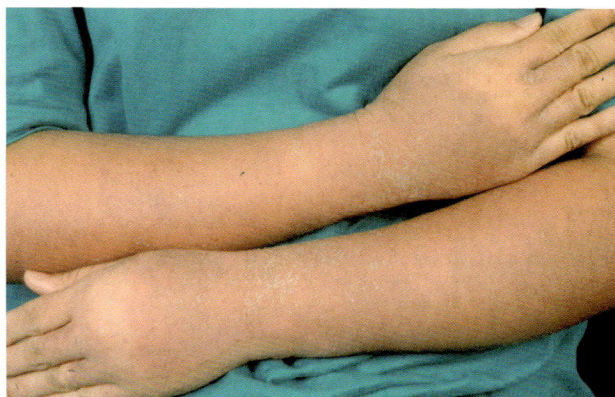

Figure 2–2 □ Subacute eczema. This patient has a non-vesicular form of irritant contact dermatitis from coolants. There is subacute eczematous involvement of both forearms. Subacute eczema has features midway between acute and chronic forms of eczema. Rather than seeing florid erythema and weeping, the erythema of subacute eczema is less intense than that seen in acute eczema. Scales and crusting are often seen as the acute eczema heals and subacute features become more prominent.

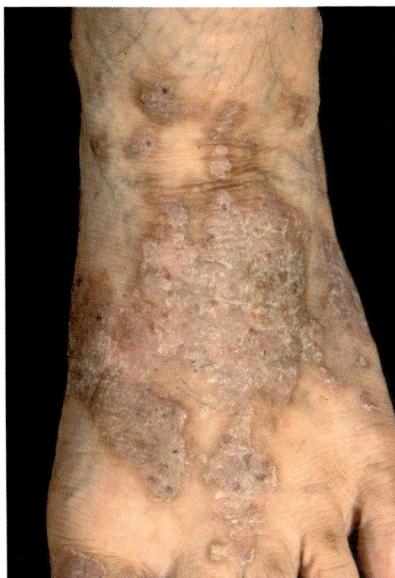

Figure 2–3 □ Chronic eczema – lichen simplex chronicus. This is an example of chronic eczema that has failed to resolve. Frequent rubbing and scratching have produced textural changes in the skin, elevation of the surface, and accentuation of the skin lines (lichenification). This patient has lichen simplex chronicus. In contrast to lesions of acute eczema, there is little or no erythema or weeping. Instead dryness, scaling, lichenification, and post-inflammatory hyperpigmentation are prominent features.

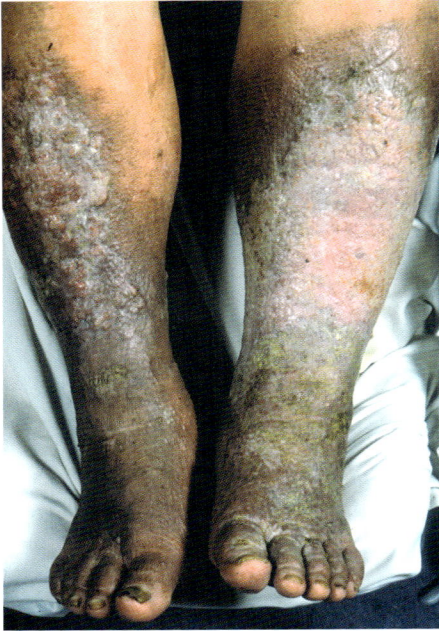

Figure 2–4 □ Chronic eczema – stasis dermatitis. The features of chronic eczema are shown in this patient who has stasis dermatitis involving the lower legs. There is widespread involvement of the anterior and medial surfaces of the legs with extension onto the dorsa of the feet. There is crusting of much of the anterior surface of the legs, suggesting secondary bacterial infection. Chronic features that are present include post-inflammatory hyperpigmentation and dyspigmentation as a result of the hemosiderin deposition that typically occurs in stasis eczema.

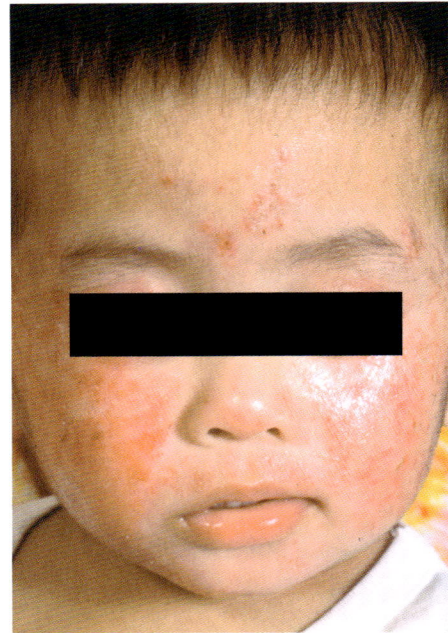

Figure 2–5 □ Atopic eczema – cheeks. Infected acute eczema on the cheeks and the forehead in a child. Eczema in infancy and young children often involves the convex surfaces such as the cheek, forehead, or scalp as well as the trunk and extensor surfaces.

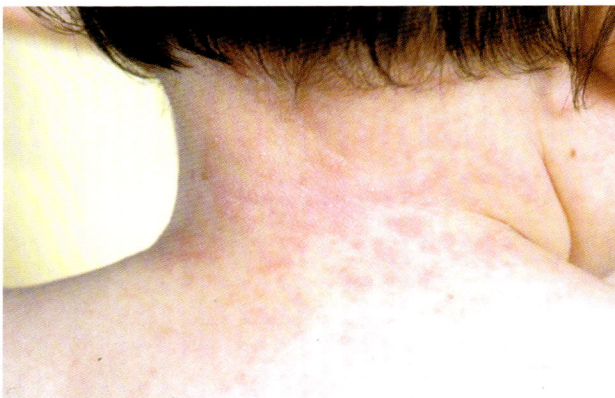

Figure 2–6 □ Atopic eczema – neck. Subacute eczema affecting the posterior neck in a young child with atopic eczema. Erythematous papules and macules can be seen. In this child, there is no evidence of lichenification, however the nuchal area is known to be a common site of lichenification, which may develop if the eczema is poorly controlled and repeated rubbing continues over many years.

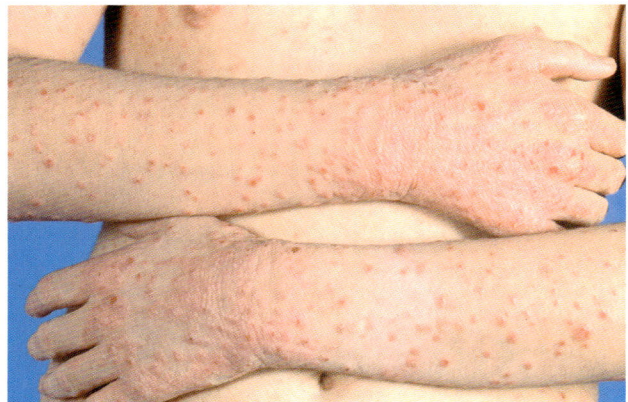

Figure 2–7 □ Atopic eczema – forearms. The dorsal surfaces of both forearms are affected in this patient. Here the acute eczema is present as discrete erythematous, excoriated papules scattered on the arms and forearms. The intense pruritus associated with atopic eczema leads to extensive excoriations, a common feature in atopic eczema.

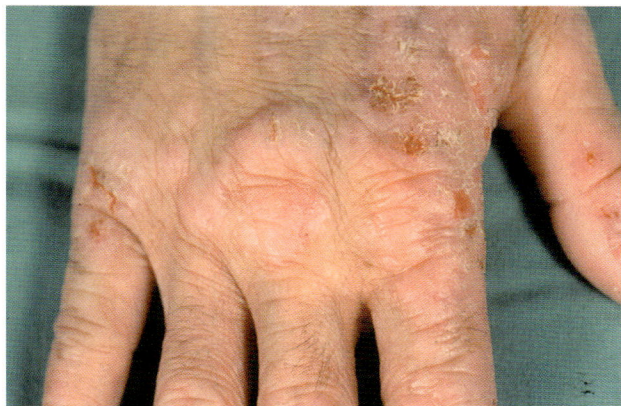

Figure 2–8 □ Atopic eczema – dorsum hand and knuckles. Chronic eczema involving the skin of the dorsum of the hand. Excoriation and lichenification are evidence of frequent rubbing and scratching due to pruritus. Recent trauma from rubbing or scratching has left an area of eroded skin. There is also some crusting visible.

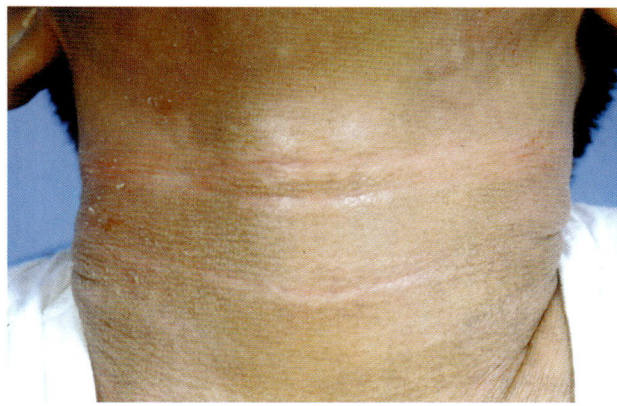

Figure 2–9 □ Atopic eczema – anterior neck. The anterior neck is a common site of involvement in atopic eczema. Care should be taken when treating flexural eczema. Note the mild eczema and reticulate pigmentation seen on the neck. This pigmentation is sometimes referred to as "dirty neck syndrome".

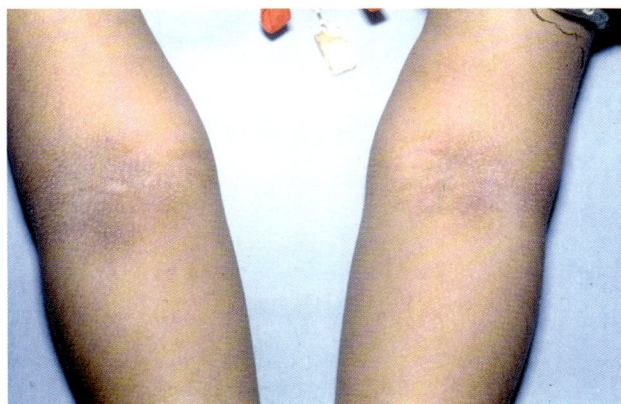

Figure 2–10 □ Atopic eczema – antecubital fossae. Flexural involvement of the antecubital fossae is frequently seen in older patients with atopic eczema. Note the chronic eczema manifesting as erythema, edema, scaling, and lichenification.

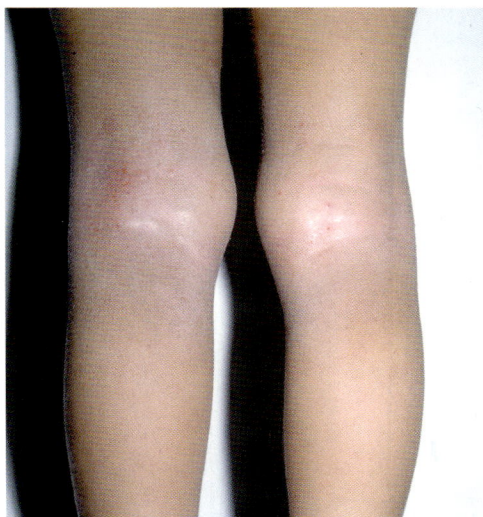

Figure 2–11 □ Atopic eczema – popliteal fossae. This patient has chronic flexural eczema on both popliteal fossae. Note the lichenification, scaling, and pigmentation that are present. The popliteal fossae, along with other flexural areas, such as the antecubital fossae, neck, wrists, and ankles, are commonly affected in atopic eczema in both childhood and adulthood. These areas are less frequently affected during infancy.

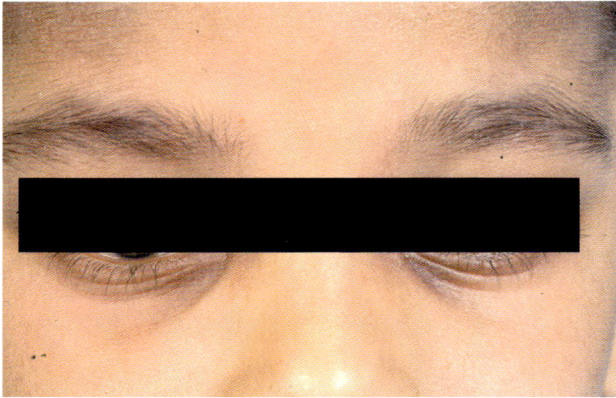

Figure 2–12 □ Atopic eczema – infraorbital fold. This patient with chronic atopic eczema has Dennie-Morgan folds present on both lower eyelids. In addition, the periorbital skin has a slightly darkened appearance. This "double fold" appearance to the lower lid skin is common in patients with eczema who rub their eyes repeatedly.

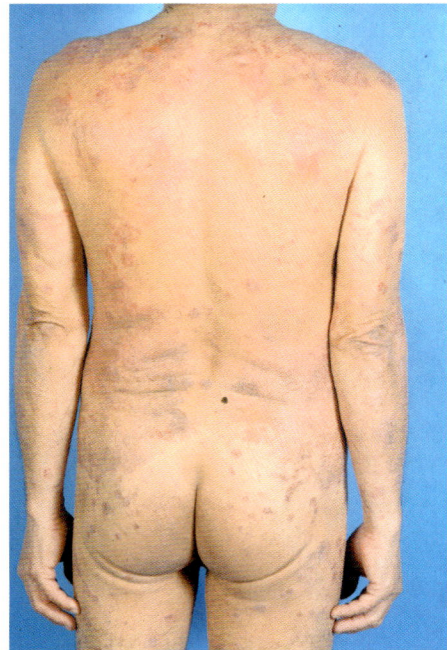

Figure 2–13 □ Atopic eczema – extensive. This patient has widespread eczema. There are papules and patches of erythema affecting the limbs, trunk, shoulders, waist and buttocks. Atopic eczema may involve the whole body and eventually lead to generalized exfoliative dermatitis.

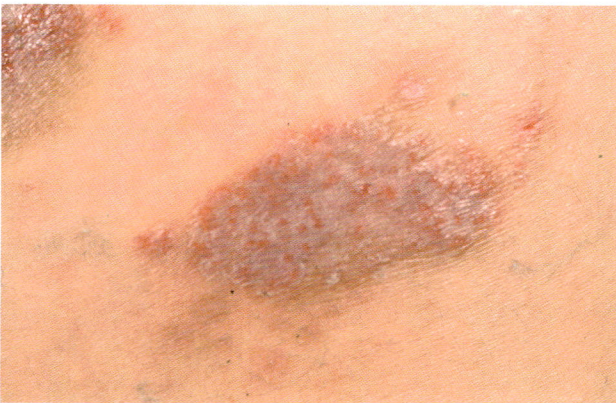

Figure 2–14 □ Endogenous discoid eczema. Discoid eczema is characterized by circumscribed, slightly moist erythematous patches of eczema consisting of papules and vesicles. Lesions are often coin-shaped, and are also referred to as "nummular eczema". This condition typically occurs in adolescents and middle-aged individuals with dry skin. The legs and arms are most commonly affected but lesions may also be seen on the trunk.

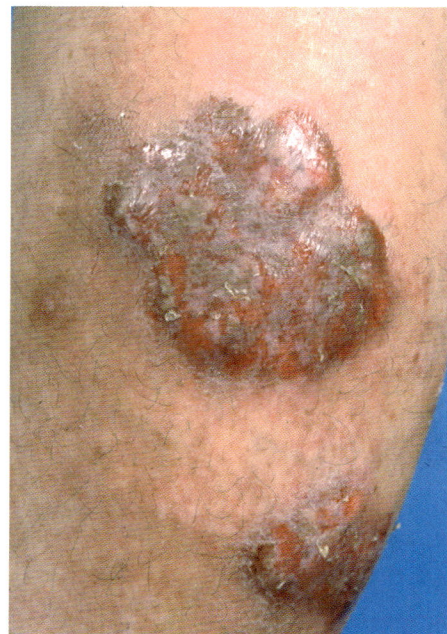

Figure 2–15 □ Endogenous discoid eczema. A large coin-shaped patch of discoid eczema is seen in this patient. The surface of this well-established lesion is elevated and partially eroded. Repeated scratching and rubbing produce the moist eroded appearance. These lesions may frequently be complicated by secondary bacterial infection. Dry scaly lesions may be misdiagnosed as psoriasis or even tinea corporis.

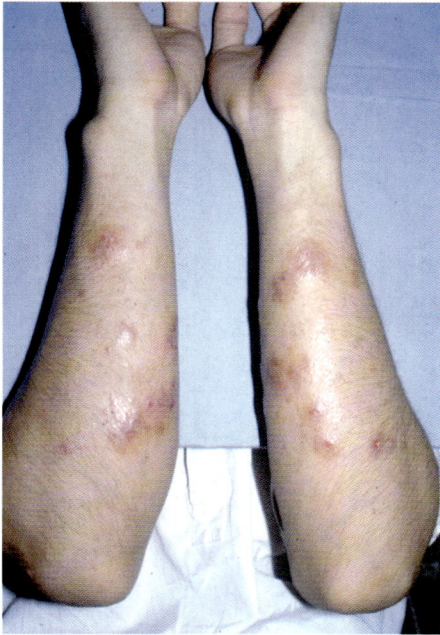

Figure 2–16 □ Endogenous discoid eczema. This patient has multiple discrete lesions of discoid eczema located on the forearms. Discoid eczema may present initially as a single lesion but may be followed by more lesions. In more severe cases, generalized discoid eczema may be present where there are multiple lesions affecting the trunk and limbs.

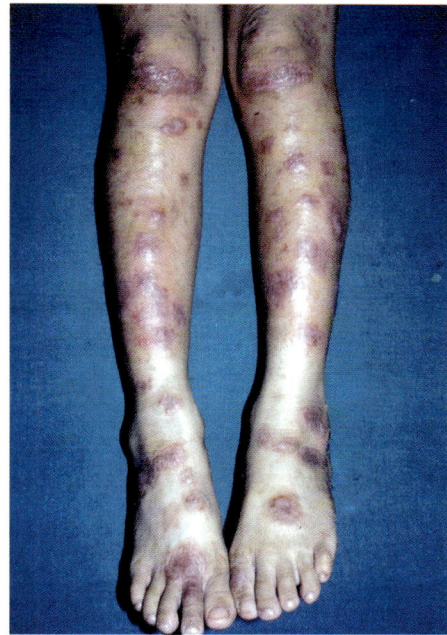

Figure 2–17 □ Endogenous discoid eczema. Numerous lesions of discoid eczema are present on the legs of this patient. Flares of discoid eczema may be followed by periods of remission. New lesions occur in areas of previous involvement or in unaffected skin. Active lesions may be slow to heal and resolved lesions can still remain identifiable for long periods of time as areas of post-inflammatory hyperpigmentation.

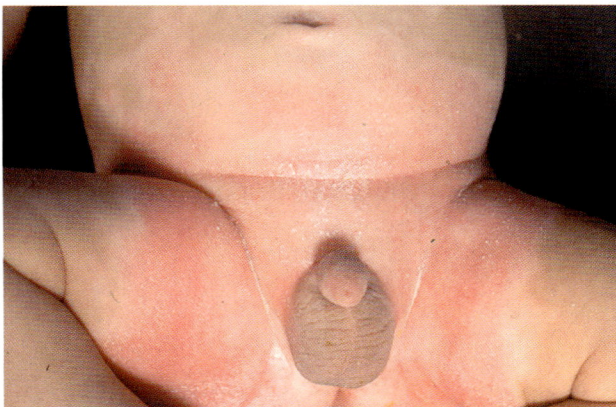

Figure 2–18 □ Infantile seborrheic eczema – diaper area. Seborrheic dermatitis in infancy often affects the diaper area. Sebaceous glands are found in high numbers in the diaper area as well as the face and scalp, hence the predilection of this condition in these sites. There is greasy bright erythematous involvement of the convex surfaces of the napkin area with sharp demarcation of the margins. A frequent complication is maceration of the diaper region. The presence of satellite pustules just beyond the margin may suggest coexisting candidal infection.

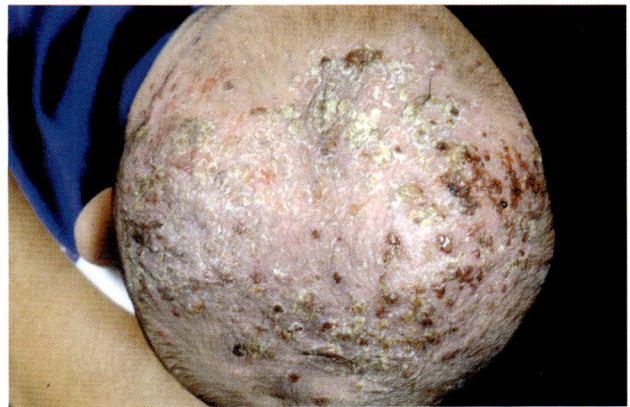

Figure 2–19 □ Infantile seborrheic eczema – scalp. Scalp seborrheic dermatitis in infancy is also known as cradle cap. In this infant, there is diffuse scalp involvement with thick greasy scales and underlying erythema. Liberal application of olive oil helps to remove the scales gradually and gently.

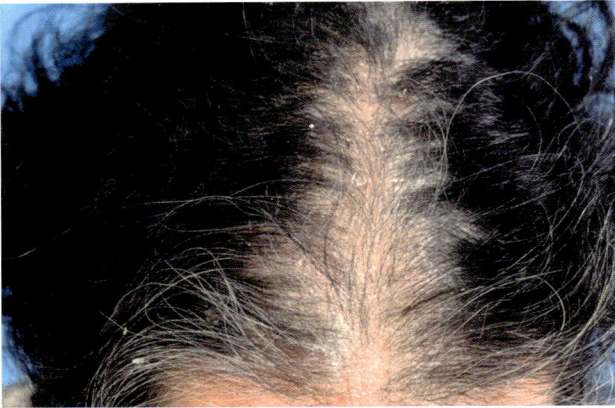

Figure 2–20 □ Adult seborrheic dermatitis – scalp. In adults, scalp seborrheic dermatitis leads to flaking of greasy scales. It is more commonly referred to as dandruff. Other regions of the head, including the eyebrows, nasolabial folds, and beard may similarly be affected. Eyelashes may be involved as well (blepharitis). The eczema may or may not be pruritic.

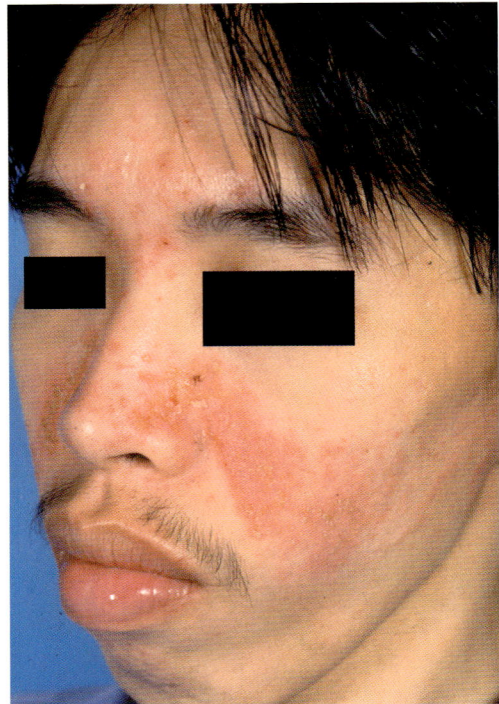

Figure 2–21 □ Adult seborrheic dermatitis. This man has seborrheic dermatitis with symmetrical involvement of the cheeks, nose, nasolabial folds, and central forehead. There are discrete and confluent yellowish red macules, plaques, and characteriztic greasy yellowish scales. Other commonly affected areas of the body include the retroauricular fold, the external auditory meatus, and scalp. Presternal involvement is common. Body folds, such as the axilla, submammary area, and groin, are also frequently involved.

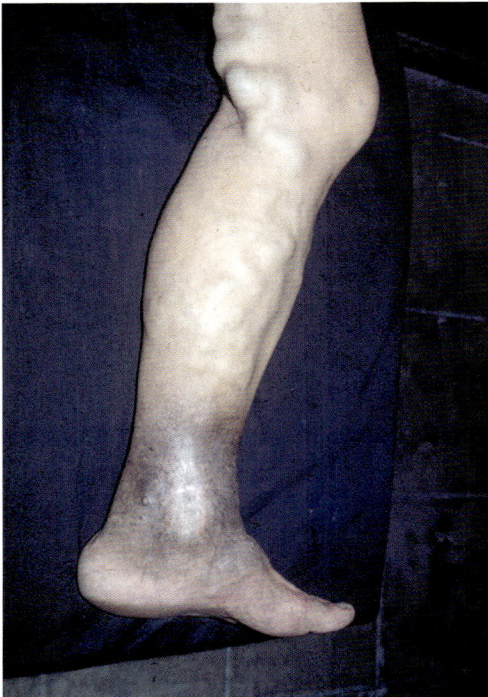

Figure 2–22 □ Stasis eczema. The left leg of this patient shows prominent features of stasis eczema affecting the medial shin and ankle regions. Features of stasis eczema seen here include pigmentation, edema, lichenification, and scaliness. Stasis eczema may develop in patients with chronic venous insufficiency of the lower legs. This man has visibly enlarged varicose veins above the affected area. Associated lipodermatosclerosis is present as well.

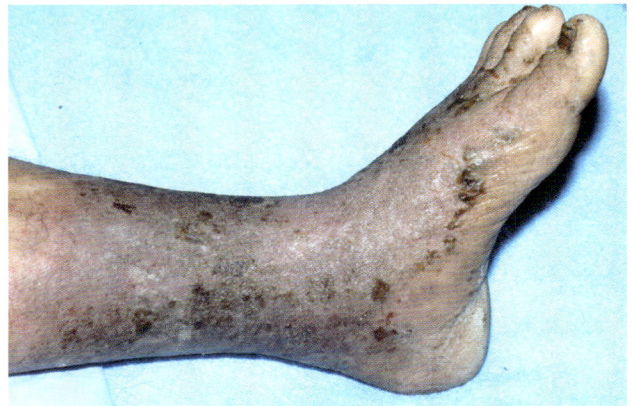

Figure 2–23 □ Stasis eczema. The medial aspect of the left shin and ankle shows pronounced changes of stasis eczema and areas of superficial ulceration. Post-inflammatory hyperpigmentation contributes to the appearance. Also, extravasation of blood results in the deposition of hemosiderin in the skin which imparts a brown discoloration to the affected areas. A patient with stasis eczema may have had a history of deep venous thrombosis as well as varicose veins. Chronic venous ulcers may develop.

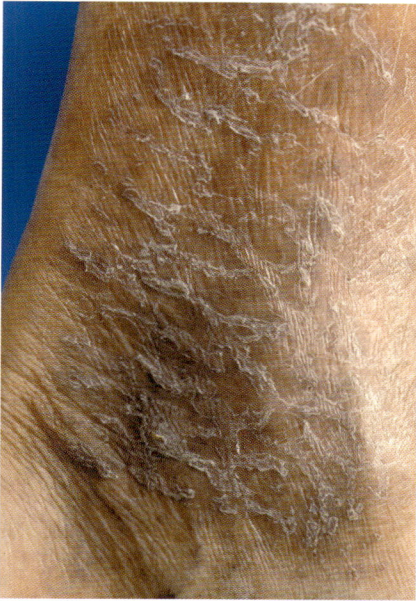

Figure 2–24 □ Asteatotic eczema. This form of eczema is commonly seen in the elderly and typically occurs on dry pretibial skin of the legs. The hands and forearms may also be involved. The lesion shows dry, erythematous, flaky skin with superficial fissuring. The skin is prone to trauma and may bleed easily. Asteatotic eczema is often referred to as eczema craquelé. Topical emollients and mild topical corticosteroids are the mainstay of treatment.

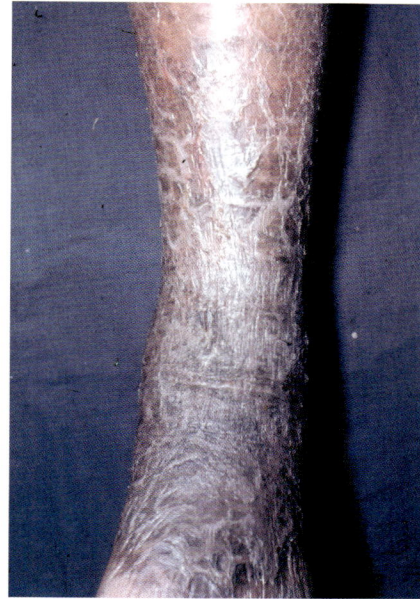

Figure 2–25 □ Asteatotic eczema. This patient has a severe form of asteatotic eczema. The entire leg has a cracked porcelain appearance. The anterior tibial region is a common site of involvement as this region has less sebaceous and eccrine gland activity. The stratum corneum and epidermis in this region are prone to dehydration which may occur as a consequence of continual use of harsh soaps and frequent washing.

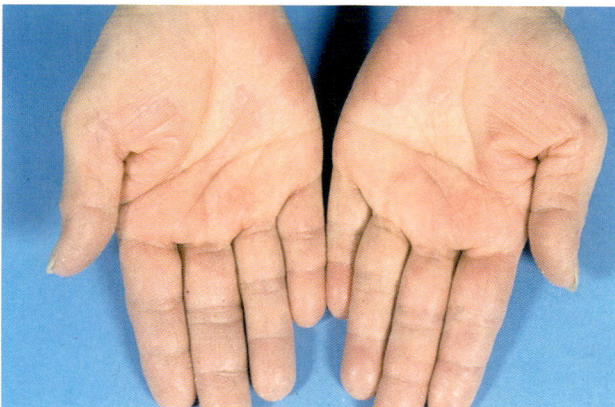

Figure 2–26 □ Endogenous hand eczema. Hand eczema affecting both palms of a patient. There is patchy eczematous involvement of the finger as well as thenar and hypothenar eminences of the palms. The fingertips are fissured and xerotic. The involved surfaces have a glazed appearance with fine scaling and hyperlinearity of markings on the palms.

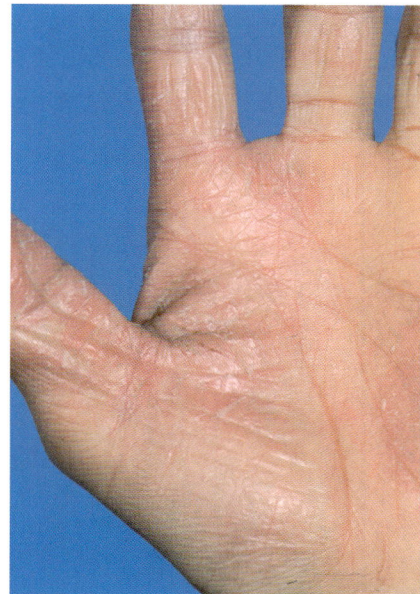

Figure 2–27 □ Hand eczema. Eczema affecting the thenar eminence, thumb, and digits of a patient on long-term topical corticosteroid use. The skin in the affected areas has a glazed erythematous appearance, and looks atrophic. Patients with hand eczema should be questioned about occupational exposure to irritants. Irritants such as detergents in the household setting may also contribute to hand eczema. Protection of the hands with emollients and gloves should be recommended. Patch testing can help determine concomitant contact allergy.

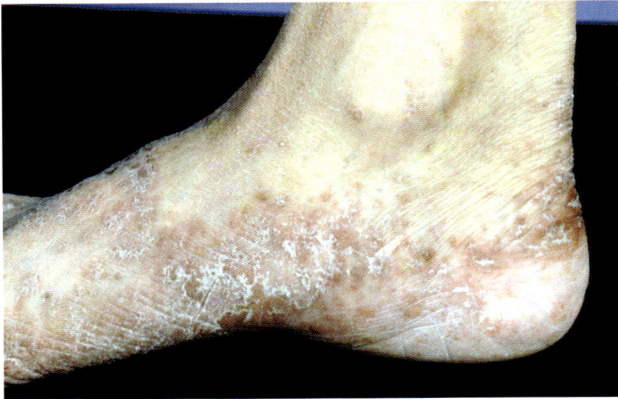

Figure 2–28 □ Endogenous feet eczema. Erythematous papules, post-inflammatory hyperpigmentation, and scaling are prominent features in this patient with endogenous feet eczema. Scaling and itch are also cardinal features of tinea pedis and microscopy of skin scrapings should be done to exclude the presence of fungal elements.

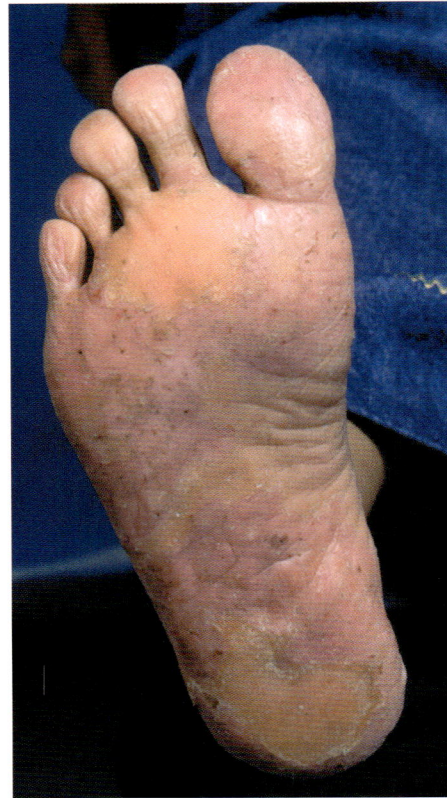

Figure 2–29 □ Foot eczema. There is chronic eczema on much of the sole of the right foot. This patient has endogeneous hands and feet eczema. The skin of the palms and soles are lichenified and scaly.

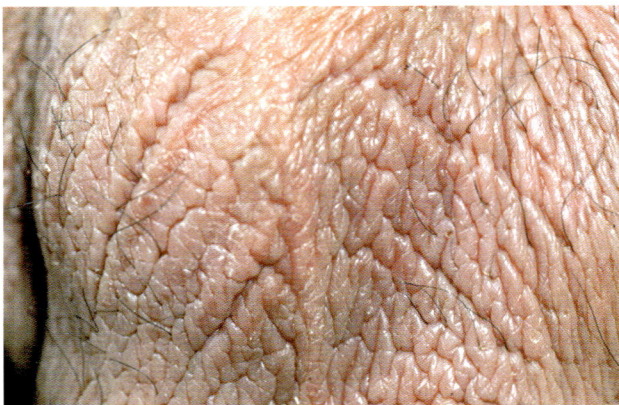

Figure 2–30 □ Lichen simplex chronicus – scrotum. Lichen simplex chronicus presents as localized, well-demarcated chronic eczematous patches and plaques. Lichen simplex chronicus of the scrotum accentuates the rugosity of the scrotal skin. Lichenified skin can become firm and thickened. Common areas of involvement include scrotal and vulval skin, as well as the posterior neck, legs, and feet. Lichenification occurs after prolonged rubbing or scratching of an area of any primary dermatosis.

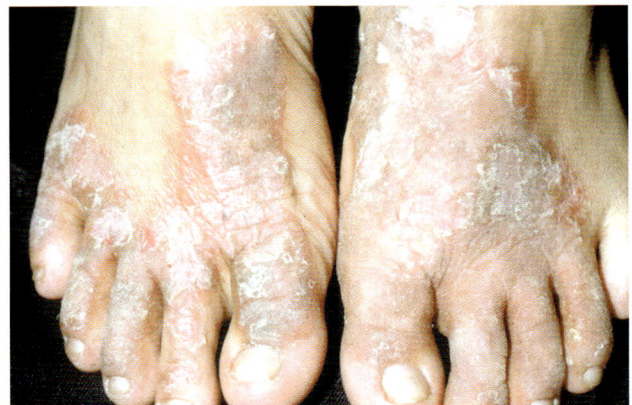

Figure 2–31 □ Lichen simplex chronicus. Lichen simplex chronicus presenting as well-demarcated, chronic eczema on the dorsa of both feet. Affected skin is often intensely pruritic. Habitual scratching over long periods produces established lesions that become difficult to treat. The term lichenification is descriptive and appropriate in that lesions are said to resemble lichen growth on the bark of a tree.

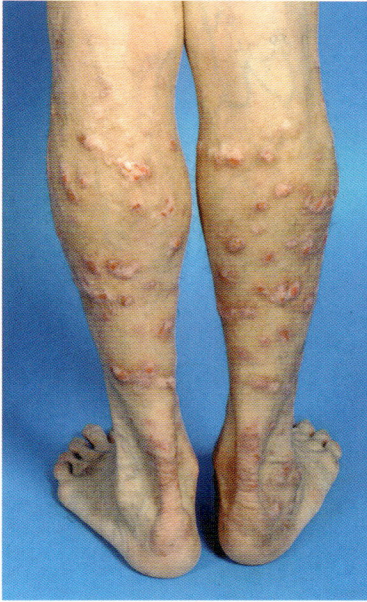

Figure 2–32 □ Prurigo nodularis. Prurigo nodularis in an adult with long-standing endogenous eczema. Repeated scratching, picking, and rubbing of the skin may lead to the development of prurigo nodules. Here, multiple discrete scaly large nodules affect the lower limbs. They are erythematous, keratotic, hyperpigmented, and firm to palpation. The surfaces of some of the lesions are excoriated and eroded from scratching. Prurigo nodules are often located on the extensor surfaces of the arms and legs and are usually symmetrically distributed. They are fairly resistant to topical steroid therapy and respond better to intralesional steroid therapy.

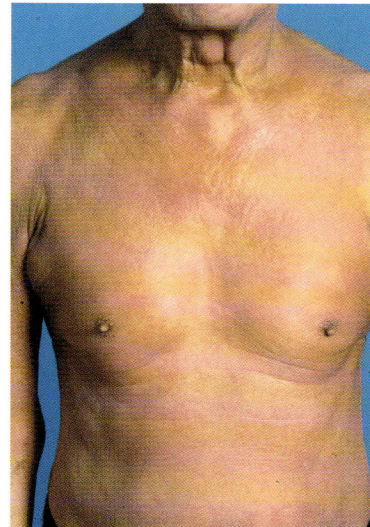

Figure 2–33 □ Generalized exfoliative dermatitis – body. Generalized exfoliative dermatitis (GED), also known as erythroderma, in a 77-year-old man with endogenous eczema. In GED, more than 95% of the total body skin surface area is affected. There are many causes of GED, including underlying systemic diseases. This man has widespread erythema affecting the entire surface of the body, including the face. Scaling was more prominent on the scalp and face than the chest. Fluid balance and body temperature should be closely monitored in GED.

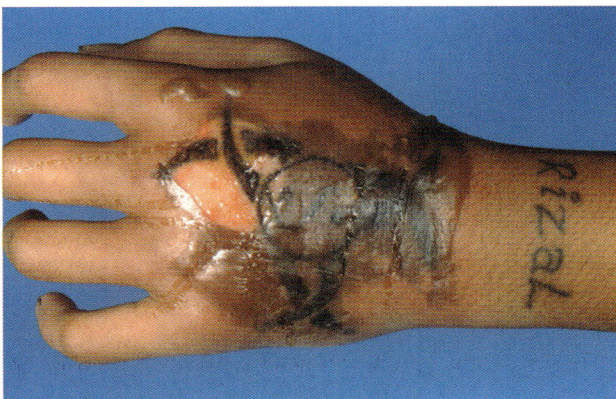

Figure 2–34 □ Acute irritant reaction – chemical burns. This usually occurs after a single contact with a strong irritant. Erythema, edema, bulla formation, and erosions occurred after the patient attempted to remove the tattoo on the dorsum of his left hand by applying onion juice and vinegar.

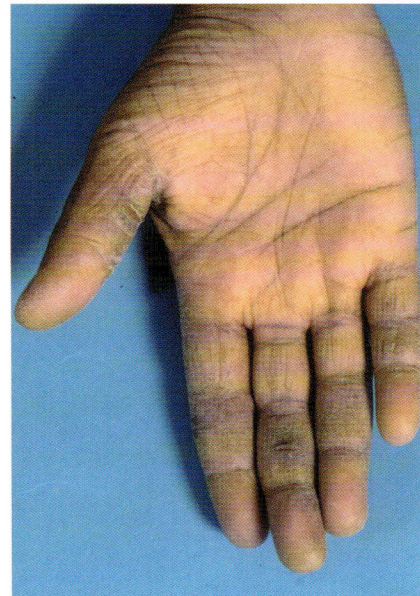

Figure 2–35 □ Cumulative irritant contact dermatitis. This occurs on susceptible skin (e.g. on patients with atopic diathesis) after repeated exposure to mild irritants (e.g. detergents and water). Scaling and lichenification indicate chronic eczema due to repeated chemical irritation and friction to the palmar aspects of the fingers and palm of the right hand. These changes were more obvious over the middle finger.

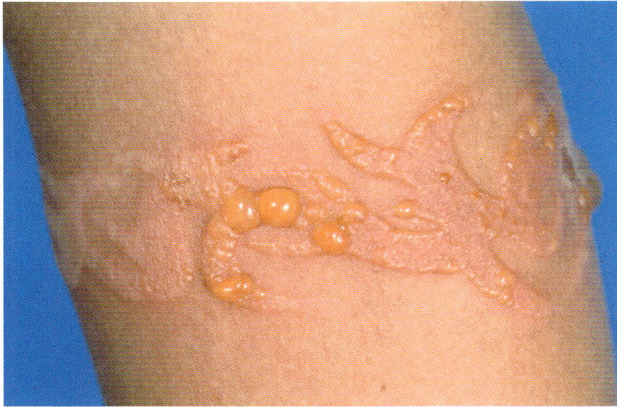

Figure 2–36 □ Acute allergic contact dermatitis. Erythema, edema, and blister formation confined to the shape of a temporary tattoo which had already faded. Many temporary tattoos contain para-phenylenediamine, the allergen that commonly causes hair dye dermatitis. This allergen is favored by many temporary tattoo artists because it imparts a clear black color which is rarely achievable with other substitutes.

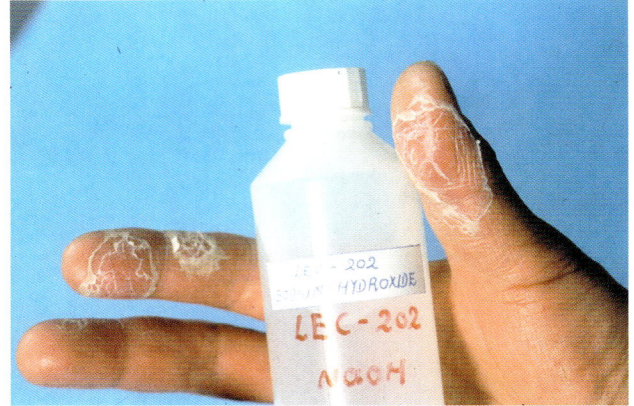

Figure 2–37 □ Cumulative irritant contact dermatitis – acids and alkalis. Erythema and scaling are seen on the tips of the thumb and index finger. This patient worked with strong acids and alkalis. Acute irritant dermatitis occurred whenever there had been accidental contact with any of these substances. In this instance, the offending irritant was sodium hydroxide.

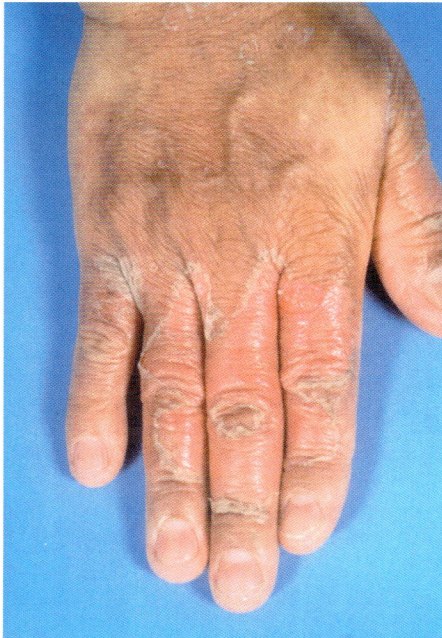

Figure 2–38 □ Acute irritant reaction – solvents. Erythema and scaling are obvious on the fingers of the right hand. The patient had worn rubber gloves when he used a cloth to wipe some aluminum plates with thinner. Severe irritant contact dermatitis resulted when some thinner had contaminated the inner surface of one of his gloves.

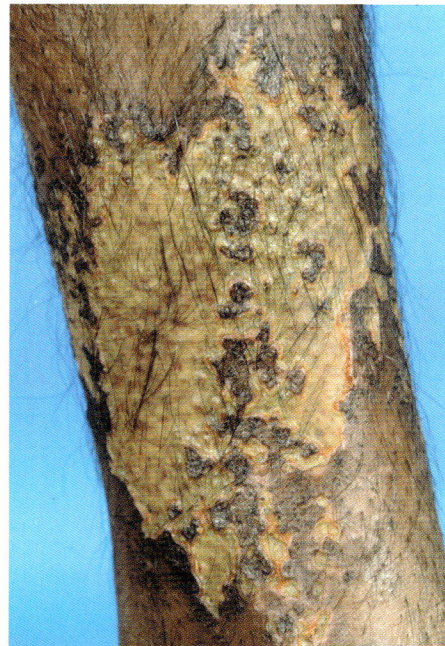

Figure 2–39 □ Acute irritant reaction – cement burns. Cement burns may occur hours after contact with wet cement. The calcium hydroxide and alkalinity of wet ready-mixed cement lead to caustic burns. Although often initially asymptomatic, severe necrosis and ulceration may occur. The scarring and pain may be persistent.

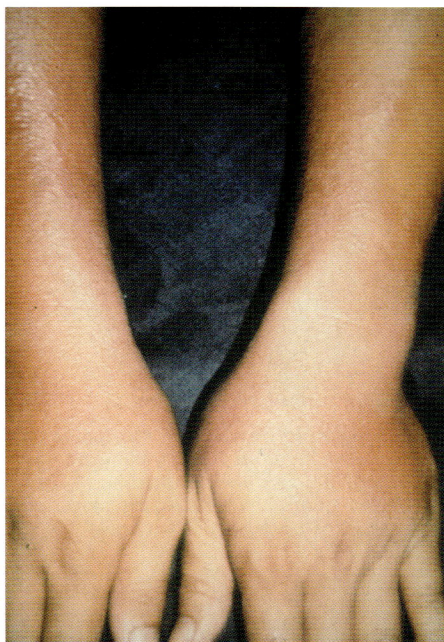

Figure 2–40 □ Irritant contact dermatitis – cement. Erythema and edema of the hands and forearms can be seen in this patient who had prolonged contact with cement. Although cement commonly causes allergic contact dermatitis, irritant contact dermatitis may also occur in non-sensitized patients with susceptible skin.

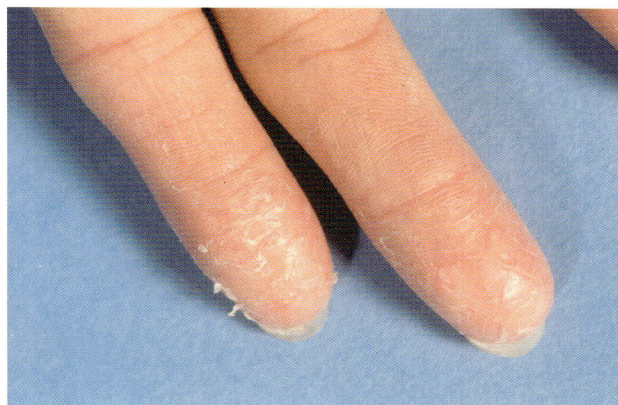

Figure 2–41 □ Frictional dermatitis. Short, sharp frictional forces, such as repetitive rubbing, whilst performing domestic chores may cause cumulative insult irritant contact dermatitis. Erythema, scaling, and a shiny appearance can be seen on the distal parts of the index and middle fingers.

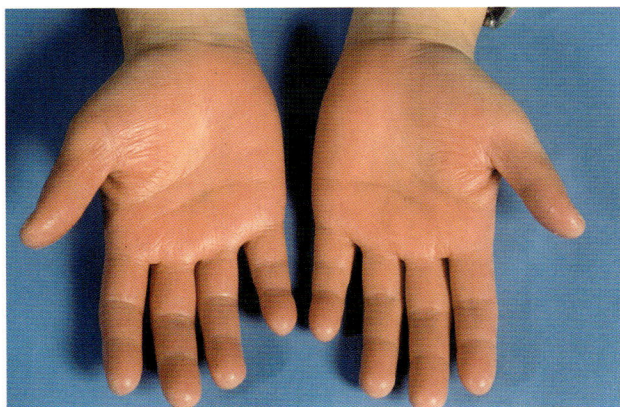

Figure 2–42 □ Irritant contact dermatitis – wet work. Erythema and edema are seen on both palms. The patient worked in a drinks stall and her job required much exposure to water and detergents. Wet work is one of the most common causes of irritant contact dermatitis in Singapore.

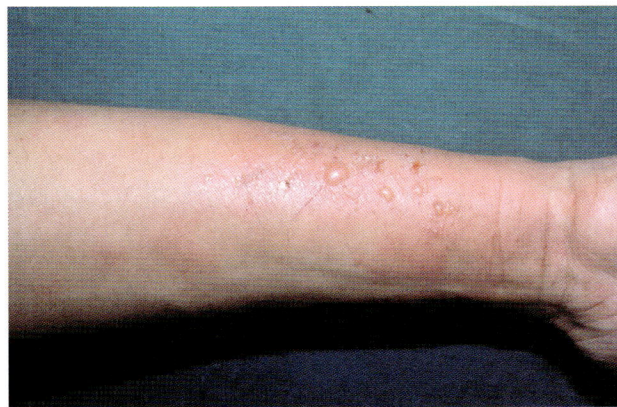

Figure 2–43 □ Acute irritant contact dermatitis – soldering flux. Erythema, edema, and bulla formation are seen on the wrist and forearm of this patient who had occupational exposure to soldering flux. A negative patch test reaction to colophony excluded allergic contact dermatitis from colophony in the soldering flux.

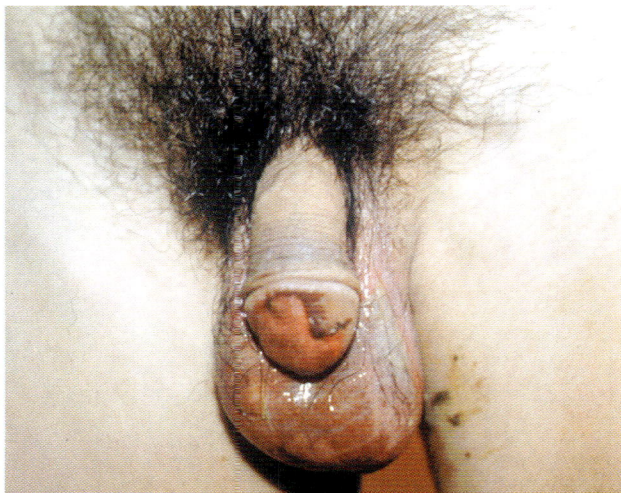

Figure 2–44 □ Acute irritant contact dermatitis – herbicide (paraquat). After working with the weed-killer paraquat, this patient did not ensure thorough washing of his hands before visiting the toilet. Erythema, swelling, and exudation of the glans penis and scrotum are features of acute irritant contact dermatitis from paraquat.

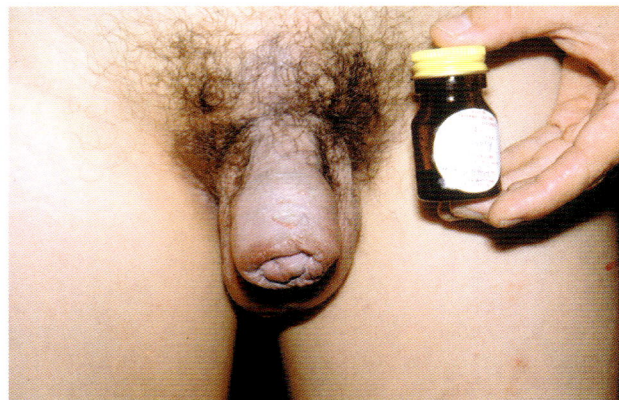

Figure 2–45 □ Acute irritant from topical medicament – podophyllin paint. Redness and swelling on the prepuce in a patient who had applied podophyllin paint for the treatment of his genital warts. Acute irritation is a well-known side effect of podophyllin therapy.

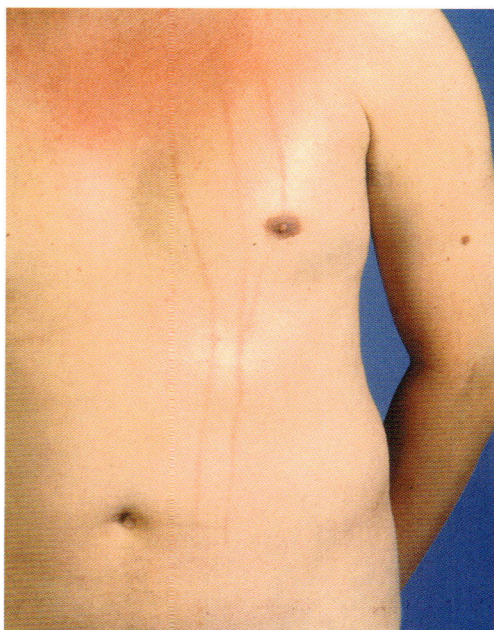

Figure 2–46 □ Irritant contact dermatitis – antiseptics (Dettol). After washing his upper chest with Dettol (a widely available antiseptic solution containing 4-chloro-3-xylenol), this patient developed irritant contact dermatitis. Streaks of dermatitis where the solution had flowed down his trunk can be seen. Allergic contact dermatitis was excluded, as the patch test for 4-chloro-3-xylenol was negative.

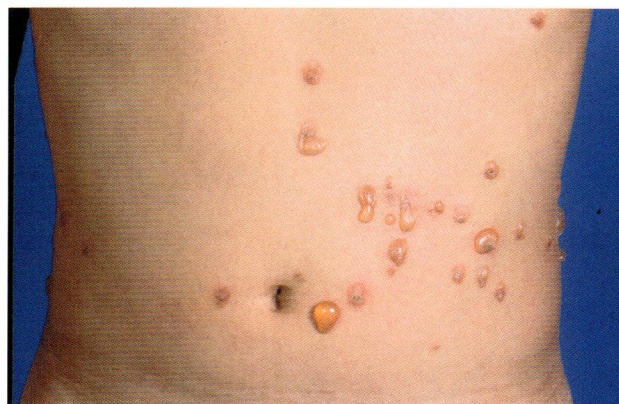

Figure 2–47 □ Acute irritant contact dermatitis from medicament – cantharidine. Multiple erythematous papules and bullae were seen after the application of cantharidine paint for the treatment of molluscum contagiosum on this patient's abdomen. This was the intended effect of this treatment.

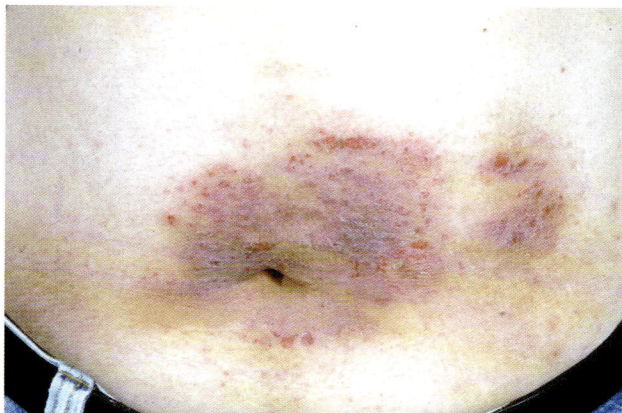

Figure 2–48 □ Allergic contact dermatitis from nickel – belt buckle. Erythematous papules and plaques due to allergic contact dermatitis in this man who was allergic to the nickel in his metal belt buckle. Small amounts of nickel are present in most metallic objects and nickel is the most common cause of allergic contact dermatitis in most countries.

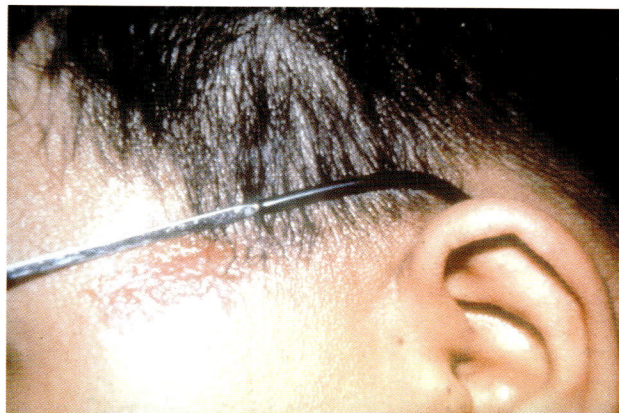

Figure 2–49 □ Allergic contact dermatitis from nickel – spectacle frame. This patient had an erythematous weepy plaque on his temple due to allergic contact dermatitis from nickel in the spectacle frame. The rash resolved once he substituted it with a non-metallic frame.

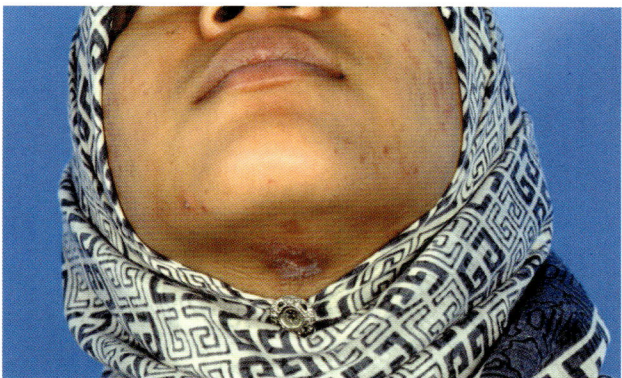

Figure 2–50 □ Allergic contact dermatitis from nickel – scarf brooch. This lady developed an allergic contact dermatitis from nickel in the metal clip which she used to fasten her scarf. Nickel dermatitis from metal scarf clips have so far been reported only in Southeast Asia.

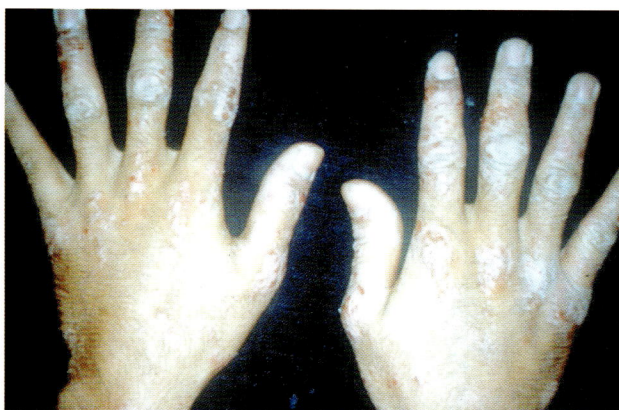

Figure 2–51 □ Allergic contact dermatitis from chromate – cement. Erythematous plaques and scaling on the dorsal aspects of the fingers and hands of a construction worker who had been sensitized to chromates in cement. Chromate is the most common occupational allergen in Singapore.

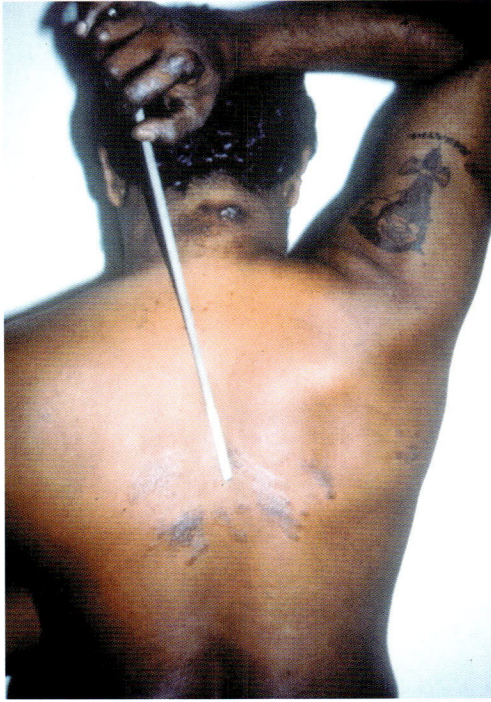

Figure 2–52 □ Allergic contact dermatitis from chromate – welding rod. Erythematous lichenified plaques on the back of a welder who had been scratching his back with a metal rod which contained chromate. Besides cement, other causes of allergic contact dermatitis from chromate include metal objects and leather.

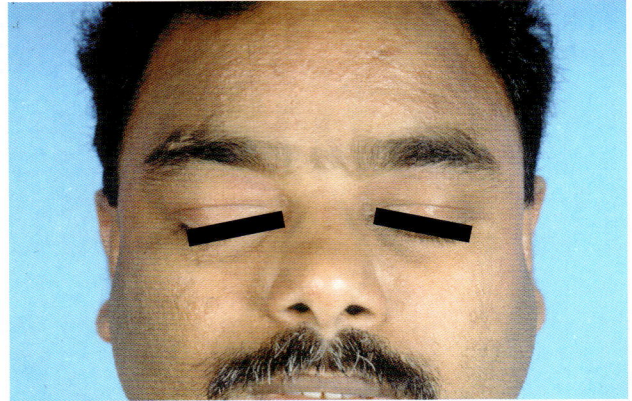

Figure 2–53 □ Allergic contact dermatitis from fragrance – airborne. Lichenification and scaling on the forehead and eyelids of a man who had allergic contact dermatitis from his car perfume. Airborne allergic contact dermatitis usually affects the forehead, cheeks, eyelids, ears, jaws, nostrils, lips, neck, and uncovered parts of the arms.

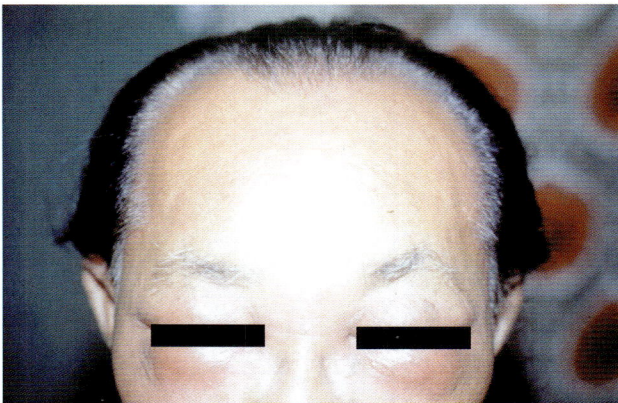

Figure 2–54 □ Allergic contact dermatitis from para-phenylenediamine – hair dye. Symmetrical bilateral redness and swelling of the eyelids of a man who had allergic contact dermatitis from para-phenylenediamine in hair dyes. Para-phenylenediamine is found in almost all permanent black hair dyes.

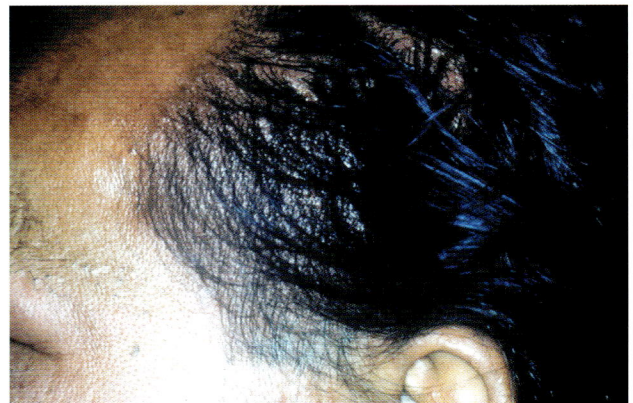

Figure 2–55 □ Allergic contact dermatitis from para-phenylenediamine – hair dye. Erythema and edema of the scalp and forehead in another patient who also had allergic contact dermatitis from para-phenylenediamine in black permanent hair dye. This is another pattern of hair dye dermatitis that is commonly seen.

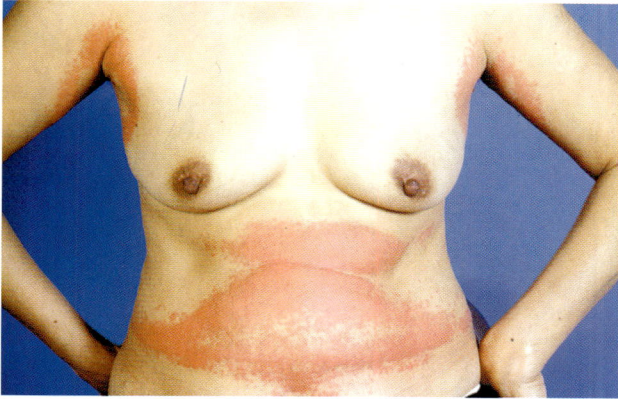

Figure 2–56 □ Allergic contact dermatitis from para-phenylenediamine – clothing dye. A patient who had erythema and edema over her axillae and abdomen after wearing new clothes dyed black. The allergen is para-phenylenediamine.

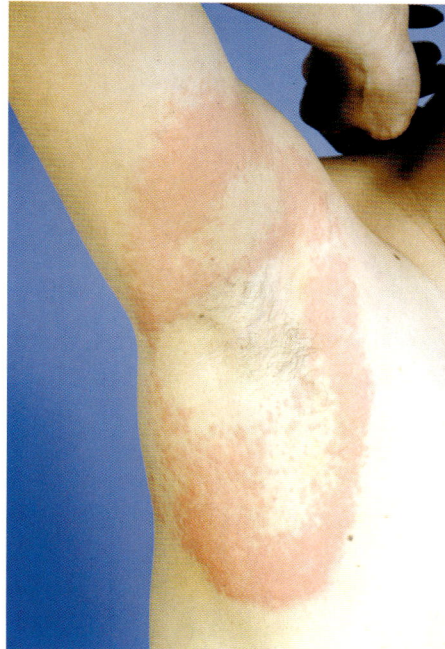

Figure 2–57 □ Allergic contact dermatitis from para-phenylenediamine – clothing dye. The right axilla of the patient in Figure 2–56 shows the characteriztic pattern of textile dermatitis with erythema and edema around the axilla with sparing of the vault region.

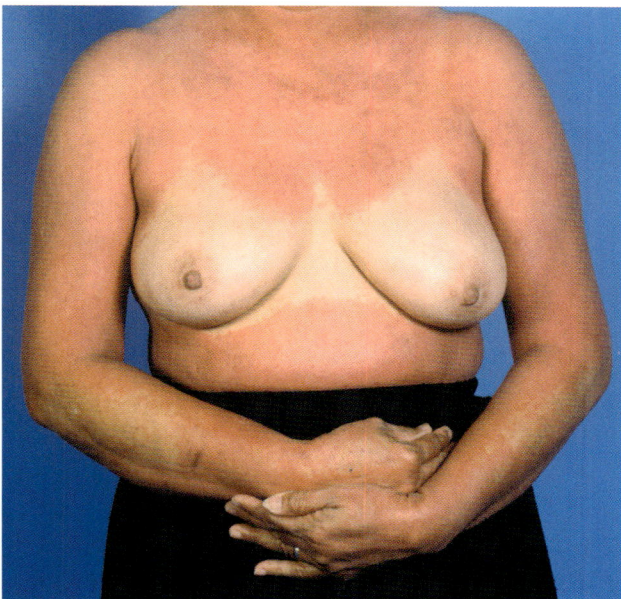

Figure 2–58 □ Allergic contact dermatitis from para-phenylenediamine – clothing dye. Widespread truncal and upper limb erythema due to allergic contact dermatitis from the black clothing worn at Chinese funerals. Note the sparing of the areas protected by the patient's brassiere. Patch test was positive to her black clothing and para-phenylenediamine.

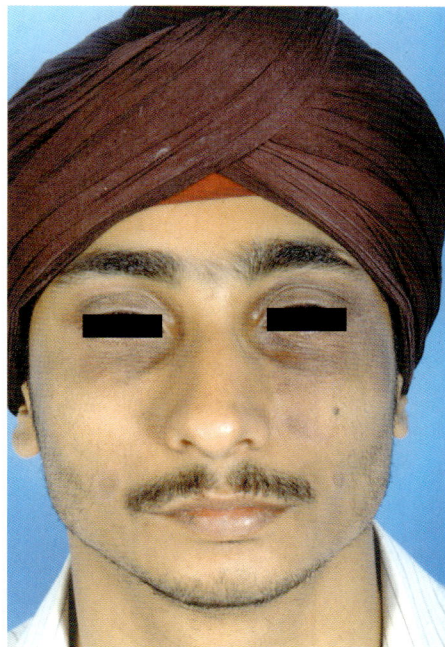

Figure 2–59 □ Allergic contact dermatitis from neomycin – eyedrop medicament. Lichenification of the eyelids and cheeks in a man who had been sensitized to neomycin in eyedrops. Neomycin is one of the most common topical medicaments associated with allergic contact dermatitis.

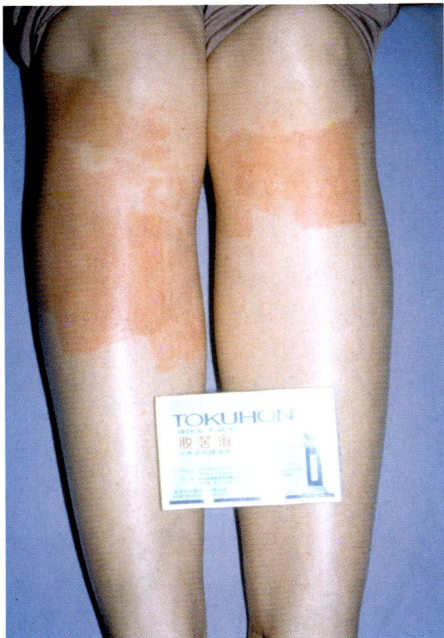

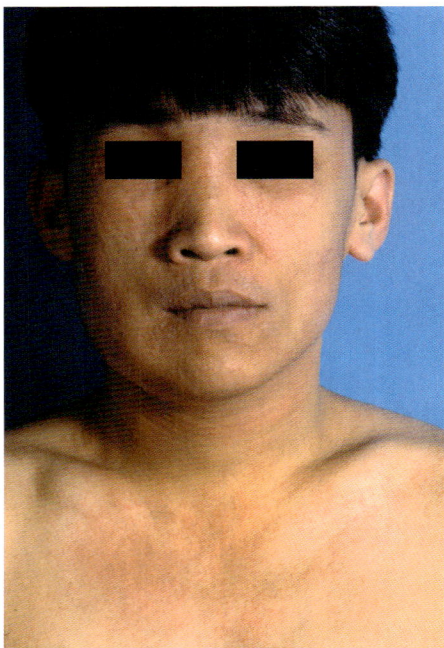

Figure 2–61 □ **Allergic contact dermatitis from clotrimazole.** This patient had applied clotrimazole cream to his groin and lower abdomen. He subsequently developed pruritic erythema and edema over the area of application. Patch testing confirmed allergy to clotrimazole. Other common allergens in medicaments include preservatives.

Figure 2–60 □ **Allergic contact dermatitis from colophony – medicated plaster.** Erythema and edema with distinct edges, corresponding to areas where this medicated plaster had been applied to the patient's shins. Common allergens in medicated plasters include colophony and topical non-steroidal anti-inflammatory drugs (NSAIDs).

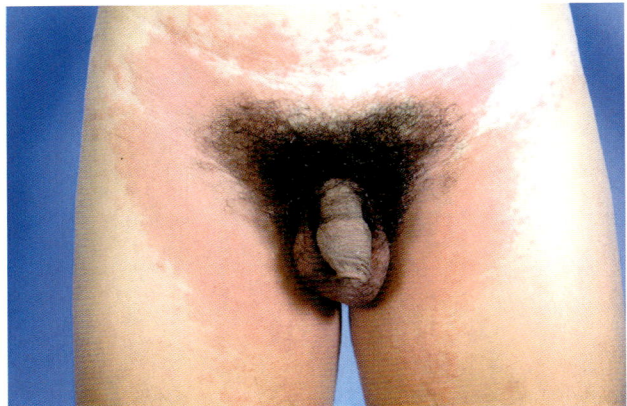

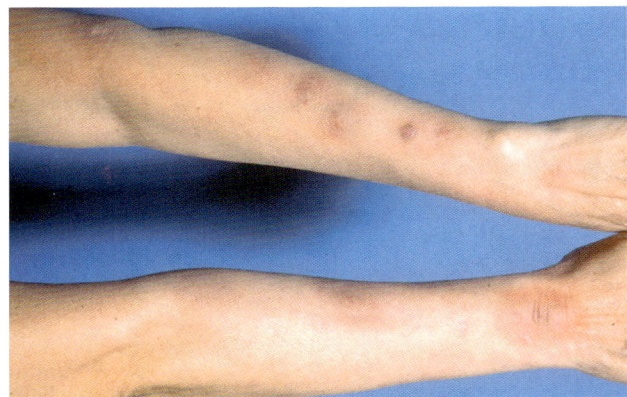

Figure 2–63 □ **Allergic contact dermatitis from a corticosteroid cream.** Another patient who had a worsening of his rash after applying a corticosteroid cream. There are multiple eczematous plaques on both forearms, where he had applied the medication.

Figure 2–62 □ **Allergic contact dermatitis from beta-methasone valerate.** This man developed a worsening of his pruritic eczematous lesions after applying betamethasone cream. The rash was more prominent in the periorbital region. He is allergic to the topical steroid betamethasone valerate.

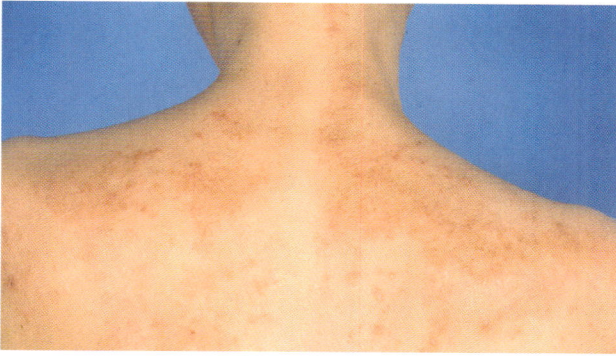

Figure 2–64 □ **Allergic contact dermatitis from squaric acid dibutylester (SADBE).** This patient developed an eczematous eruption over her nape and upper back whilst undergoing treatment with SADBE. This agent was being used as topical immunotherapy for extensive alopecia areata. The goal of this treatment was to therapeutically induce localized allergic contact dermatitis in order to stimulate hair regrowth on her bald areas.

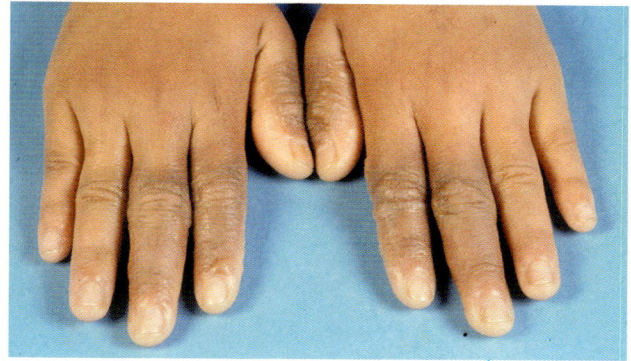

Figure 2–65 □ **Allergic contact dermatitis from rubber chemicals – finger cots.** Lichenification and scaling on the thumbs, index and middle fingers where this patient had been wearing rubber finger cots at work in an electronics factory. Rubber dermatitis is usually caused by accelerators, antioxidants, and other chemicals used in the manufacture of rubber. Common rubber chemicals include constituents of para-phenylenediamine mix, carba mix, and thiuram mix.

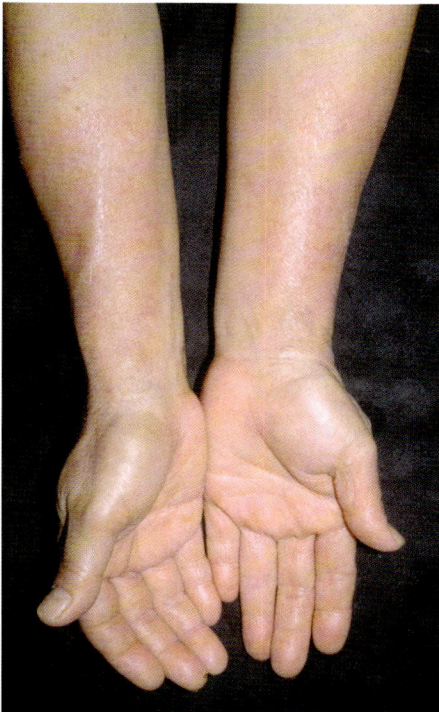

Figure 2–66 □ **Allergic contact dermatitis from rubber chemicals – rubber gloves.** Erythema and edema of the hands and forearms, with a sharp demarcation on the forearm, indicating the areas of contact with the patient's rubber gloves. Rubber glove dermatitis is seen in domestic as well as in industrial settings.

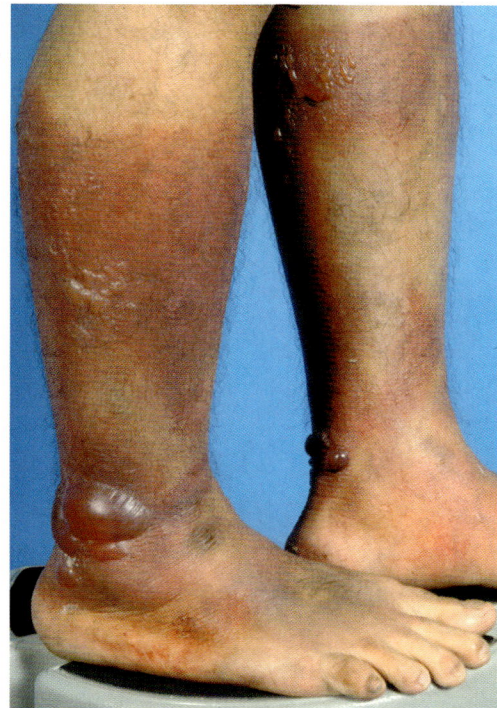

Figure 2–67 □ **Allergic contact dermatitis from rubber chemicals – boots.** Erythema, edema, and bulla formation on the legs and feet of a patient with allergic contact dermatitis from rubber chemicals in his rubber boots.

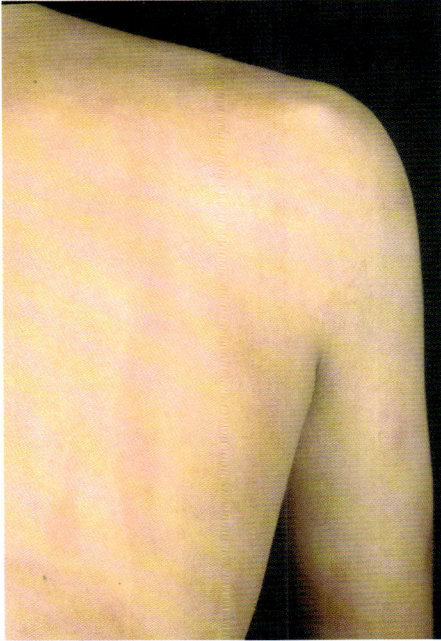

Figure 2–68 □ Phytodermatitis. Streaky erythema and post-inflammatory hyperpigmentation on the back of a national serviceman who had trained in a jungle area. Contact dermatitis to plants is typically streaky in appearance. The exact causative plant was not identified.

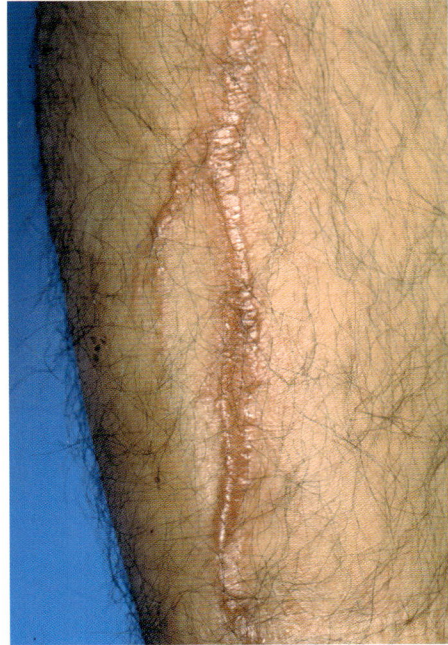

Figure 2–69 □ Phytodermatitis. Another patient with streaky erythema and induration after contact with plants. Resin from Rengas (*Anacardiaceae*) wood, which is commonly used in Southeast Asia to make furniture, is a common cause of phytodermatitis in this region.

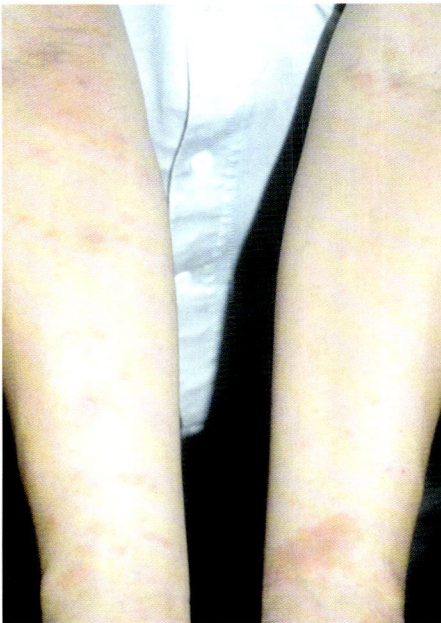

Figure 2–70 □ Phytodermatitis – mango. Erythematous plaques on the arms of a patient who had allergic contact dermatitis from mango sap. The mango plant (*Mangiferae indica*), which is related to poison ivy (*Anacardiaceae*), is a very common cause of allergic contact dermatitis in Southeast Asia. Urushiol is the allergen contained in plants of this family.

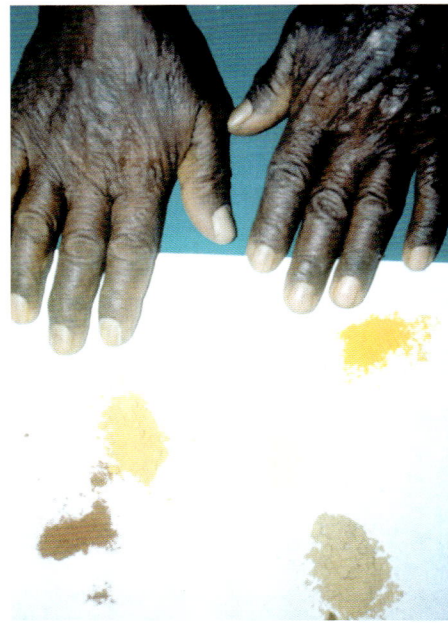

Figure 2–71 □ Allergic contact dermatitis – turmeric spice. Lichenified plaques on the hands of an Indian cook who handled turmeric powder at work. Turmeric (*Curcuma domestica*) is an ingredient in all curry powders and is used extensively in Indian cooking. Allergic contact dermatitis from turmeric has also been reported in several other countries.

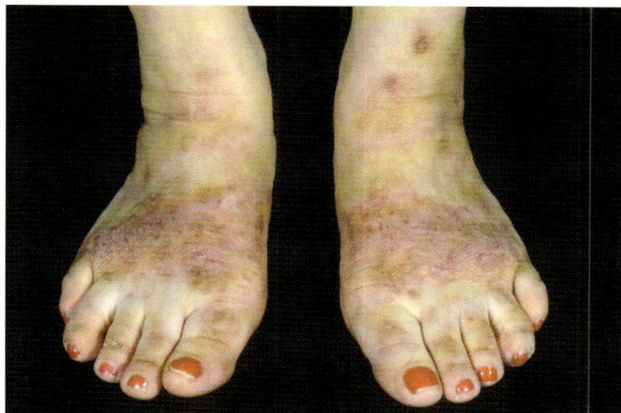

Figure 2–72 □ Allergic contact dermatitis from butylphenol formaldehyde resin – shoes resin. This lady developed eczematous plaques on the dorsa of both feet soon after wearing a pair of new shoes. Patch test was positive to butylphenol formaldehyde resin and the inner lining of her upper shoes. Butylphenol formaldehyde resin is commonly found in the glue in leather shoes.

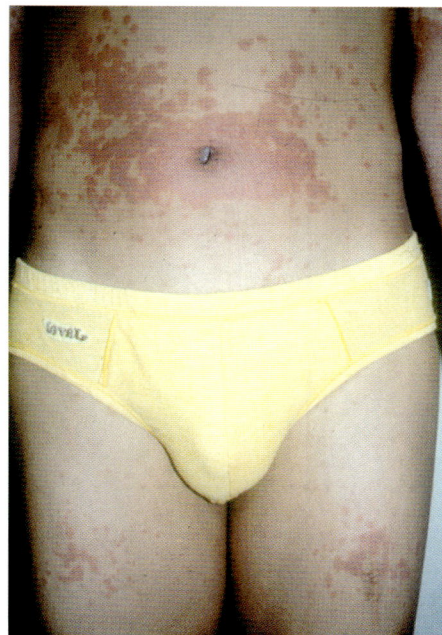

Figure 2–73 □ Allergic contact dermatitis – trinitro-toluene. Confluent erythematous papules and plaques on the abdomen and thighs of a man who worked in a munitions factory. Such an urticarial eruption is a manifestation of a non-eczematous allergic contact reaction.

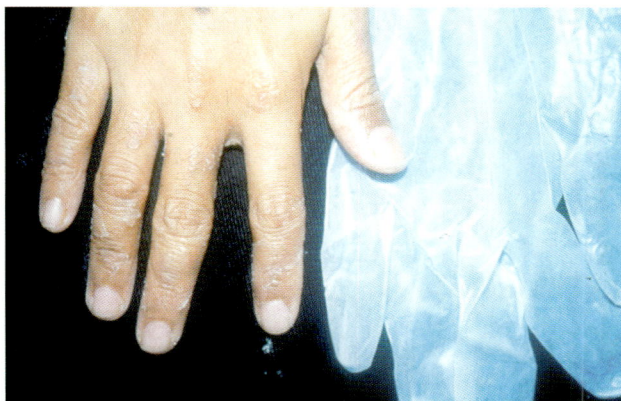

Figure 2–74 □ Allergic contact dermatitis from plastic gloves. Lichenification and scaling of the fingers of a cook who had developed allergic contact dermatitis from his plastic gloves. The exact causative allergen is unknown. Allergy to plastic gloves is rare, compared to rubber and latex gloves.

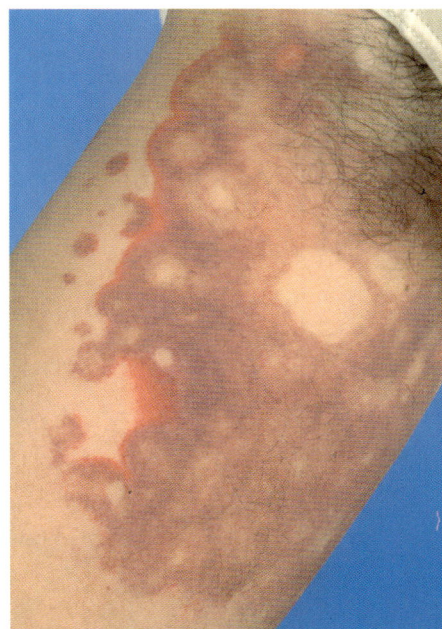

Figure 2–75 □ Erythema multiforme-like allergic contact dermatitis – proflavin. This man developed red and dusky targetoid lesions on his thigh. He had allergic contact dermatitis from proflavin. The initial lesion at the point of origin is usually eczematous but the lesions that radiate outward appear urticarial and target-like. These peripheral lesions may appear after the initial reaction has subsided.

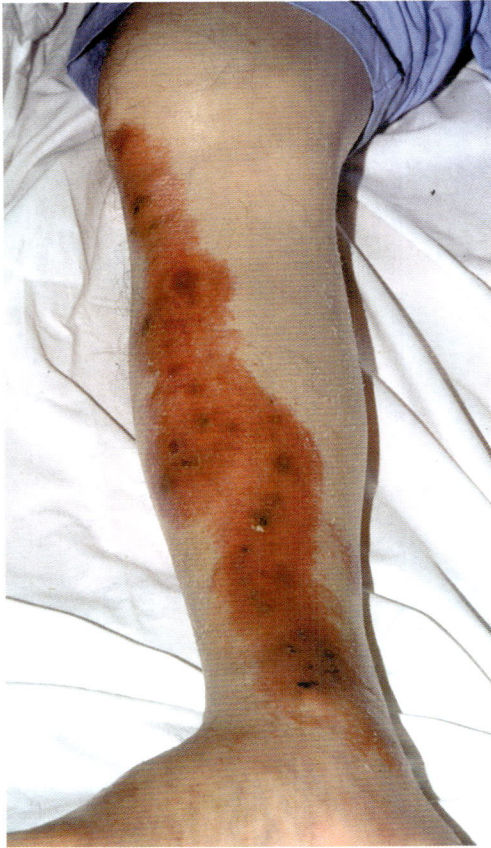

Figure 2–76 □ Purpuric contact dermatitis – iodine. Purpuric plaques on the right lower leg. Most of such cases are allergic in nature but some may be irritant reactions. In this patient, iodine was the offending agent. Other reported causes of purpuric contact dermatitis include black rubber, Disperse Blue 85 dye, proflavine, bonesetter's herbs, and EMLA cream.

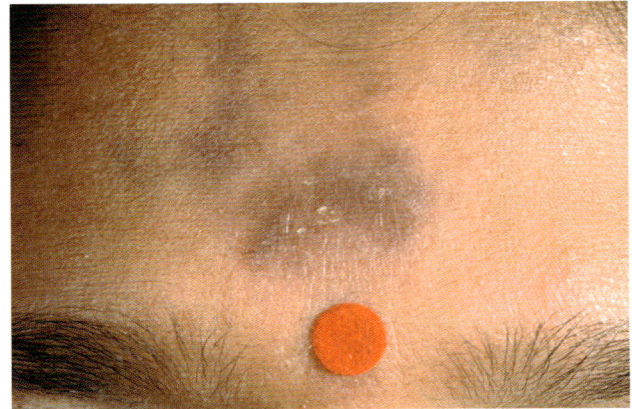

Figure 2–77 □ Pigmented contact dermatitis – "Kumkum". Hyperpigmentation of the skin due to "Kumkum" – colorful cosmetics that are applied to the center of the forehead of Hindu women. Contact allergy occurs gradually, often without any preceding eczema or itch. Causative allergens include Sudan I and other azo dyes.

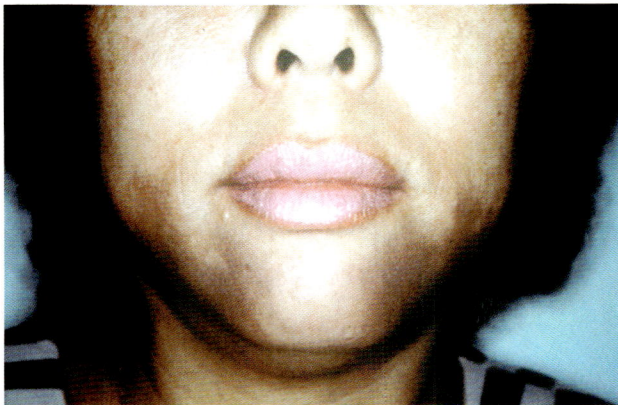

Figure 2–78 □ Pigmented contact dermatitis – cosmetics. Pigmented contact dermatitis presenting as hyperpigmentation on the face of a woman after prolonged use of certain cosmetics. The offending agent was an azo dye, Sudan I. Other causes of pigmented contact dermatitis include textile dyes and fragrances.

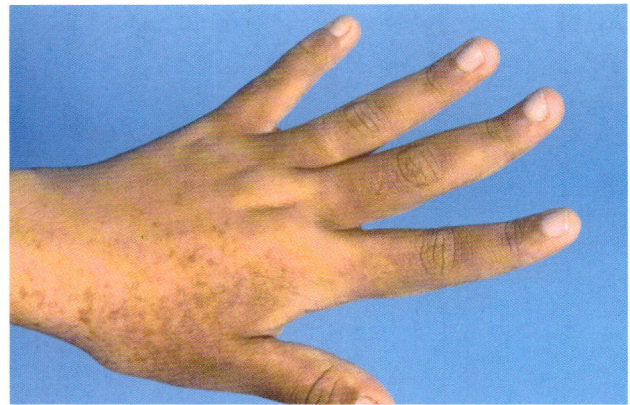

Figure 2–79 □ Phototoxic contact dermatitis – lime. Specks of brown hyperpigmented macules usually not preceded by erythema are commonly seen on the dorsum of hands of people squeezing lime (*Citrus aurantifolia*) in sunlight. This hyperpigmentation persists for months but will eventually resolve.

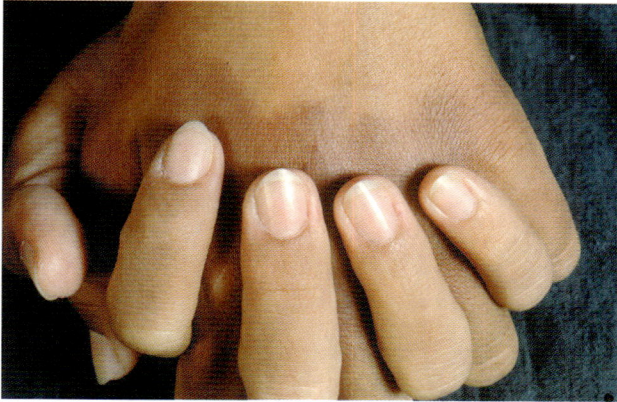

Figure 2–80 □ Phototoxic contact dermatitis – lime. Larger patches of hyperpigmentation on the hands of a cook who had squeezed lime followed by exposure to sunlight. The phototoxic agents are furocoumarins (plant psoralens) found in lime and other citrus fruits. Other common causes of phototoxic contact dermatitis include tar and dyes.

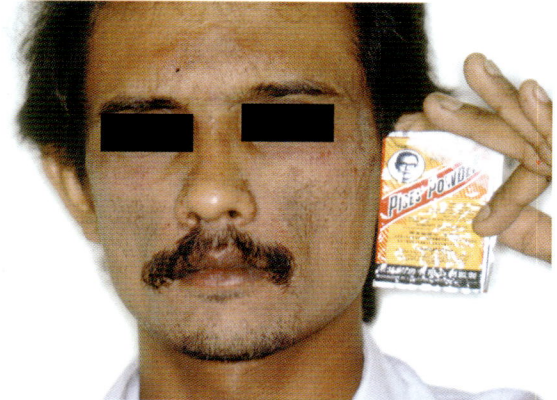

Figure 2–81 □ Photo-allergic contact dermatitis – medicament. Erythema and scaling on the face of a man who had used topical traditional Chinese medication. Other frequently implicated drugs include chlorpromazine and Phenergan cream.

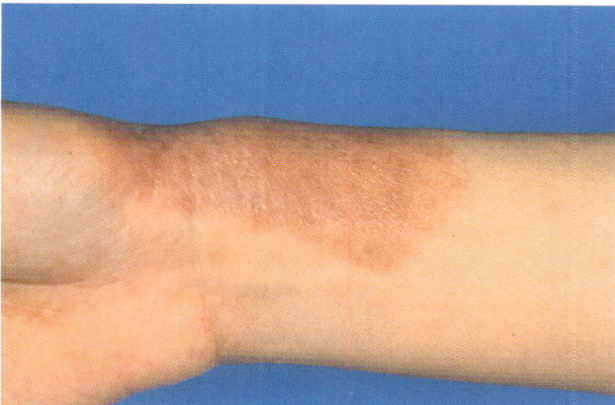

Figure 2–82 □ Photo-allergic contact dermatitis – medicament. A well-demarcated erythematous indurated plaque where a medicated plaster containing a non-steroidal anti-inflammatory drug (NSAID) had been applied. The most common NSAID causing such problems is ketoprofen.

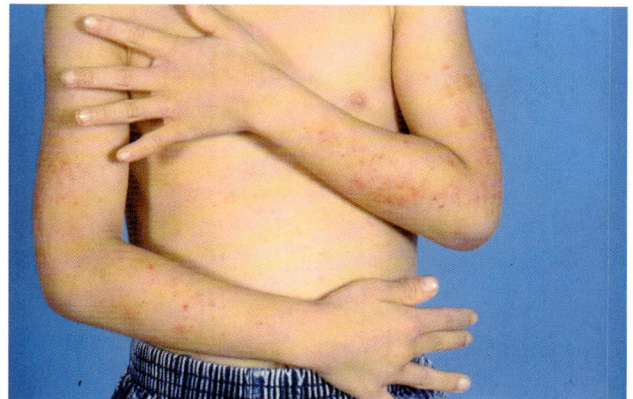

Figure 2–83 □ Photo-allergic contact dermatitis – insect repellant. Erythematous papules on the arms, where this patient had applied a herbal insect repellant. The photopatch test to the patient's insect repellant was positive.

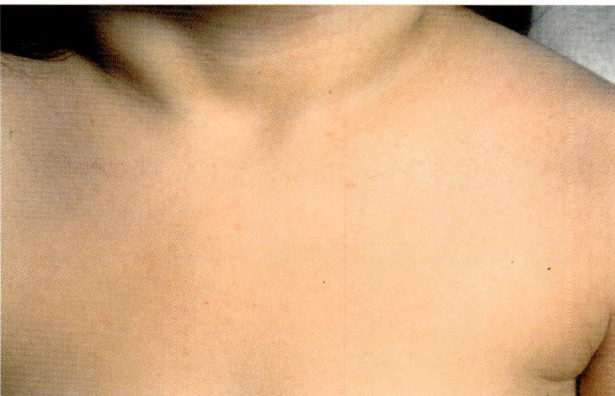

Figure 2–84 □ Pigmented photo-allergic contact dermatitis – sunscreen. Specks of pigmentation on the chest due to photo-allergic contact dermatitis from sunscreen. The most important allergens are the chemical sunscreens. These allergens are also found in moisturizers, shampoos, and lipsticks.

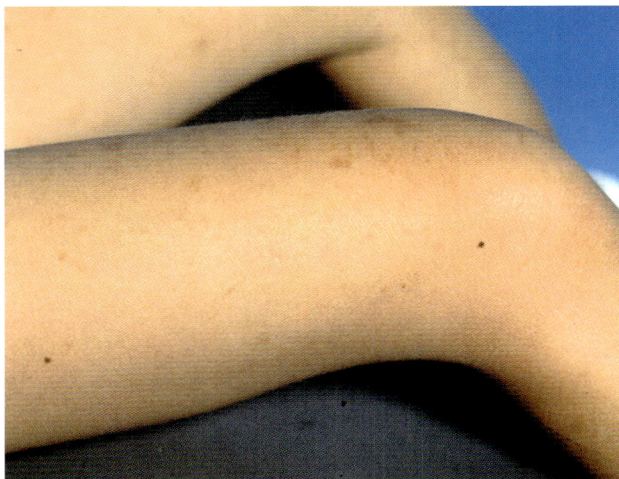

Figure 2–85 □ **Pigmented photo-allergic contact dermatitis – sunscreen.** Specks of pigmentation on the thigh of the patient in Figure 2–84. The main chemical sunscreens implicated are benzophenones, dibenzoyl-methanes, PABA and its esters, and the cinnamates.

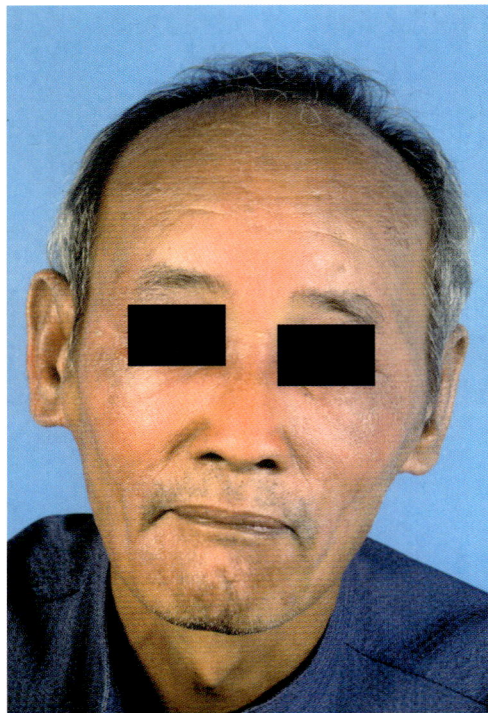

Figure 2–86 □ **Photo-allergic contact dermatitis – musk ambrette.** Erythema and lichenification of the face due to photo-allergic contact dermatitis from musk ambrette. This was common in the 1970s and 1980s due to musk ambrette in male colognes. The use of musk ambrette has been restricted since then.

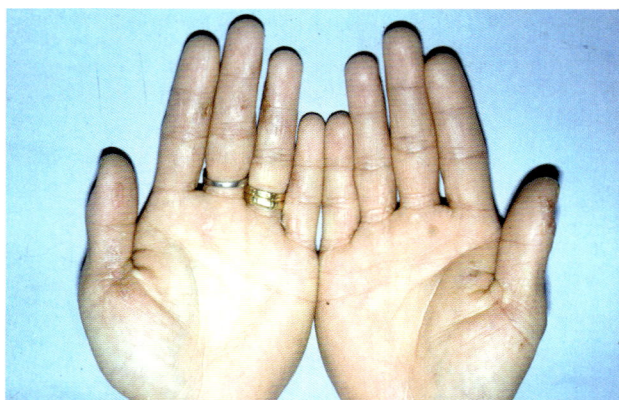

Figure 2–87 □ **Contact urticaria – seafood.** Urticarial lesions on the fingers of a chef who had a type I allergy to seafood. The itch and lesions usually begin within 20 minutes after contact with the allergen. The allergens are the proteins in raw foods. This condition may present as an eczematous rash, especially when it is more chronic.

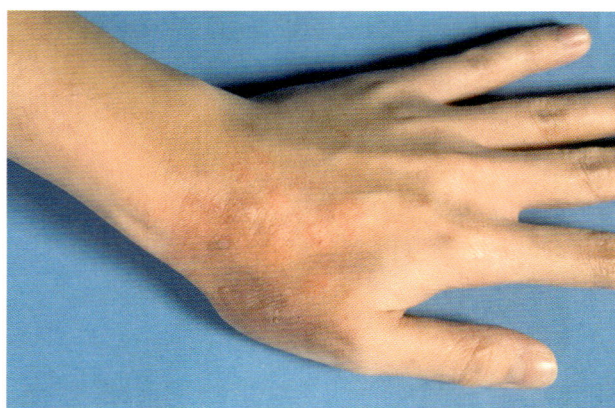

Figure 2–88 □ **Contact urticaria – latex gloves.** Urticaria and post-inflammatory hyperpigmentation on the left hand of a dental nurse. Skin prick test was positive for natural rubber latex. The allergens are the latex proteins hevein and prohevein. Healthcare workers are at special risk of acquiring latex allergy. Latex allergy cross-reacts with fruits such as banana, kiwi fruit, and avocado.

Papulosquamous Disorders
Khoo L.S.W. and Foo C.C.I.

Papulosquamous disorders are a group of common dermatoses characterized by primary lesions of scaly papules. The clinical conditions in this group include psoriasis, lichen planus, lichen amyloidosis, pityriasis rosea, secondary syphilis, pityriasis lichenoides chronica, and pityriasis lichenoides acuta.

PSORIASIS (Figures 3–1 to 3–16)

Psoriasis is one of the most common dermatoses in this group. This is an inflammatory cutaneous disorder with important genetic predisposition. There are a number of clinical variants, of which psoriasis vulgaris (plaque-type psoriasis) is the most common. It is characterized by reddish scaly plaques distributed commonly on the scalp, extensor surfaces of elbows and knees, umbilicus, and gluteal cleft. Although often described as non-pruritic, most patients find the condition itchy and lesions are often lichenified and excoriated. The other variants of psoriasis include flexural psoriasis (often presents with smooth, glazed, erythematous, well-defined plaques on flexural surfaces), guttate psoriasis (presents with abrupt eruption of small lesions the size of water drops (2 to 5 mm in diameter) following acute upper respiratory tract infection), erythrodermic psoriasis (which is an important differential for patients with generalized exfoliative dermatitis), and pustular psoriasis (which can either be localized or generalized).

Inflammatory arthritis occurs in 6 to 10% of moderate to severe psoriatic patients. The arthritis usually takes the form of oligoarthritis with swelling and tenosynovitis of one or few hand joints (in about 70% of psoriatic arthritis). The other patterns of arthritis include asymmetrical distal interphalangeal joint involvement, arthritis mutilans, rheumatoid arthritis-like polyarthritis and ankylosing spondylitis. Nail changes may be seen in up to 50% of patients. Individual morphologic alteration seen in a nail unit is not specific or diagnostic of the disease unless there is associated cutaneous psoriasis of the proximal and lateral nailfolds or volar finger pads. However, the constellation of nail changes taken together is strongly suggestive of psoriasis. Some of the common nail changes seen in psoriasis patients are pitting, red spots in the lunula, transverse ridges, nail thickening, onycholysis, yellow-brown spot on the nail bed ("oil droplet" sign), and splinter hemorrhages.

LICHEN PLANUS (Figures 3–17 to 3–27)

Lichen planus is characterized by pruritic papules that are often flat-topped, polygonal, and purplish in color. On the surface of the papules, grayish or whitish puncta or streaks (Wickham's striae) may be seen. In Asian patients, especially those with darker skin, the lesions are often pigmented and associated with intense post-inflammatory hyperpigmentation. The lesions typically affect the flexor surface of wrists, trunk, medial thighs, shins, dorsal hands, and glans penis. A number of variants of lichen planus are seen, including the hypertrophic form (where the confluent lesions may mimic lichen simplex chronicus), erosive form (especially on the genitals and scalp), annular form (on genitalia and lips), linear form (commonly seen on limbs), atrophic form, and bullous form.

Nail changes are seen in about 5 to 10% of patients and may take the form of longitudinal grooving, proximal and distal onycholysis, ridging, splitting, midline fissure, pterygium and total obliteration, and loss of nails. About 20% of patients with mucous membrane involvement also have cutaneous lesions. The oral lesions may be reticulate, atrophic, or ulcerative.

Although the condition of most patients spontaneously improves after 12 to 18 months, mucous membrane and hypertrophic lesions tend to be more persistent. Rare cases of squamous cell carcinoma occurring on the lower leg in hypertrophic lichen planus and in erosive oral lichen planus have been reported.

LICHEN AMYLOIDOSIS (Figures 3–41)

Lichen amyloidosis is a common primary cutaneous amyloidosis. Although uncommon in the West, it is fairly common amongst Asian patients. Patients often present with mildly scaly, skin-colored or brownish papules on the calves, forearms, and upper back. The lesions are often secondarily eczematized due to severe pruritus. Occasionally, the macular form of lichen amyloidosis is seen where patients present with macular brownish lesions instead

of the typical papular eruption.

PITYRIASIS ROSEA (Figures 3–28 to 3–33)

Pityriasis rosea is a fairly common, self-limiting papulosquamous eruption seen in young healthy adults. Patients may recall prodromic, flu-like symptoms one to two weeks prior to the onset of a rash. The initial lesion often takes the form of an annular patch, slightly scaly around the lesion ("collarette scaling") located on the trunk (known as the "herald patch"). This is followed by subsequent development of smaller scaly annular lesions formed along the longitudinal axis of the trunk, giving rise to the typical fir-tree appearance. New lesions may then form centrifugally on the limbs. The rash typically lasts between 8 to 12 weeks before complete resolution. A number of variants of pityriasis rosea are observed – the inverse pattern spares the covered parts of body, the papular variant may be seen in children, and the inflamed variant may be rather eczematized or purpuric.

PITYRIASIS LICHENOIDES CHRONICA (Figures 3–36 to 3–38)

Patients with pityriasis lichenoides chronica present with recurrent crops of erythematous, scaly macules and lichenoid papules. The lesions are typically found on sides of trunk, thighs, and upper arms. Asian patients tend to have prominent post-inflammatory hypopigmentation after resolution of the rash. This is a benign condition that clears spontaneously after a few months to years.

PITYRIASIS LICHENOIDES ET VARIOLIFORMIS ACUTA (Figures 3–39 to 3–40)

Pityriasis lichenoides et varioliformis acuta (PLEVA) occurs with a sudden appearance of a polymorphous eruption consisting of macules, papules, and occasional vesicles. The papules tend to form crusting, necrosis, and hemorrhage. The vesicles tend to be deep seated and varicelliform. The papulonecrotic lesions have brownish crusts and hemorrhagic excoriations. The rash usually heals leaving pigmented, depressed, varioliform scars. However, a new crop of lesions will then

appear. The rash commonly involves the anterior trunk, flexor surfaces of upper limbs, and the axillary areas. Although usually resolving after months to years, rare cases of PLEVA developing into cutaneous T-cell lymphoma have been reported.

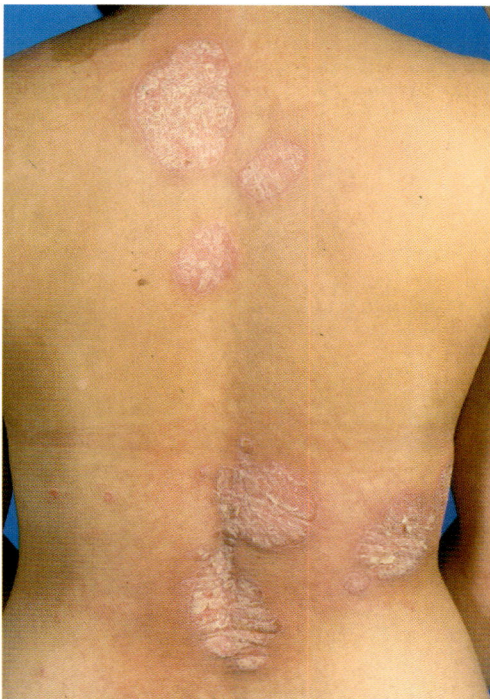

Figure 3–1 □ Psoriasis. This picture shows typical psoriatic plaques on the back of a 30-year-old Chinese male. The plaques are red, indurated, and scaly.

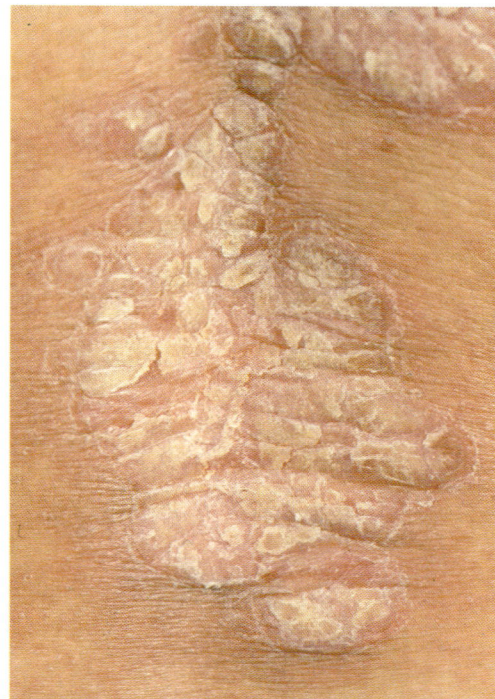

Figure 3–2 □ Psoriatic plaque – close up. The psoriatic plaque has silvery white scales and well-defined borders.

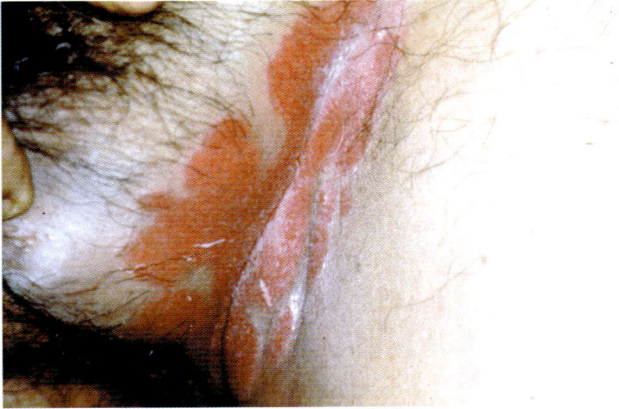

Figure 3–3 □ Flexural psoriasis. Psoriatic plaques on flexures appear differently from the usual indurated scaly lesions. Flexural lesions tend to appear as well-defined, glazy, reddish plaques.

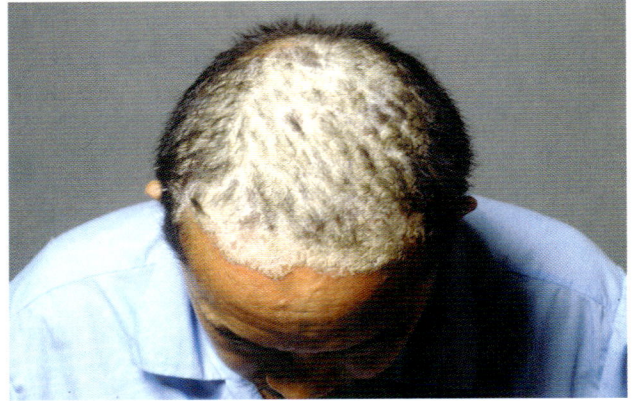

Figure 3–4 □ Scalp psoriasis. This 54-year-old Chinese male has extensive psoriasis involving the scalp. The scalp lesions can be better appreciated if the hairs are short. The well-demarcated borders may extend beyond the hairline to the adjacent skin. Patients tend to pick on the scales, resulting in köebnerisation of the lesions.

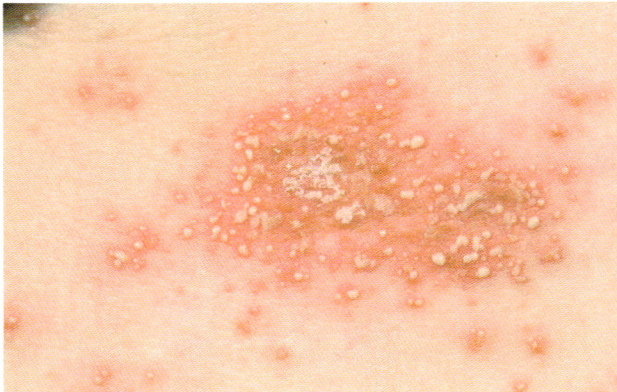

Figure 3–5 □ Pustular psoriasis. Pustular psoriasis may be localized or generalized. The localized lesions may appear as a collection of pustules over well-defined, red plaques. The generalized variant may present as generalized erythema with extensive pustules covering the whole body surface ("Von Zumbush" type).

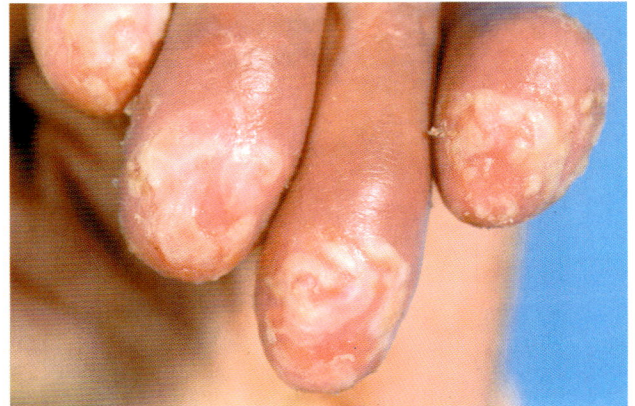

Figure 3–6 □ Localized pustular psoriasis – acral. Localized pustular psoriasis may take the form of acral pustulosis affecting the digits. Pustular eruptions occur on the digits, with the resultant collection of pustules, yellowish crusting, and destruction of nails.

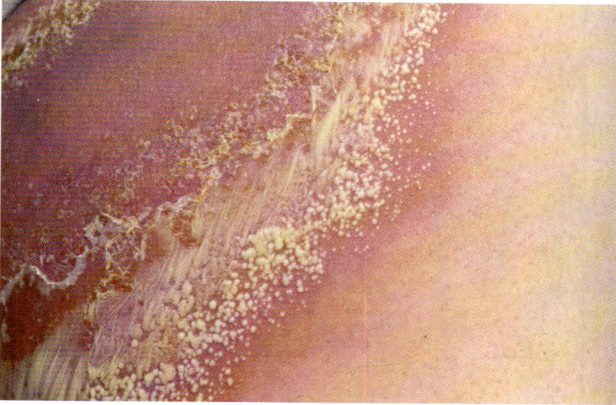

Figure 3–7 □ Generalized pustular psoriasis. Generalized pustular psoriasis is one of the rare dermatological emergencies that patients may present with. The patient is usually febrile and toxic-looking. The skin is erythematous and covered with lakes of pustules. Elderly patients are particularly prone to hemodynamic instability and heat loss. Treatment includes careful management of the associated fluid and electrolyte imbalance. Systemic retinoids or methotrexate given under close monitoring can be used to hasten the resolution of the pustules.

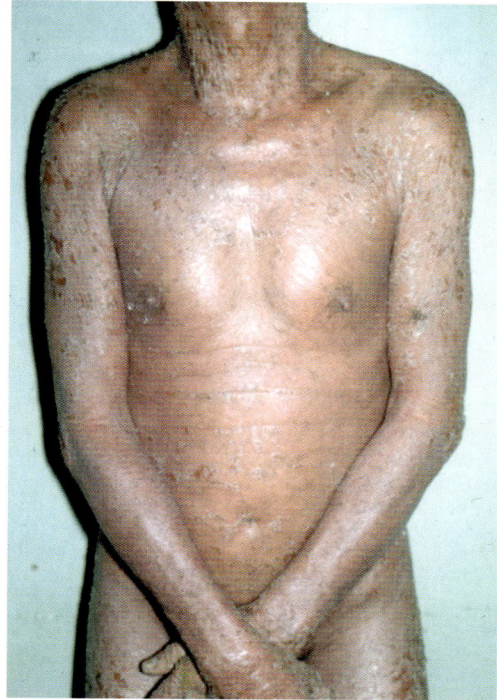

Figure 3–8 □ Erythrodermic psoriasis. This 56-year-old Chinese male presents with erythroderma or generalized exfoliative dermatitis secondary to psoriasis. Erythrodermic psoriasis is associated with significant hemodynamic and temperature regulation problems. The clues to this diagnosis include a prior history of psoriasis and presence of other psoriatic lesions such as nail changes and joint involvement.

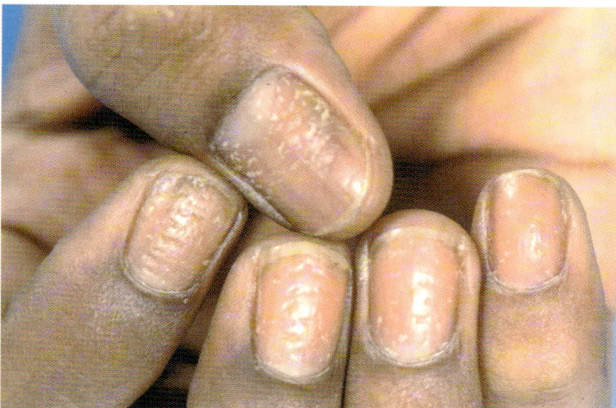

Figure 3–9 □ Psoriatic nail changes. This picture shows typical mild psoriatic nail changes of pitting and onycholysis which are seen in about 50% of patients.

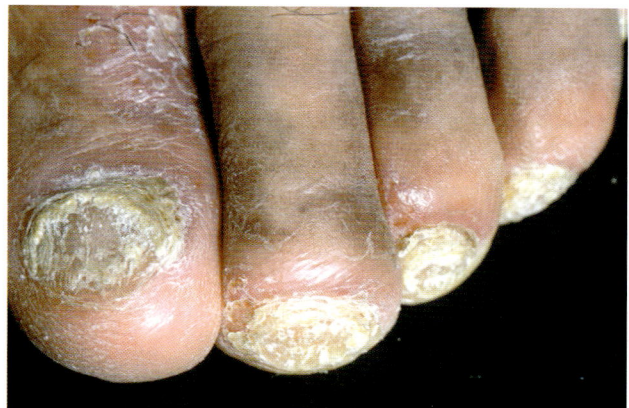

Figure 3–10 □ Psoriatic nail changes. In a more severe form of nails involvement, total dystrophy of nails may be seen. The nails are thickened, with a roughened and crumbled surface.

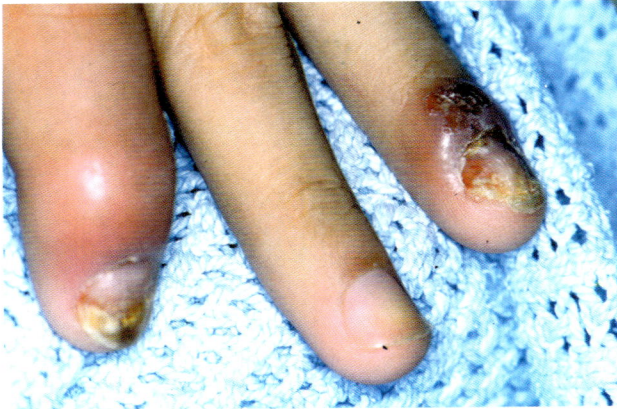

Figure 3–11 □ Psoriatic arthritis. Inflammatory arthritis occurs in about 10% of patients. The types of arthropathy may be oligoarthropathy, osteoarthritis-like, rheumatoid arthritis-like, ankylosing spondylitis-like or arthritis mutilans. The diagram shows an osteoarthritis-like involvement of the distal interphalangeal joint.

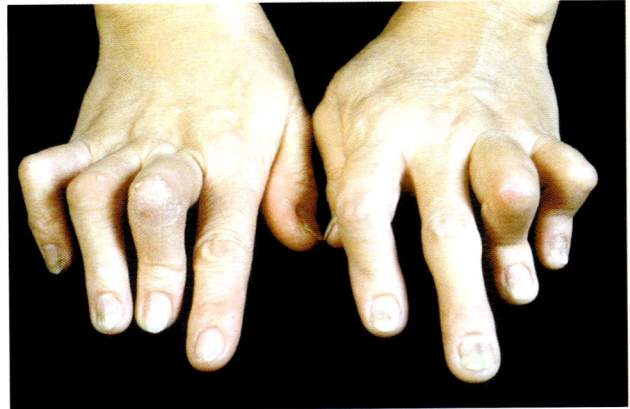

Figure 3–12 □ Psoriatic arthritis. A rheumatoid arthritis-like type of joint involvement is shown in this picture.

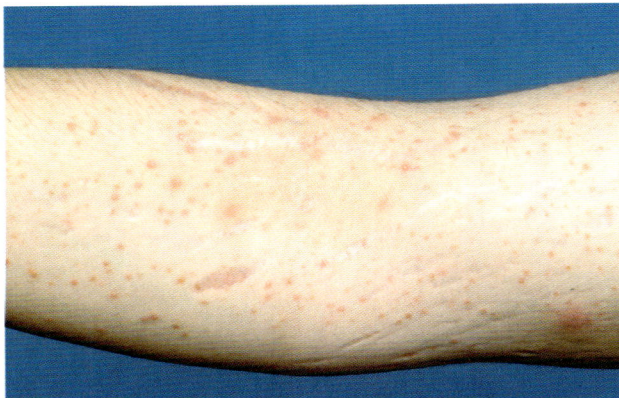

Figure 3–13 □ Psoriasis therapy – complications. Various types of topical agents are used in the treatment of psoriasis. Topical steroid is often used for its quick effect. However, inappropriate, excessive, prolonged use of potent topical steroids may result in prominent steroid atrophy as shown in the picture.

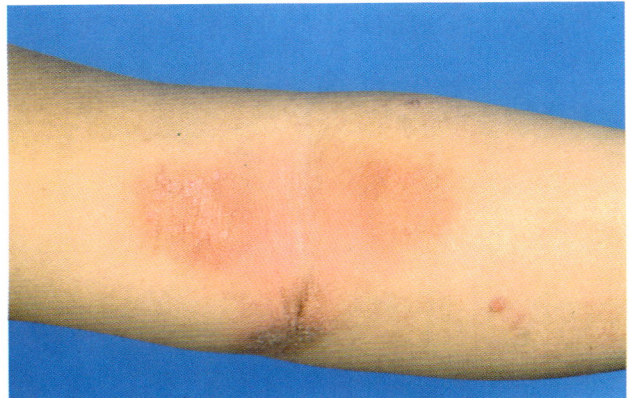

Figure 3–14 □ Psoriasis therapy – complications. Dithranol is commonly used to treat localized psoriatic plaques. It is often used as short contact therapy where dithranol is carefully applied on psoriatic lesions for 15 to 20 minutes and washed away after the period of contact. Accidental contact of dithranol on the surrounding normal skin may result in irritation of the normal skin.

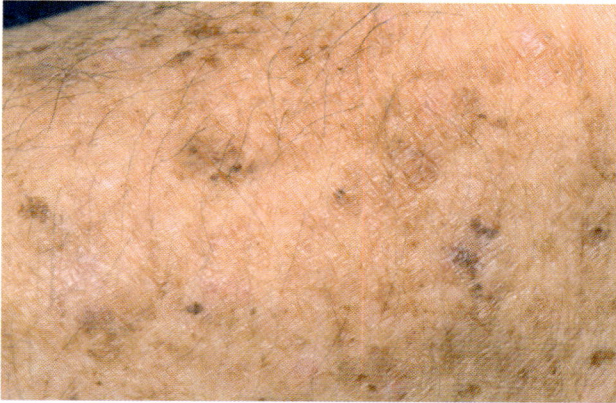

Figure 3–15 □ PUVA keratosis. For patients who have received many courses of PUVA photochemotherapy, PUVA keratosis may develop due to excessive UV exposure. These are pigmented macules and papules which may be slightly scaly.

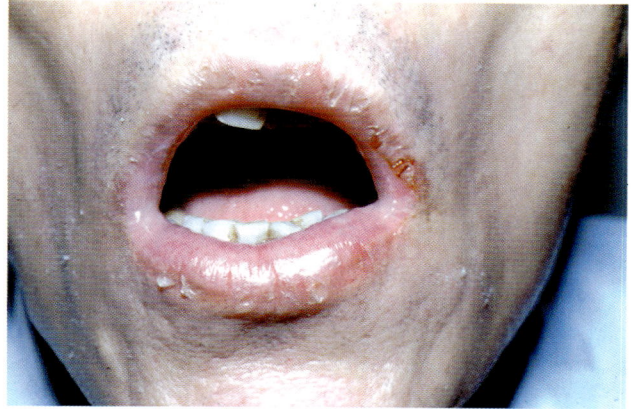

Figure 3–16 □ Acitretin-induced cheilitis. Acitretin is a commonly used systemic retinoid for patients with extensive psoriasis. Cheilitis is a common side effect.

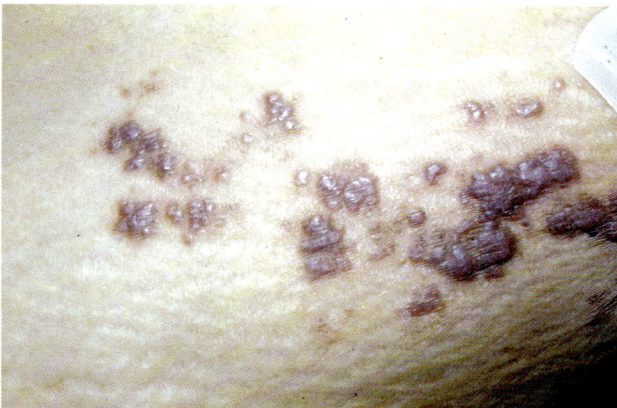

Figure 3–17 □ Lichen planus. Lichen planus is typically a papular eruption which is purplish, flat-topped, and extremely pruritic.

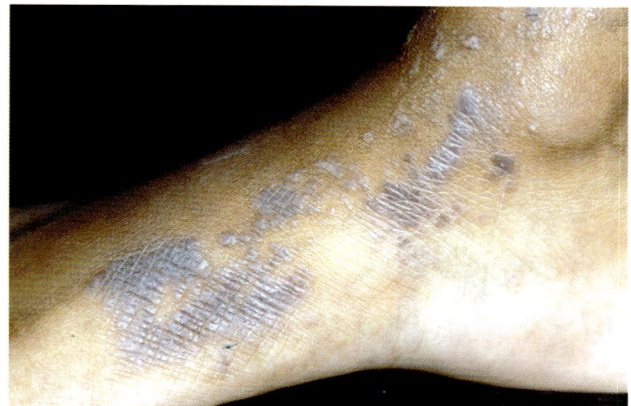

Figure 3–18 □ Lichen planus. In patients with darker skin, lichen planus eruption may be more pigmented rather than purplish in color. This is often confused with post-inflammatory hyperpigmentation.

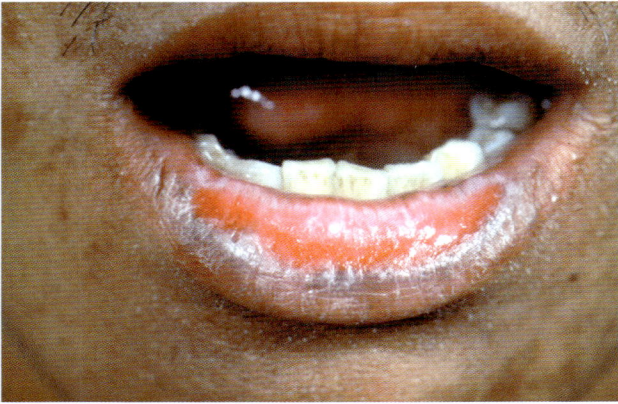

Figure 3–19 □ Lichen planus – lip. Lichen planus involving the lips may present as whitish patches or superficial erosions.

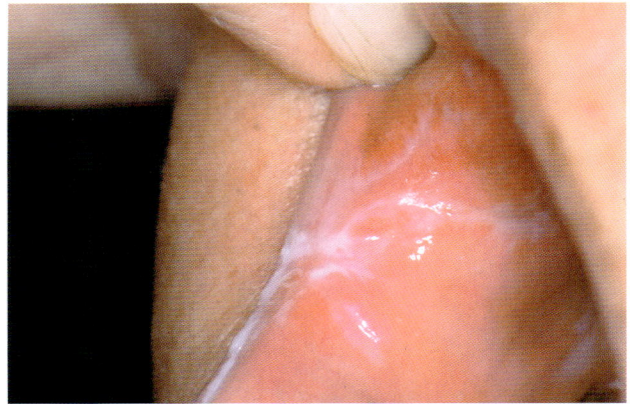

Figure 3–20 □ Lichen planus – buccal mucosa. Lichen planus involving the buccal mucosa often presents as typical whitish lacy patches.

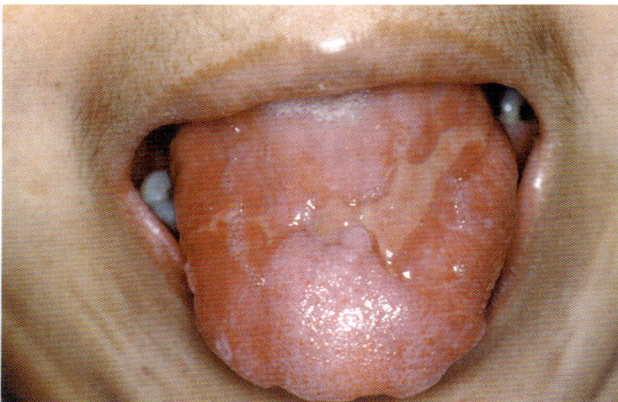

Figure 3–21 □ Lichen planus – tongue. Lichen planus of the tongue presenting as painful erosions and ulcers. It is important to rule out infective causes (such as herpetic infection) and immunobullous eruption involving the tongue.

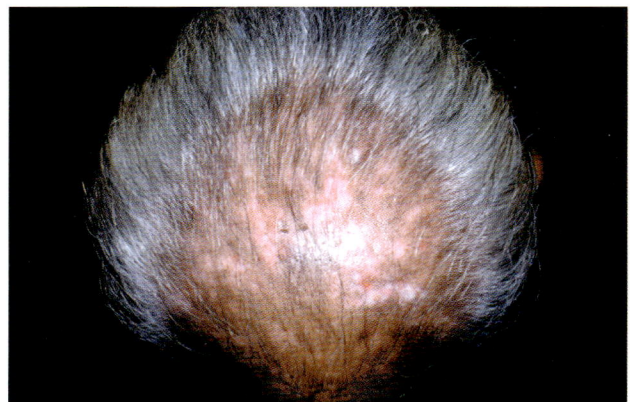

Figure 3–22 □ Lichen planus – scalp. Lichen planus involving the scalp may present as erythematous patches to erosions or ulcerations. In chronic cases, these eruptions on the scalp may lead to scarring alopecia.

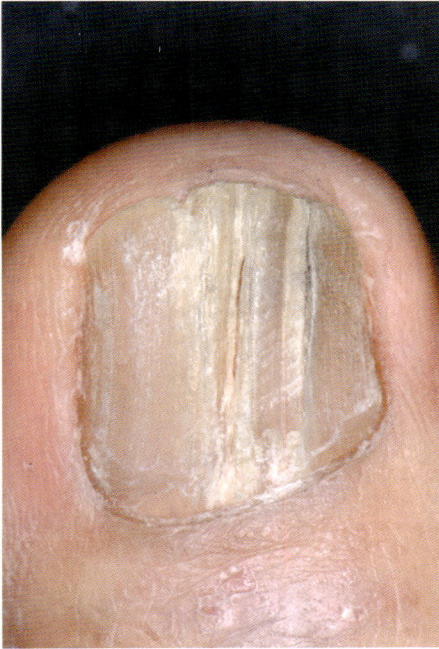

Figure 3–23 □ Lichen planus – nails. Nail changes are present in 5 to 10% of lichen planus patients. Longitudinal grooving (as seen in this picture), onycholysis, ridging, splitting, pterygium formation, and even 20 nail dystrophy may occur.

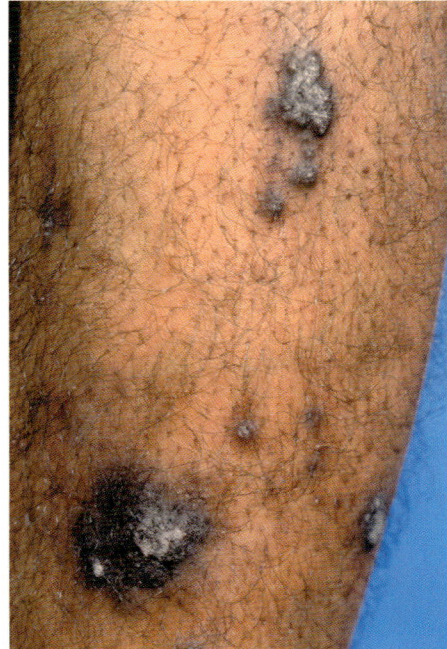

Figure 3–24 □ Hypertrophic lichen planus. This is most commonly seen on the shins and is thought to represent lichen planus with simultaneous changes of lichen simplex chronicus. The lesion is typically a verrucous, violaceous plaque with variable degrees of scaling. In patients with darker skin, the lesion may be heavily pigmented.

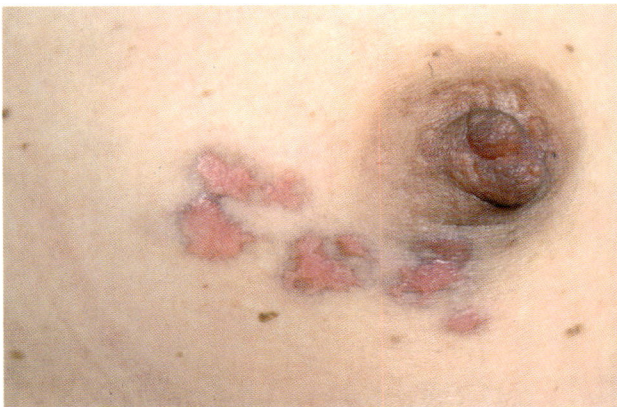

Figure 3–25 □ Atrophic lichen planus. The lichen planus lesions appear as thin, atrophic, erythematous macules, sometimes associated with post-inflammatory hyper-pigmentation.

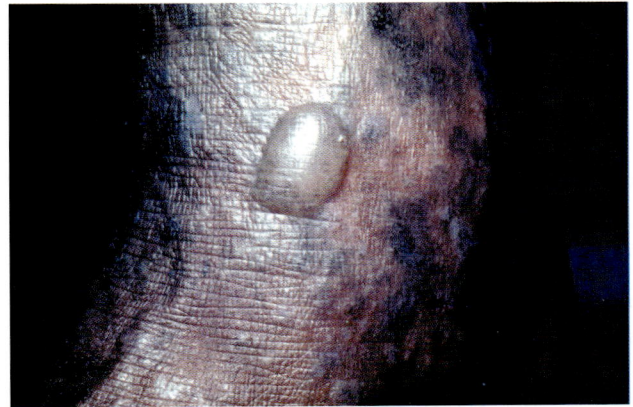

Figure 3–26 □ Bullous lichen planus. Bullous eruptions may occur as a result of intense inflammation in the typical lichen planus lesions or may occur in lichen planus pemphigoides where blistering eruptions may develop on pre-existing lichen planus lesions and on normal skin.

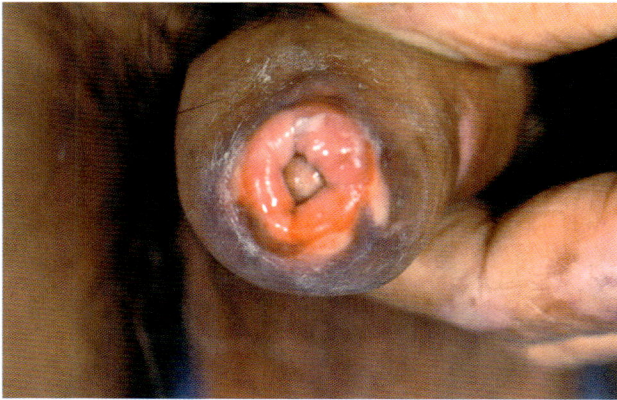

Figure 3–27 □ Erosive lichen planus. Intense inflammation in the genital area may result in superficial, painful erosions. This has to be differentiated from other erosive conditions such as herpes genitalia and fixed drug eruption.

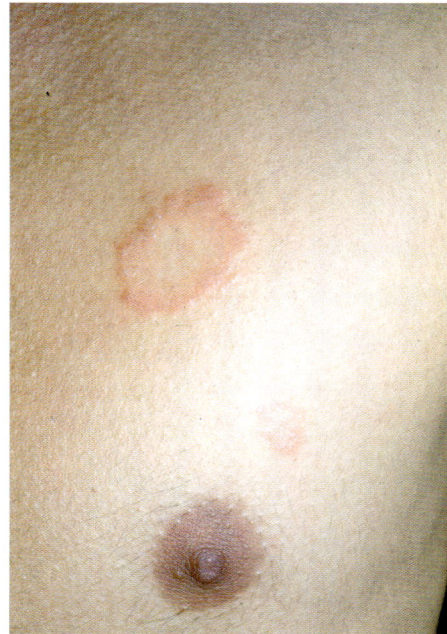

Figure 3–28 □ Pityriasis rosea – herald patch. The herald patch of pityriasis rosea on the left upper trunk is present. This is often remembered as the earliest, largest, annular lesion in a patient with pityriasis rosea. The herald patch may precede the eruption of multiple papulosquamous lesions by several weeks.

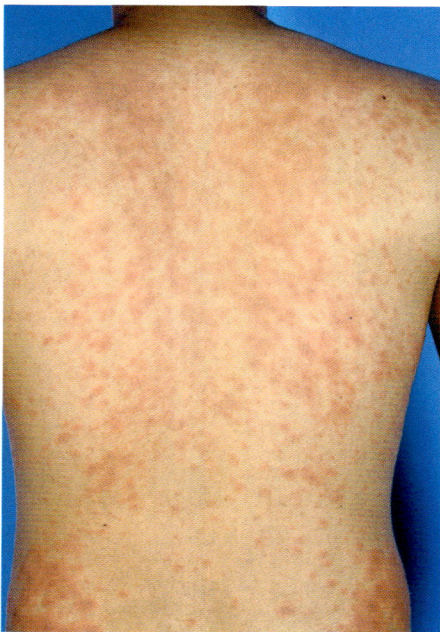

Figure 3–29 □ Pityriasis rosea. In established pityriasis rosea, the patient develops extensive, scaly, erythematous papules on the trunk. The truncal lesions typically have a "fir-tree" distribution, with the long axis of individual lesions orientating along the skin cleavages.

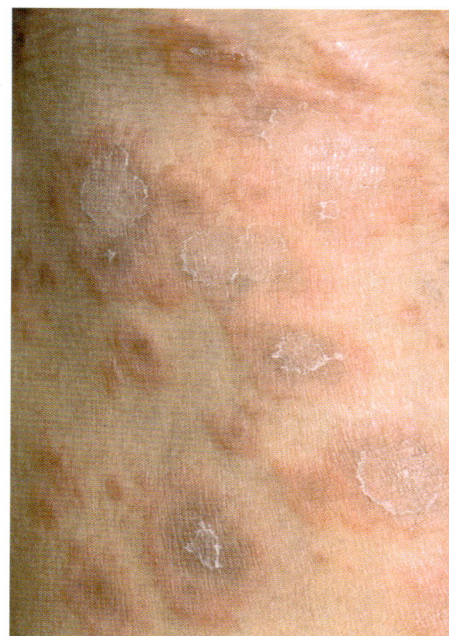

Figure 3–30 □ Pityriasis rosea. Individual lesions in pityriasis rosea often have fine scales that desquamate, leaving behind fine, collarette scaling around the papular eruptions.

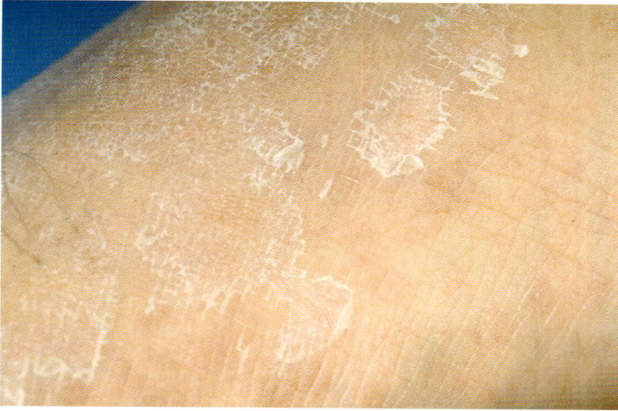

Figure 3–31 □ Pityriasis rosea. Patients are often prescribed calamine lotion which enhances the annular nature of the lesions.

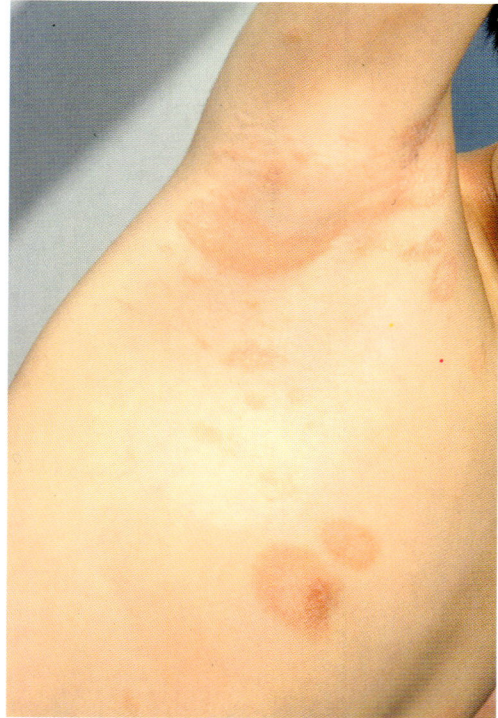

Figure 3–32 □ Pityriasis rosea – inverse pattern. Some patients with pityriasis rosea have lesions concentrated on flexural surfaces such as the axillae and groins, giving rise to the inverse pattern of distribution of lesions.

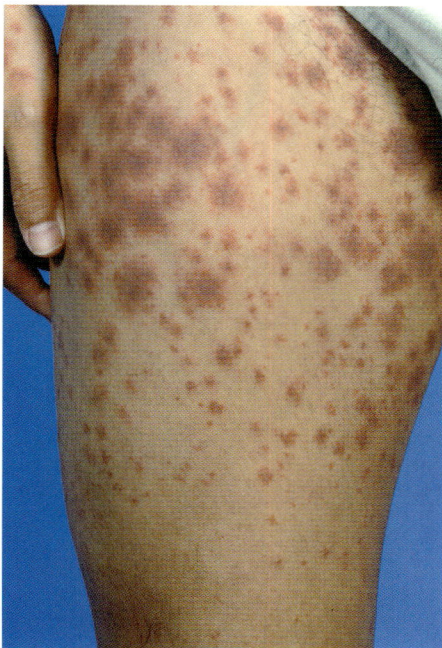

Figure 3–33 □ Pityriasis rosea – inflammatory variant. The typical lesions may sometimes be intensely erythematous in the inflamed type of pityriasis rosea.

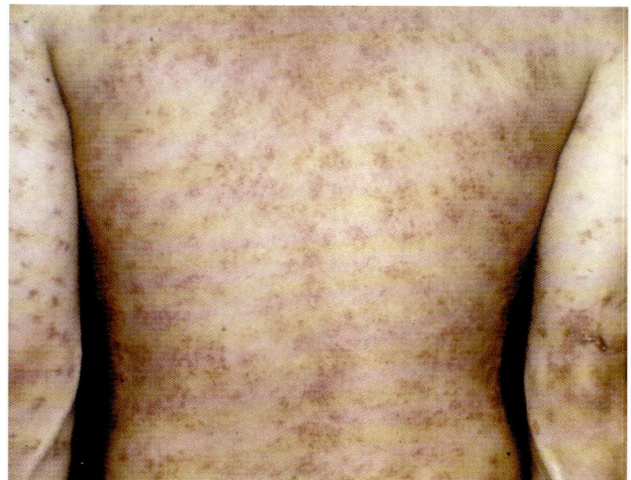

Figure 3–34 □ Secondary syphilis. Pityriasiform lesions occur in secondary syphilis. It is always important to rule out secondary syphilis in a patient with pityriasis rosea-like lesions who also has a history of sexual exposure. The lesions in secondary syphilis are usually more uniform in size, more brownish, less scaly, and less pruritic.

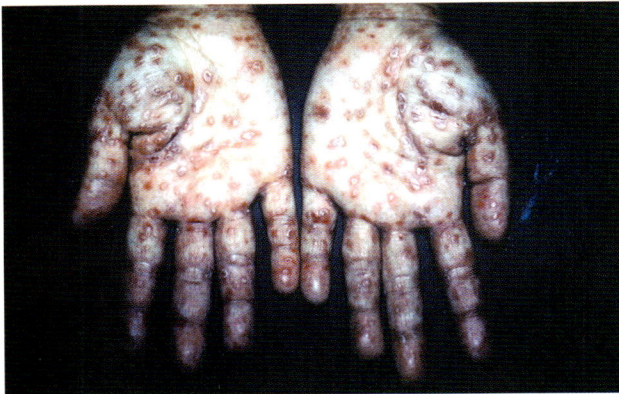

Figure 3–35 □ Secondary syphilis. Brownish-orange macular rash on the palms of a patient with secondary syphilis. Palmer involvement is not common in patients with pityriasis rosea and sexually active young adults presenting with pityriasiform lesions and palmo-plantar involvement should have a VDRL screen to exclude secondary syphilis.

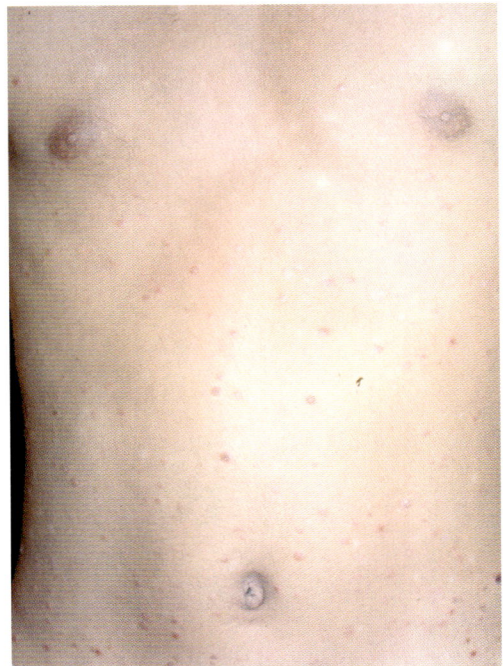

Figure 3–36 □ Pityriasis lichenoides chronica. This patient has the characteriztic erythematous scaly macules and lichenoid papules that are found mainly on the trunk, thighs, and upper arms.

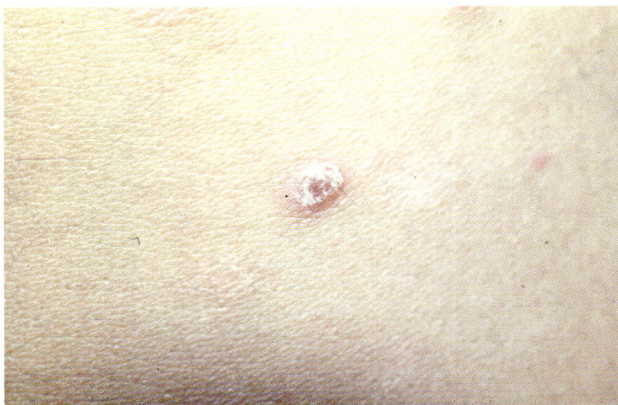

Figure 3–37 □ Pityriasis lichenoides chronica – close up. A thin piece of scale ("mica" scale) may cover the erythematous papule in pityriasis lichenoides chronica.

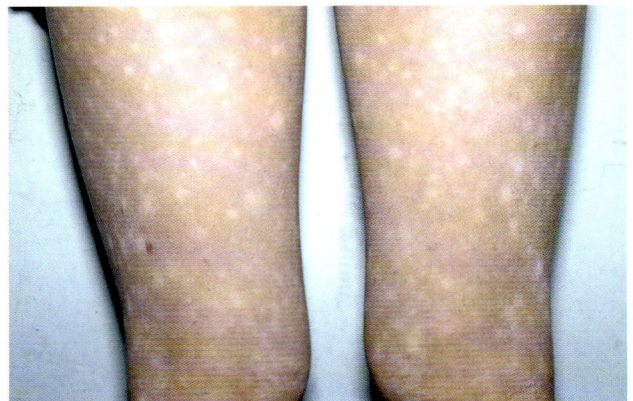

Figure 3–38 □ Pityriasis lichenoides chronica – hypopig-mentation. In Asian patients, resolving pityriasis lichenoides chronica lesions often result in hypopigmentation which may persist for months.

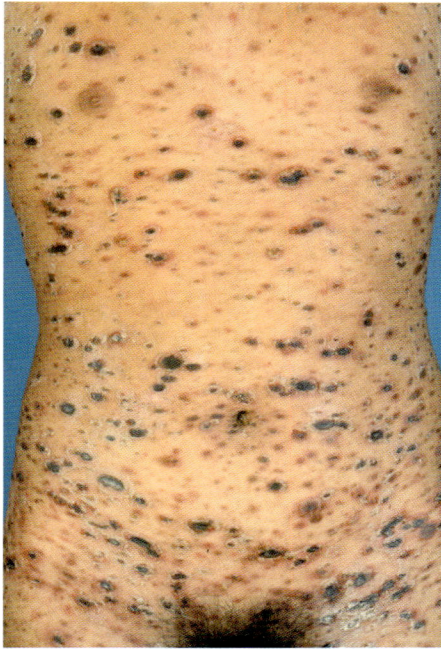

Figure 3–39 □ Pityriasis lichenoides et varioliformis acuta (PLEVA). This patient presents with a sudden appearance of a polymorphous eruption comprising macules, papules, and occasional vesicles. The papules are brownish-red, rounded lesions with associated crusting, necrosis, and hemorrhage. The rash commonly involves the anterior trunk, flexor surfaces of the upper extremities, and axillary regions.

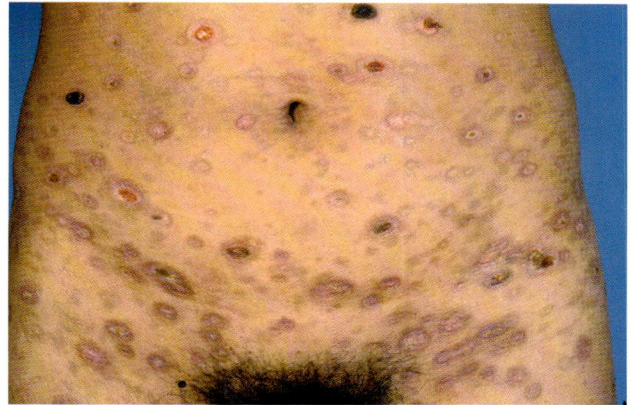

Figure 3–40 □ Pityriasis lichenoides et varioliformis acuta. Vesicular lesions in PLEVA may be deep seated and varicelliform. The papulonecrotic lesions may be covered with brown crusting and hemorrhagic excoriations. The lesions may then heal, leaving behind smooth, pigmented, depressed, varioliform scars.

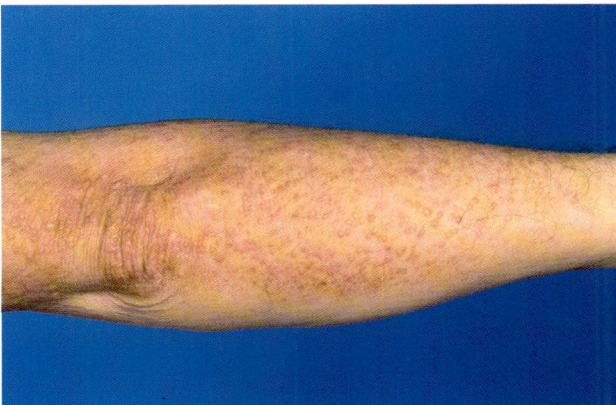

Figure 3–41 □ Lichen amyloidosis. Lichen amyloidosis occurs secondary to cutaneous amyloid deposits. The rash may be macular or papular, is brownish in color and is usually pruritic. Common sites of involvement are the extensor surfaces of forearms and lateral calves.

Pigmentary Disorders
Kumarasinghe P. and Chio M.T.W.

Asia is home to billions of people with "pigmented skin". Pigmentary disorders are more visible on the Asian skin, and are of great cosmetic concern to the Asian patient. A significant proportion of patients attending most dermatology clinics in Asia have pigmentary disorders.

Certain pigmentary disorders occur more frequently in Asians than in Caucasians; these include Mongolian blue spot, Hori's nevus, nevus of Ota, progressive macular confluent hypomelanosis and reticulate acropigmentation of Kitamura. Post-inflammatory hyperpigmentation arising from a diversity of skin insults and injuries is also more frequent, pronounced, and persistent on the Asian skin.

Pigmentary disorders are a complex group of dermatoses which may be genetically determined or acquired. Much progress has been made in the last two decades in pigment cell research, molecular biology and genetic studies: now clinicians and scientists are able to understand many of these conditions better.

MELANIN: ITS ROLE IN PIGMENTARY DISORDERS

Melanin plays a central role in most pigmentary disorders. It is the melanin content in the epidermal prickle cell layer that gives the distinct color to an individual. Hemoglobin, bilirubin, and beta-carotene play additional but minor roles in visible pigmentation. The number of melanocytes does not vary amongst different races. It is the amount of melanin in the melanosomes and the distribution of the pigment and the melanosomes that make the difference amongst the different ethnic groups and races.

In most Caucasians, Indians, and Africans, the predominant pigment is eumelanin. In Mongoloids and red-headed Caucasians, the predominant pigment is pheomelanin. However, in a given individual of any race, there may be a mixture of eumelanin and pheomelanin. Other than genetic encoding, factors such as pH changes within the melanosomes can shift the melanogenesis towards eumelanin and pheomelanin.

The melanocyte is the key cellular player in most pigmentary disorders. Melanocytes are influenced by many factors including cytokines produced by keratinocytes, lymphocytes, fibroblasts, hormones, and ultraviolet radiation. In addition, melanocytes also possess an ability to control melanogenesis in an autocrine manner. The inherent genetic encoding expressed by the melanocyte is the most important determinant in a given person's general pigmentation. Tyrosinase is the most important rate-limiting enzyme in melanogenesis.

Visible pigmentation due to melanin may be altered due to lack of or excess in the production of melanin, defects in transport of melanosomes within the melanocytes, defects in melanin uptake by keratinocytes, or defects in the spread of melanin granules within keratinocytes or their turnover time.

EVALUATING A PIGMENTARY DISORDER

Clinical features are very important in evaluating disorders of pigmentation. The morphology, pattern, distribution, and other characteristics all serve as clues to the diagnosis. As melanocytes are embryologically derived from the neural crest cells, many congenital disorders of pigmentation have associated neurologic, ocular, auditory, endocrinologic, or other anomalies which should be actively looked for and screened. The patients should be examined in good light (preferably natural light or simulated natural light) to detect subtle changes of pigmentation.

Investigations become necessary in some conditions. Routine skin biopsy for histopathology with or without special stains may be required to confirm whether the pigment is melanin or some other pigment (e.g. hemosiderin), and to identify the distribution of the pigment and the melanocytes. The absence of melanocytes suggests vitiligo, melanophages in the dermis suggests post-inflammatory hyperpigmentation (which can be due to numerous causes), melanocytes in the dermis suggests conditions such as Mongolian blue spot and Hori's nevus, deeper nevoid cells suggest lesions such as a blue nevus. Electron microscopy may be necessary to assess the melanosomes and the dendrites of melanocytes. Genetic studies have also become very useful in understanding some of the pigmentary disorders.

CLASSIFICATION

Classification of pigmentary disorders can be based on etiology, pathology, genetics or clinical morphology. Of these, the morphological classification appears to be most useful in guiding the dermatologist in the routine evaluation of a pigmentary disorder.

A morphological classification of the more common and medically relevant disorders with pigmentary abnormalities is presented in Table 4.1. This table categorizes pigmentary disorders according to their main clinical presentation and pattern. Pigmentary disorders are first broadly divided into two groups: hyperpigmented and hypopigmented. The conditions in these two groups are not mutually exclusive as hyper and hypopigmented lesions can occur together in some conditions. Morphological subdivision is based on whether the lesion is single or if the lesion has a specific pattern such as guttate or small macules, patchy or large macules, whorled, linear, reticulated or diffuse or generalized. Under each subcategory, the conditions are listed in alphabetical order to facilitate a search. Melanocytic naevi, pigmented tumors, such as malignant melanoma and pigmented basal cell carcinoma, have been excluded from this table as they are listed in Chapter 6.

Table 4–1   Morphological classification of pigmentary disorders

A.   Hyperpigmented lesions

I.   Single lesion (Figures 4–1 to 4–5)
Becker's nevus
Mongolian blue spot
Nevus of Ito
Nevus of Ota
Nevus spilus (speckled lentiginous nevus)

II.   Guttate or small macules (Figures 4–6 to 4–22)
Dyschromatosis universalis
Freckles
Flat seborrheic keratosis
Hori's nevus
Idiopathic eruptive macular pigmentation
Lentigines (syndromes: LEOPARDS, NAME, LAMB,
   Peutz-Jegher's)
Post-inflammatory, e.g. following injury, lichen planus, infection
Prurigo pigmentosa
Solar lentigo
Urticaria pigmentosa

III.   Patchy or large macules (Figures 4–23 to 4–38)
Ashy dermatosis (erythema dyschromicum perstans, lichen
   planus pigmentosus)
Café-au-lait macules
Dermatomyositis
Drugs, e.g. minocycline, cyclophosphamide, amiodarone,
   phenothiazine, etc.
External ochronosis due to prolonged use of hydroquinone
Fixed drug eruption
Frictional melanosis
Hori's nevus
Macular amyloidosis
Melasma
Morphea
Pellagra
Periorbital hyperpigmentation
Phakomatosis pigmentovascularis
Sunburns

IV.   Whorled (Figures 4–39 and 4–40)
Incontinentia pigmenti
Linear and whorled hypermelanosis

V.   Linear (Figures 4–41 and 4–47)
Berloque dermatitis
Flagellate pigmentation due to bleomycin
Flagellate pigmentation due to injury resulting from jellyfish
   contact
Melanonychia
Phytophotodermatitis
Pigmentary demarcation lines

VI.   Reticulate (Figures 4–48 to 4–55)
Confluent and reticulate papillomatosis
Dowling-Degos disease
Ichthyosiform erythroderma
Livedo reticularis
Pigmented purpura
Reticulate acropigmentation of Kitamura

VII.   Diffused/Generalized (Figures 4–56 to 4–62)
Acanthosis nigricans
Cachexia associated with terminal malignancy and lymphoma
Carotenemia
Chronic liver disease
Chronic renal failure
Drugs, e.g. clofazimine
Endocrine abnormalities, e.g. Addison's, ACTH therapy,
   hyperthyroidism
Generalized exfoliative dermatitis
Kala-Azar

B.   Hypopigmented lesions

I.   Single lesion (Figures 4–63 to 4–67)
Ash leaf macule of tuberous sclerosis
Lymphangioma circumscriptum associated
Nevus anemicus
Nevus depigmentosus (achromic nevus)

II.   Guttate or small macules (Figures 4–68 to 4–77)
Acropigmentation of Dohi
Chronic arsenic poisoning
Clear cell papulosis
Darier's disease-associated guttate leucoderma
Halo nevus
Idiopathic guttate hypomelanosis
Pityriasis versicolor
Post-inflammatory, e.g. following psoriasis, pityriasis lichenoides
   chronica, insect bites
Punctate leucoderma

III.   Patchy or large macules (Figures 4–78 to 4-90)
Leprosy
Mycosis fungoides – hypopigmented type
Piebaldism
Pityriasis alba
Post-inflammatory
Post-Kala-Azar dermal leishmaniasis
Progressive macular (confluent) hypomelanosis
Pseudoleucoderma angiospasticum
Submucous fibrosis
Vitiligo
Vogt-Koyanagi-Harada syndrome
Waardenburg's syndrome

IV.   Whorled (Figure 4–91)
Hypomelanosis of Ito

V.   Linear (Figures 4–92 to 4–93)
Post-inflammatory (following lichen striatus, abrasions)
Segmental vitiligo

VI.   Reticulated (Figure 4–94)
Goltz syndrome (focal dermal hypoplasia)

VII.   Diffused/Generalized (Figures 4–95 to 4–96)
Albinism
Vitiligo

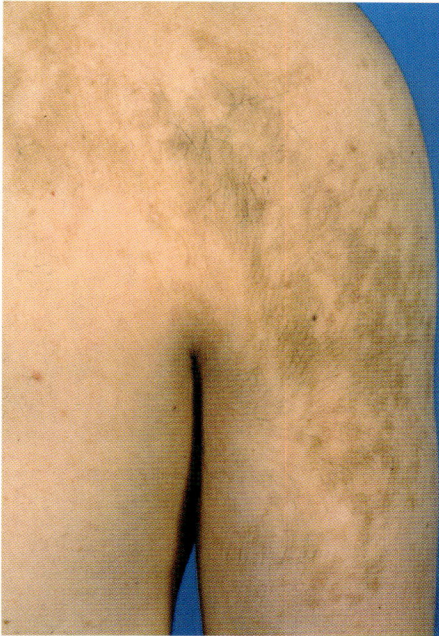

Figure 4–1 □ Becker's nevus. A typical Becker's nevus in the shoulder area is shown here. These are hyperpigmented lesions associated with smooth muscle hamartomas around hair follicles. They usually become apparent around puberty. Hairs within the nevus are usually coarser than the normal surrounding skin. It is usually not associated with any other serious systemic disease.

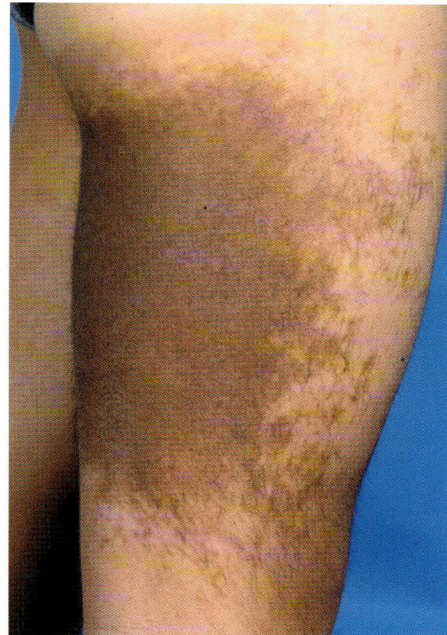

Figure 4–2 □ Becker's nevus. Although Becker's nevus typically occurs around the deltoid region, lesions may occur in other parts of the body. A Becker's nevus on the back of the right thigh is shown here.

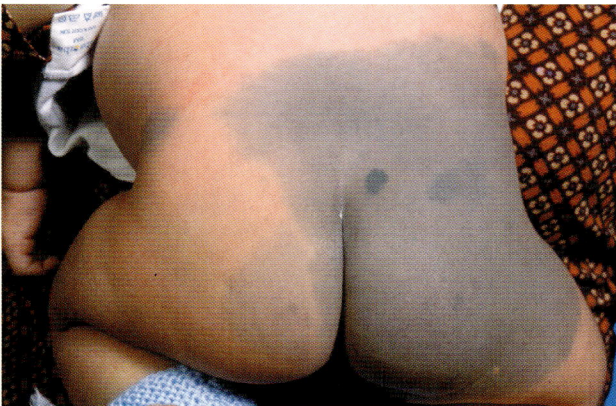

Figure 4–3 □ Mongolian blue spot. A large Mongolian blue spot occupies the right buttock and the lumbosacral area of this baby. These are very common in Asian newborns; in fact they can be considered a "normal" transient event in the lives of most Asian babies. They are due to dermal melanocytosis. They usually disappear as the child grows. Typically, they occur in the sacral area and the buttocks. Extensive aberrant Mongolian spots may be associated with other pigmentary disorders such as phakomatosis pigmentovascularis.

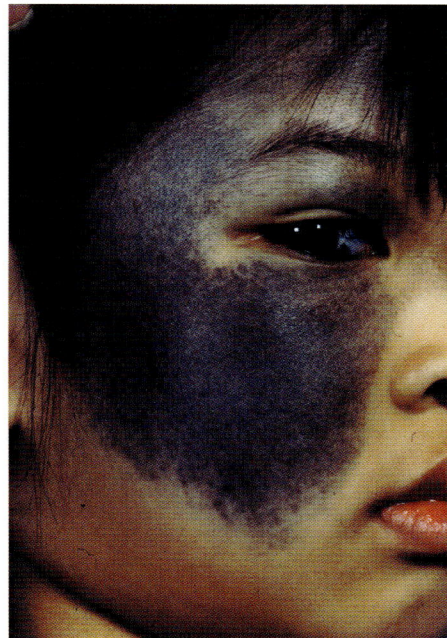

Figure 4–4 □ Nevus of Ota. This Chinese female has a typical nevus of Ota involving most of the right cheek. Unilateral pigmentation around an eye is characteristic. It is due to dermal melanocytosis. It may be associated with scleral and retinal hypermelanosis as well as glaucoma. Nevus of Ota is sometimes associated with several multi-system syndromes such as phakomatosis pigmentovascularis. Although uncommon, nevus of Ota may occur bilaterally around both eyes.

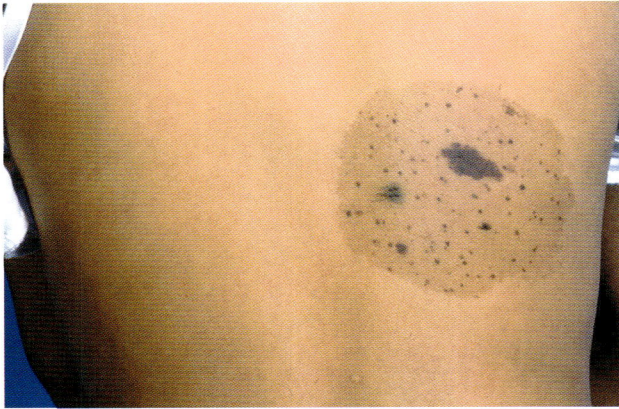

Figure 4–5 □ Nevus spilus (speckled lentiginous nevus). In this condition, hyperpigmented macules, like lentigines, occur in a speckled fashion in the background of a light brownish café-au-lait macule of variable size. Nevus spilus may be single or multiple, and may also occur in a zosteriform distribution. Sometimes, speckled lentiginous pigmentation may occur without a background of a café-au-lait macule.

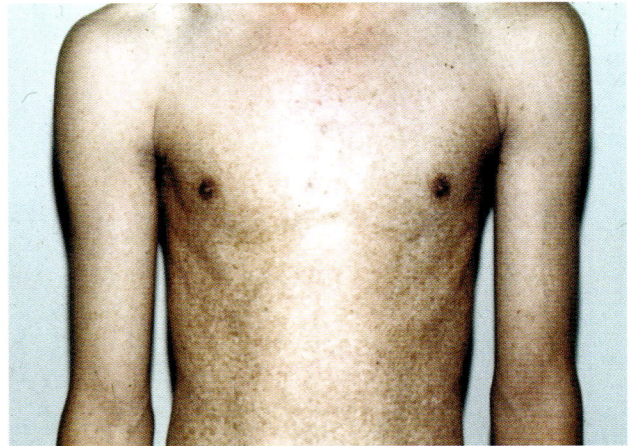

Figure 4–6 □ Dyschromatosis universalis. This Chinese patient has hyperpigmented and hypopigmented macules characteristic of dyschromatosis universalis. It is an autosomal dominant disorder. Two main variants of familial dyschromatosis are seen in Asians: dyschromatosis universalis (involving the whole body) and dyschromatosis symmetrica (limited to the limbs).

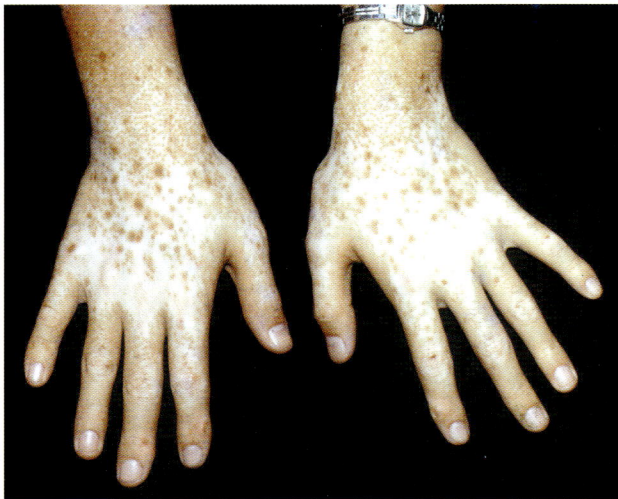

Figure 4–7 □ Dyschromatosis symmetrica. This patient has hyperpigmented and hypopigmented macules limited to the limbs. Dyschromatosis symmetrica has phenotypical features similar to the condition described as acropigmentation of Dohi.

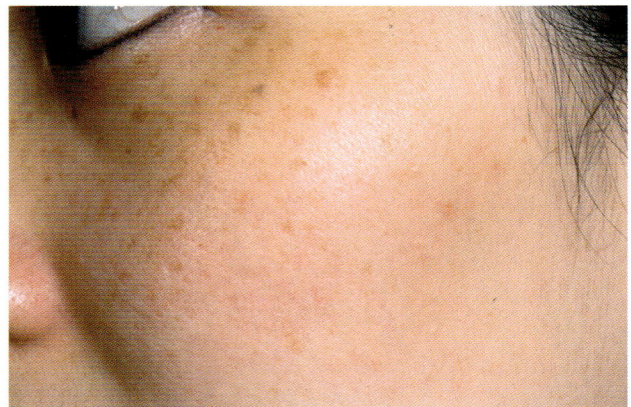

Figure 4–8 □ Freckles. Small well-demarcated light brown macules, particularly on the sun-exposed areas, are characteristic of freckles, as seen in this Chinese female. Freckles are generally less common in Asians as compared to Caucasians. Freckling may be present in several dermatological syndromes such as xeroderma pigmentosum and Bloom's syndrome.

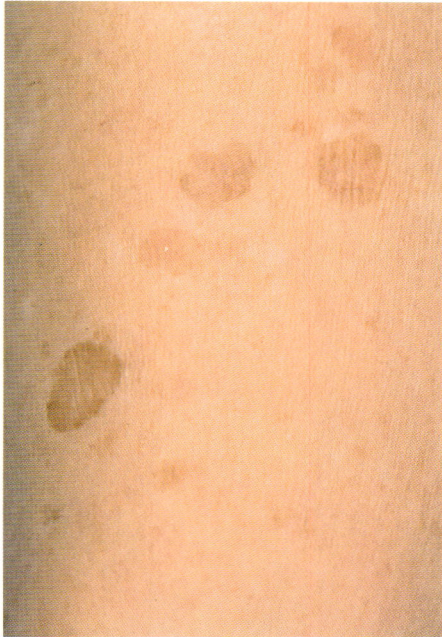

Figure 4–9 □ Flat seborrheic keratosis. Small flat seborrheic keratoses may be difficult to distinguish from solar lentigo on the sun-damaged skin. However, in these lesions, the texture of the skin is altered – the epidermis is slightly thickened and the borders are well-demarcated, as seen in this picture.

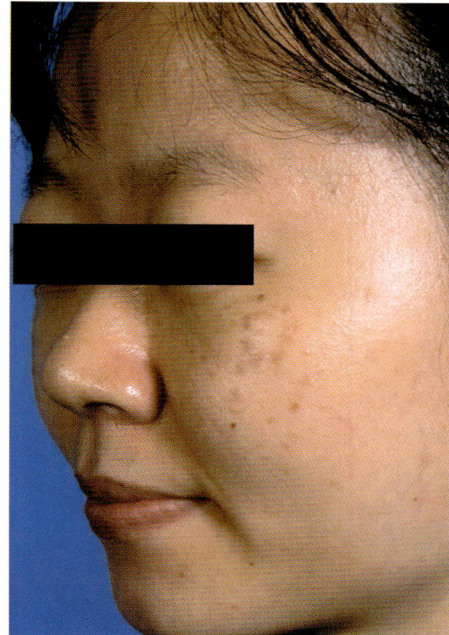

Figure 4–10 □ Hori's nevus. This Chinese female has multiple grayish-brown macules on her upper cheeks. These acquired nevus of Ota-like pigmented macules occur predominantly in Oriental races, e.g. Chinese, Korean and Japanese. They tend to affect women in their 30s to 40s and result from melanin in dermal dendritic cells.

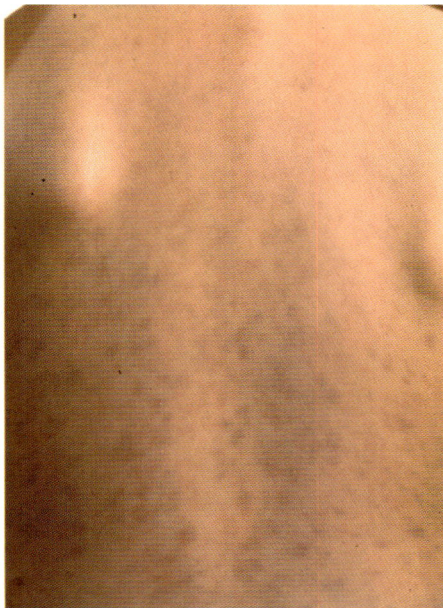

Figure 4–11 □ Idiopathic eruptive macular pigmentation. Numerous hyperpigmented macules appear without any history of preceding inflammation, injury, or pruritus as shown in this case. It is more common in children and young adults. The trunk is the most prominently affected area. Pathology is similar to that of ashy dermatosis. It is not clear whether this is part of the same disease spectrum or whether this is a form of post-inflammatory pigmentation following subclinical inflammation.

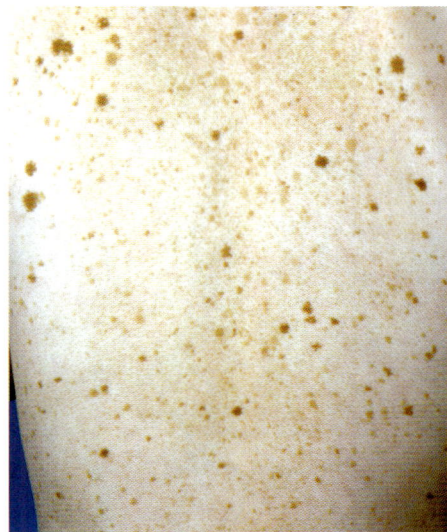

Figure 4–12 □ LEOPARD syndrome – multiple lentiginosis syndrome. This patient has numerous lentigines which are a characteristic feature of LEOPARD syndrome. Although multiple lentigines may be a benign normal variation, if excessive or concentrated over a particular area, it may indicate an underlying syndrome. Multiple lentigines occur in several syndromes including LEOPARD, NAME, LAMB, and Peutz-Jegher's syndrome. LEOPARD syndrome is characterized by lentigines, electrocardiographic abnormalities, ocular hypertelorism, pulmonary hypertension, abnormal genitalia, growth retardation, and sensorineural deafness.

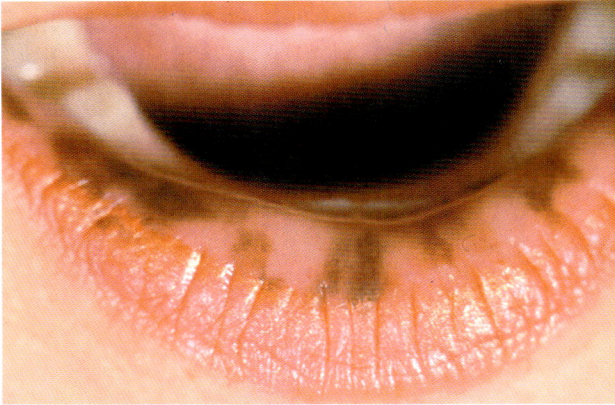

Figure 4–13 □ Peutz-Jegher's syndrome. Labial melanotic macules as seen here are characteristic of Peutz-Jegher's syndrome. Perioral and buccal lentigines may be the initial clinical sign. Intestinal obstruction due to intestinal polyps may be another presentation. Recently, this condition has attracted the attention of many researchers due to its association with LKB 1 gene (also called STK 11 gene), which is associated with multiple neoplasms.

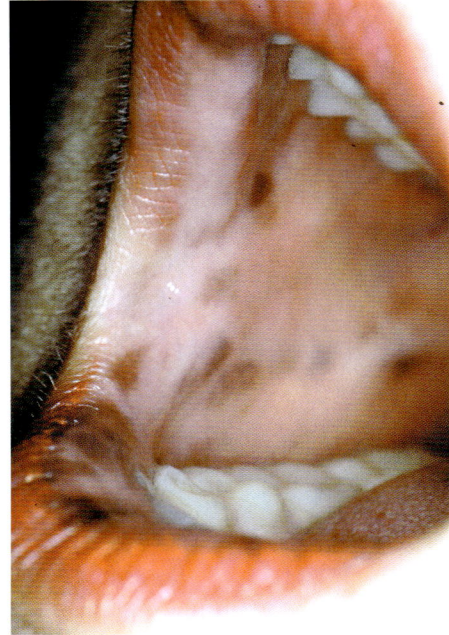

Figure 4–14 □ Peutz-Jegher's syndrome. This figure shows melanotic macules affecting the lateral buccal mucosa of a patient with Peutz-Jegher's syndrome.

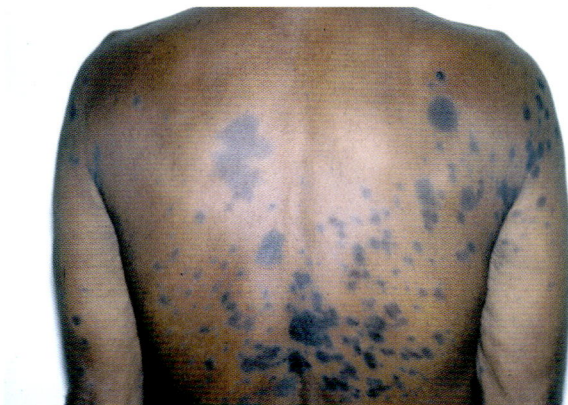

Figure 4–15 □ Post-lichen planus hyperpigmentation. Pigmentation on the posterior trunk appeared in this Indian patient as a sequel to lichen planus. Inflammation of the skin, regardless of the cause, often leads to prominent hyperpigmentation in the Asian skin. Post-inflammatory hyperpigmentation is usually transient but may take several months to years to gradually resolve. The probability of long-lasting pigmentation is greater when there is an interphase dermatitis leading to basal cell degeneration and appearance of melanophages in the dermis.

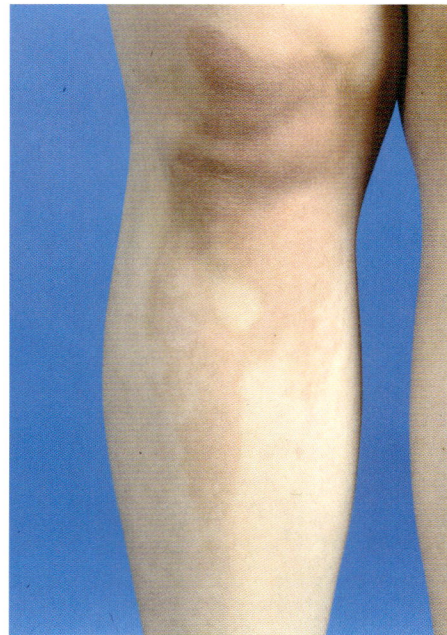

Figure 4–16 □ Post-injury hyperpigmentation. A patterned hyperpigmentation due to accidental scalding injury is seen in this patient. Gradual resolution over the next several weeks and months is to be expected.

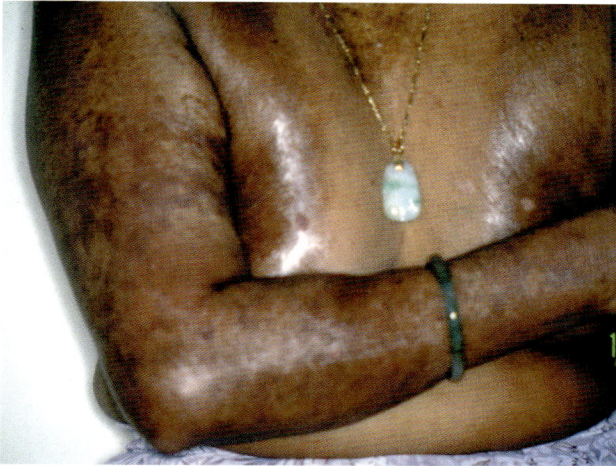

Figure 4–17 □ Porphyria cutanea tarda. This patient with porphyria cutanea tarda has increased pigmentation and thickening of skin on the forearms and some parts of the chest. Porphyrias are uncommon in the Asia-Pacific region.

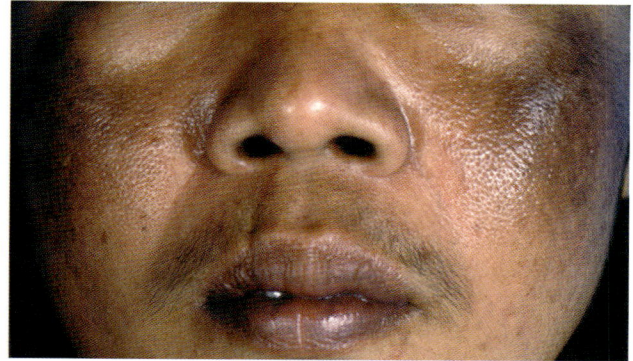

Figure 4–18 □ Post-inflammatory hyperpigmentation due to contact dermatitis. This patient's hyperpigmented macules on the cheeks followed irritant contact dermatitis due to the use of facial cosmetics. Facial cosmetics may cause irritant, allergic, or "pigmented" contact dermatitis.

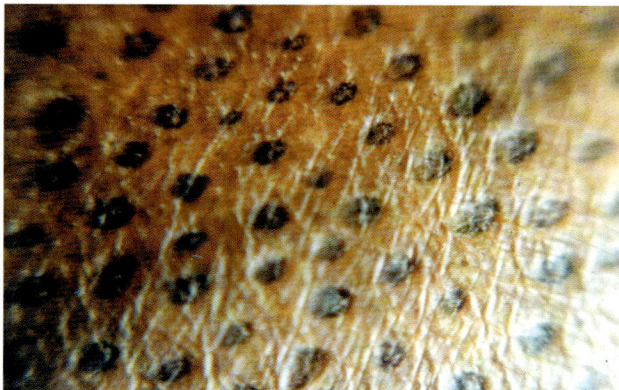

Figure 4–19 □ Chronic folliculitis. The leg of this Sri Lankan patient shows typical "dot-like" pigmentation following chronic folliculitis of the legs after the hairs have been shed through the disease process. It is a common sequel to this condition. Chronic folliculitis of the legs is more commonly found in the Indian subcontinent, Sri Lanka, and some African countries. It is also known as epilating folliculitis, dermatitis cruris pustulosis et atrophicans, or sycosis cruris. Some cases with this condition also have concurrent sycosis barbae or scalp folliculitis.

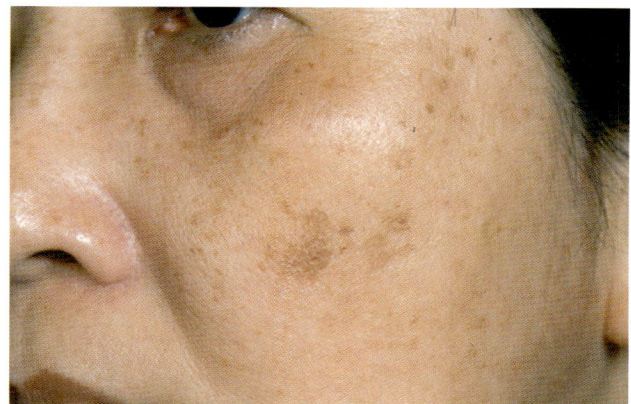

Figure 4–20 □ Solar lentigines. These are small macules of pigmentation without any textural change, on sun-exposed areas, as seen on this patient's cheek. Sometimes, a lesion may grow up to about 10 mm, and multiple lesions may coalesce to give rise to a larger area of pigmentation. These are more common in lighter-skinned Asians.

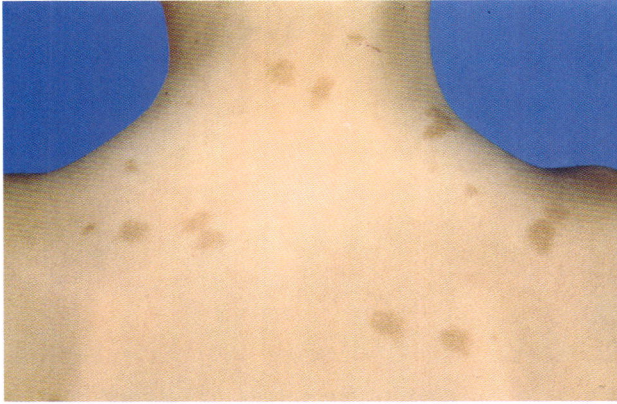

Figure 4–21 □ Urticaria pigmentosa. This Eurasian child shows several pruritic reddish-brown plaques and nodules on the upper trunk and neck, typical of urticaria pigmentosa which is the prototype of cutaneous mastocytosis. When an area adjacent to a lesion is rubbed, one can demonstrate a pruritic, urticarial response with an erythematous flare (Darier's sign). The pigmentation results from excess melanin in the epidermal basal cell layer. Most cases of cutaneous mastocytosis improve with time, though rarely it may transform into mast cell leukemia.

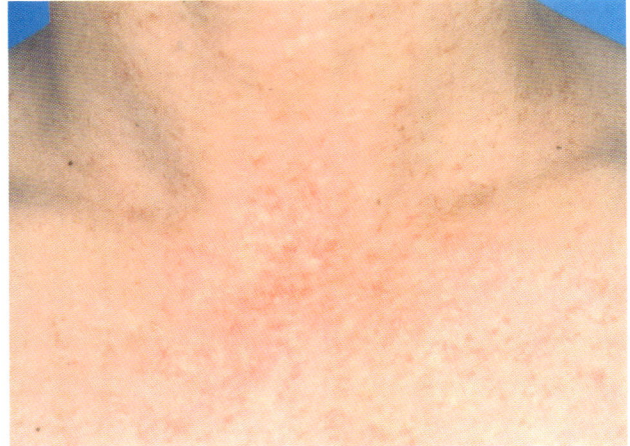

Figure 4–22 □ Telangiectasia macularis eruptiva perstans. This Chinese patient has multiple non-pruritic reddish brown macules on the anterior upper chest and the lower neck. Skin biopsy showed an excess of mastocytes in the dermis. The site of involvement and the clinical picture shown here are typical of telangiectasia macularis eruptiva perstans. Darier's sign is usually absent in this condition.

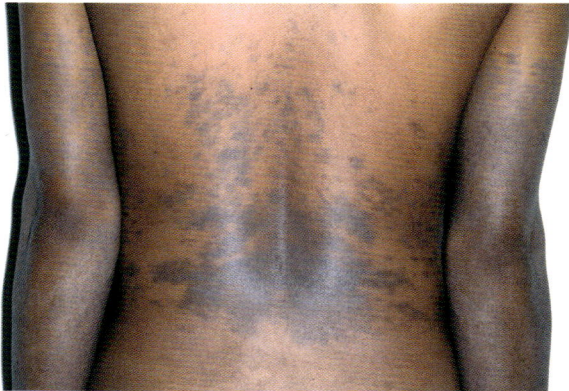

Figure 4–23 □ Ashy dermatosis (erythema dyschromicum perstans). An Indian male with ill-defined, hyperpigmented patches involving the trunk is shown here. In this condition, ill-defined, blotchy hyperpigmentation occurs on the face as well as trunk and less commonly on the limbs, without any history of preceding inflammation. In darker-skinned people, there is often no evidence of an erythematous rim at the periphery of the lesion, described in initial publications on erythema dyschromicum perstans. Skin biopsy reveals melanophages in the dermis with thinned out epidermis. The condition described as lichen planus pigmentosus in Indian patients and idiopathic eruptive macular pigmentation also appear to be within the spectrum of the same condition.

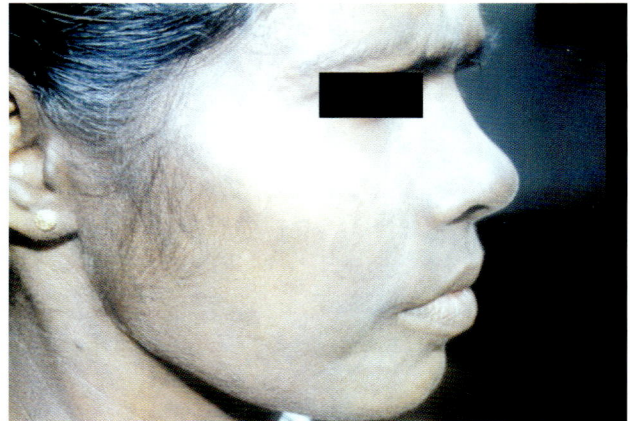

Figure 4–24 □ Ashy dermatosis (erythema dyschromicum perstans). A 30-year-old Sri Lankan female with ill-defined ashy discoloration of the facial skin is shown here, depicting another presentation of this condition. The etiology of this type of pigmentation is not known. Pigmentation following extensive lichen planus may also give rise to a similar clinical picture. In the latter, however, there will be a history of a pruritic lichenoid rash preceding the onset of pigmentation.

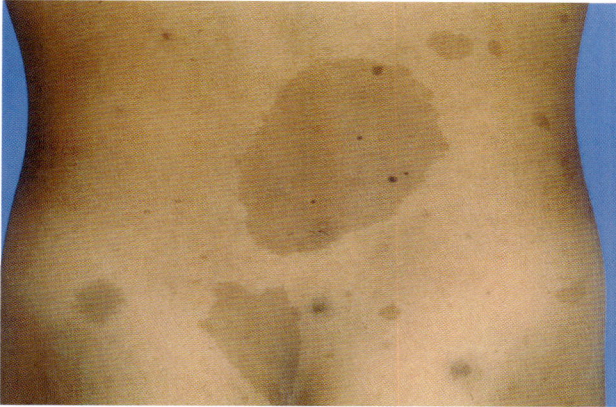

Figure 4–25 □ Café-au-lait macules. This patient with Neurofibromatosis type I has numerous café-au-lait macules of varying sizes. These are brownish nevoid macules which are present from birth before the cutaneous fibromas become evident. Axillary freckling is also characteristically present in Neurofibromatosis type I. Multiple café-au-lait macules are also seen in other syndromes such as Bloom's and McCune-Albright syndromes.

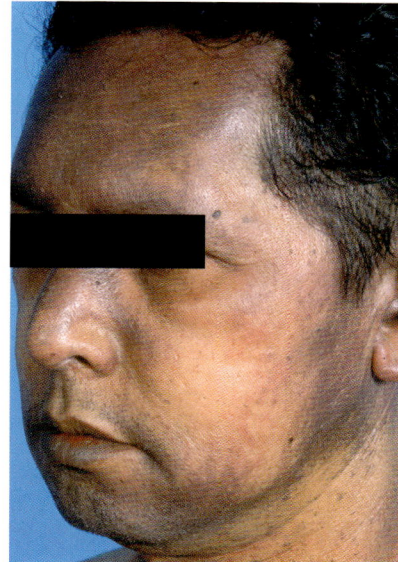

Figure 4–26 □ Dermatomyositis. This Malay patient with dermatomyositis with associated hepatocellular carcinoma shows patchy hyperpigmentation of the face, icterus, and mild swelling of eyelids. The cutaneous lesions of dermatomyositis are characterized by the presence of a heliotrope facial rash, Gottron's papules, photodistributed rash, and poikiloderma. Pigmentation may follow the skin inflammation. In darker-skinned Asian patients, as in this patient, the pigmentation may be very prominent and may be persistent for months to years.

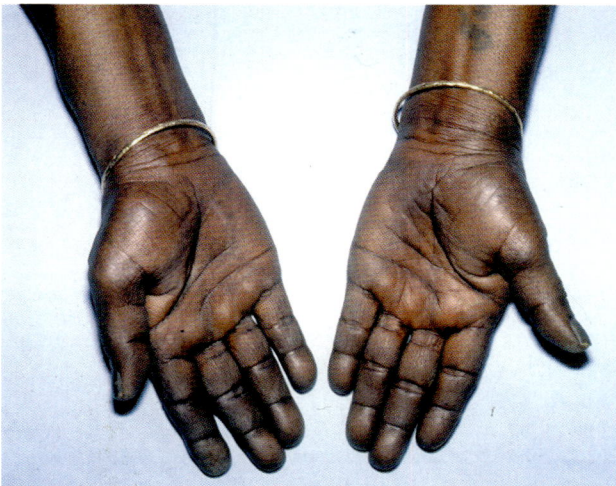

Figure 4–27 □ Drug-related hyperpigmentation. This Indian patient developed hyperpigmentation of the hands whilst on cyclophosphamide. Many drugs, including minocycline, busulphan, cyclophosphamide, amiodarone, and phenothiazine can lead to various types of pigmentation. Minocycline causes ill-defined blotchy hyperpigmentation anywhere on the body as well as on previous scars, whilst drugs like amiodarone and phenothiazines tend to cause pigmentation on sun-exposed areas.

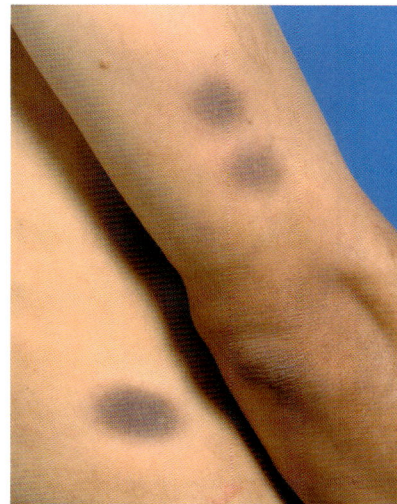

Figure 4–28 □ Fixed drug eruption. The Chinese patient shown here developed a fixed drug eruption to sodium valproate given for epilepsy. Three darkly pigmented circumscribed macules are clearly visible on the right flank and the arm. In fixed drug eruption, distinct hyperpigmented macules occur exactly over the same sites after the same drug is ingested again. Common drugs causing fixed drug eruption include antibiotics such as cotrimoxazole and tetracyclines. In the active stage of the eruption, there may be vesicles or bullae in the center of the lesion and erythema at the periphery. The resultant hyperpigmentation may last for many years.

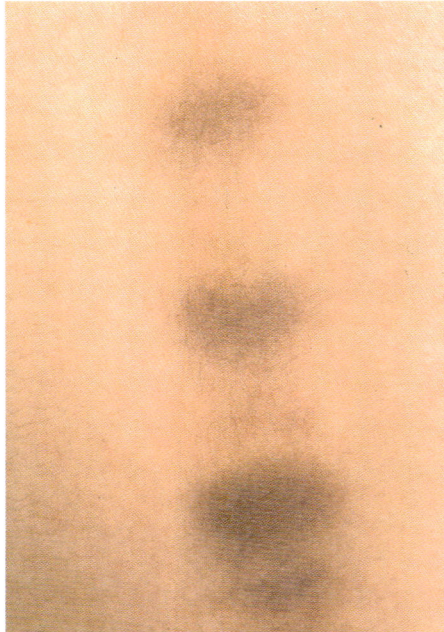

Figure 4–29 □ Frictional melanosis. This 21-year-old Eurasian female has frictional melanosis in the lumbar region, on the skin overlying the bony prominences of the spine. This is commonly seen on extensor surfaces and other areas where there is frequent or constant friction. It is more prominent in more pigmented races. In some cases, it may be associated with cutaneous amyloidosis.

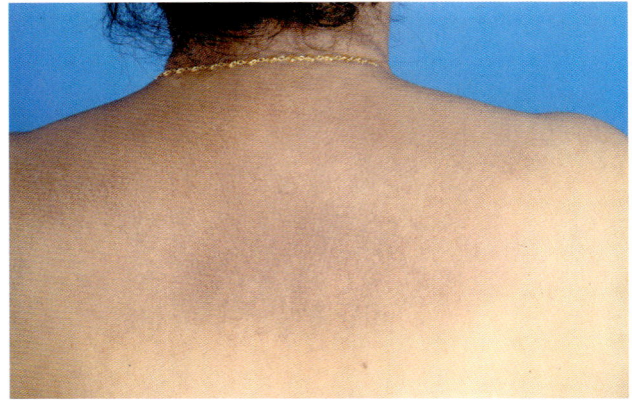

Figure 4–30 □ Macular amyloidosis. A large area of macular amyloidosis is seen on the upper back of this 47-year-old Indian patient. This condition is more common in Asians. The site of involvement on the upper back is typical. The borders are relatively ill-defined and blend gradually with the surrounding unaffected skin.

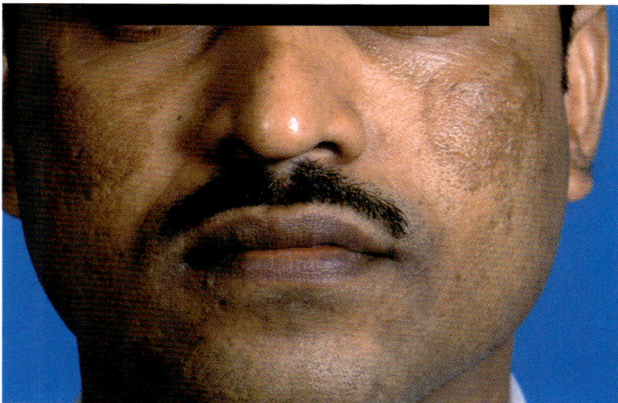

Figure 4–31 □ Melasma. Both cheeks of this Indian man show typical brownish patches of melasma. Melasma is a common acquired pigmentary disorder affecting more women than men. Typically, it occurs on the cheeks, but lesions on the forehead and nose are also common. Epidermal melasma is accentuated with exposure to ultraviolet (Wood's) light. Aggravating factors include sun exposure, pregnancy, and oral contraceptives.

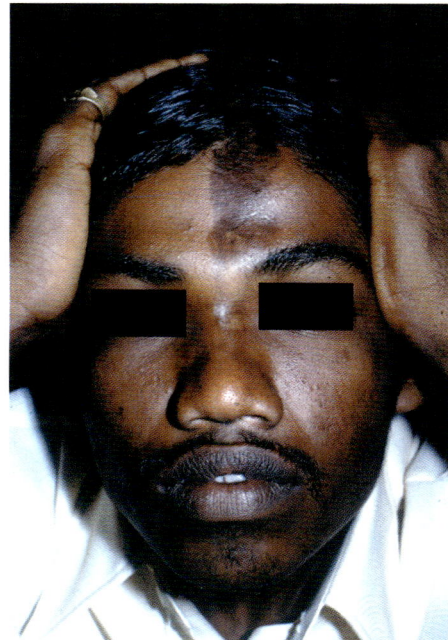

Figure 4–32 □ Morphea. A patient with *en coup de sabre* type of morphea with obvious hyperpigmentation is shown here. The sclerosis results in a bound down appearance. The overlying skin is shiny and hyperpigmented.

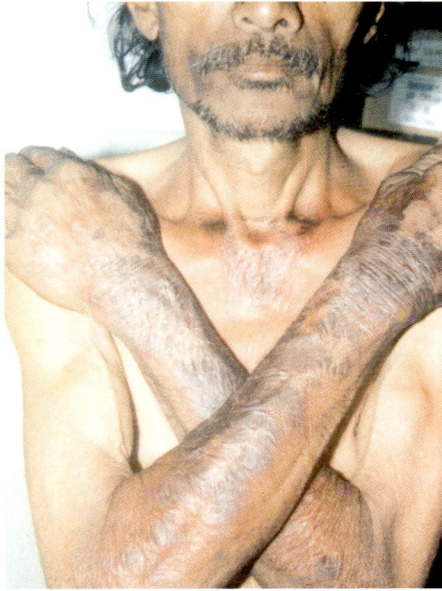

Figure 4–33 □ Pellagra. Scaly hyperpigmented lesions on sun-exposed areas of upper limbs and the "V" of the upper chest (Casal's necklace) are characteristic of pellagra. Niacin (vitamin B₃) deficiency leads to pellagra. Although the triad of dermatitis, diarrhoea, and dementia are classical clinical features, all three features may not be present in mild cases. Pellagra is more common in alcoholics who neglect their diet and in certain conditions where there are derangement of tryptophan metabolism.

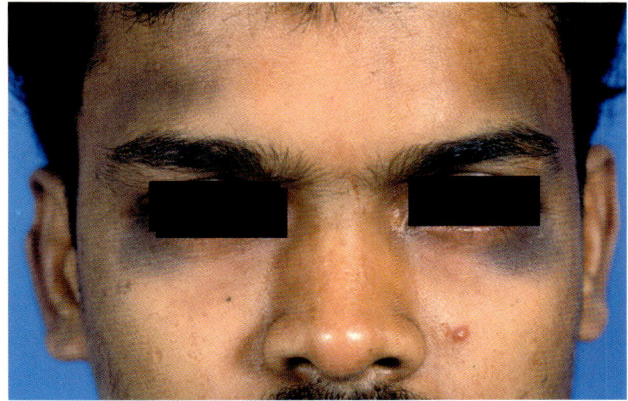

Figure 4–34 □ Periorbital hyperpigmentation. A darker pigmentation of the lower eyelid region is clearly visible in this patient. This is particularly common amongst pigmented Asians, especially Indians. Pigmentation of the lower eyelid area is characteristic. There appears to be a familial tendency and an association with obesity and atopic eczema. Occasionally, similar hyperpigmentation is seen around the mouth.

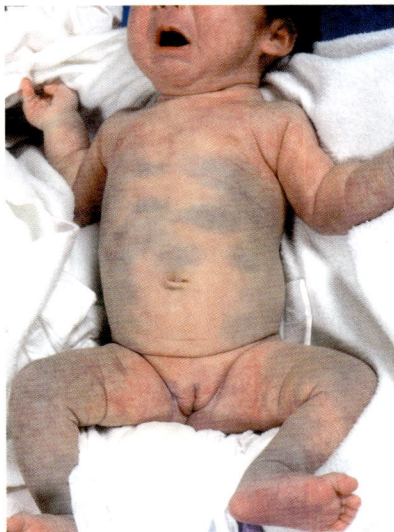

Figure 4–35 □ Phakomatosis pigmentovascularis. An infant with multiple port wine stains and large areas of dermal melanocytosis characteristic of phakomatosis pigmentovascularis is shown here. Most reported cases have concerned Asians. There are pigmentary as well as associated vascular anomalies. Dermatological features include multiple Mongolian spots, nevus of Ota, port wine stains, nevus spilus, and nevus anemicus. Four major types have been described, the most common being type II. Type III is associated with multiple granular cell tumors.

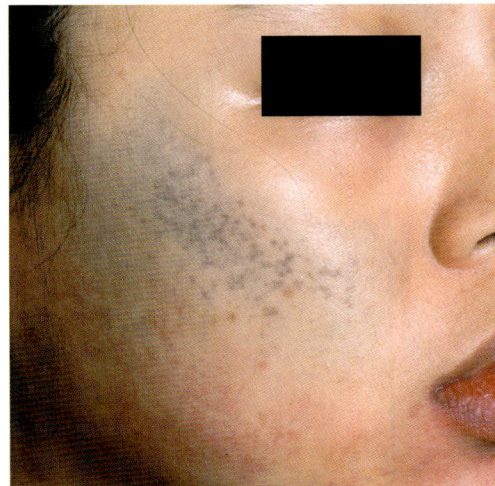

Figure 4–36 □ Phakomatosis pigmentovascularis. This 23-year-old Chinese female with phakomatosis pigmentovascularis has nevus of Ota and multiple port wine stains. On the trunk, the port wine stains are distributed in a checkerboard pattern.

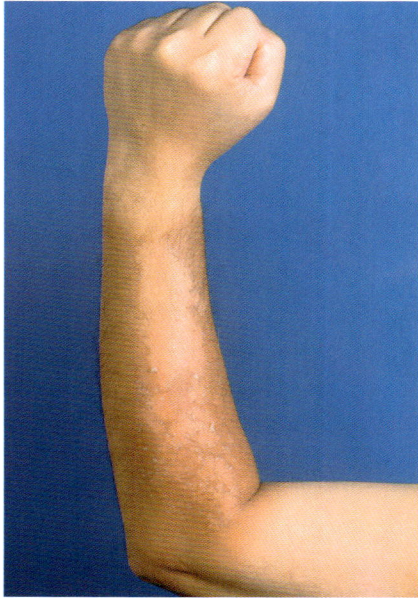

Figure 4–37 □ Sunburns. This 19-year-old Chinese man developed sunburns on the exposed areas of limbs and face after spending several hours in the sun without protection. The skin in the affected area is exfoliating and the contrast of the sun-tanned area is clearly visible in this picture. Although sunburns are more common amongst fair-skinned Caucasians, many fairer Asians also get sunburns, especially if they are not accustomed to exposure to strong sun. It causes hyperpigmentation of the exposed areas (immediate and delayed response).

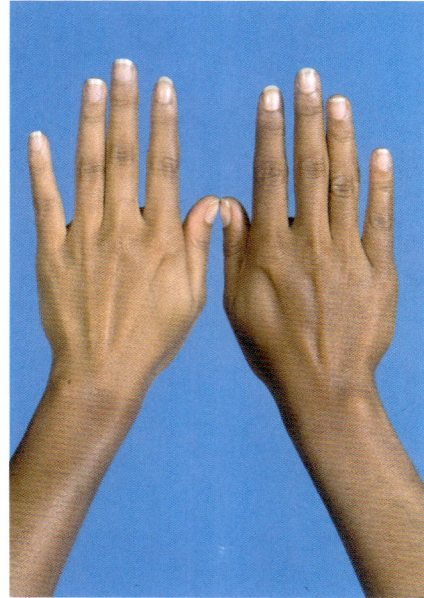

Figure 4–38 □ Sun tan. This avid female golfer's right hand, which is usually not gloved, is more tanned, compared to the left hand which is always gloved ("Golfer's hands"). Prolonged exposure to the sun causes the skin to tan in persons with pigmented skin, without acute burns, as is clearly visible here.

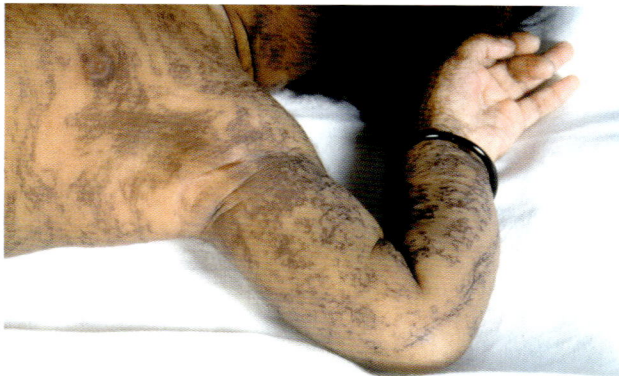

Figure 4–39 □ Incontinentia pigmenti. Whorled streaky hyperpigmentation seen in this female child is characteristic of incontinentia pigmenti. This condition is transmitted as an X-linked dominant trait and is almost exclusively seen in girls. It is characterized by linear and whorled lesions and systemic features. Typically, the lesions pass through a vesicular stage, a verrucous stage, and a longer-lasting whorled hypermelanotic stage.

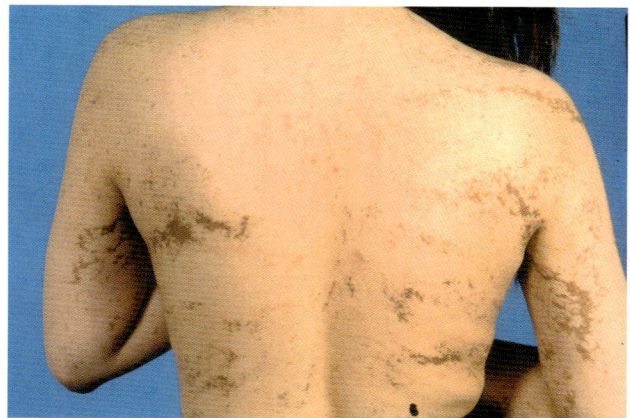

Figure 4–40 □ Linear and whorled hypermelanosis. This nevoid condition may be present at birth or developed shortly thereafter. Upper trunk and proximal limbs are usual areas of involvement. The lesions may follow lines of Blaschko as seen in this patient. This is generally not associated with any other systemic abnormalities or incontinentia pigmenti.

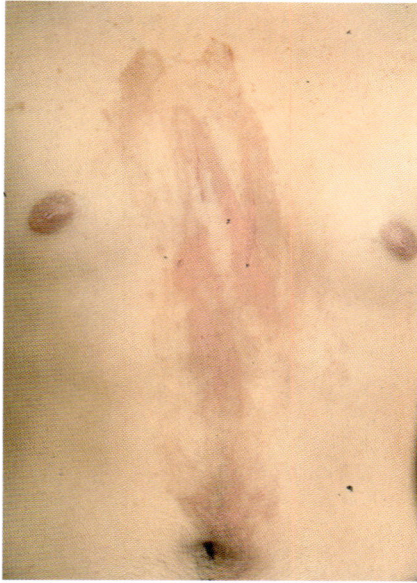

Figure 4–41 □ Berloque dermatitis. This patient noticed streaky areas of hyperpigmentation several days after applying some perfume. The perfume contained oil of bergamot, a member of the citrus family, whose principal phototoxic agent is bergapten (5-MOP). In this condition, linear or streaky hyperpigmented lesions occur following photoactivation and secondary pigmentation due to psoralen containing perfumes.

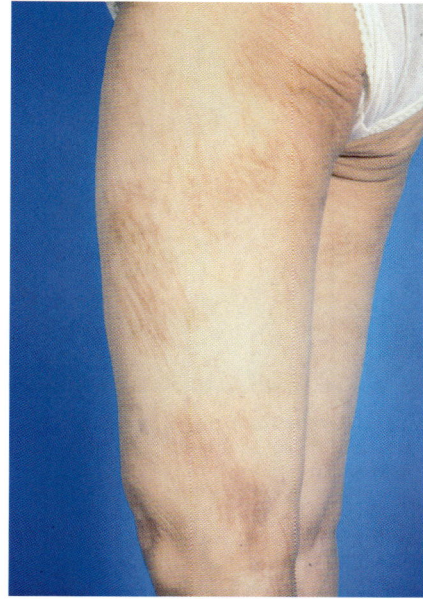

Figure 4–42 □ Bleomycin-associated flagellate pigmentation. This 60-year-old Chinese female developed flagellate and streaky lesions of dark brown pigmentation on the lower limbs, buttocks, and trunk several weeks after starting cancer chemotherapy with systemic bleomycin. Bleomycin-associated flagellate hyperpigmentation is usually seen after systemic administration of this drug although cases of similar pigmentation occurring after intralesional bleomycin have been reported.

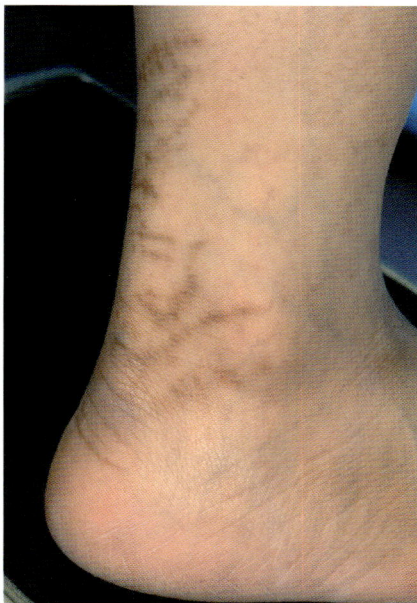

Figure 4–43 □ Flagellate pigmentation after jellyfish contact. Post-inflammatory hyperpigmentation in a flagellate and streaky pattern is seen in this patient who came in contact with jellyfish several weeks before. In the tropical seas, a variety of jellyfish is found. Sometimes, a patient may not recall the contact with less toxic jellyfish and may present to the clinician these characteristic skin lesions several days to weeks later.

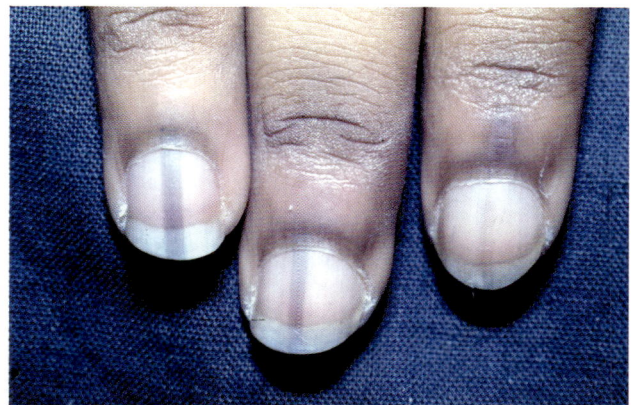

Figure 4–44 □ Melanonychia – linear. This Indian patient has linear melanonychia involving several finger nails. In pigmented Asian races, linear melanonychia is not uncommon. This condition is totally benign, and unlike malignant melanoma involving the nail, hyperpigmentation of the nail fold skin (Hutchinson's sign) is absent. Linear melanonychia may involve one or more nails.

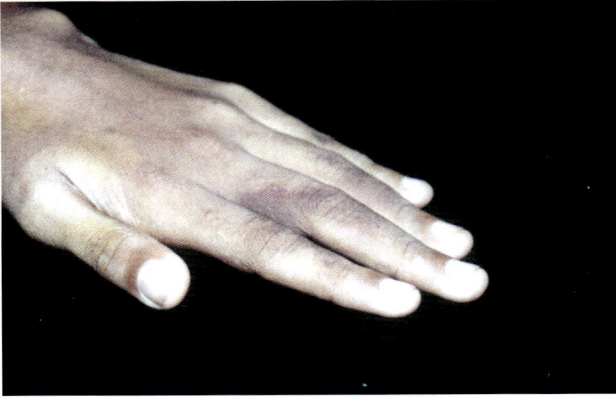

Figure 4–45 □ Phytophotodermatitis. This Sri Lankan patient developed these pigmented patches on the hands several days after squeezing lime. Many plants have been identified to contain furocoumarins, including limes, lemons, and celery. For limes and lemons, the furocoumarins are present primarily in the rind rather than the pulp. Reactions are usually mild, showing erythema, although severe blistering reactions can occur. The reaction resolves with prominent post-inflammatory hyperpigmentation that may take months to gradually disappear.

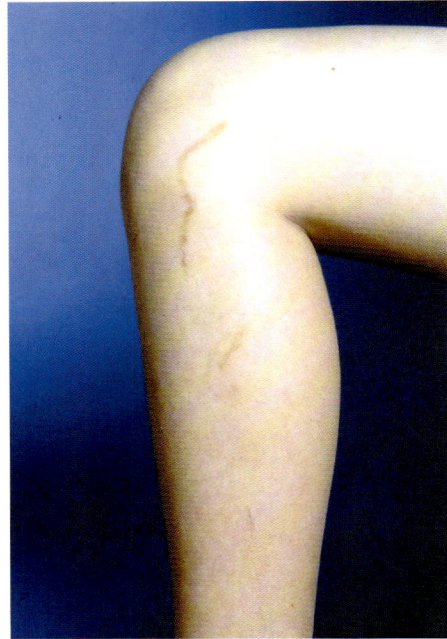

Figure 4–46 □ Phytophotodermatitis. This Chinese child presents with hyperpigmented brownish streaks over the lower leg several days after squeezing lime. The streaky or spotty pigmentation over the hands and other exposed areas of recent onset is most typical. Often, patients do not relate the skin pigmentation to contact with fruit juice or plant material; direct questioning is often needed to elicit contact history. Psoralen-like substances in some plant material lead to phytophotodermatitis and pigmentation.

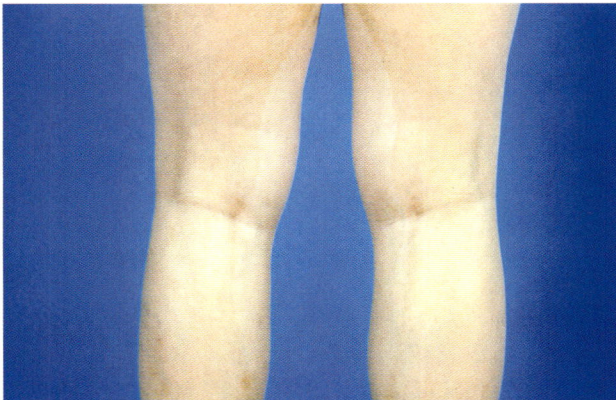

Figure 4–47 □ Pigmentary demarcation lines. This Chinese female shows clear pigment demarcation lines on the posterior thighs. These lines are more common amongst the dark-skinned Asian races. Several types have been described. Pregnancy may make the demarcation lines more prominent. These lines are not associated with any significant medical consequences.

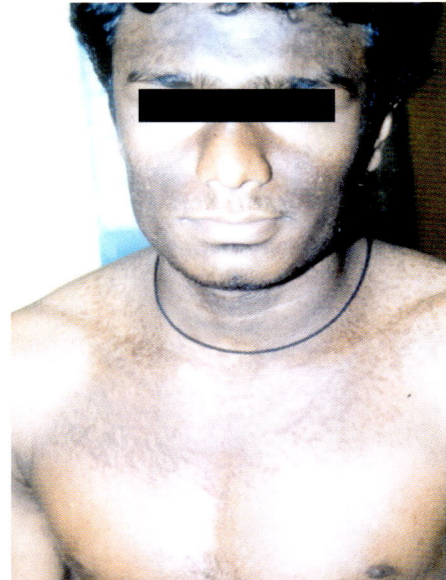

Figure 4–48 □ Confluent and reticulate papillomatosis. This Sri Lankan patient shows hyperpigmented, erythematous, confluent, and reticulate papules on the face and upper trunk. Typically, skin lesions occur on the upper chest, both anteriorly and posteriorly. Involvement of the face is uncommon. These scaly, reticulated confluent lesions are more common amongst young adults.

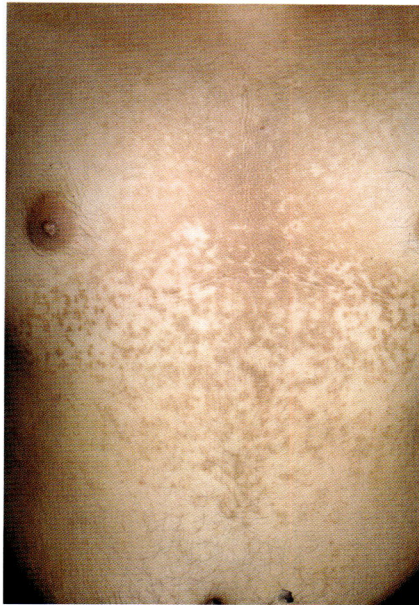

Figure 4–49 □ Confluent and reticulate papillomatosis. This Chinese patient shows the typical hyperpigmented reticulate pigmentation (CRP) on the chest. At present, the etiology and pathogenesis of CRP remain unknown. The two prominent theories are an abnormal host response to fungi such as *Malassezia furfur* and a keratinisation defect. Response to treatment is variable with isolated case reports citing successful treatment using oral itraconazole, oral minocycline, oral azithromycin, topical tretinoin, and topical calcipotriol.

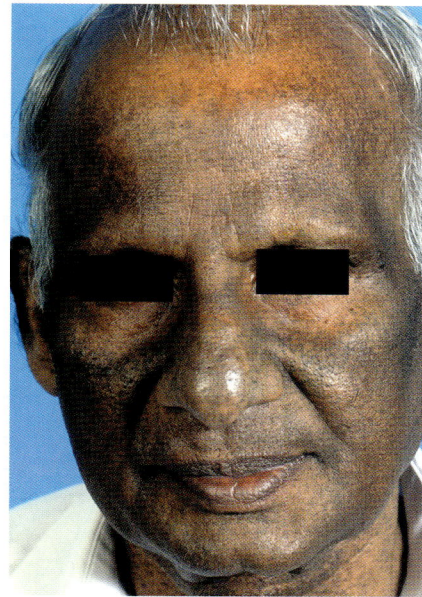

Figure 4–50 □ Dowling-Degos disease (reticular pigmentary anomaly of the flexures). This Indian patient has depressed, pigmented, comedo-like lesions on the nose and cheeks. In this autosomal dominant condition, hyperpigmented reticulated macules classically occur in the flexures. It usually afflicts those who are in their 30s or 40s and is progressive. There may be an overlap of the features with reticulate acropigmentation of Kitamura. Some believe that these two are different phenotypic expressions of the same disease.

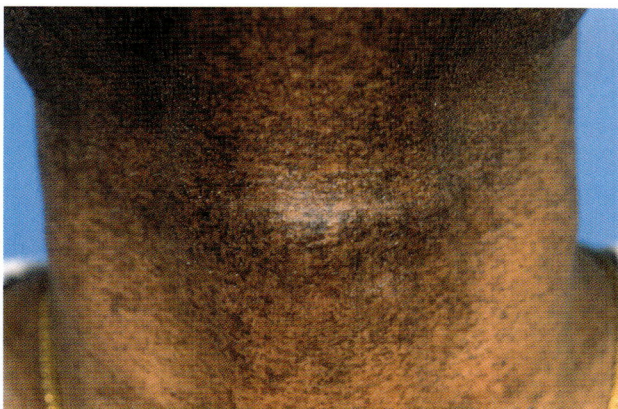

Figure 4–51 □ Dowling-Degos disease (reticular pigmentary anomaly of the flexures). The anterior neck of the patient in Figure 4–50 shows the typical reticulate pigmentation of the flexures. Dowling-Degos disease is generally not associated with any significant medical consequences.

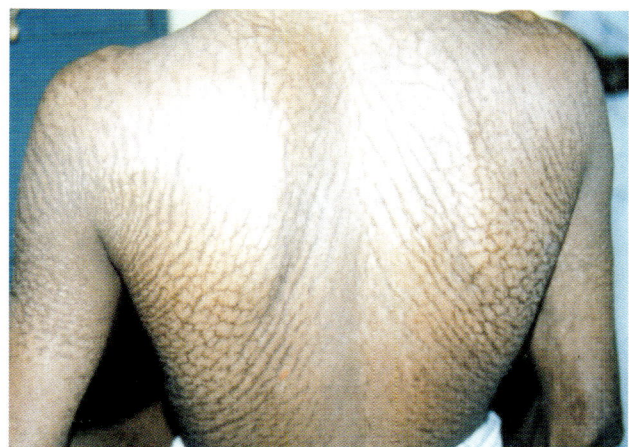

Figure 4–52 □ Ichthyosiform erythroderma. This Sri Lankan patient with severe congenital ichthyosis (ichthyosiform erythroderma) has rippled pigmentation. Ichthyoses cause a darkening of the skin due to slow removal of the scales rather than from primary hypermelanosis. X-linked ichthyosis is traditionally associated with dark brownish larger scales, and severe ichthyoses, such as lamellar ichthyosis, often show hyperpigmented scales. Bullous ichthyosiform erythroderma sometimes gives rippled pigmentation between scaly areas.

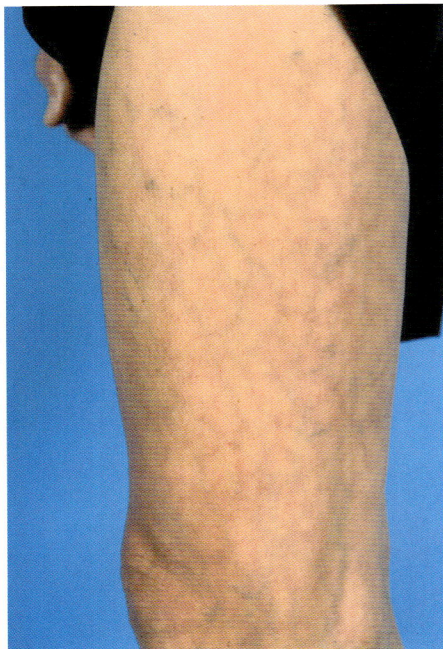

Figure 4–53 □ Livedo reticularis. This patient shows a reticulated, erythematous, lace-like pattern on the lower limbs. In this condition, ill-defined mottled or reticulated hyperpigmented lesions occur on the limbs, sometimes in response to cold weather. This may be benign or may be associated with a connective tissue disorder, cold agglutinins, cryoglobulinaemia, or certain drugs.

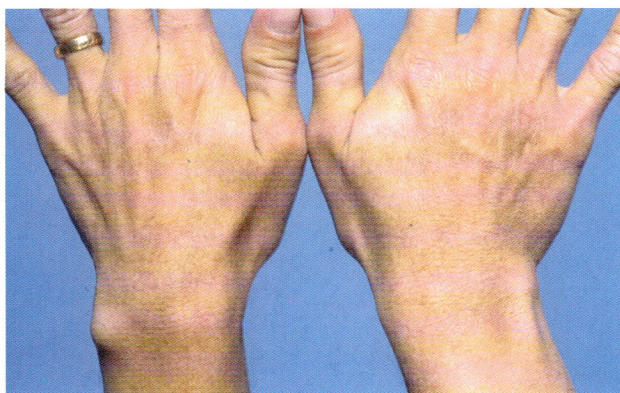

Figure 4–54 □ Pigmented purpuric dermatosis. This patient has non-pruritic pigmented purpura of the legs, particularly around the ankles. There are several types of pigmented purpura. Brownish, pigmented reticulate, or blotchy lesions commonly occur on the legs. Other areas are less involved. Some lesions coalesce whilst others remain discrete. The spectrum of pigmentation can range from reddish-brown to black. This condition may be pruritic and appear lichenoid. Rarely, mycosis fungoides can mimic pigmented purpura.

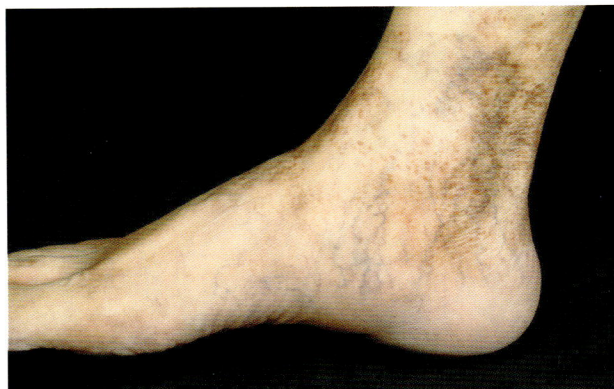

Figure 4–55 □ Reticulate acropigmentation of Kitamura. The dorsa of the hands of this patient shows symmetrical hyperpigmented macules. In this condition, there are multiple small pigmented macules scattered on the limbs, particularly on the dorsal aspect of the hands and feet. There is an overlap of the clinical features of reticulate acropigmentation of Kitamura (RAPK) and Dowling-Degos disease. There may be keratotic pits on the palms in RAPK.

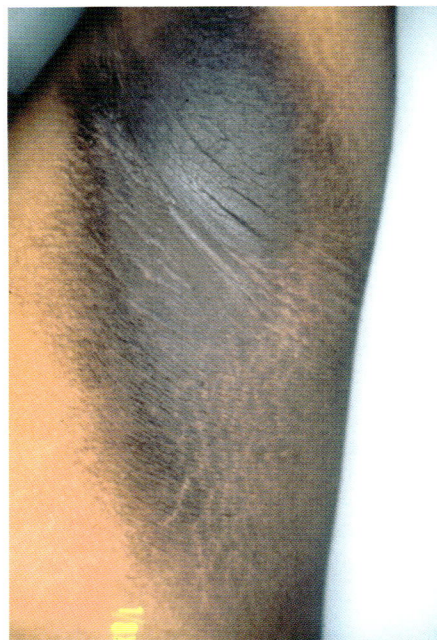

Figure 4–56 □ Acanthosis nigricans. The axilla of this Malay patient shows velvety thickening and hyper-pigmentation characteristic of acanthosis nigricans. There are several types of acanthosis nigricans. Flexural involvement is characteristic in all types. It may be familial, drug-related, part of a genetic syndrome, associated with obesity, or associated with an underlying malignancy. Acanthosis nigricans is often associated with insulin resistance. Very severe, rapidly progressive acanthosis nigricans with papillomatosis is often associated with internal malignancy.

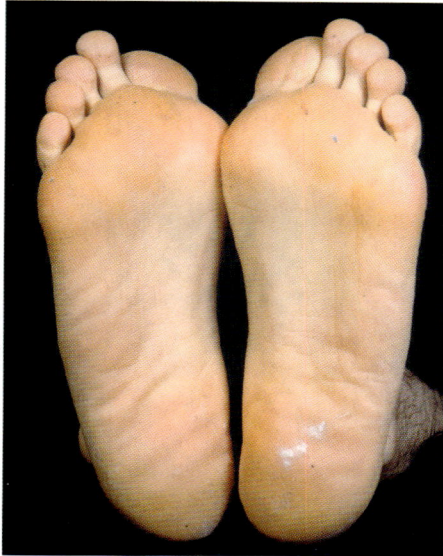

Figure 4–57 ▫ Carotenemia. The feet of this patient shows a yellowish hue. His palms also show a similar color but the sclera is normal. If too much carotene-laden foods (e.g. mangoes, carrots) are consumed, the serum and tissue carotene levels may rise and give a yellowish hue to the skin. This does not stain the sclera, unlike in hyperbilirubinemia (icterus). Palms and soles are common areas where carotenemia becomes evident.

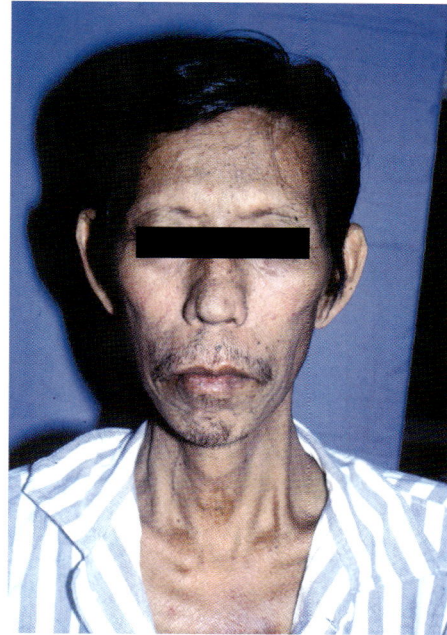

Figure 4–58 ▫ Chronic liver disease. The skin of this patient with hemochromatosis associated with chronic liver disease has gradually become diffusely darker in color. There is increased melanogenesis in chronic liver disease. The exact mechanism is not known.

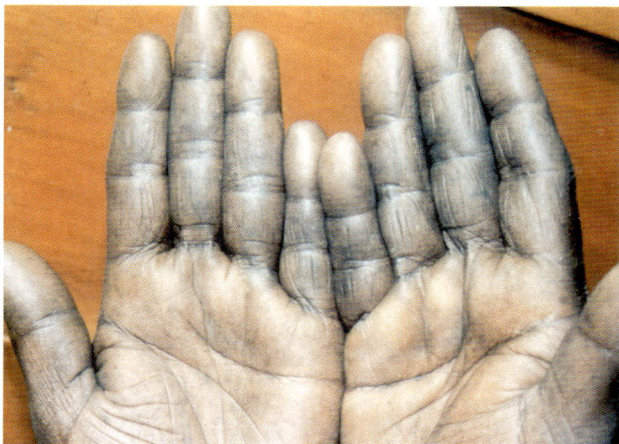

Figure 4–59 ▫ Addison's disease. This Sri Lankan patient has Addison's disease. There is diffuse darkening of his hands, with pigmentation of the skin creases. Addison's disease is the prototype of generalized increased pigmentation amongst systemic diseases which cause hyperpigmentation. Increased pigmentation is particularly seen on palmar creases, buccal mucosa, finger nails, and friction points. The figure shows typical pigmentation of the buccal mucosa, nails, and palms.

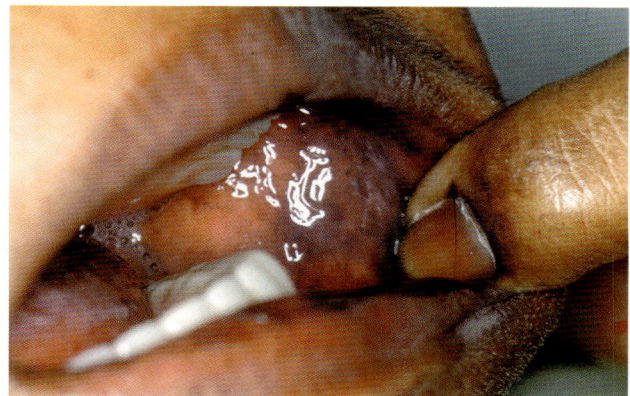

Figure 4–60 ▫ Addison's disease. This patient with Addison's disease has increased pigmentation of the buccal mucosa. This developed at the same time as the diffuse hyperpigmentation of the skin. In dark-skinned Asians, isolated buccal mucosal pigmentation is not uncommon and is physiological and benign.

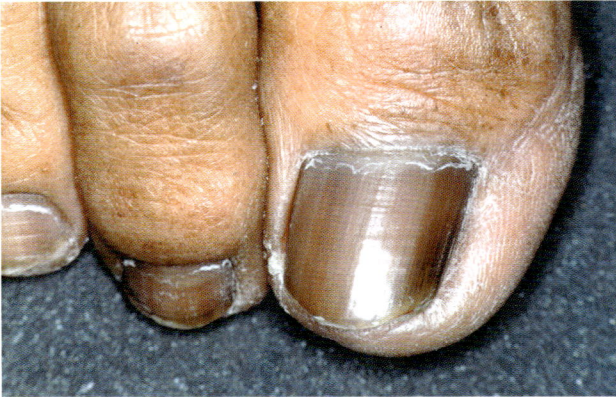

Figure 4–61 □ Addison's disease. Increased pigmentation of toe nails is clearly seen in this patient with Addison's disease.

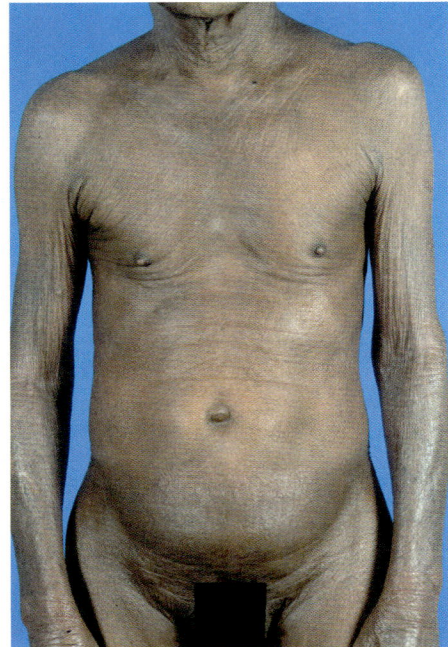

Figure 4–62 □ Generalized exfoliative dermatitis. This patient with generalized exfoliative dermatitis shows hyperpigmentation secondary to chronic dermatitis. Inflammation may cause areas of hyperpigmentation, hypopigmentation or both types in the same patient.

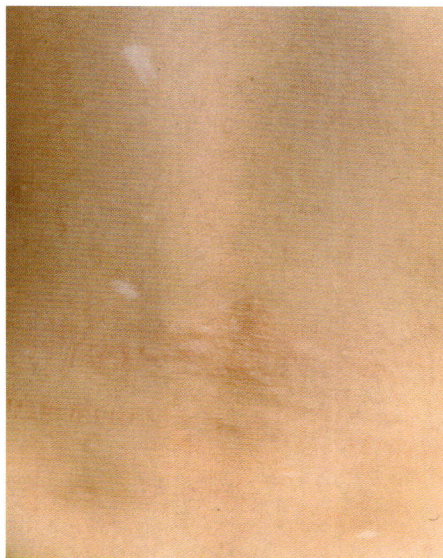

Figure 4–63 □ Ash leaf macule of tuberous sclerosis. A hypopigmented macule or macules, usually on the back, as seen in this child, may be noted at birth or infancy. Usually they occur on the trunk. The macule is highlighted when examined with a Wood's lamp. The size ranges from one to several centimeters, and lesions may be numerous in some cases. The defect is due to abnormal melanin synthesis and impaired melanosome transfer from melanocytes to keratinocytes. A shagreen patch is also present in this patient.

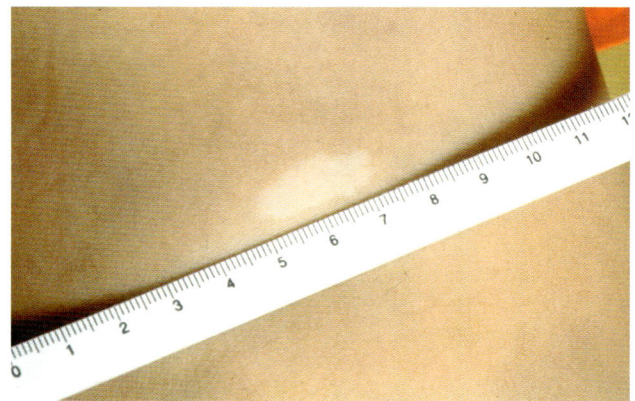

Figure 4–64 □ Ash leaf macule of tuberous sclerosis. This is a close-up view of a typical ash leaf depigmentation in a patient with tuberous sclerosis. The well-demarcated, irregular border is clearly visible.

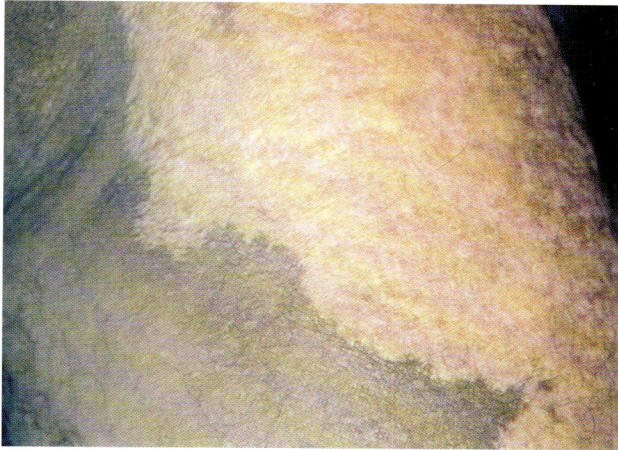

Figure 4–65 □ Lymphangioma circumscriptum. Most lymphangioma circumscriptum lesions are small. In the larger lesions, as in this Sri Lankan patient's lower limb, hypopigmentation is clearly evident. The exact mechanism for this phenomenon is not known.

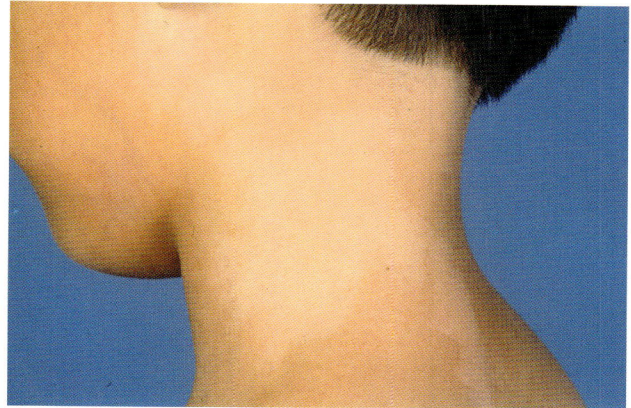

Figure 4–66 □ Nevus anemicus. This eight-year-old boy has a large hypopigmented lesion on the neck with irregular borders, which has been present from birth. The lesion is demarcated by irregular margins with occasional satellite macules and it commonly occurs on the neck or chest. When rubbed, the lesional skin does not get flushed, compared to the surrounding skin. When pressed with a glass slide, the difference between the lesional and perilesional skin gets obscured. Nevus anemicus is a result of a localized vascular disorder rather than a true hypomelanosis.

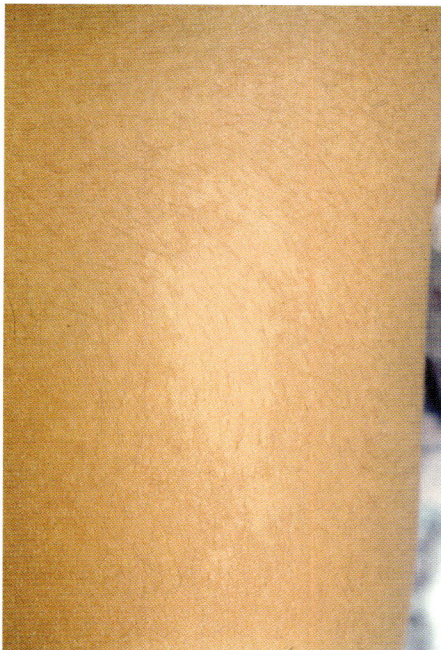

Figure 4–67 □ Nevus depigmentosus (achromic nevus). This picture shows a normosensitive, hypopigmented, irregular macule which was present from birth. Rubbing on the macule elicits an erythematous response, unlike in the case of nevus anemicus. Nevus depigmentosus is usually a quasi-dermatomal unilateral macule on the trunk or proximal limbs, with irregular, serrated, or geographic margins. It is usually solitary and is not associated with any other abnormalities.

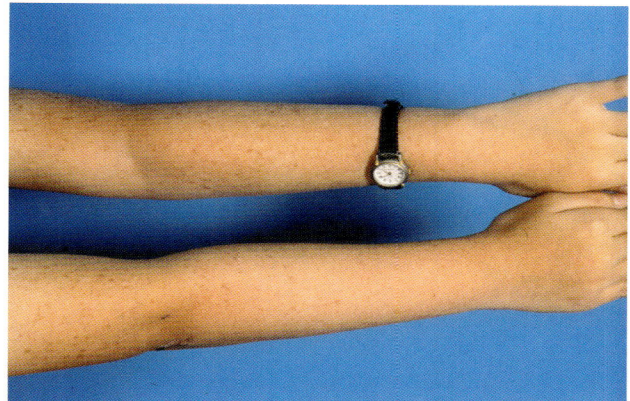

Figure 4–68 □ Acropigmentation of Dohi. This patient has coexisting hyperpigmented and hypopigmented small macules without textural change, on the extremities. Some authors believe that acropigmentation of Dohi and the condition described as dyschromia heriditaria symmetrica of the limbs are similar. However, the latter phenotype has more severe dyschromatosis. This condition is autosomal dominant in inheritance.

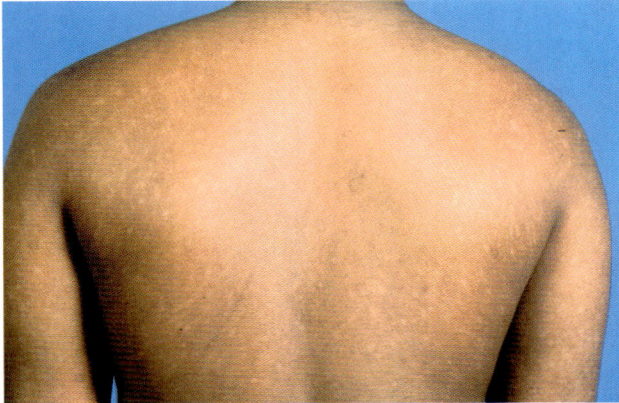

Figure 4–69 □ Chronic arsenic poisoning. This Bangladeshi patient has confetti-like hypopigmented macules on the trunk characteristic of chronic arsenic poisoning. In some parts of Asia, especially Bangladesh, arsenic poisoning is endemic due to drinking from arsenic contaminated ground water from wells. In the past, consumption of traditional Chinese medications containing arsenic for treatment of asthma was a common cause as well.

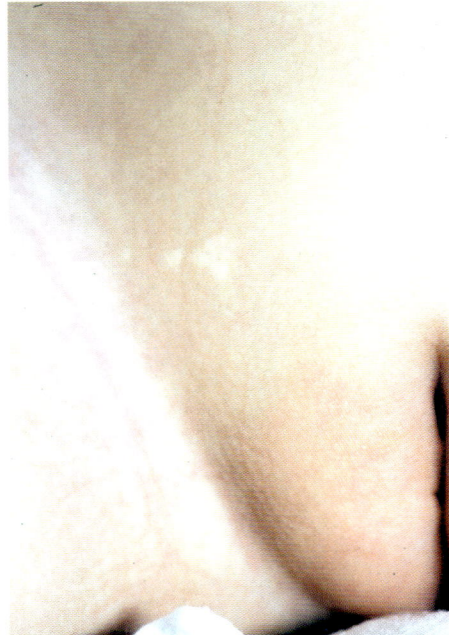

Figure 4–70 □ Clear cell papulosis. This eight-month-old girl has slightly elevated hypopigmented lesions on both sides of the pubic region. There is no history of injury, inflammation, or vitiligo. Symmetrical small oval and circular macules along the "milk line" and pubic region are characteristic of clear cell papulosis. Histology showed scattered clear cells that stain positive for AE 1, gross cystic fluid protein, and carcinoembryonic antigens. Most cases have been reported in Asian Orientals.

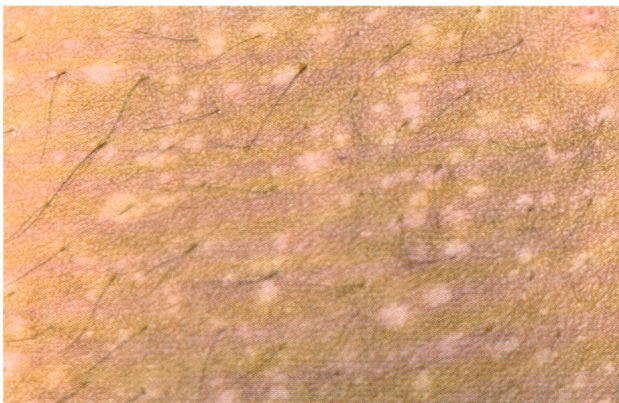

Figure 4–71 □ Darier's disease-associated guttate leukoderma. Characteristic hypopigmented macules on the anterior chest are seen in this Malay patient with Darier's disease. These confetti-like leucodermic macules are more visible on the trunk. Decreased numbers of melanocytes are seen on histological sections from these macules. They are mostly reported in dark-skinned individuals. They may arise in perifollicular or inter-follicular areas.

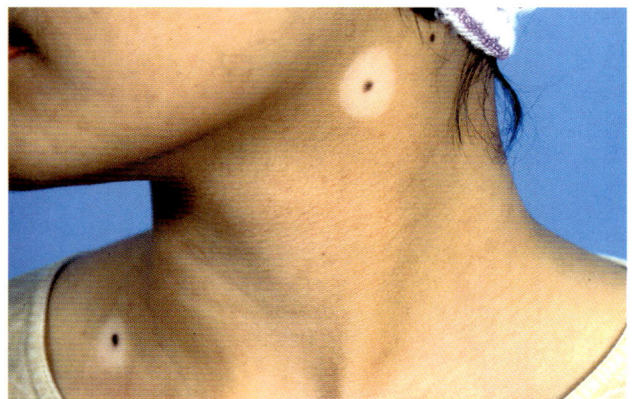

Figure 4–72 □ Halo nevus. A white depigmented halo surrounds two compound melanocytic nevi in this Malay lady. Pigmentation usually returns after a variable period. In some cases, the nevus may spontaneously undergo complete involution leaving a white macule. Vitiligo or other autoimmune conditions may be associated with halo nevi. It is important to critically evaluate the lesion, as a malignant melanoma rarely shows a halo phenomenon.

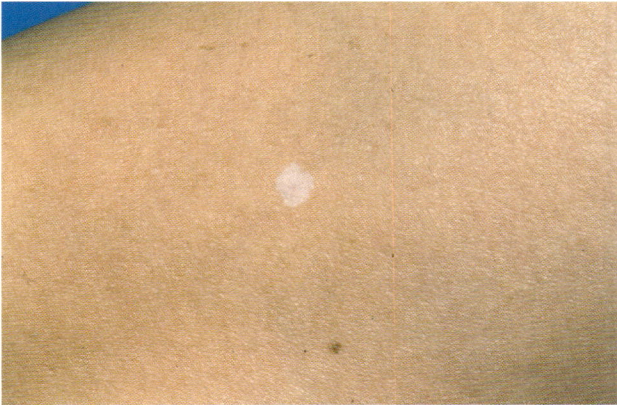

Figure 4–73 □ Idiopathic guttate hypomelanosis. An ivory white, well-demarcated solitary lesion of idiopathic guttate hypomelanosis (IGH) is shown here. Clinically, IGH often presents as hypopigmented, well-demarcated macules in the background of sun-damaged skin. The dorsum of the arms are most commonly affected, followed by the lower limbs and trunk. These lesions are benign and may be misdiagnosed as vitiligo. The lesions are generally small, ranging from a few millimeters to about 10 mm.

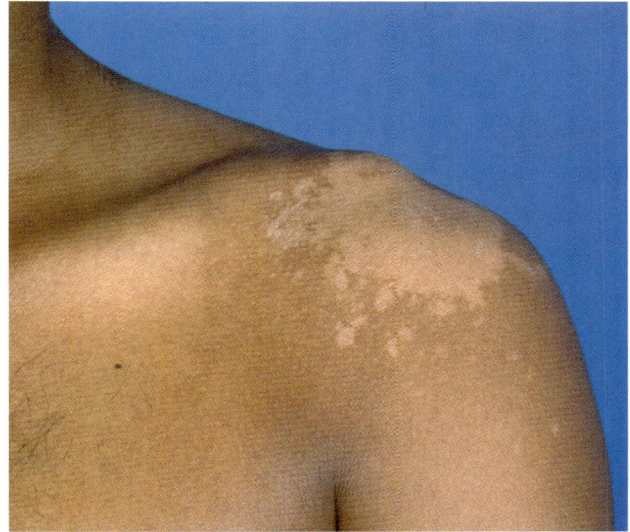

Figure 4–74 □ Pityriasis versicolor. This Indian patient has hypopigmented scaly lesions coalescing into a larger patch over the left shoulder area. The KOH mounts of skin scrapings have a typical "spaghetti and meat ball" appearance, confirming the clinical diagnosis of pityriasis versicolor. This condition is very common in the tropics. The causative yeast *Malassezia furfur* produces azelaic acid which inhibits the tyrosinase enzyme and results in the reduction of pigmentation in affected skin. The resultant hypopigmentation may persist for months after elimination of the yeast.

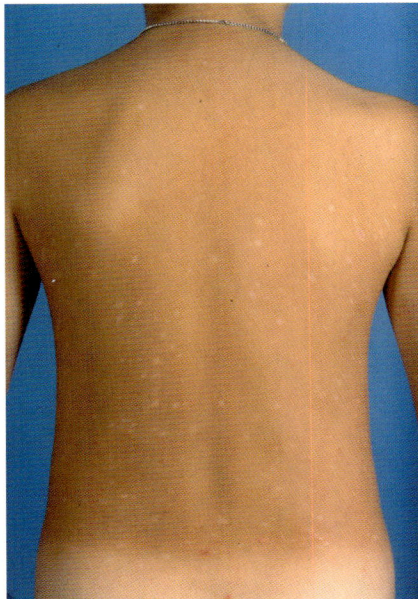

Figure 4–75 □ Pityriasis lichenoides chronica. In Asian skin, hypopigmented macules following pityriasis lichenoides chronica are common. Certain inflammatory mediators elevated in inflammatory disorders have been shown to inhibit melanization. Usually, post-inflammatory hypopigmentation improves and normal pigmentation returns after a variable length of time. Severe damage to melanocytes may, however, impair complete repigmentation.

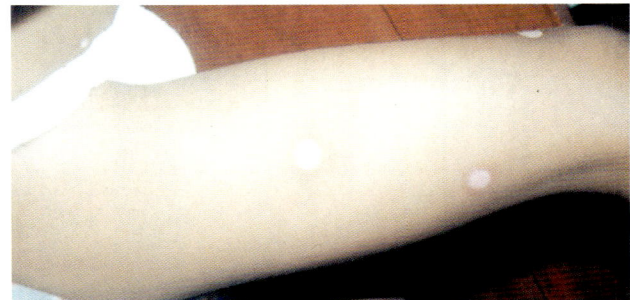

Figure 4–76 □ Post-bullous insect bite hypopigmentation. These well-demarcated circumscribed macules occurred in this Sri Lankan child as a sequel to bullous insect bite reactions. Depigmented macules following bullous insect bite reactions are, however, uncommon; usually only mild hypopigmentation or hyperpigmentation occurs.

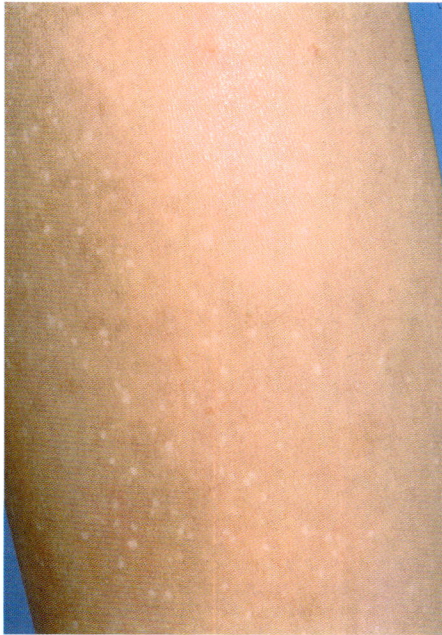

Figure 4–77 □ Punctate leukoderma. Punctate depigmented lesions are seen on the leg of this Chinese female patient. There is no history of inflammation or injury. This form of punctate leukoderma is traditionally described in patients treated with prolonged ultraviolet light therapy, although the etiology may be idiopathic as in this case. This condition is benign with no medical consequence.

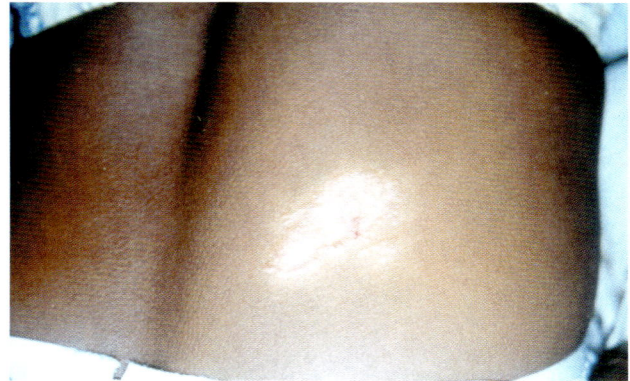

Photograph courtesy of *Dr Sunil Settinayake*

Figure 4–78 □ Leprosy. Pigmentary changes in tuberculoid leprosy may be very prominent in dark-skinned persons as shown in this Sri Lankan patient. This lesion in the lumbar region is semi-anesthetic. This chronic infectious disease caused by *Mycobacterium leprae* may present with semi-anesthetic hypopigmented patches with thickened peripheral nerves. Lesions may repigment slowly following appropriate anti-leprosy therapy.

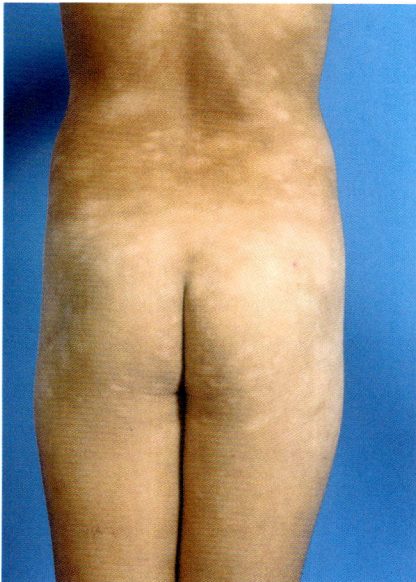

Figure 4–79 □ Hypopigmented mycosis fungoides. This variant of mycosis fungoides affecting a 14-year-old Chinese boy, who presents with multiple hypopigmented lesions involving the posterior trunk and the buttocks, is shown here. The hypopigmented patches tend to be of varying sizes, slightly scaly with indistinct borders, and associated with poikilodermatous changes. Hypopigmented mycosis fungoides is increasingly being recognized and described in Asians.

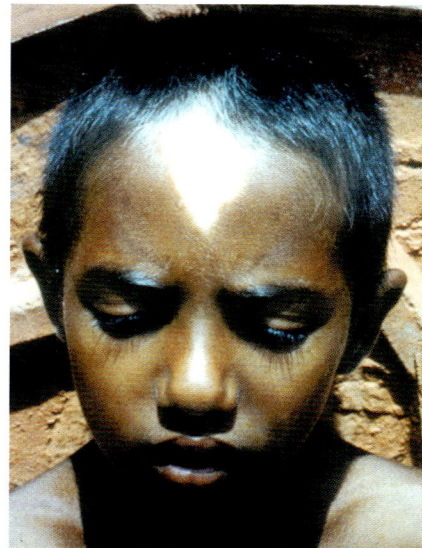

Photograph courtesy of Associate Professor Binod Khaitan, All India Institute of Medical Sciences.

Figure 4–80 □ Piebaldism. An Indian boy with a white forelock, a triangular depigmented macule on the forehead and partial poliosis of eyebrows, is shown here. Piebaldism, a rare autosomal dominant disorder, is characterized by a white forelock and depigmented macules (usually on the forehead and trunk), with small areas of hyperpigmented macules within them. These patients are not hard of hearing, which is a characteristic feature of Waardenburg's syndrome.

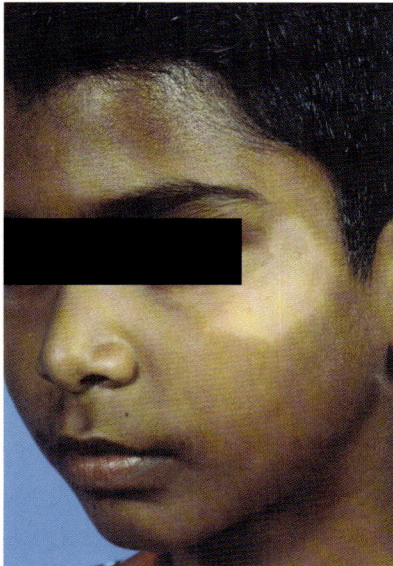

Figure 4–81 □ Pityriasis alba. A hypopigmented scaly macule is clearly visible in this Indian boy. Skin scrapings were negative for fungi and there was no sensory impairment. Pityriasis alba presents as scaly, whitish single, or multiple lesions. This condition usually appears on the face of young children but it can occur on the limbs and trunk as well. The pathogenesis is unknown but it appears to be a form of eczema. Pityriasis alba is more prominent in dark-skinned races as seen in this picture.

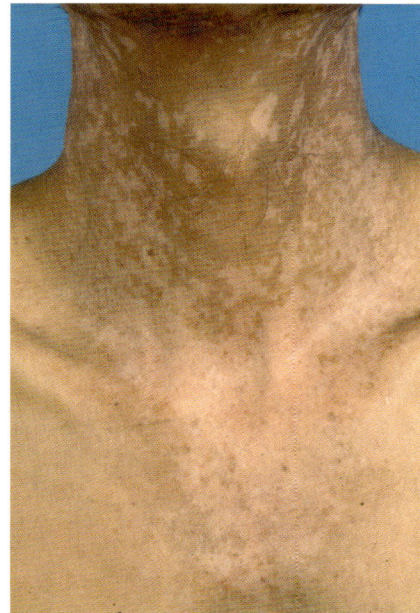

Figure 4–82 □ Post-drug eruption hypopigmentation. This picture shows a patient with post-inflammatory hypopigmentation following a photosensitive drug eruption due to thiazides. Depending on the area of inflammation, various shapes and sizes of hypopigmented lesions may become visible. Most cases of hypopigmentation following inflammation revert to normal color after a variable period of months to years.

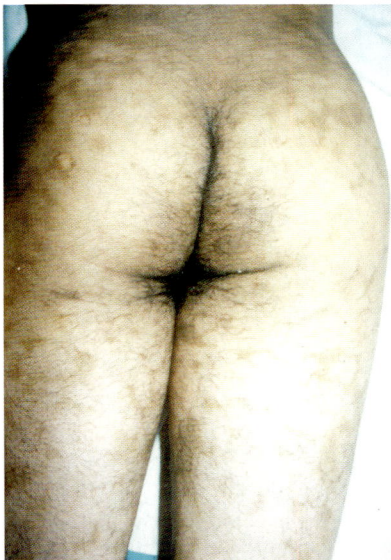

Photograph courtesy of Associate Professor Binod Khaitan, All India Institute of Medical Sciences

Figure 4–83 □ Post-Kala-Azar dermal leishmaniasis. This Indian patient with post-Kala-Azar dermal leishmaniasis (PKDL) has widespread hypopigmented macules. He also has granulomatous, infiltrated lesions of cutaneous leishmaniasis on the penis. Leismaniasis is found in several Asian, African, and South American countries. It is due to infection by the intracellular protozoa belonging to the genus Leishmania. PKDL is a sequel of visceral leishmaniasis. It may cause the more common hypopigmentation, or hyperpigmentation.

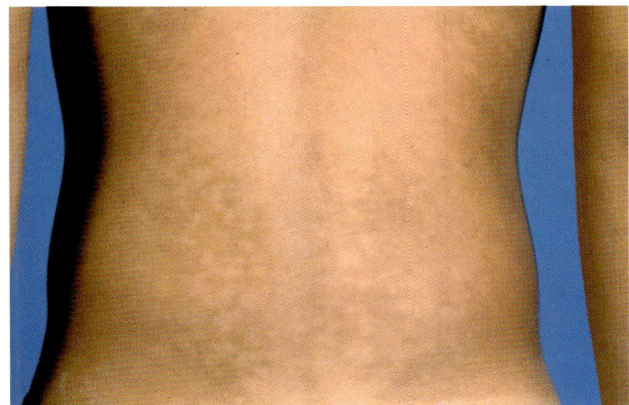

Figure 4–84 □ Progressive macular hypomelanosis. Hypopigmented discrete and coalescing lesions are seen in the lumbar region and on the loins of this Chinese patient. Skin fungal scrapings were negative for fungi and the biopsy did not show any significant pathology. This benign condition was first described in the French West Indies afflicting racially mixed, colored individuals. It was later described in The Netherlands, Sri Lanka, and Singapore. Typically, hypopigmented discrete and confluent macules develop insidiously in young adults without any preceding history of pityriasis versicolor or other forms of inflammation. The lumbar region, loins, and abdomen are the commonly affected areas.

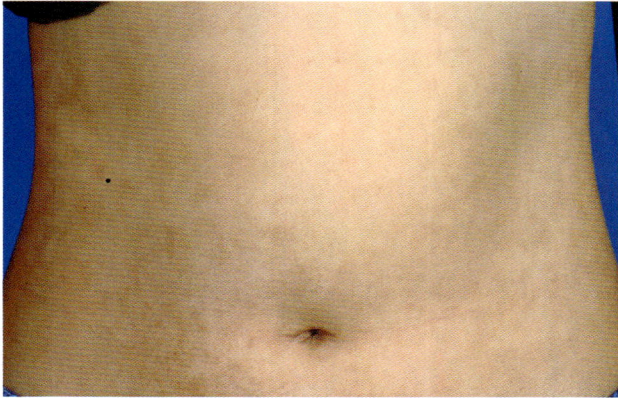

Figure 4–85 □ Progressive macular hypomelanosis. The anterior abdomen of a 20-year-old patient with multiple coalescing ill-defined hypopigmented macules of this benign idiopathic pigmentary disorder. Hypopigmented mycosis fungoides is a differential diagnosis that needs to be excluded. An ultrastructural examination of these macules showed less mature melanosomes when compared to the normal skin of the same patient. The hypopigmented areas also appear to tan less than the normal skin. Though the name implies a "progressive" course, this condition is often "self-limiting" and may regress after several years.

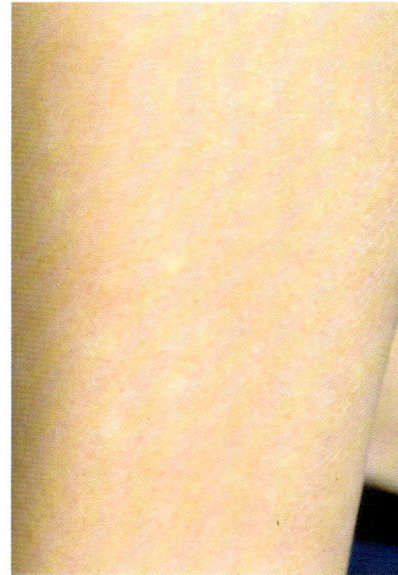

Figure 4–86 □ Pseudoleucoderma angiospasticum. Mottled "apparently hypopigmented" lesions are seen in a background of "flushed skin" in this fair-skinned Chinese patient. This condition is due to a benign vasospastic phenomenon. It is not due to a reduction of melanin pigment. This condition is not noticeable in dark-skinned individuals due to the dark constitutive pigmentation. The lesions become clearer after exercise or when the area is well-perfused. For example, if the upper limbs are affected, when the limbs are raised, the distinction between the "hypopigmented" and the normal skin becomes less obvious. No treatment is required for this benign condition.

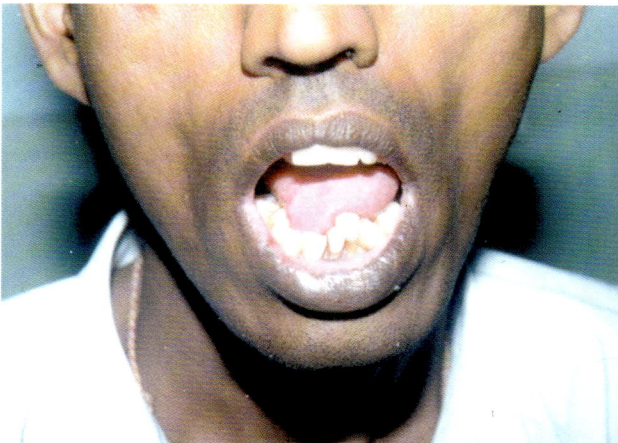

Figure 4–87 □ Submucous fibrosis. This Sri Lankan patient, with a history of betel (areca) nut chewing, presents with loss of papillae on the tongue, hypopigmentation of the lips, tongue and buccal mucosa with complaints of a burning sensation in the mouth when chilli or other strong spices are consumed. The chewing of betel nut is a common practice in some Asian communities (especially the Indian subcontinent). A toxin in the areca nut is suspected to be the cause of this condition. In severe cases, opening of the mouth is restricted due to sclerosis of the subcutaneous tissue of the lips and surrounding tissues and lips become depigmented. Squamous cell carcinoma may occur on the tongue or the buccal mucosa in long-standing cases.

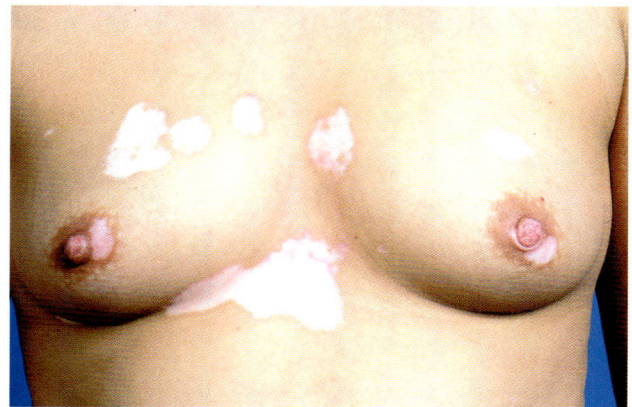

Figure 4–88 □ Vitiligo – patchy. This patient shows several well-demarcated, irregular depigmented macules on the chest. Vitiligo is an acquired depigmentary disorder, with a familial tendency, whereby there is destruction or dysfunction of melanocytes. Sometimes it is associated with other autoimmune conditions like Addison's disease and autoimmune thyroiditis.

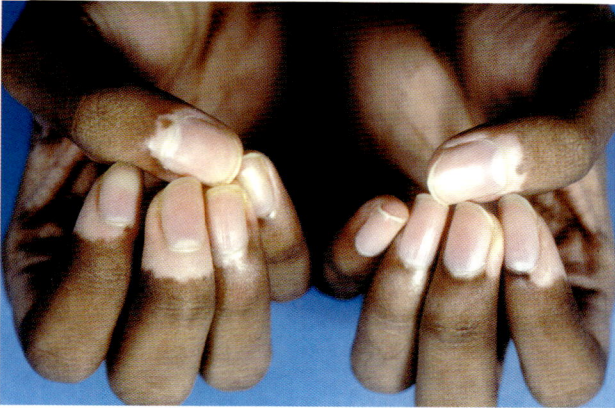

Figure 4–89 □ Vitiligo – lip-tip pattern. This patient has developed depigmentation on the finger tips, toes, around the eyes, on the lips, and ears which is characteristic of "lip-tip (periorificial) pattern" vitiligo. This acral pattern of vitiligo is generally more resistant to treatment.

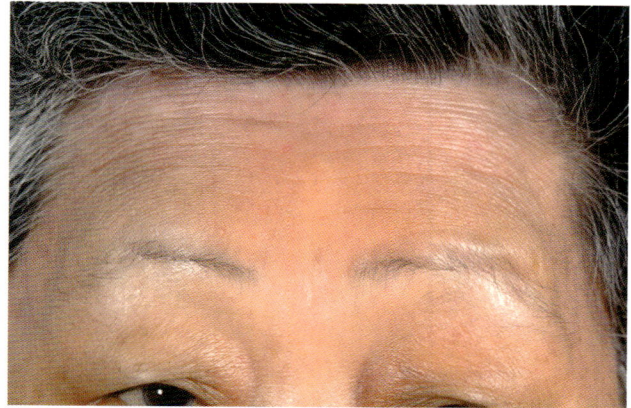

Figure 4–90 □ Vogt-Koyanagi-Harada syndrome. This 70-year-old lady, with a history of inflammatory uveitis, has depigmentation on the forehead, eye brow region, and alopecia. Vogt-Koyanagi-Harada syndrome is a multi-system, inflammatory disease characterized by vitiligo, poliosis of the eyebrows, uveitis, dysacousia, and alopecia. It occurs in three phases: meningoencephalitic phase, ophthalmic-auditory phase, and convalescent phase. Many patients first develop uveitis-related symptoms. Systemic steroids are effective in arresting the progression of the disease.

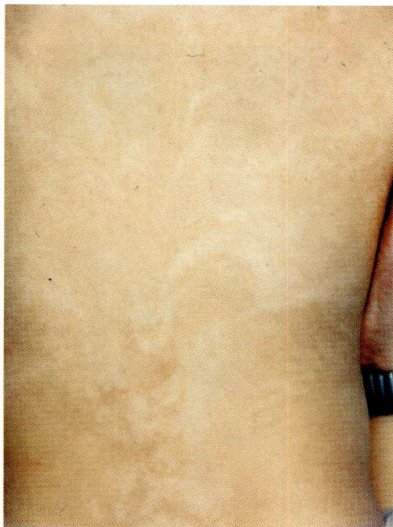

Figure 4–91 □ Hypomelanosis of Ito. Whorled hypopigmentation in the posterior trunk of this patient is characteristic of hypomelanosis of Ito. This is a rare disorder characterized by bizarre, bilateral, irregularly patterned leukoderma affecting the trunk and extremities. Whorled or streaky "marbling" often occurs in parallel arrays and along Blaschko's lines. Margins of lesions may be serrated and blurred or sharply outlined. It may be associated with other neurological and musculoskeletal abnormalities.

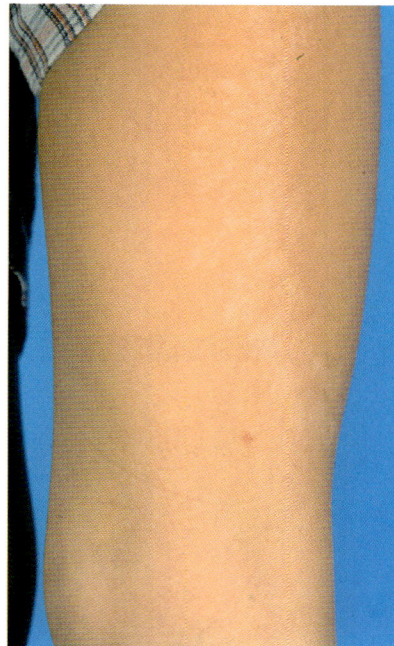

Figure 4–92 □ Lichen striatus. This patient presented with lichen striatus involving the upper left limb. The linear hypopigmentation lasted for several years before it faded. The nature and the distribution of the original condition dictate the area of hypopigmentation. Occasionally, the original insult or injury may be forgotten, but the patient may present with an acquired linear pigmentary anomaly.

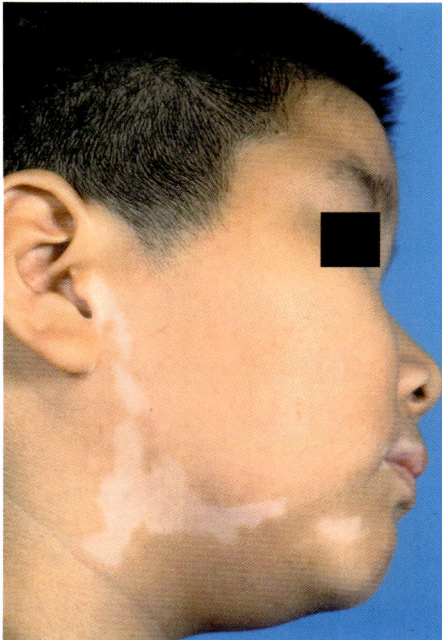

Figure 4–93 □ Vitiligo – segmental. This child has segmental vitiligo of the right mandibular region. Distribution is usually unilateral and quasi-dermatomal. This condition usually does not lead to generalized vitiligo. It is thought to be a subset aetiologically different to generalized vitiligo.

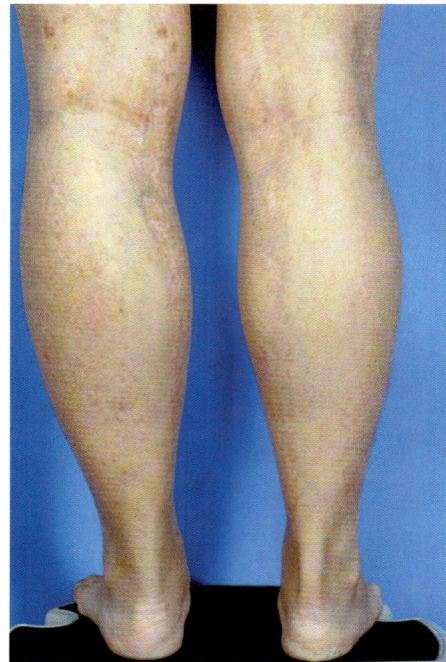

Figure 4–94 □ Goltz syndrome (focal dermal hypoplasia). Linear and reticulated hypopigmented atrophic lesions are seen on the lower limbs of this patient with Goltz syndrome. In this condition, reticulated, linear, or whorled areas of depigmentation may occur in relation to focal dermal hypoplasia. Associated neurological abnormalities may be present.

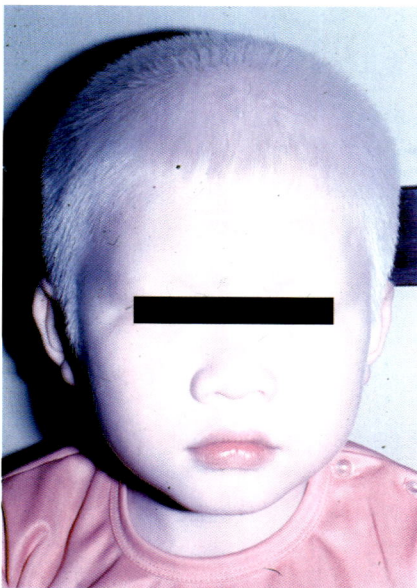

Figure 4–95 □ Albinism. A Chinese albino child with white hair is shown here. Albinism usually presents as hypopigmented or depigmented skin and hair. This may be associated with decreased visual acuity, photophobia, and nystagmus. There are several types of albinism. The prototype is the tyrosinase negative, oculocutaneous albinism. In tropical countries, albinos are at a greater risk of developing sun-related dermatoses such as actinic keratoses and squamous cell carcinoma.

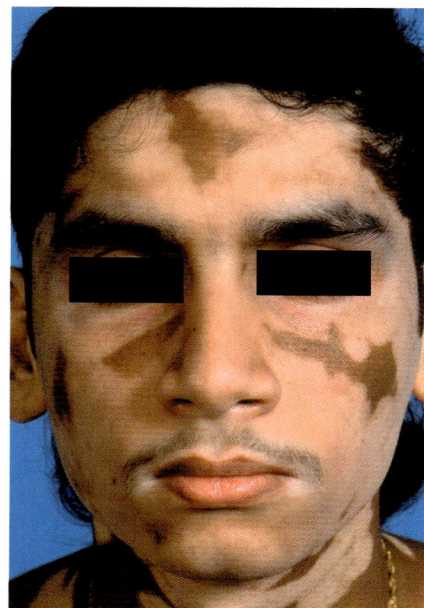

Figure 4–96 □ Vitiligo – generalized. This young Indian patient has extensive disfiguring vitiligo. In pigmented Asian races, vitiligo has a great psycho-social impact on affected persons as it is more clearly visible and areas of depigmentation have historically been associated with leprosy which still carries with it much social stigma. The vitiligo areas are more vulnerable to the effects of sun-damage compared to normal pigmented skin.

Infections and Infestations, Bites and Stings

Tan H.H. and Tan A.W.H.

Cutaneous infections are one of the most common reasons for attending a dermatology clinic. The normal skin of healthy individuals is highly resistant to invasion by microorganisms, but it only requires a minor breach in skin integrity for these agents to establish an infection. The immunocompromised patient also presents a particular challenge, especially when classical features of an infection are altered. In such a patient, infectious diseases of the skin represent the most extensive, and in their medical significance, one of the most important groups of all dermatoses.

BACTERIAL INFECTIONS (Figures 5–1 to 5–20)

Bacterial infections are common clinical problems encountered in most fields of clinical medicine. *Staphylococcus aureus* and *Streptococcus pyogenes* cause both primary pyodermas such as folliculitis, furunculosis, and impetigo, but are also common invaders of eczematous, traumatized or immunocompromised skin.

S. aureus is the most common organism isolated from both primary and secondary pyodermas. It is a hardy non-spore-forming, gram-positive coccus. Humans are the primary reservoir, and at least 80% of strains in the community produce beta lactamase, which causes resistance to the natural penicillins G and V. Colonization, which is the presence of the organism without producing disease, is important in both acquisition and spread of infection. In neonates, the umbilical stump, skin, gastrointestinal tract, and perineal areas are rapidly colonized. About 30% of adults are nasal carriers and 10% or more females are vaginal carriers with the percentage increasing at menses. Amongst hospital personnel, colonization is more prevalent.

Many infections originate in hair follicles. These infections are almost always due to *S. aureus*, but folliculitis associated with hot tubs and whirlpools caused by *Pseudomonas aeruginosa* can occasionally occur. Some patients present with the problem of recurrent furunculosis. In this situation, a search for an underlying cause is often initiated. However, screening for underlying diabetes mellitus, blood dyscrasias, low serum iron levels, defects in neutrophil function, and immune deficiency states is often unrewarding. Specific predisposing factors such as poor hygiene, pressure from occlusive clothing, and industrial exposure to oils and grease should be looked for, and a nasal swab for carriage of *S. aureus* should be done.

When assessing more serious infections, such as erysipelas and cellulitis, predisposing conditions, such as diabetes, venous and lymphatic obstruction, and tinea pedis, should be managed as well. The limbs are the most commonly affected sites, although it can occur anywhere on the body. The treatment of staphylococcal infections is usually with cloxacillin, erythromycin, or cephalexin. Penicillin combinations with clavulanate are also increasingly being used. The carrier state of the patient should be treated routinely too. This includes bathing with an antibacterial skin cleanser and application of mupirocin to anterior nares. The key issue in treating bacterial infections is the need to be vigilant regarding changing trends in antibiotic resistance, which should be monitored regularly.

Pyodermas that do not respond to the usual course of antibiotics may be due to unusual organisms. Occasionally, typical presentations, such as abscesses, can be due to less commonly encountered organisms. In such situations, non-tuberculous mycobacteria have to be considered as a possible cause. In Southeast Asia, cutaneous melioidosis (Figures 5–19 and 5–20) is a fairly recently described infection that also warrants consideration. Unlike systemic infections with *Burkholderia pseudomallei*, which can present as a fulminant septicemia and also with cutaneous features, this infection is primarily a skin infection with no systemic features. Affected individuals tend to be younger, and there is often a history of recreational or occupational contact with contaminated water or soil. *B. pseudomallei* has a characteristic antibiogram, showing resistance to aminoglycosides, many beta-lactam antibiotics, and fluoroquinolones. Combinations of at least two antibiotics including tetracyclines, amoxycillin/clavulinic acid, and trimethoprim-sulfamethoxazole have proven useful in our local experience. The choice of antibiotics should be guided by antibiotic sensitivity of the isolates.

MYCOBACTERIAL INFECTIONS
(Figures 5–21 to 5–48)

Leprosy (Figures 5–21 to 5–32) is still a prevalent disease, particularly in the Asian continent. There are many aspects of M. *leprae* that still elude the scientist, not least the fact that it cannot be cultured, and routes of transmission are still not well-known although the nasal mucosa is probably the most important source of bacillary emission. It is possible that the incubation period is longer in multibacillary forms and that the route of infection may differ. Clinical aspects of leprosy differ depending on the immunological status of the host although the agent is always the same. Susceptibility to leprosy shows considerable variation, from absolute refractoriness to complete absence of resistance. It is estimated that only less than 10% of any population is susceptible, and amongst these, only a few are prone to develop the disease. Environmental factors, such as poor nutrition and sanitation, also play a role. With the advent of multi-drug therapy (MDT), a cure for leprosy is possible. During a 24-month regimen, rifampicin, dapsone, and clofazimine are given for multibacillary forms of leprosy, whilst the paucibacillary types require rifampicin and dapsone for six months. On completion of MDT, patients are followed up for several years for relapse.

Pulmonary TB remains a problem in many countries, but cutaneous forms of TB (Figures 5–33 to 5–39) are relatively uncommon. Over the past two decades, there has been an increase in the number of cutaneous infections caused by non-tuberculous mycobacteria (NTM), or the so-called "atypical mycobacteria" (Figures 5–40 to 5–48). NTM with dermatological interest include M. *marinum*, M. *hemophilum*, M. *fortuitum*, M. *chelonae*, and M. *avium intracellulare* complex, amongst others. These are not usually transmitted by person to person contact, but are acquired from environmental sources such as water, soil, and vegetation, and their occurrence reflects their natural distribution. Diagnosis often requires a high index of suspicion. An appropriate history and clinical picture, with compatible histology are suggestive; proof is obtained from cultures and subsequent treatment should be guided by in-vitro sensitivity tests as far as possible.

VIRAL INFECTIONS (Figures 5–49 to 5–66)

Many viral diseases present with cutaneous lesions. Viral exanthems and enanthems are common, and can present in several forms, of which the most frequent are macular and papular eruptions, or morbilliform rashes. These and other exanthems will be discussed in the chapter on pediatric conditions (Chapter 7). Viral skin infections also present as bullous lesions as well as growths.

Bullous viral eruptions can be caused by *Herpes simplex virus* (HSV) types 1 and 2, *Varicella zoster virus* (VZV), and *Coxsackieviruses*, amongst others. The clinical entities include herpes labialis, herpes genitalis, chickenpox, herpes zoster, and hand-foot-mouth disease.

Patients with underlying skin conditions, such as atopic dermatitis, may develop generalized lesions (eczema herpeticum) with HSV infection, regardless of whether their eczema is active.

Human papilloma virus (HPV) infections are widespread and can infect the skin and mucous membranes and lead to benign or malignant epithelial tumors. More than 80 HPV types are known. Predisposing host factors to the development of warts include frequent trauma (nail biting, scratching), smoking, hyperhidrosis, chronic use of topical steroids and immunosuppression (HIV, renal transplant recipients). In immunosuppressed patients, particularly renal transplant recipients, cutaneous and unusual HPV infection is more likely to undergo malignant transformation.

Human herpesvirus 8 (HHV 8) is the cause of Kaposi's sarcoma, as well as rare conditions such as Castleman's disease and primary body cavity lymphoma. There are still questions with regards to its mode of transmission, but it seems clear that the presence of this virus coupled with severe immunosuppression from HIV infection or iatrogenic causes are the settings which cause the vascular tumor.

FUNGAL INFECTIONS (Figures 5–67 to 5–99)

Dermatophytes (Figures 5–67 to 5–94) are dependent on a favorable environment for their continuing success as pathogens. As the environment constantly changes, it is the ability of the fungi to adapt that determines their ability to survive. *Trichophyton rubrum* has been established in humans worldwide and is the most common cause of tinea corporis, cruris, and pedis. More patients are also seeking treatment for onychomycosis. *Malassezia furfur* is an important agent in tropical regions, causing pityriasis versicolor. Although easily treated, recurrences are not uncommon. Even after the infection has been treated, the pigmentary changes in the skin may take several weeks to normalize, and a pseudo-vitiliginous state may appear. The deep mycoses (Figures 5–95 to 5–99) are an important cause of morbidity and mortality in many regions. Systemic fungal infections are common in immunocompromised patients, while the agricultural worker is at risk of developing mycetoma in endemic areas. Certain infections, such as those caused by *Penicillium marneffei*, are found mainly in Southeast Asia, and are AIDS-defining illnesses in this region.

Developments in antifungal drugs have increased therapeutic options for the dermatologist, but compared to antibiotics, the number of drugs is still small. Superficial fungal infections are easily treated, but onychomycosis and many deep fungal infections remain therapeutically challenging.

PARASITIC INFECTIONS AND INFESTATIONS (Figures 5–100 to 5–110)

There are many parasitic infections of medical importance, which can produce both systemic disease as well as skin lesions. Parasitic infections and infestations by arthropods are caused by scabies and lice. Scabies is transmitted by close and prolonged contact with afflicted persons and affects all races and social classes worldwide. Pediculosis is an infestation caused by lice, which are bloodsucking, wingless insects. Lice are very host-specific and are only transmitted from human to human. Infestations are common in all parts of the world, including Asia, and do not spare any socio-economic class. Helminthic infections presenting with dermatologic signs include cutaneous larva migrans and cercarial dermatitis (swimmer's itch). Cutaneous leishmaniasis is a disease occurring in certain geographical zones. Although it is not endemic in many areas in Asia, one must constantly be aware of the different infections that are prevalent in specific locales.

BITES AND STINGS (Figures 5–111 to 5–119)

Insect bite reactions are cutaneous responses to a biting or stinging arthropod that usually causes itching. The problem occurs worldwide. Sources include domestic pets, birds, bedding and furniture, travel, and military training.

Patients are often reluctant to accept the diagnosis of insect bite reactions; they may feel slighted at the suggestion that their homes or their pets are infested. A tactful approach is required.

The dermatologist may also encounter cutaneous reactions to stings from jellyfish and other marine creatures, which can produce bizarre patterns. A full description of this subject is beyond the scope of this atlas.

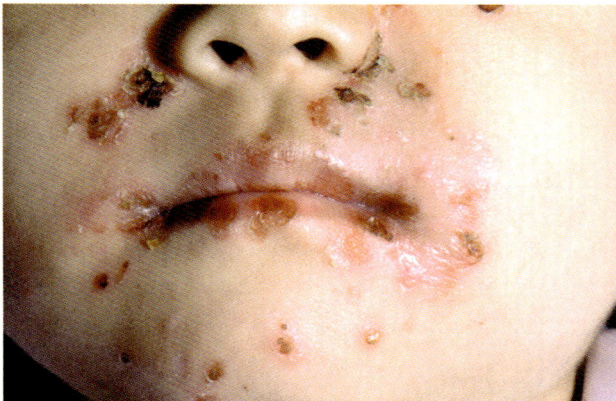

Figure 5–1 □ Impetigo. The face, especially of infants and children, is a common location for impetigo. Note the characteristic "stuck-on" dirty-yellow crusts. Either *Staphylococcus aureus* or *Streptococcus pyogenes* causes this infection, with *S. aureus* more commonly found.

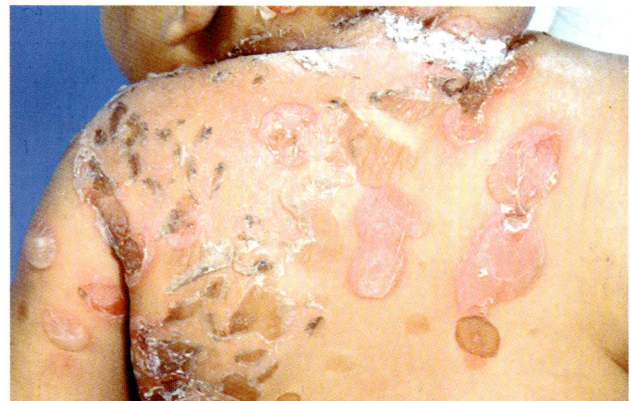

Figure 5–2 □ Bullous impetigo. In this child, large flaccid bullae are seen, some of which have ruptured to form shallow erosions and crusted lesions. This form is produced by an extracellular exotoxin released by *S. aureus*. Recommended treatments include a course of cloxacillin or cephalexin, with erythromycin as an alternative in penicillin-allergic patients.

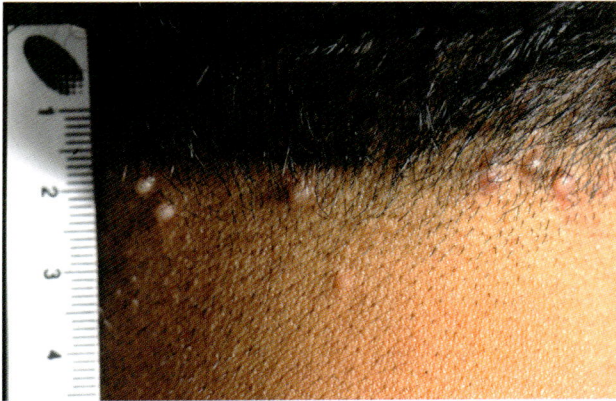

Figure 5–3 □ Folliculitis. Erythematous papules and pustules are noted around follicular openings at the posterior hairline. This staphylococcal infection is usually non-tender or slightly tender, and patients may complain of pruritus. The superficial form seen here heals without scarring, but chronic, recurrent, deep folliculitis can occur on the scalp and in the beard area, with resultant scarring.

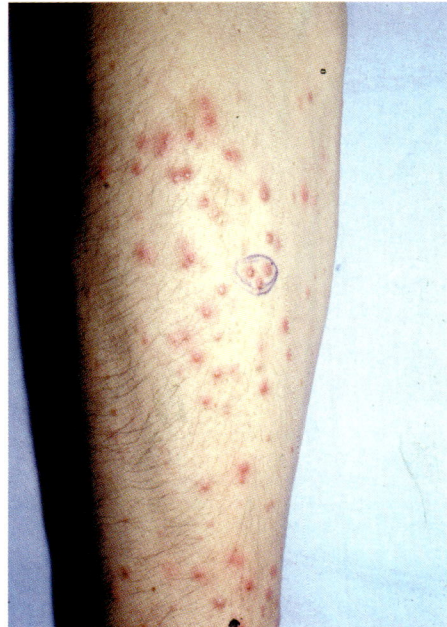

Figure 5–4 □ Folliculitis. Discrete dome-shaped papules and pustules occurring in the ostia of the hair follicles of the arm. In this patient, exposure to mineral oils was a contributing cause.

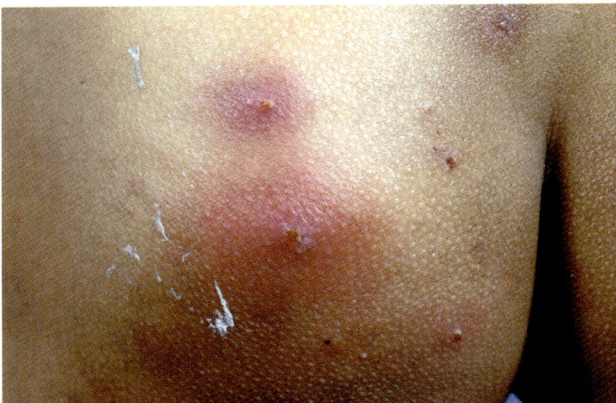

Figure 5–5 □ Furunculosis. Tender discrete erythematous firm nodules on the buttocks. These boils represent deep-seated infections that evolve from a staphylococcal folliculitis. Systemic antibiotics are often indicated and incision and drainage are occasionally required.

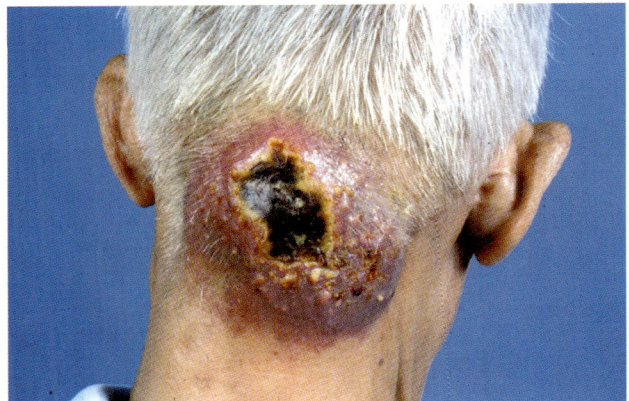

Figure 5–6 □ Carbuncle. A large, tender, erythematous indurated plaque with a necrotic, ulcerated portion is seen on the nape of the neck of this diabetic patient. A carbuncle is formed by multiple coalescing furuncles, often accompanied by severe constitutional symptoms such as fever and malaise. Systemic antibiotics and surgical intervention are required.

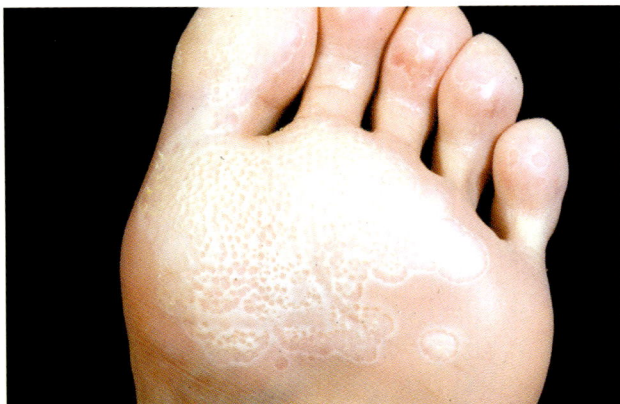

Figure 5–7 □ Pitted keratolysis. These are multiple, confluent, small, reticulated pits with an annular pattern occurring on macerated skin of the toe pulps and sole. The causative agent is usually a corynebacterium. Hyperhidrosis is a predisposing factor. Treatment with topical erythromycin is effective.

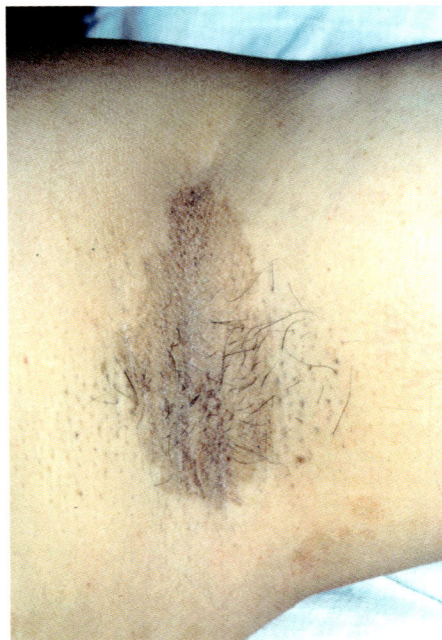

Figure 5–8 □ Erythrasma. A well-defined, mildly scaly, brownish patch on the axilla is seen. This is a bacterial infection of the intertriginous areas caused by *Corynebacterium minutissimum*. A characteristic "coral-red" fluorescence due to porphyrins produced by the bacteria, can be seen when viewed with a Wood's lamp. Topical or systemic erythromycin is effective.

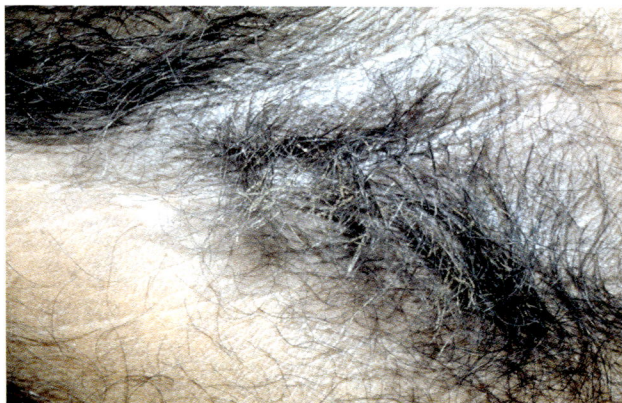

Figure 5–9 □ Trichomycosis axillaris. Yellowish concretions are seen on the axillary hair. These lesions are due to bacterial colonization of the hair. It is usually asymptomatic. Shaving the hair is an effective treatment.

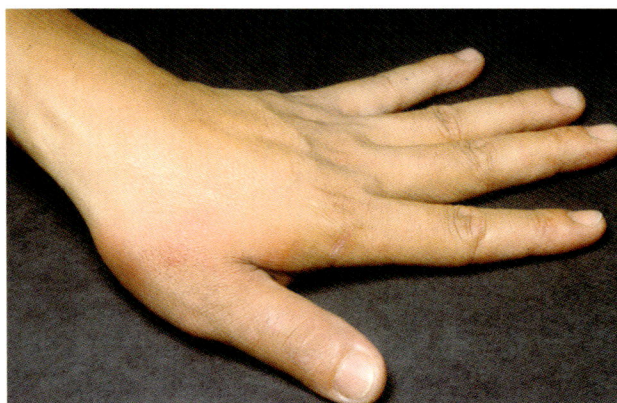

Figure 5–10 □ Erysipeloid. Erythematous, tender, well-defined macules and plaques are seen on the hand, thumb and index finger. This is an infection of traumatized skin caused by *Erysipelothrix rhusiopathiae*, a gram-positive rod. It is often an occupational disease, associated with the handling of fish, shellfish, or meat. Systemic symptoms are uncommon. Treatment with penicillin or erythromycin is effective.

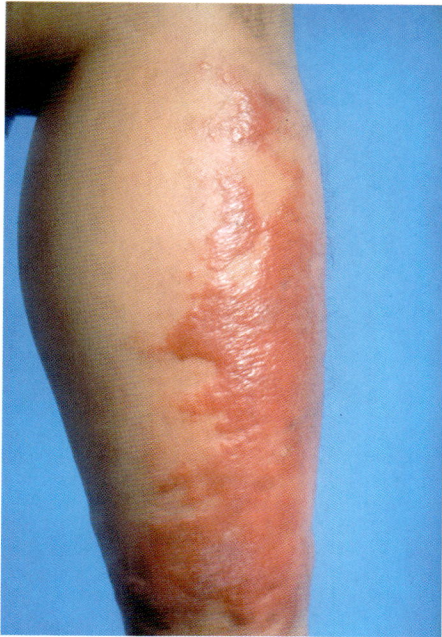

Figure 5–11 □ Erysipelas. A febrile patient with a tender erythematous plaque on the leg. Vesicles are seen in the advancing margin. The causative organism is *Streptococcus pyogenes*. In adults, the lower leg is affected in about 50% of the cases.

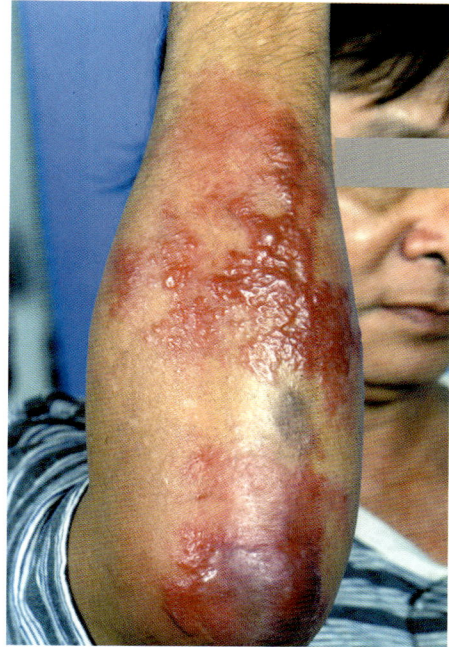

Figure 5–12 □ Erysipelas. Involvement of the upper limb is seen here. Bacteria may gain entry through a superficial wound in the skin. Treatment with penicillin or erythromycin if the patient is allergic to penicillin, should be started without delay.

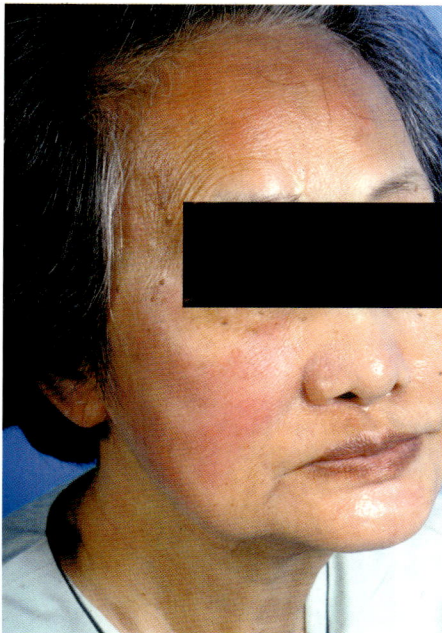

Figure 5–13 □ Erysipelas. In this elderly patient, there is early involvement of the right cheek. Note the less intense erythema and lack of edema. Erysipelas in the elderly and immunocompromised patients may present with more subtle features.

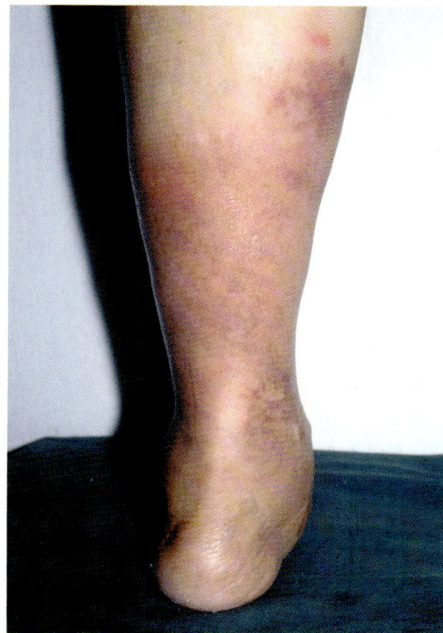

Figure 5–14 □ Cellulitis. Painful, warm, tender, erythematous swelling of the leg associated with edema. The demarcation between normal and affected skin is not as distinct as in erysipelas. The patient presents with marked constitutional symptoms and intravenous antibiotics (a combination of penicillin and cloxacillin is recommended) are required.

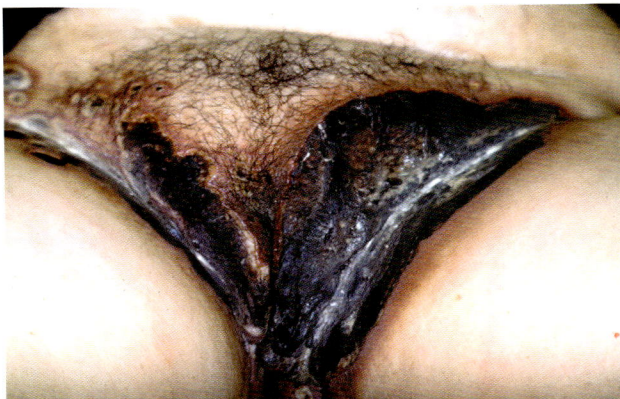

Figure 5–15 □ Necrotizing fasciitis. This woman presents with a rapidly developing erythematous and painful swelling over the vulval region which progressed to frank necrotic ulceration within a few days. This is a potentially life-threatening infection of the skin, most commonly associated with *Streptococcus pyogenes*, but *Staphylococcus aureus*, gram-negative organisms and anaerobes may also be found, and synergistic infection also occurs. Early aggressive surgical treatment with extensive tissue debridement and systemic antibiotics are required.

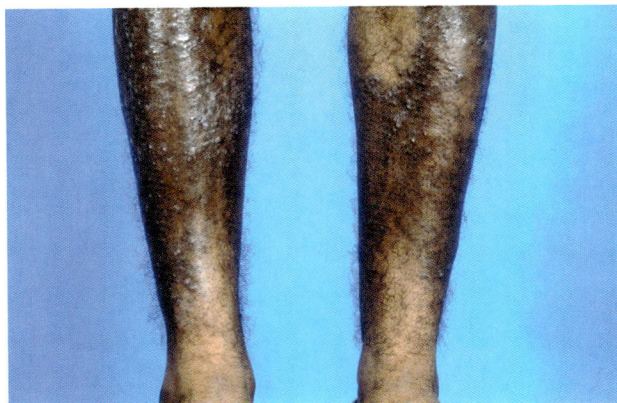

Figure 5–16 □ Dermatitis cruris pustulosa et atrophicans. Bilateral, symmetrical, superficial, and deep follicular pustular lesions on the legs of an Indian patient. The lesions heal with atrophic scarring. *Staphylococcus aureus* was isolated from a swab culture. This condition is common in the Indian subcontinent, especially in the rural population. The cause is unknown. The usual treatment involves long courses of systemic antibiotics, but a tendency to recur is a feature.

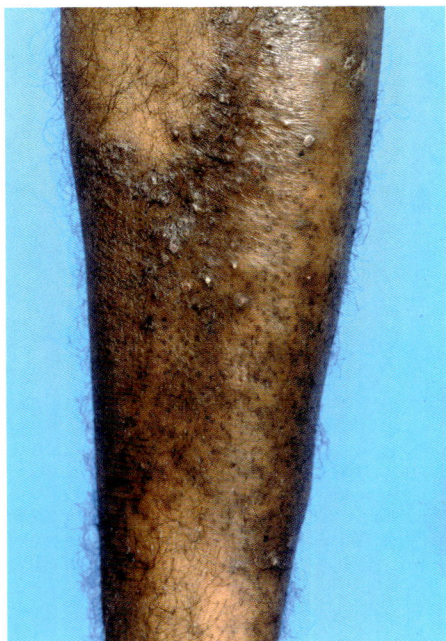

Figure 5–17 □ Dermatitis cruris pustulosa et atrophicans. A close-up view of active follicular pustules on the legs, with previously healed areas showing hair loss following the development of atrophic scarring. This patient was treated with extended courses of anti-staphylococcal antibiotics.

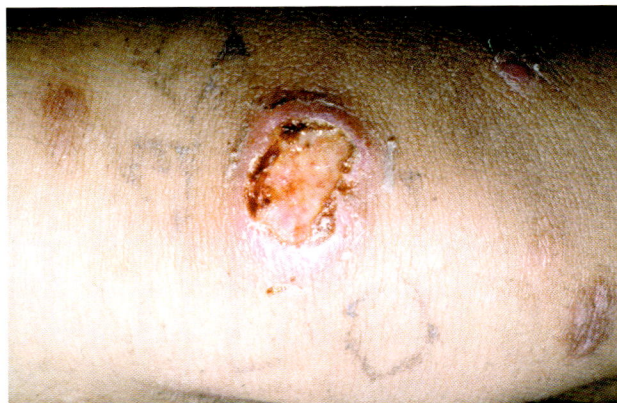

Figure 5–18 □ Ecthyma. Following an insect bite, this patient developed a deep-seated pyoderma, which had a thick, adherent crust that revealed a shallow ulceration on removal. In this patient, *Streptococcus* was isolated, although mixed infections are also common.

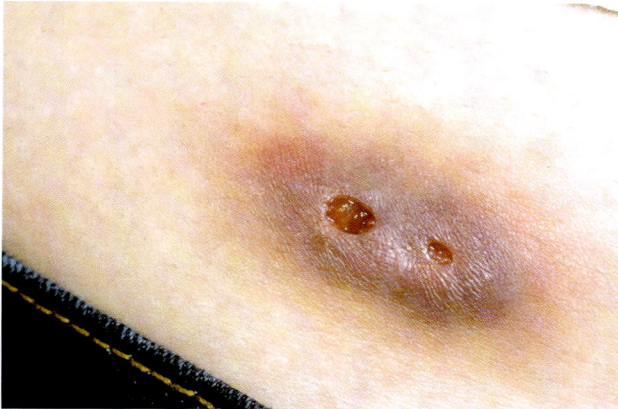

Figure 5–19 □ Cutaneous melioidosis. An abscess, with discharging sinuses, had developed on the abdomen of a female teenager following minor trauma. She did not respond to an extended course of cephalexin prescribed by her family doctor. *Burkholderia pseudomallei* was isolated. Investigations did not reveal any systemic infection and she responded to a six-month course of cotrimoxazole and doxycycline.

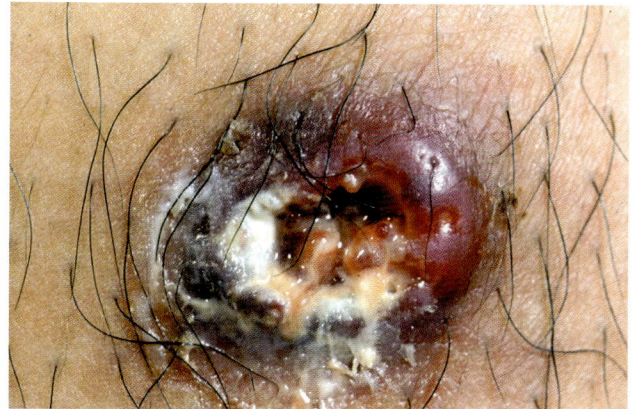

Figure 5–20 □ Cutaneous melioidosis. An enlarging ulcerated plaque with slough and discharging sinuses developed on the posterior thigh of this patient who had fallen into a drain several weeks before. This patient responded to a six-month course of clavulanate-potentiated amoxicillin and doxycycline. In this case, *Burkholderia pseudomallei* isolated on swab culture was resistant to cotrimoxazole. This patient also did not have any evidence of systemic involvement.

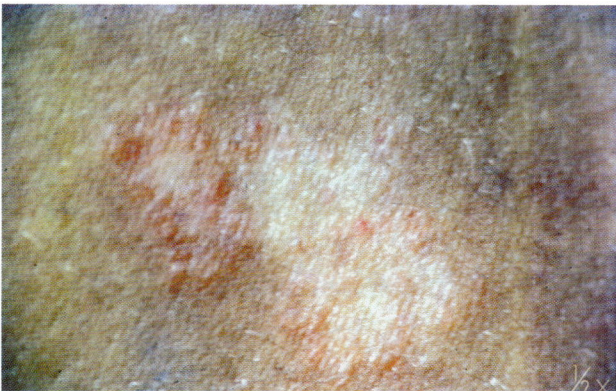

Figure 5–21 □ Hansen's disease – tuberculoid (TT) leprosy. A single, well-defined, anesthetic, hypopigmented patch is seen here. In this form of leprosy, the immunity of the host is good. The lepromin skin test was strongly positive. Slit-skin smears did not reveal presence of acid-fast bacilli (AFB). Lesions are typically solitary or few in number, and histology revealed well-defined tuberculoid granulomas, with local destruction of the nerves and appendages. No AFB was seen on histology. Tuberculoid and borderline tuberculoid leprosy represent the paucibacillary forms of Hansen's disease.

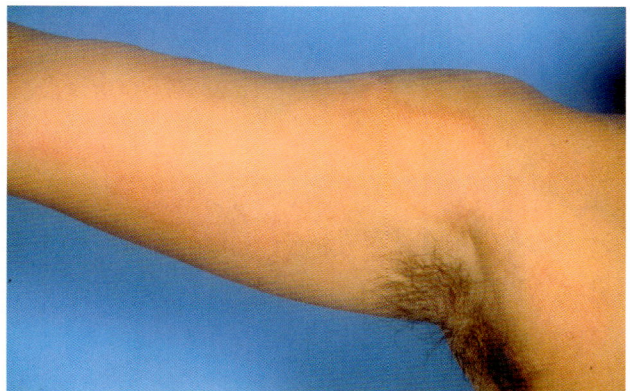

Figure 5–22 □ Hansen's disease – borderline tuberculoid (BT) leprosy. This male has a large, annular, hypo-pigmented patch on the arm, with peripheral erythema and a margin that is mildly infiltrated. There is loss of sensation and anhidrosis over the lesion. The borderline group of leprosy is divided into three forms, intermediate between the two polar types: borderline tuberculoid (BT), borderline borderline (BB), and borderline lepromatous (BL) are designated based on clinical, histological, and bacteriological parameters. BT leprosy is closer to the TT form, but if untreated may relapse toward the other spectrum of the disease.

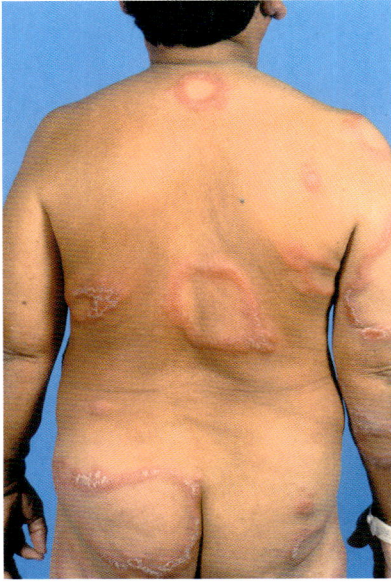

Figure 5–23 □ **Hansen's disease – borderline lepromatous (BL) leprosy.** Multiple annular plaques, with infiltrated erythematous borders are seen on the back, arms and buttocks of this patient. BL leprosy represents the multibacillary form of Hansen's disease, and is similar to lepromatous leprosy (LL). Sensory loss tends to occur later. The lepromin test was negative. Histology revealed a picture closer to that of LL, with AFB readily identifiable. A 24-month course of multi-drug therapy (MDT) is required.

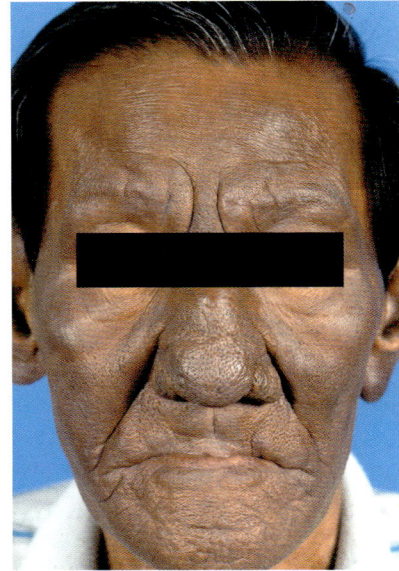

Figure 5–24 □ **Hansen's disease – lepromatous (LL) leprosy.** This male has developed the typical "leonine" facies, characterized by infiltration of the supraorbital ridges, earlobes, and the nose, as well as a depressed nasal bridge, accompanied by loss of the lateral eyebrows. He has a distinctive brownish pigmentation following the administration of clofazimine, which is a dye compound. LL represents the pole of Hansen's disease where patients have no immunity against the bacteria. The disease is disseminated. Skin smears readily revealed AFB. The lepromin test was negative.

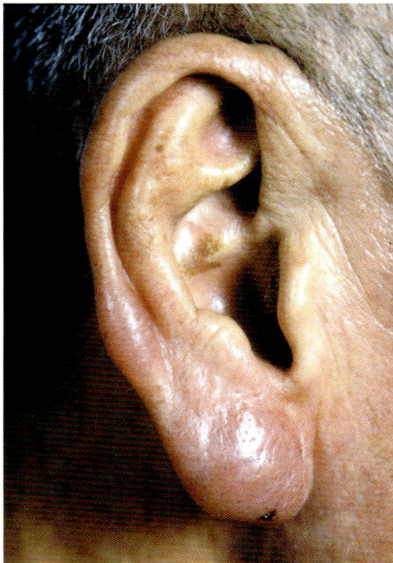

Figure 5–25 □ **Hansen's disease – lepromatous (LL) leprosy.** Infiltration of the earlobe is typical. *Mycobacterium leprae* shows a preference for the "cooler" parts of the body.

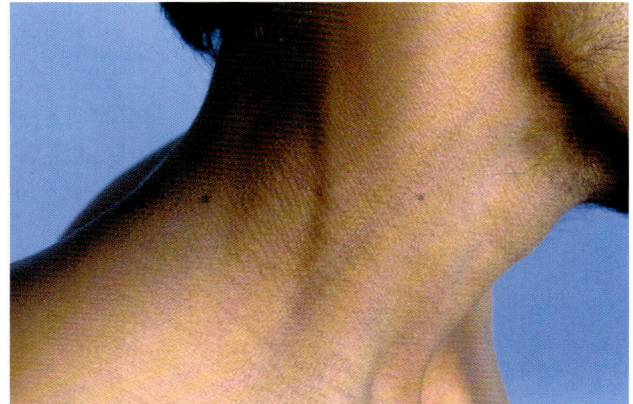

Figure 5–26 □ **Pure neural Hansen's disease.** This Indian male patient presents with a tender, thickened swelling of the right greater auricular nerve, in the absence of other skin signs. Nerve sheath biopsy confirmed Hansen's disease. The pure neural form of Hansen's disease affects only one or more peripheral nerves, and may result in sensory loss with or without motor deficit.

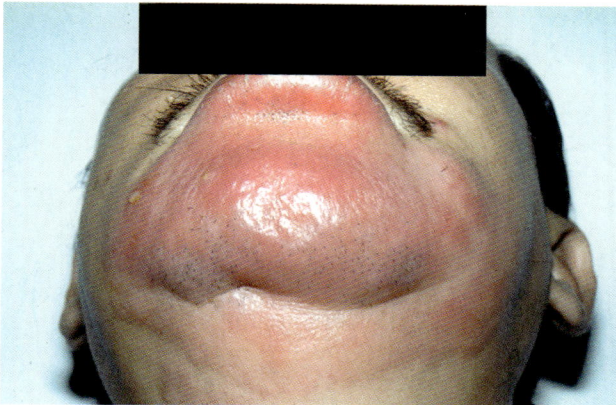

Figure 5–27 □ Type I reaction in Hansen's disease. A patient with BT Hansen's involving the chin presents with increased swelling, erythema, and tenderness over the original plaque two months after the initiation of MDT. Reactions in leprosy are acute clinical events. Type I reactions are seen in TT, BT or BB forms of leprosy. This reaction can result from a sudden deterioration (downgrading reaction) or improvement (upgrading reaction) of the immunity of the host. Systemic steroids are usually indicated to control the reaction.

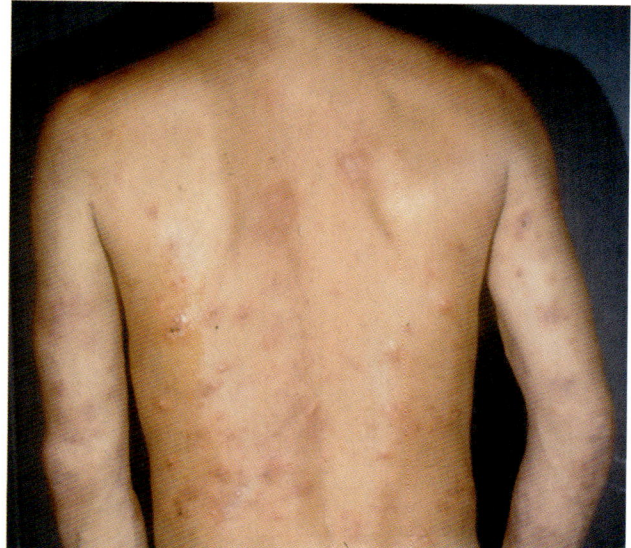

Figure 5–28 □ Type II reaction in Hansen's disease (erythema nodosum leprosum). This patient with LL Hansen's presents with a sudden onset of new multiple, tender, erythematous nodules and plaques on the trunk, which are separate from his underlying LL lesions. Type II or erythema nodosum leprosum (ENL) reactions occur in BL or LL Hansen's and is due to the deposition of immune complexes. ENL reactions are often accompanied by nerve pains and other constitutional symptoms. Urgent treatment with systemic steroids is required, and thalidomide is particularly useful in controlling ENL reactions.

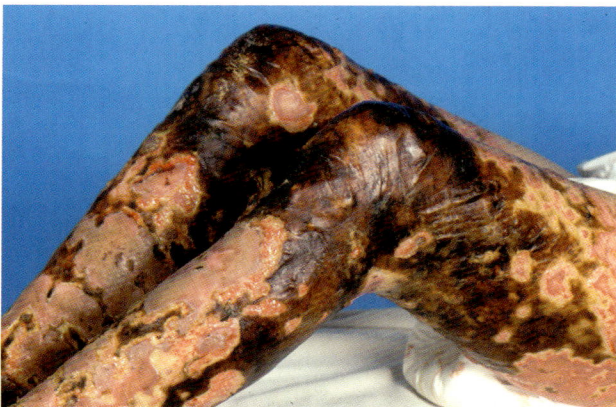

Figure 5–29 □ Lucio phenomenon. Large painful hemorrhagic infarcts, necrotic ulcers, and vasculitic lesions on the legs of an elderly Chinese man who had previously untreated leprosy. He does not have any overt nodules or plaques on presentation, but is noted to have a loss of the lateral third of his eyebrows. Skin smears from clinically normal appearing skin were strongly positive for AFB, indicating a diffuse infiltration of the skin. The Lucio phenomenon is an extreme type II reaction in untreated patients. Histology revealed epidermal necrosis, necrotizing vasculitis, and large numbers of AFB in endothelial cells.

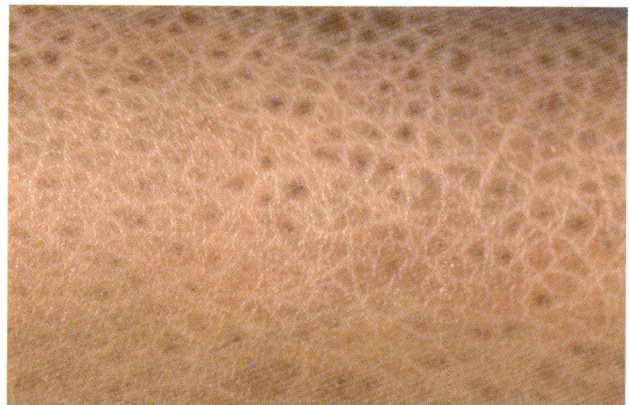

Figure 5–30 □ Hansen's disease – acquired ichthyosis. This patient has extremely dry skin with pigmented rhomboidal scales on the legs. The ichthyosis that has developed is related to damage to the peripheral and autonomic nerves.

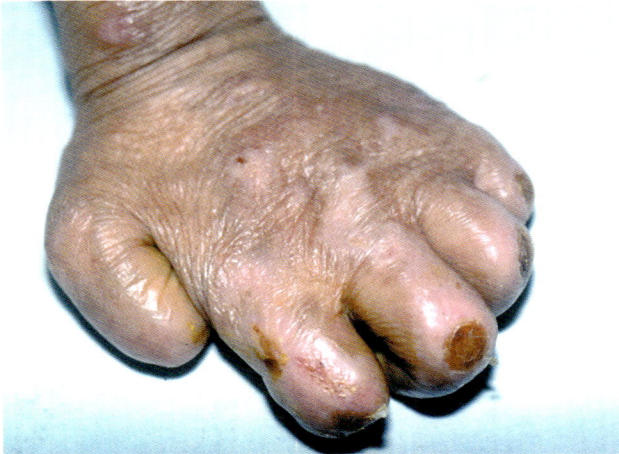

Figure 5–31 □ Complications of Hansen's disease – hand deformities. This patient with burnt-out leprosy displays stigmata of the disease, with fixed flexion deformities of the fingers, "stubby" shortened fingers due to digital resorption and ulceration on the hands, resulting from a thermal injury.

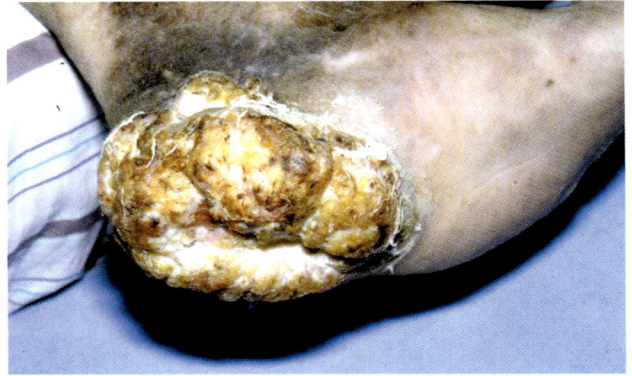

Figure 5–32 □ Complications of Hansen's disease – squamous cell carcinoma. This patient had burnt-out leprosy and a long-standing trophic ulcer on the heel, which developed a verrucous, fungating tumor due to squamous cell carcinoma. A below-knee amputation was required.

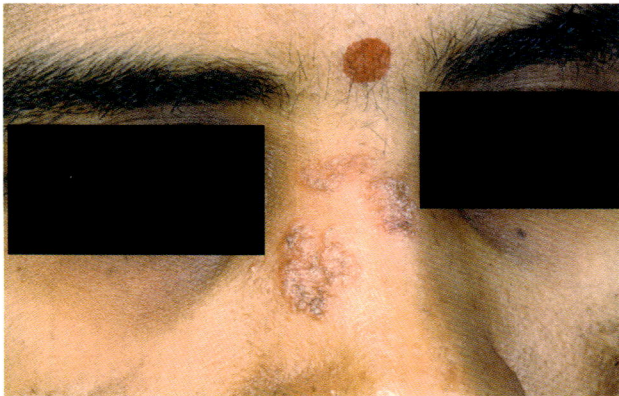

Figure 5–33 □ Lupus vulgaris. Discrete reddish-brown plaques on the nasal area of an Indian female. Diascopy reveals the characteristic "apple-jelly" yellowish-brown color. Lupus vulgaris represents a form of post-primary tuberculous infection in a person with an intact immune system. Lesions often display uniform or irregular scarring. Large lesions on the face can result in considerable mutilation. A screen for systemic tuberculosis (TB) is mandatory.

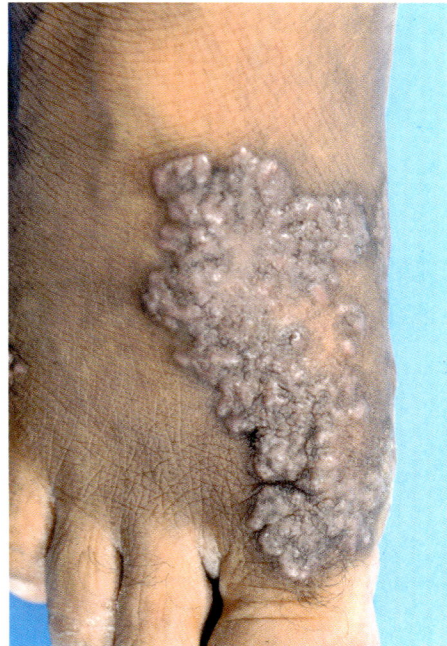

Figure 5–34 □ TB verrucosa cutis. This irregular, brown, warty plaque on the dorsum of the foot has been present for five years, and is progressing very slowly. TB verrucosa cutis results from exogenous inoculation of the skin in patients who have good immunity against TB. Spontaneous healing is unusual, and the patient has a strong Mantoux test reaction, but cultures are often negative. Treatment with standard anti-TB drugs is curative.

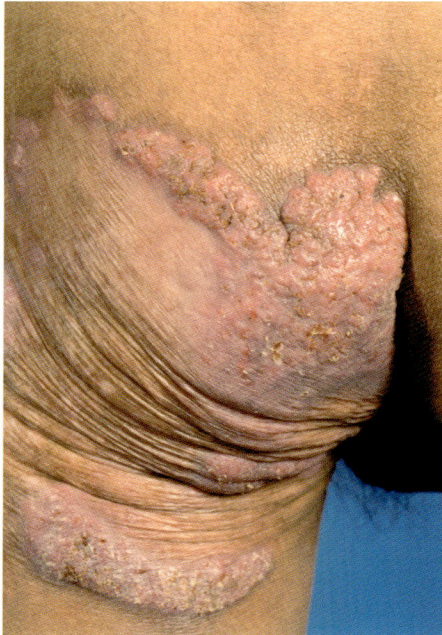

Figure 5–35 □ TB verrucosa cutis. A large, annular, erythematous warty plaque on the buttock, with an atrophic central area. The feet, hands, and buttocks are common sites for TB verrucosa cutis.

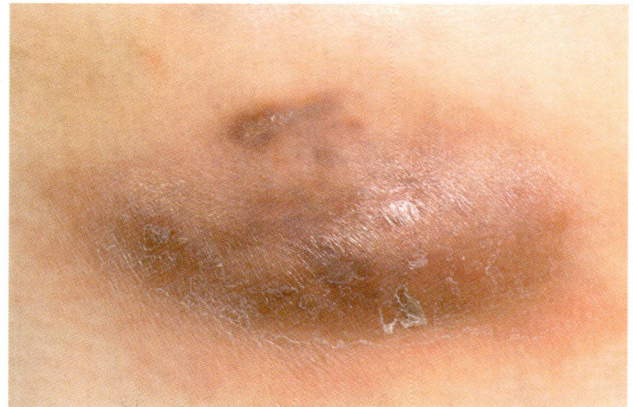

Figure 5–36 □ Tuberculous abscess. A large, fluctuant subcutaneous swelling on the flank of a woman. This is also known as a tuberculous gumma or "cold abscess" because of the lack of inflammation. Lesions can break down and form fistulas and ulcers. It represents hematogenous spread to the skin from a primary focus of TB in the body.

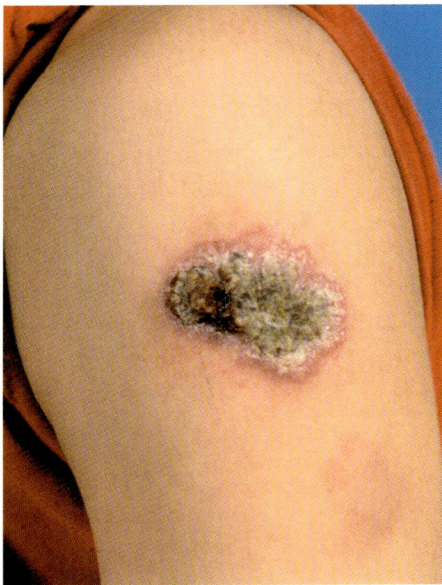

Figure 5–37 □ BCG-induced lupus vulgaris. This 12-year-old boy has developed an enlarging granulomatous plaque on the left deltoid region following BCG vaccination. This is a rare complication following vaccination with an attenuated strain of *Mycobacterium bovis*.

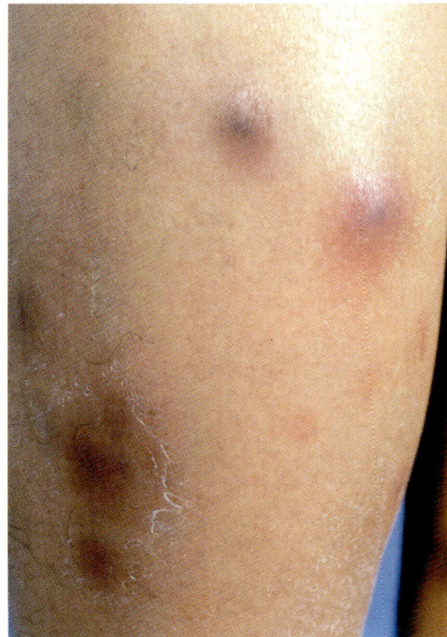

Figure 5–38 □ Erythema induratum. This woman presented with painful, dusky-red nodules on the calves, which eventually broke down to form ulcers with ragged, irregular edges. Her Mantoux test reaction was strongly positive, and histology revealed a nodular vasculitis. This condition is considered a classic example of a tuberculid. Recent investigative work using polymerase chain reaction (PCR) shows a high positive rate for detection of *Mycobacterium tuberculosis* DNA within skin biopsy specimens.

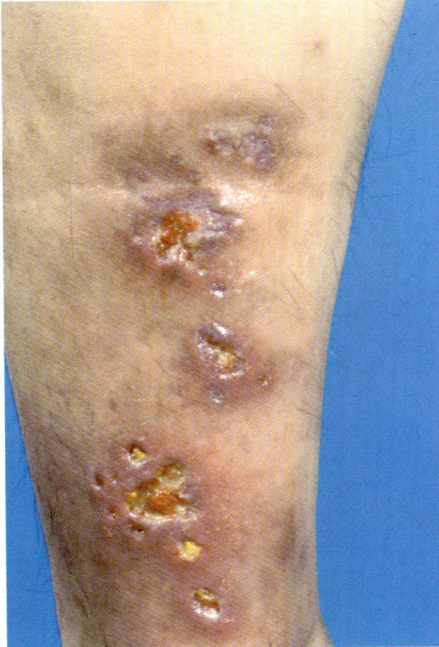

Figure 5–39 □ Erythema induratum. Multiple ragged ulcers and areas of scarring are seen on the posterior calf of this patient. Response to anti-TB treatment is excellent.

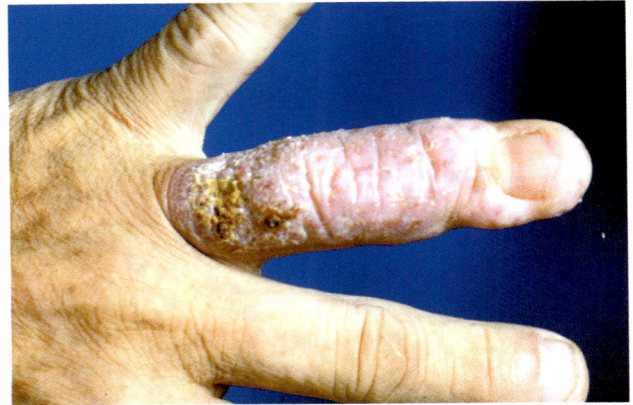

Figure 5–40 □ Non-tuberculous mycobacterial infection by *Mycobacterium marinum*. A fish-tank granuloma developed on the ring finger of this man several months after he cut his finger whilst cleaning his aquarium. A variety of "atypical" or non-tuberculous mycobacteria can infect the skin. *Mycobacterium marinum*, which causes fish-tank granulomas, is probably the most common. This type of infection usually responds to prolonged antibiotic therapy with cotrimoxazole. Alternatives include minocycline, doxycycline, clarithromycin, or a combination of rifampicin and ethambutol.

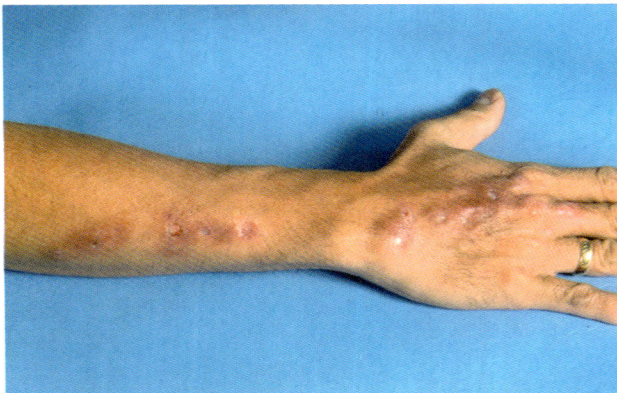

Figure 5–41 □ Non-tuberculous mycobacterial infection by *Mycobacterium marinum*. Erythematous ulcerated nodules are present on the dorsum of the hand, with dissemination of tender inflamed nodules progressing proximally up the arm, showing a sporotrichoid pattern. Culture revealed *Mycobacterium marinum*. Up to 20% of infections with *M. marinum* can show a sporotrichoid spread.

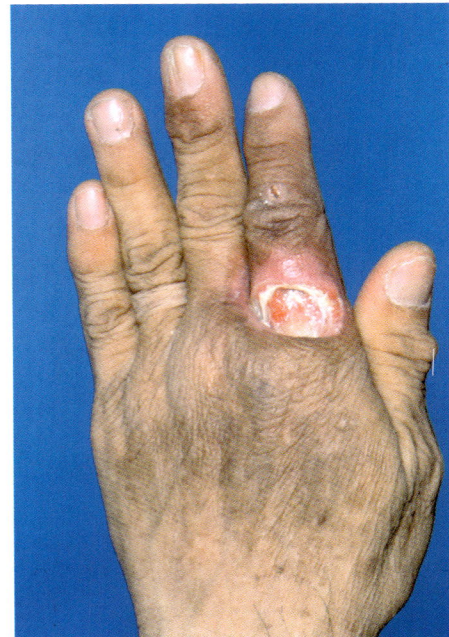

Figure 5–42 □ Non-tuberculous mycobacterial infection by *Mycobacterium abscessus*. An ulcerated erythematous plaque on the dorsum of the hand and index finger is seen. This infection was due to *Mycobacterium abscessus*. In the evaluation of a possible infective granuloma, biopsy for histopathology, special stains, and cultures should be done.

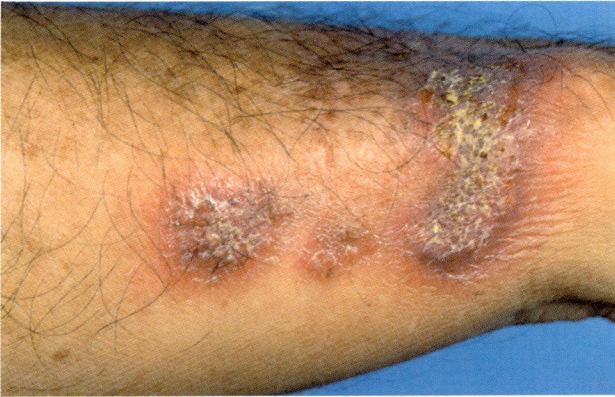

Figure 5–43 □ **Non-tuberculous mycobacterial infection by *Mycobacterium fortuitum*.** This elderly gentleman developed an expanding ulcer and inflamed plaques on the forearm. Culture revealed *Mycobacterium fortuitum*, which is a rapidly growing non-tuberculous mycobacteria. He responded to an antibiotic combination of clarithromycin, ciprofloxacin, and doxycycline.

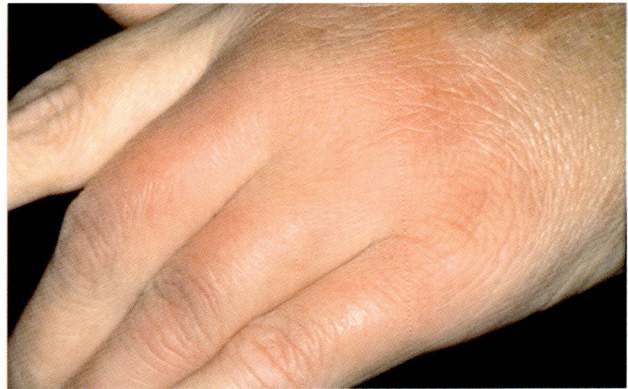

Figure 5–44 □ **Non-tuberculous mycobacterial infection by *Mycobacterium hemophilum*.** This patient with systemic lupus erythematosus presented with cellulitis over the hand, which failed to respond to intravenous penicillin and cloxacillin. Culture revealed *Mycobacterium hemophilum*. This is one of the newer non-tuberculous mycobacteria first described in 1978. It is a blood-loving organism, and requires hemin as a growth factor for its culture.

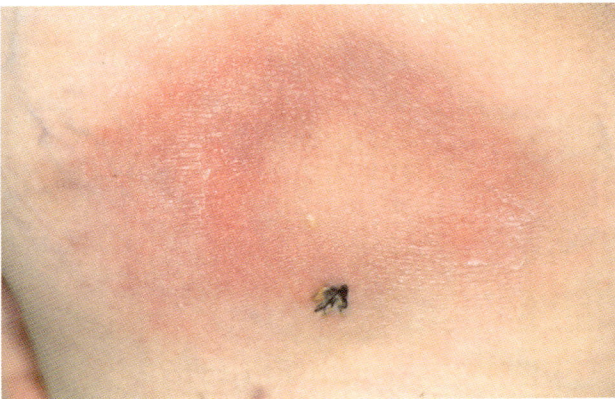

Figure 5–45 □ **Non-tuberculous mycobacterial infection by *Mycobacterium hemophilum*.** The patient in Figure 5–44 later developed an annular erythematous expanding plaque on the posterior thigh. *Mycobacterium hemophilum* was also isolated from this lesion, demonstrating that it can cause a myriad of cutaneous presentations, particularly in immunocompromised individuals.

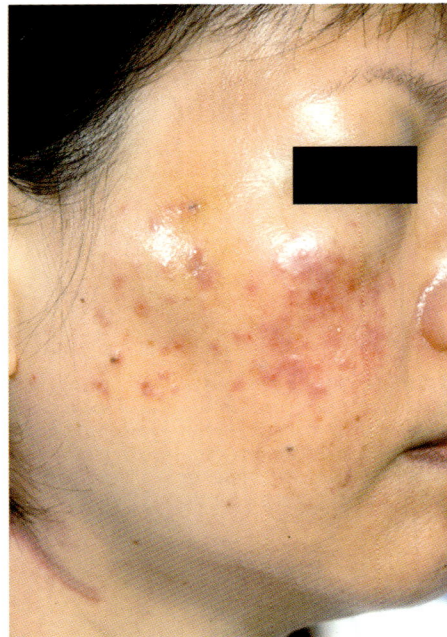

Figure 5–46 □ **Non-tuberculous mycobacterial infection by *Mycobacterium hemophilum*.** This lady presents with erythematous inflamed papules on the right cheek due to *Mycobacterium hemophilum* infection. Histology showed a granulomatous dermatitis with a few AFB seen.

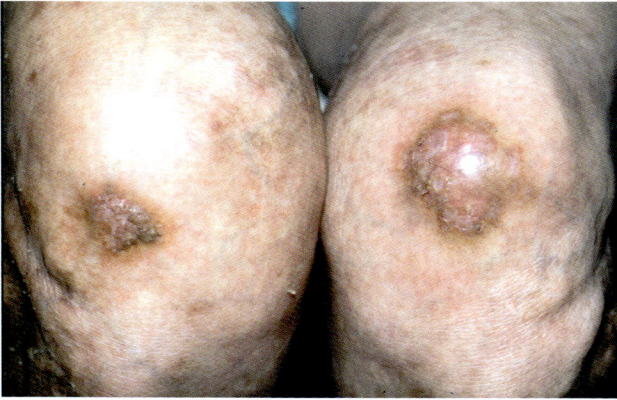

Figure 5–47 □ **Non-tuberculous mycobacterial infection by _Mycobacterium hemophilum_.** An elderly lady with a problem of recurrent vasculitis requiring long-term systemic corticosteroids, developed tender abscesses on both knees several weeks after azathioprine was added. Cultures revealed _Mycobacterium hemophilum_.

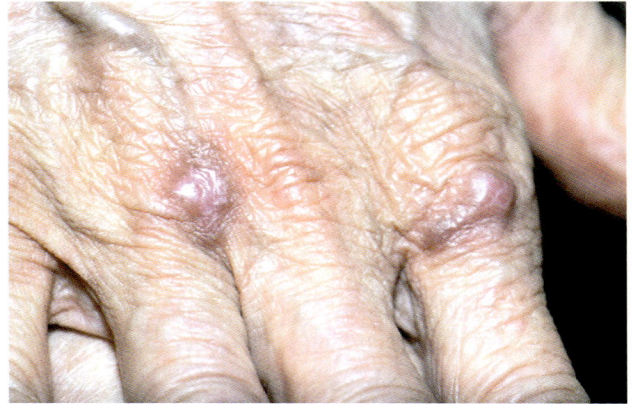

FIGURE 5–48 □ **Non-tuberculous mycobacterial infection by _Mycobacterium hemophilum_.** The lady in Figure 5–47 also developed erythematous nodules on the dorsum of her hand. Biopsy showed a granulomatous dermatitis with the presence of AFB. _Mycobacterium hemophilum_ was cultured.

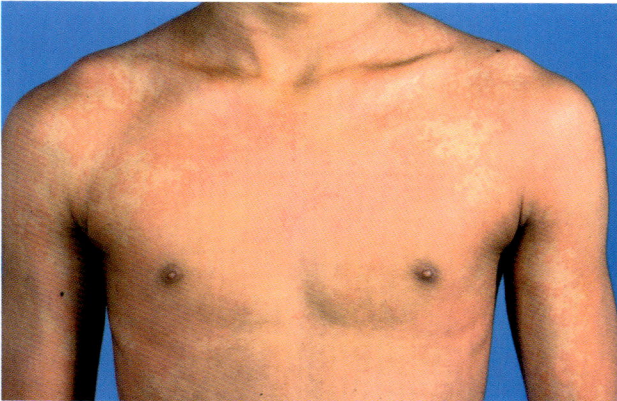

Figure 5–49 □ **Viral exanthem.** This young man has a diffuse, erythematous, confluent, maculopapular eruption associated with mild constitutional symptoms of fever and sore throat. Viral exanthems can result from infection by several common viruses. An important differential to consider here will be that of a drug eruption.

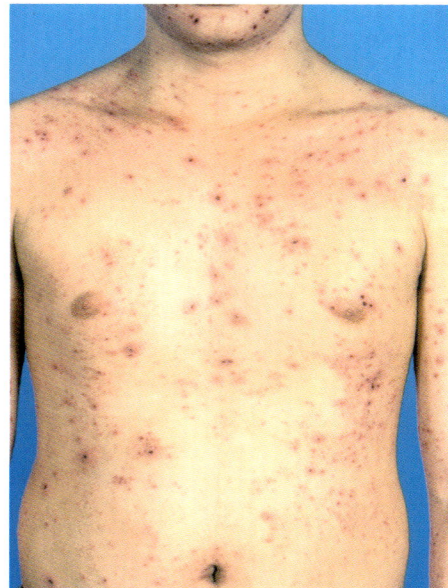

Figure 5–50 □ **Chickenpox.** Chickenpox results from infection by the varicella zoster virus. Patients present with crops of vesicles on an erythematous base. The face, trunk, oral mucosa, and extremities are typically affected. Besides the vesicular rash, erosions and scabbed lesions are also present. Patients may benefit from the use of acyclovir or its analogs if treatment is started early. Patients are infectious during the prodromal phase, and are only non-infectious when vesicles have stopped forming.

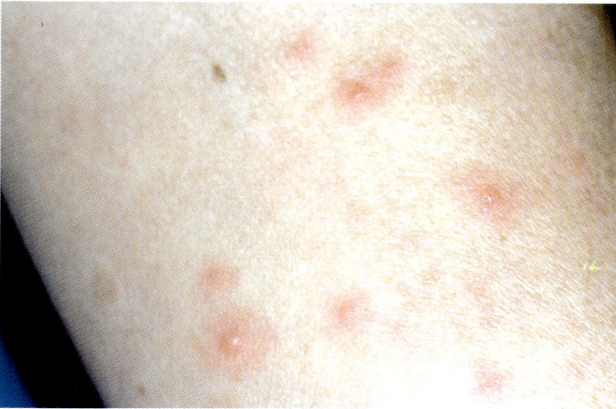

Figure 5–51 □ Chickenpox. A close-up view of the characteristic vesicles, each like a dewdrop on an inflamed red base.

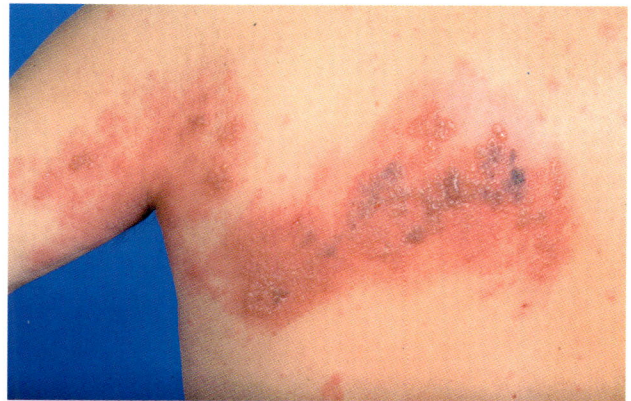

Figure 5–52 □ Herpes zoster. Erythematous, band-like, inflamed lesion with hemorrhagic vesicles and erosions occurring over a thoracic dermatome. This is due to the reactivation of the varicella zoster virus that had previously been dormant in the dorsal root ganglia following a previous occurrence of chickenpox.

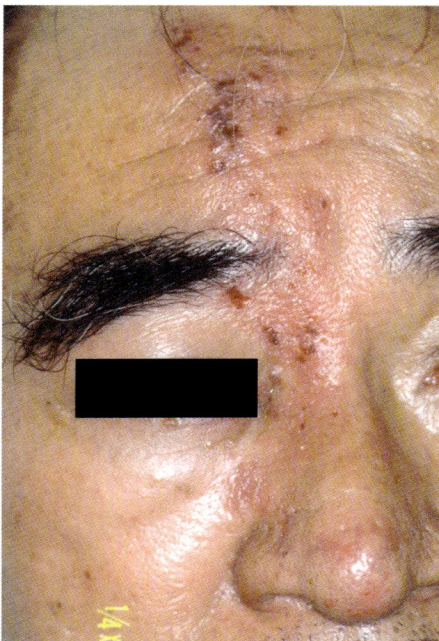

Figure 5–53 □ Herpes zoster opthalmicus. A vesicular rash with crusting and severe conjunctival erythema is seen in this patient with herpes zoster involving the eye. An urgent opthalmological referral is required, as ocular scarring and blindness can result.

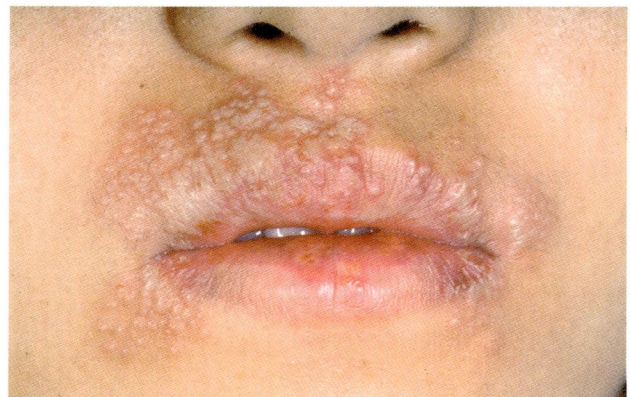

Figure 5–54 □ Herpes gingivostomatitis. Diffuse crusting and vesiculation of the lips and perioral region are seen here. They represent a severe, primary infection of the lips by herpes simplex virus (HSV-1). After this initial bout, patients may subsequently have bouts of herpes labialis triggered by factors such as local trauma, concurrent infections, and mental stress as well as sun exposure.

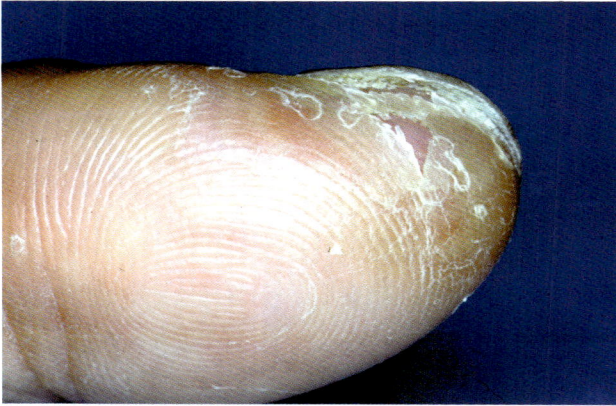

Figure 5–55 □ Herpetic whitlow. Herpes simplex infection of a digit, with painful grouped vesicles, that have ruptured to leave shallow erosions.

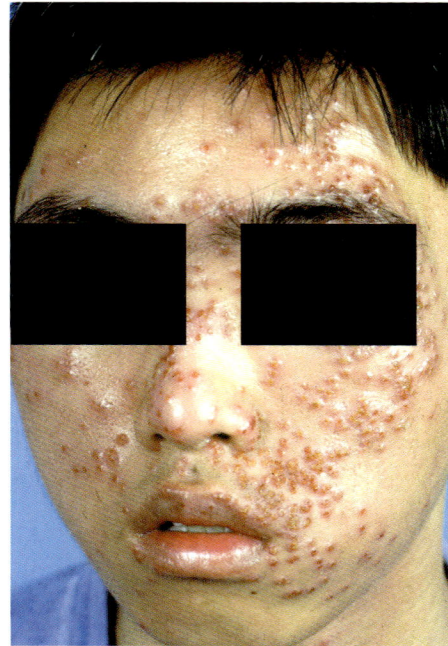

Figure 5–56 □ Eczema herpeticum (Kaposi's varicelliform eruption). Widespread erosions, vesicles, and pustules are seen on the face of this boy with atopic dermatitis. This condition is due to herpes simplex infection of eczematous skin. The clinical picture is distinct and can be supported by a positive Tzanck smear showing multinucleated giant epidermal cells and confirmed by culture. Early treatment with systemic anti-virals is needed.

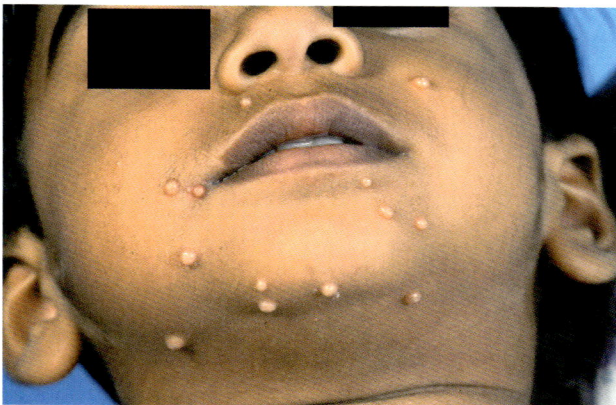

Figure 5–57 □ Molluscum contagiosum. Multiple, discrete, flesh-colored, and shiny white papules with central umbilication are seen on the face of this Indian boy. This contagious infection, caused by a pox virus, is spread by direct contact and is most commonly seen in young school-going children. Spontaneous resolution occurs in most children although treatment with a variety of destructive methods, such as cryotherapy, electrocautery, application of trichloroacetic acid or cantharidin, may be used if they can be tolerated, to hasten the resolution of the lesions.

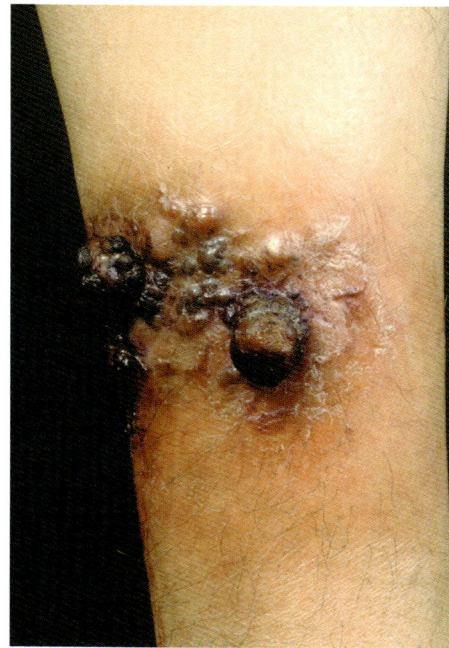

Figure 5–58 □ Kaposi's sarcoma. Numerous violaceous nodules and papules, with associated background erythema and edema, are seen on the lower leg of this AIDS patient. Kaposi's sarcoma (KS) is a multicentric vascular tumor caused by human herpes virus 8 (HHV-8).

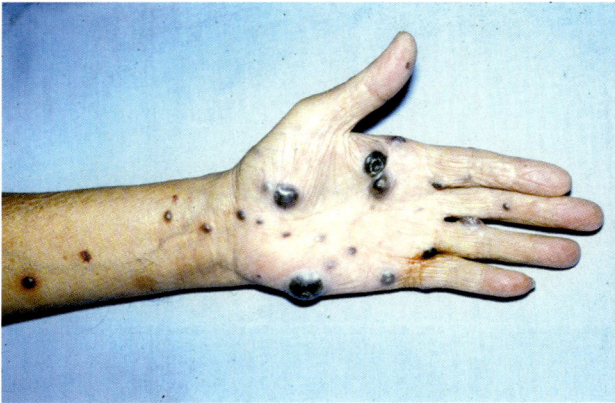

Figure 5–59 □ Kaposi's sarcoma. Large violaceous nodules on the hand, with evidence of lymphatic dissemination proximally. Cutaneous KS lesions usually begin as a bruise-like area, which is initially noted because of cosmetic disturbance. In advanced cases, such as this patient, progressive edema of the extremity can be associated with fibrosis, stricture formation, and impediment of function.

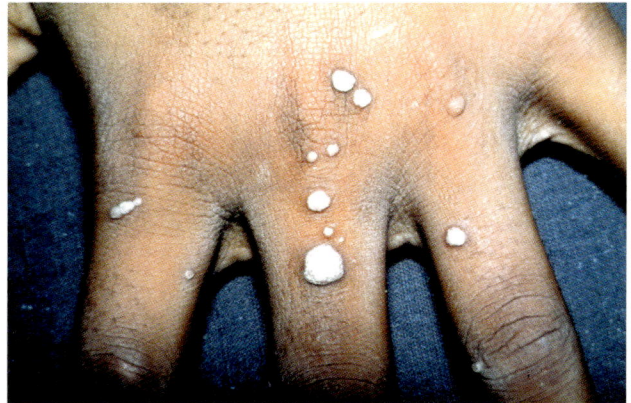

Figure 5–60 □ Verruca vulgaris. Multiple firm hyperkeratotic verrucous papules on the dorsum of the hand and fingers, due to infection by human papilloma virus (HPV). HPV types 1 to 4 cause the majority of common warts.

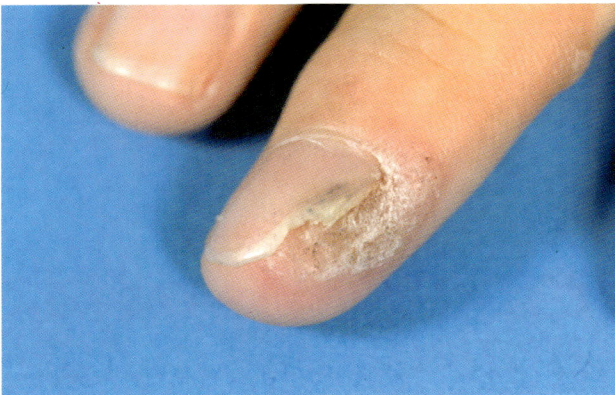

Figure 5–61 □ Periungual warts. A periungual wart extending to involve the nail bed. Periungual warts may cause nail abnormalities by compressing the nail matrix. This patient was treated with carbon dioxide laser.

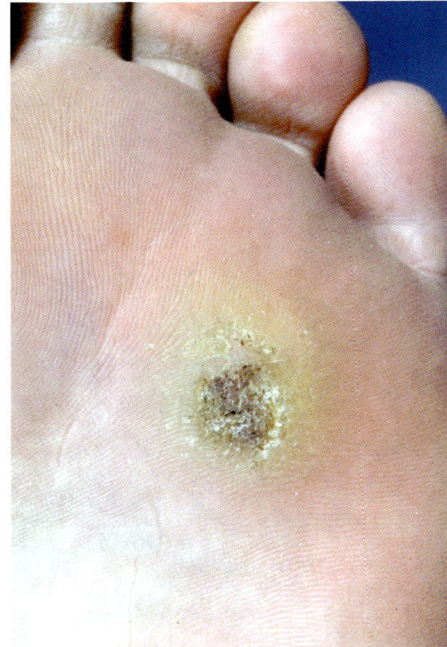

Figure 5–62 □ Plantar wart. A hyperkeratotic plaque on the sole, with multiple black dots on the surface, representing thrombosed capillaries. The normal skin lines are obscured.

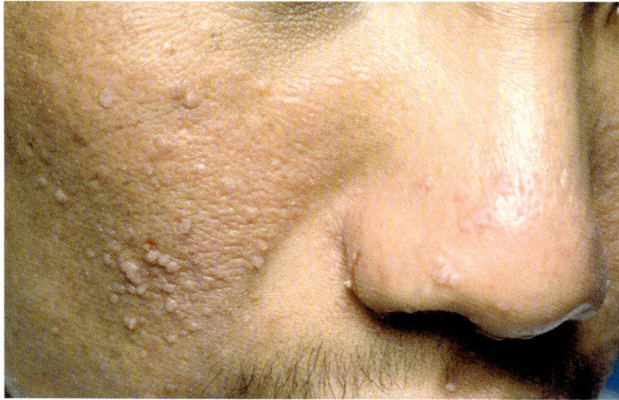

Figure 5–63 □ **Plane warts.** Multiple skin-colored papules on the face. Plane warts on the face can be challenging to treat, as destructive measures must be used with caution in this area. Topically, tretinoin or a salicylic acid preparation is usually used.

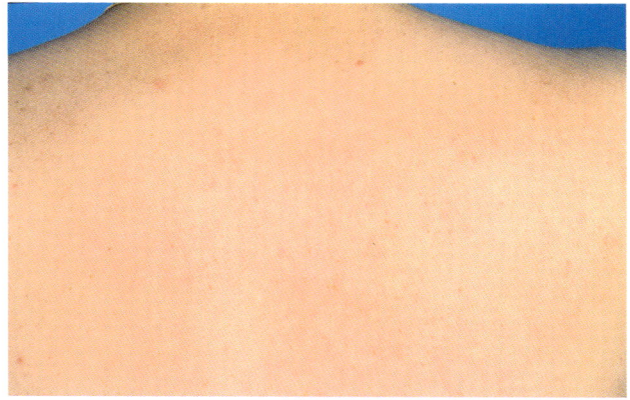

Figure 5–64 □ **Epidermodysplasia verruciformis.** Multiple plane warts and reddish macules, some resembling lesions of pityriasis versicolor, have been present on the back of this Chinese man since he was 10 years old. Epidermodysplasia verruciformis is a rare lifelong cutaneous disorder characterized by persistent refractory HPV infection, which manifest as disseminated plane warts and erythematous or hypopigmented macules. Lesions are mainly located on the face, trunk, and extensor surfaces of the limbs.

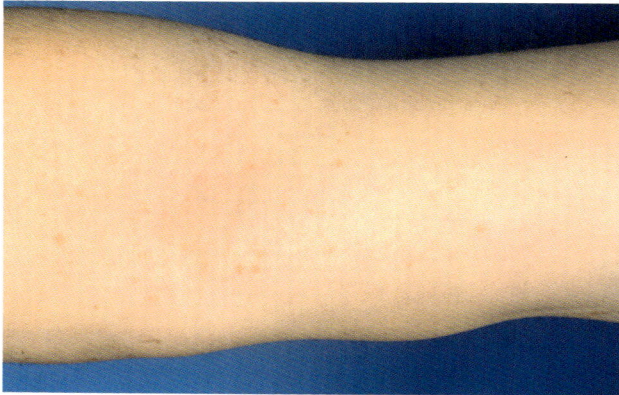

Figure 5–65 □ **Epidermodysplasia verruciformis.** Multiple plane warts are seen on the arm. Epidermodysplasia verruciformis is associated with certain HPV types. A high proportion of patients can develop skin cancers (usually Bowen's disease) at an early age. Ultraviolet radiation probably plays an important part in the development of skin cancer in these patients as well. HPV types 5 and 8 are most commonly detected in epidermodysplasia verruciformis associated skin cancer.

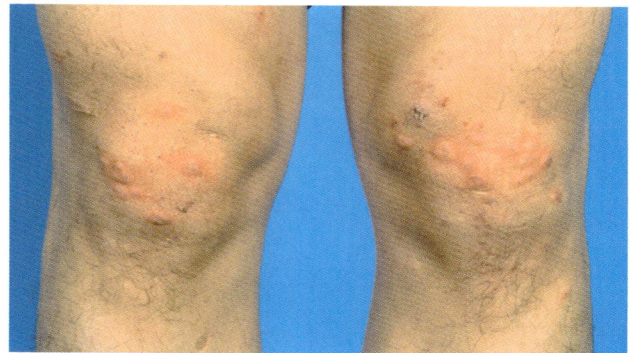

Figure 5–66 □ **Epidermodysplasia verruciformis.** Multiple lesions on the knees which had been treated with cryotherapy. Patients must be counseled on sun protection and regular skin surveillance.

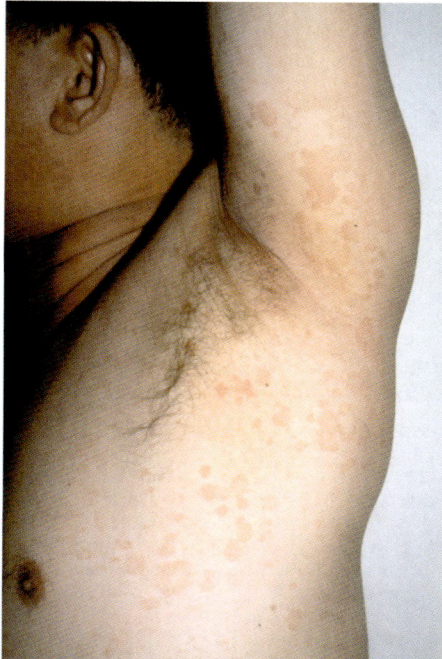

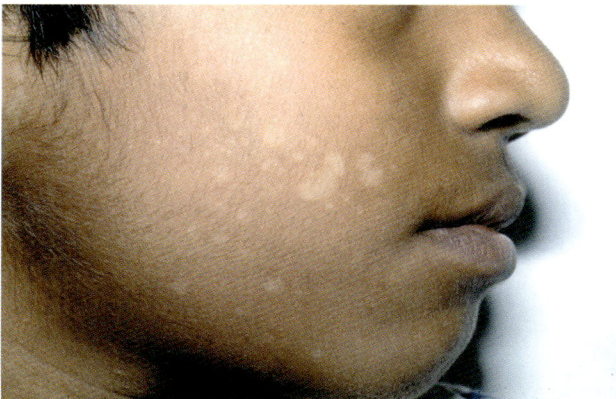

Figure 5–68 □ **Pityriasis versicolor.** The hypopigmented form is the most common. Topical treatment with 2.5% selenium sulphide or ketoconazole shampoo is effective in most cases. When there is extensive involvement, oral ketoconazole, itraconazole, or fluconazole may be utilized.

Figure 5–67 □ **Pityriasis versicolor.** Brownish scaly macules on the arm and chest. This is a common, superficial infection by the lipophilic yeast, *Malassezia furfur*. Fungal scraping with potassium hydroxide (KOH) preparation was diagnostic, showing a characteristic "spaghetti and meatballs" appearance of the hyphae.

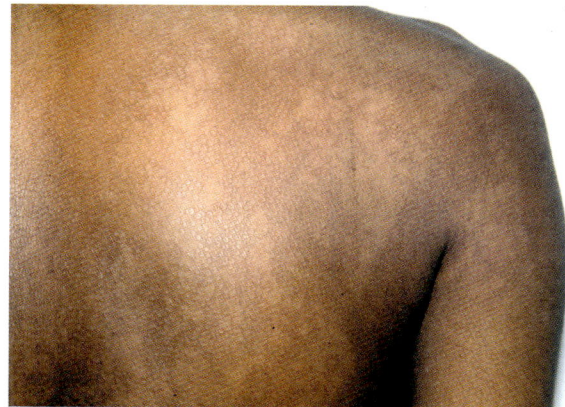

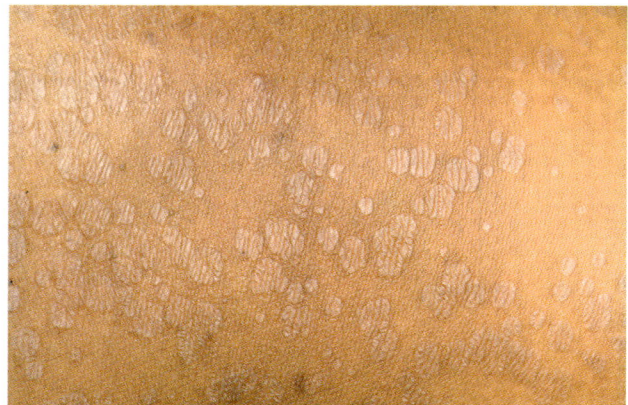

Figure 5–69 □ **Pityriasis versicolor.** Hypopigmented macules on the cheek of an Indian boy. The face is a relatively uncommon site of involvement. Differentials to consider will include pityriasis alba, post-inflammatory hypopigmentation, and early vitiligo. A topical imidazole cream can be used to treat facial lesions.

Figure 5–70 □ **Pityriasis versicolor.** A close-up view of the lesions shows the characteristic fine scale.

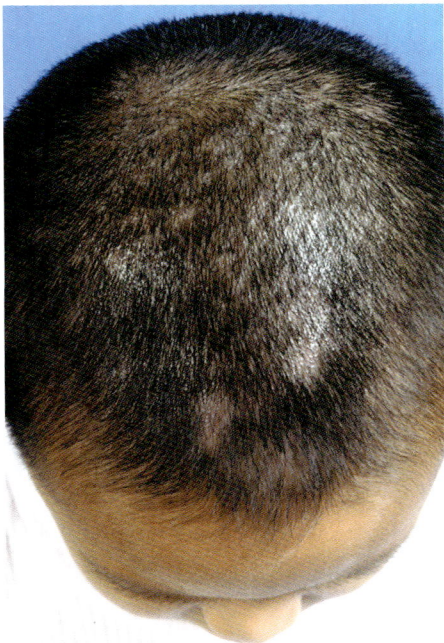

Figure reproduced with permission from *Medical Progress*.

Figure 5–71 □ **Tinea capitis – non-inflammatory.** Multiple rounded, scaly patches on the scalp. Tinea capitis is a dermatophytic trichomycosis of the scalp that affects children. In this non-inflammatory gray patch type, the brittle hair breaks off close to the scalp surface. The source of infection is another child or a young pet, such as a kitten or a puppy. *Microsporum canis*, *Trichophyton tonsurans*, or *Microsporum audouini* are the usual causes.

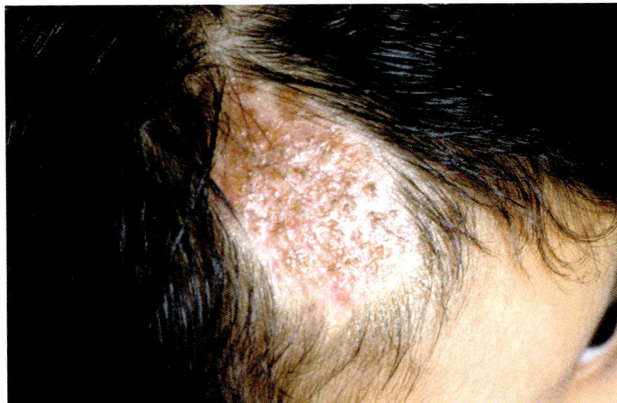

Figure reproduced with permission from *Medical Progress*.

Figure 5–72 □ **Tinea capitis – inflammatory.** Numerous follicular pustules are seen over a patch of alopecia. The inflammatory type of tinea capitis is associated with pain and tenderness, as well as cervical lymphadenopathy. It can heal with scarring alopecia. Systemic treatment with griseofulvin remains the gold standard in therapy of tinea capitis.

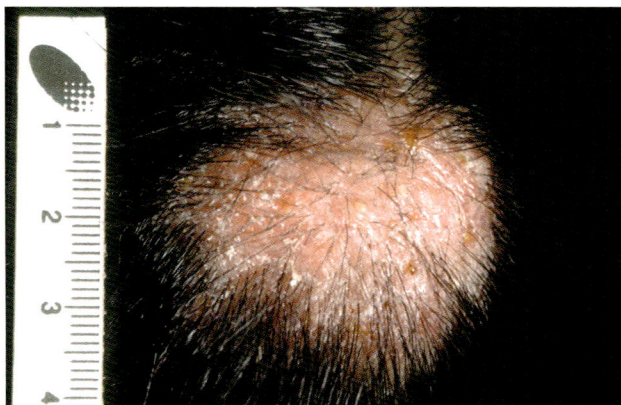

Figure reproduced with permission from *Medical Progress*.

Figure 5–73 □ **Tinea capitis.** A circular area of hair loss, with surface scaling and broken hairs. The hair shafts exhibit a greenish fluorescence under a Wood's light. *Microsporum canis* was cultured.

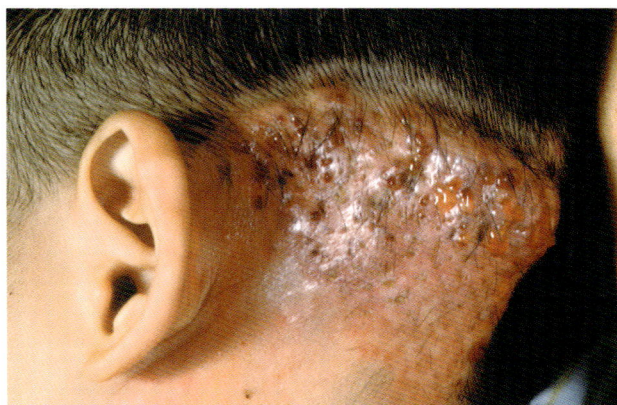

Figure 5–74 □ **Tinea capitis – kerion.** A large, tender boggy plaque with discharging pus on the occiput. The hairs can be pulled out easily. Systemic therapy with griseofulvin should be started without delay.

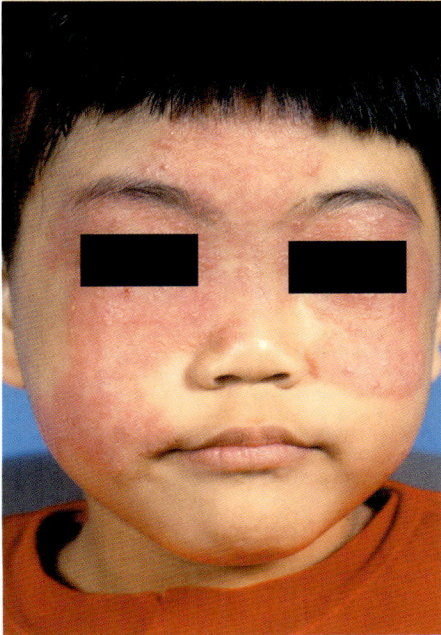

Figure 5–75 □ Tinea faciei. Extensive annular scaly patches on the face of a child. This condition is often misdiagnosed as facial dermatitis initially, and topical steroids are prescribed, which mask the appearance of the surface scales.

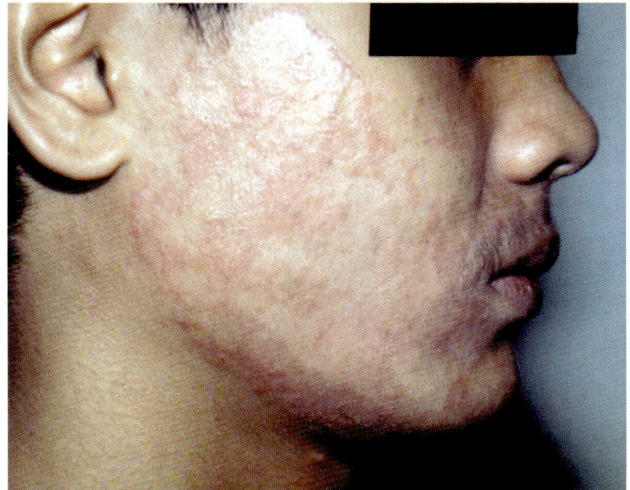

Figure 5–76 □ Tinea faciei. A large erythematous patch with a raised scaly border. The unilateral involvement and the annular margins and scales point to a superficial fungal infection.

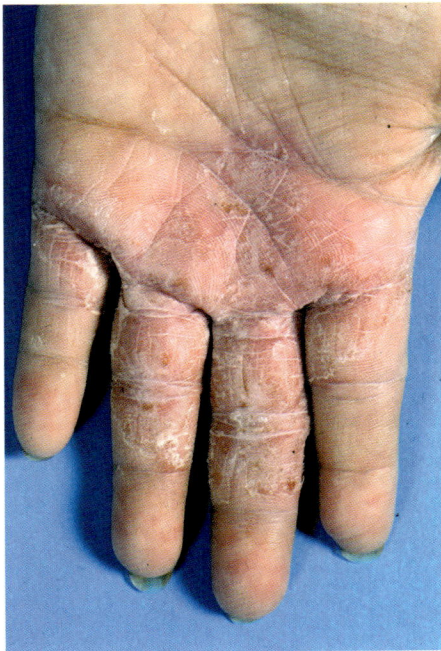

Figure 5–77 □ Tinea manuum. Erythematous, scaly rashes on the palmar aspect of the hand. When evaluating a patient with tinea manuum, the feet must also be examined. The "two feet, one hand" disease is a common pattern of infection by *Trichophyton rubrum*, where there is chronic, bilateral tinea pedis associated with tinea manuum.

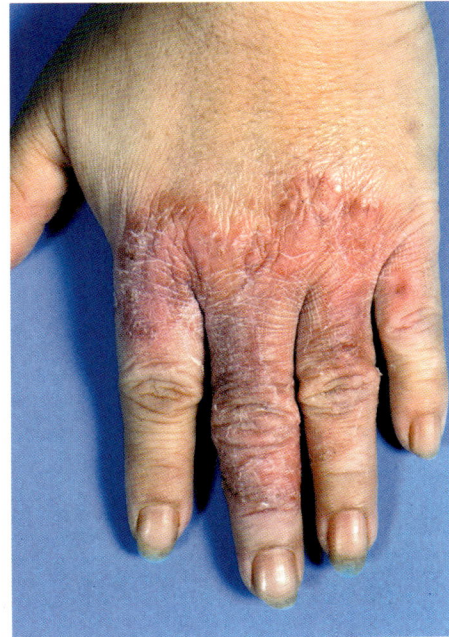

Figure 5–78 □ Tinea manuum. On the dorsal aspect of the hand, the annular scaly border is easier to discern.

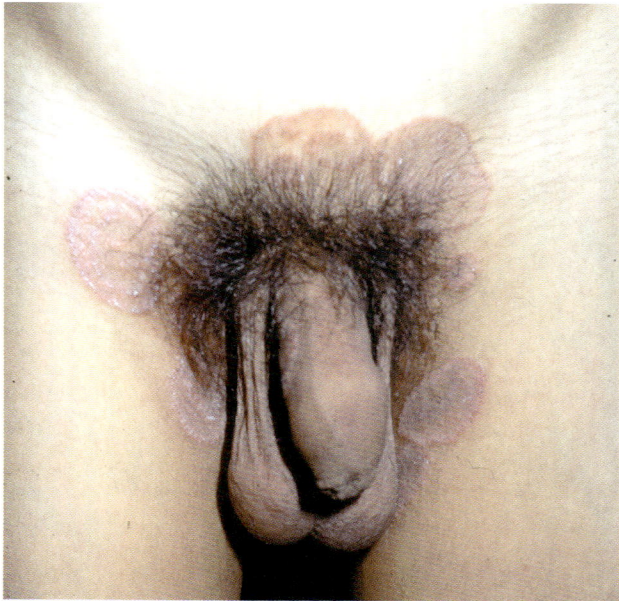

Figure 5–79 □ Tinea cruris. This is characterized by scaly, red, annular rashes. Itching may be severe. It occurs mostly in men; the warm, moist environment of the groin is conducive for fungal infection. A topical antifungal cream is usually sufficient to clear the rashes.

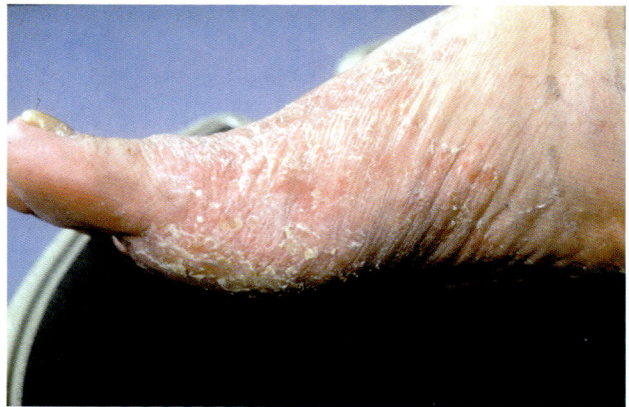

Figure 5–80 □ Tinea pedis. A red, scaly rash on the medial aspect of the foot. The infection usually begins in the toe webs before extending to the sole.

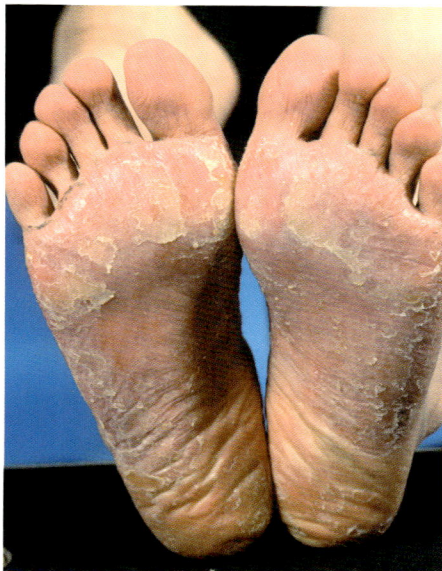

Figure 5–81 □ Tinea pedis. Bilateral involvement of both soles is seen, creating a moccasin distribution. Toe nail involvement should be excluded as this can serve as a source for reinfection. Patients with tinea pedis should be advised to continue to use antifungal cream for one to two weeks after the skin appears normal.

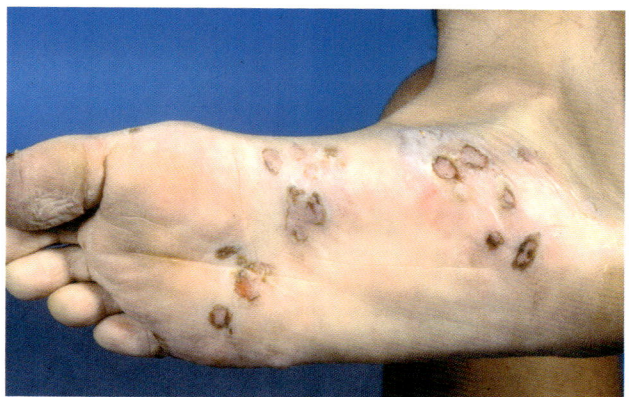

Figure 5–82 □ Tinea pedis – vesiculobullous variant. This is the vesiculobullous type of tinea pedis, characterized by an acute eruption of vesicles and bullae on the sole. It represents a very vigorous immune system response to the presence of the fungus, which is usually *Trichophyton mentagrophytes*.

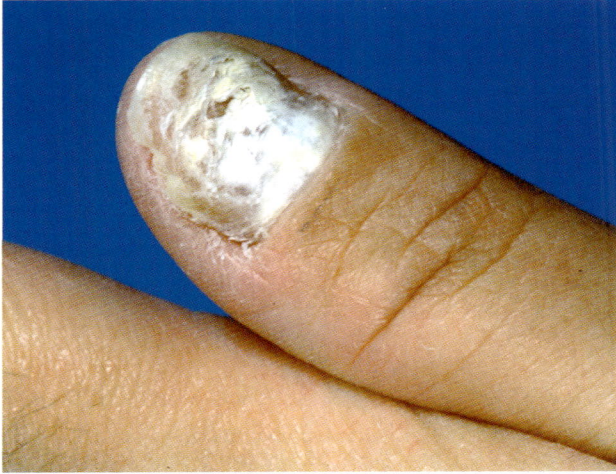

Figure 5–83 □ Onychomycosis – total dystrophic onychomycosis. Total dystrophic onychomycosis (TDO) is seen here, with the entire nail plate showing a crumbling, yellowish discoloration associated with subungual hyperkeratosis. As a general rule, topical agents are ineffective against onychomycosis. Oral antifungal agents are often required and can be given daily or in the form of pulsed therapy, depending on the drug.

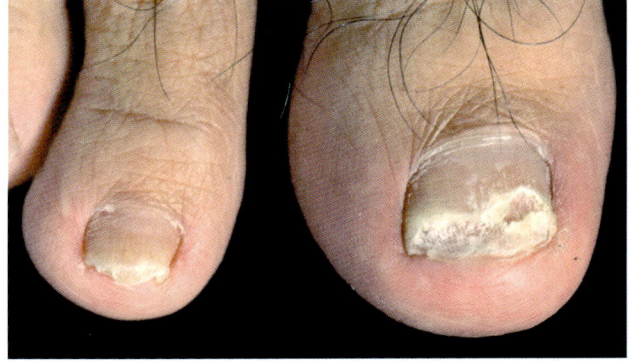

Figure 5–84 □ Onychomycosis – distal and lateral subungual onychomycosis. Distal and lateral subungual onychomycosis (DLSO), as seen here, is the most common pattern of fungal nail invasion. The fungus attacks the distal edge, and as subungual debris accumulates, onycholysis occurs and the nail thickens and becomes discolored. The causative organism here is *Trichophyton rubrum*, but besides dermatophytes, yeasts (e.g. *Candida*) and certain moulds (e.g. *Aspergillus*) can also cause this.

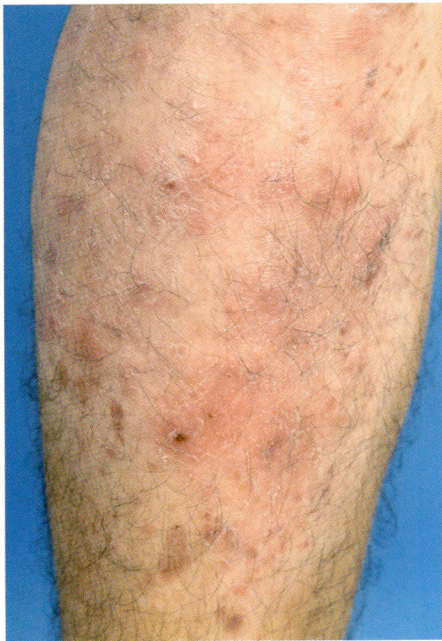

Figure 5–85 □ Majocchi's granuloma. There are numerous follicular papules, with some hair loss, occurring on a background of an erythematous patch on the leg of the patient. This represents the late stage of a hair-shaft invasion, where a persistent granuloma remains within the skin.

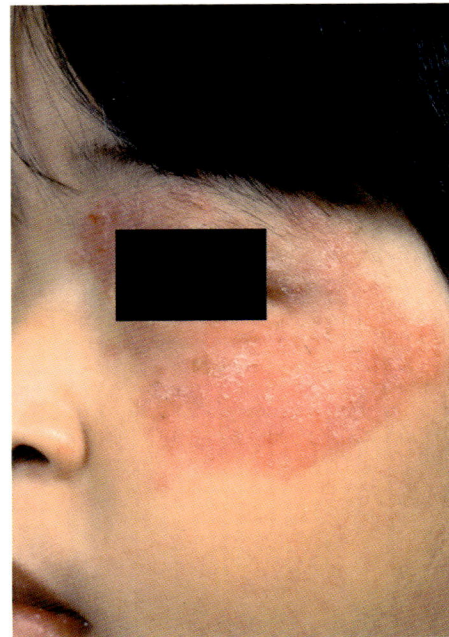

Figure 5–86 □ Tinea incognito. An erythematous patch on the right periorbital region of a young girl. This occurred after the application of potent steroids to a dermatophyte infection. Note the prominent papules and the lack of scaling and an annular rim.

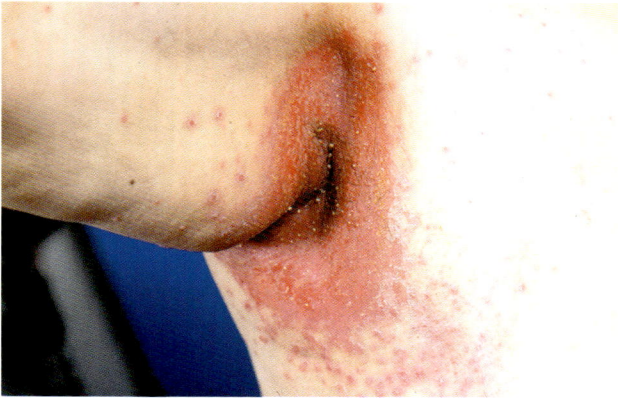

Figure 5–87 □ Candidosis. There is a prominent red rash on the axilla, with numerous discrete papules and pustules. Satellite lesions are seen slightly further away. *Candida* intertrigo occurs more commonly in obese patients exposed to hot, humid climates, as well as patients with underlying diabetes mellitus.

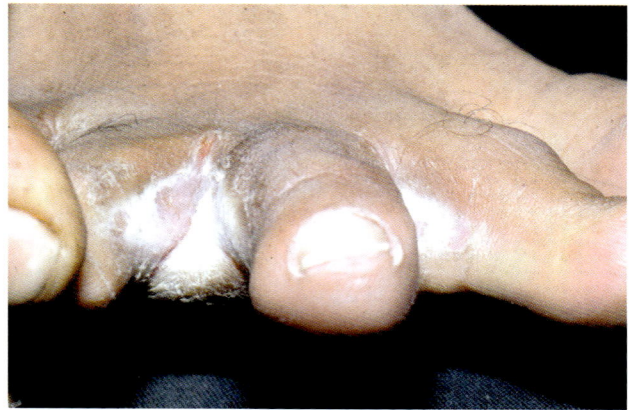

Figure 5–88 □ Interdigital candidosis. Infection of the finger web by *Candida* producing white soggy-looking skin with superficial erosions. Frequent wet work is a predisposing cause.

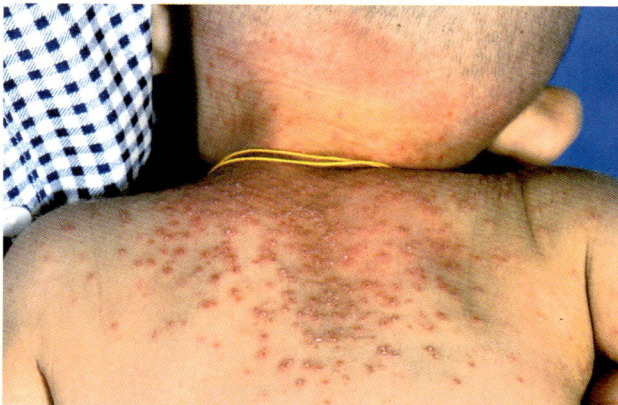

Figure 5–89 □ Candidosis. Erythematous papules and pustules on the nape of the neck and upper back of a child. Candidal growth relies heavily on occlusion, and advice regarding the thorough drying of skin folds and preventive measures to reduce maceration of the skin is required. A topical imidazole cream will clear the infection.

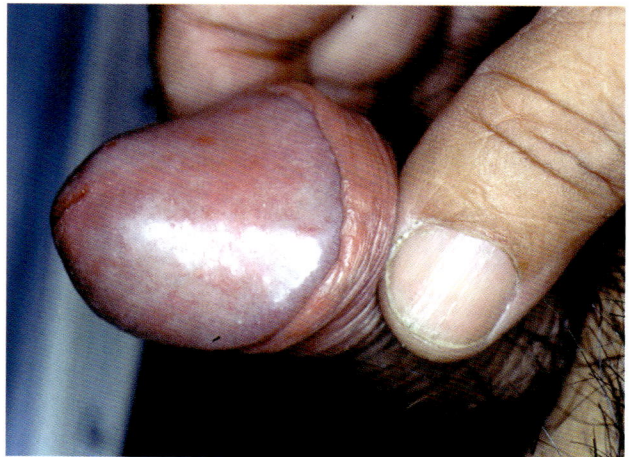

Figure 5–90 □ Candidal balanitis. There is erythema of the glans penis associated with numerous discrete small papules on the surface. This condition is more common in uncircumcised men, and the organism may have been transmitted from the sexual partner's vagina.

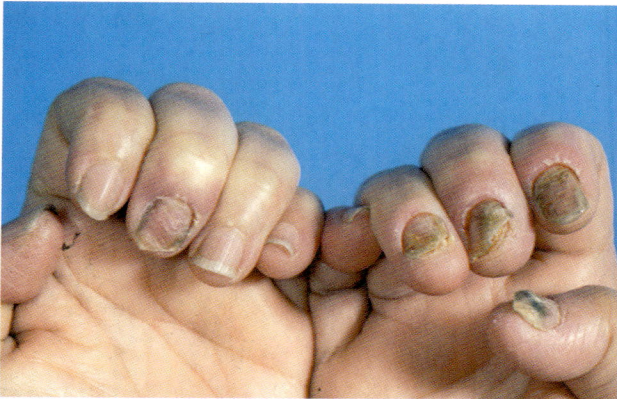

Figure 5–91 □ Chronic candidal paronychia. Swelling of the nail folds, associated with nail dystrophy, is seen in this housewife who frequently immerses her hands in water. *Candida albicans* is isolated from the intermittent discharge of pus at the nail fold. Nail plate invasion by *Candida* may occur in the presence of paronychia or in chronic mucocutaneous candidosis. Other causes of paronychia include staphylococcal and gram-negative bacterial infections.

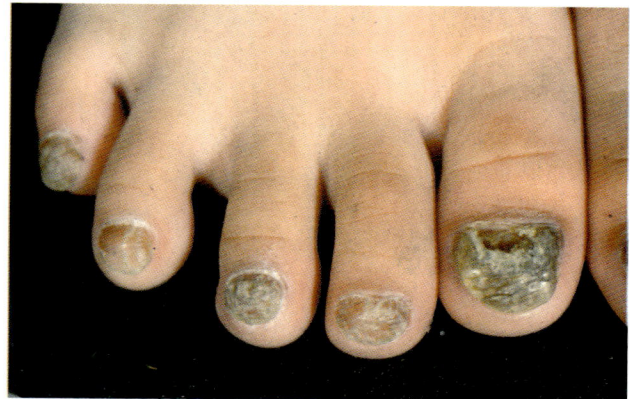

Figure 5–92 □ Chronic mucocutaneous candidosis. All the toe nails are affected due to nail plate infection by *Candida*. Chronic mucocutaneous candidosis is a rare syndrome that usually presents in childhood or infancy, with oral, nail, and cutaneous candidosis which recurs despite treatment. An adult form, which may be associated with thymoma or systemic lupus erythematosus, also exists.

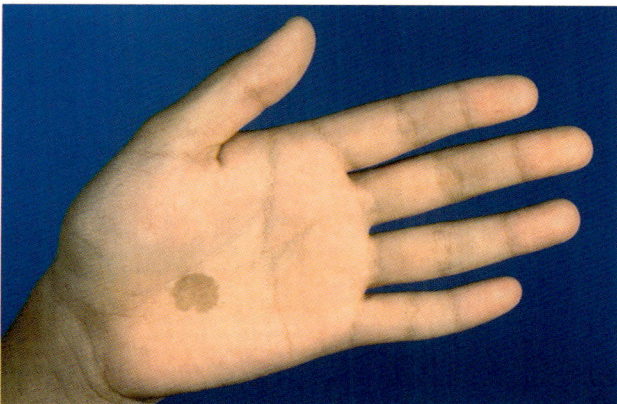

Figure 5–93 □ Tinea nigra. A discrete brown macule, resembling a lentigene, is present on the palm. This is an infection caused by *Exophiala werneckii*. It is seen mainly in the tropics and can affect the plantar skin as well.

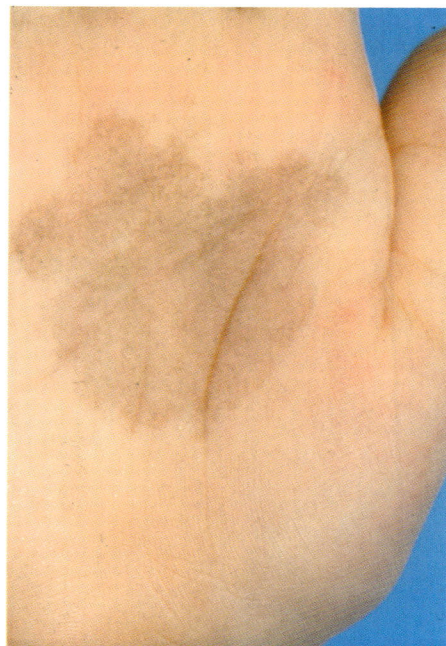

Figure 5–94 □ Tinea nigra. A flat, brown pigmented lesion is seen on the palm. When the lesion is scraped, it is shown to be scaly. Lesions of tinea nigra are usually solitary.

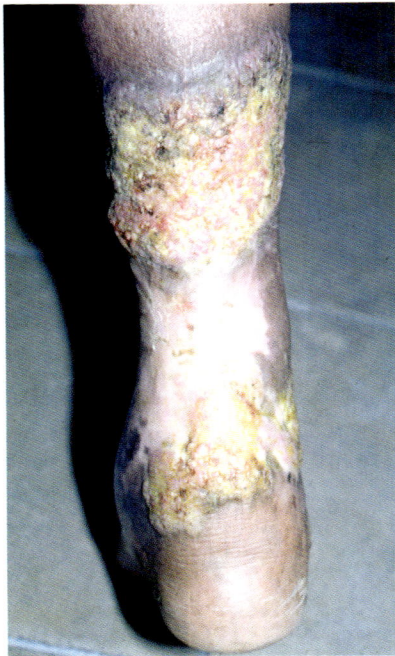

Figure 5–95 □ Chromoblastomycosis. A large ulcerated verrucous plaque on the leg of a patient. Chromoblastomycosis is a chronic deep fungal infection caused by pigmented or dematiaceous fungi. The characteristic feature is the presence of thick-walled, pigmented, rounded cells known as muriform or sclerotic cells in biopsy material. It occurs as a sporadic infection in Central and South America, Africa, and parts of Southeast Asia.

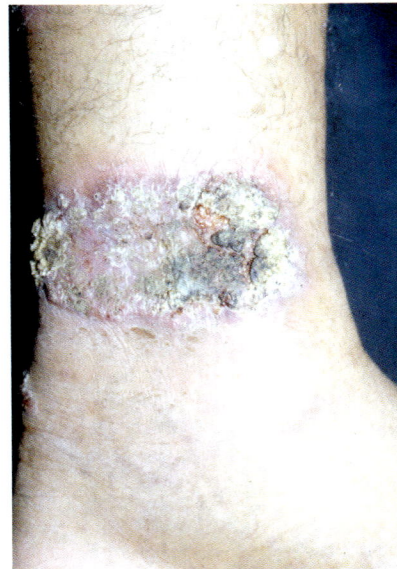

Figure 5–96 □ Chromoblastomycosis. A verrucous plaque on the lower leg that has been present for years and is extending slowly. The development of a chronic, non-healing warty plaque is characteristic of this infection. Occasionally, chromoblastomycosis can also present as atrophic annular plaques. The main organisms involved are *Fonsecaea pedrosoi*, *Cladosporium carrionii*, and *Fonsecaea compacta*.

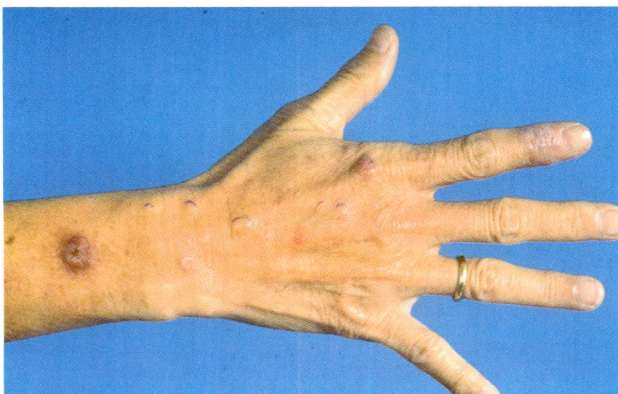

Figure 5–97 □ Sporotrichosis. Erythematous nodules occurring in a linear fashion along channels of lymphatic drainage. The ulcerated lesion on the index finger is the inoculation site. *Sporothrix schenckii* is the causative organism. Whilst this classical chronic lymphangitic type (sporotrichoid) occurs in most cases, some 40% of skin lesions in this infection may remain localized.

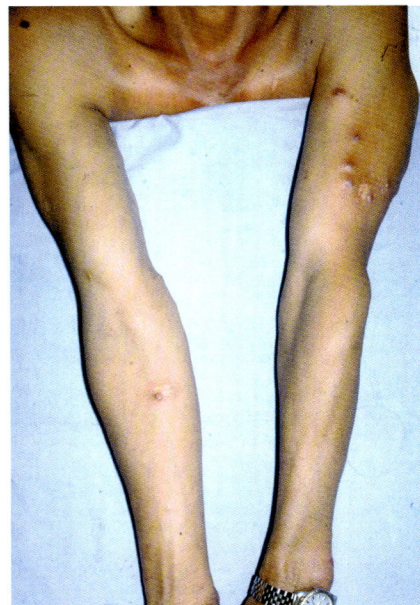

Figure 5–98 □ Histoplasmosis. Erythematous nodules caused by *Histoplasma capsulatum* on the arms of a patient with AIDS. Histoplasmosis is seen mainly in North America and Africa, where it is a relatively common systemic mycosis that usually causes lung infection in patients who are otherwise well. In HIV infection, patients with disseminated histoplasmosis may present with cutaneous lesions, which may include nodules, vegetating plaques, and ulcers on the mucosal surfaces.

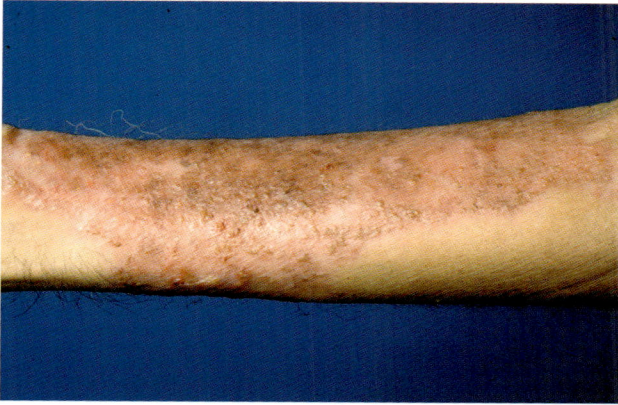

Figure 5–99 □ **Cryptococcosis.** A large, well-defined, erythematous plaque on the forearm of a patient, which initially mimicked a bacterial cellulitis. *Cryptococcus neoformans* is acquired by the respiratory route, but pulmonary symptoms are uncommon. The patient is immunocompromised, and may have underlying AIDS, lymphoma, or diabetes mellitus. Skin findings occur in 10 to 20% of these patients, and may present as disseminated papules (which may resemble molluscum contagiosum), acneiform lesions, vesicular eruptions, or as tender warm plaques.

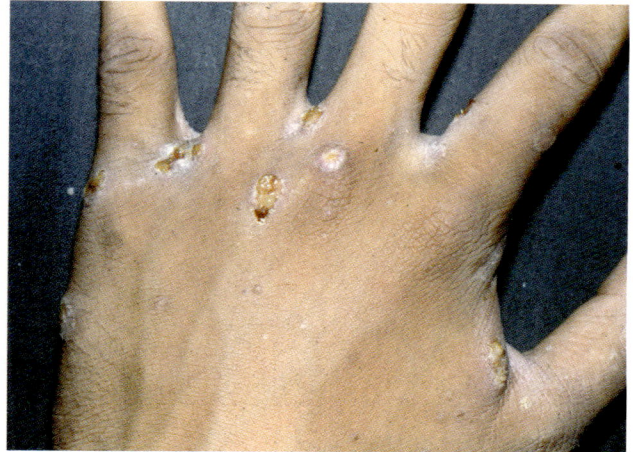

Figure 5–100 □ **Scabies.** Itchy excoriated papules and crusting are seen on the dorsum of the hands and the web spaces. They are due to a mite infestation by the female *Sarcoptes scabiei var. hominis*. It is characterized by nocturnal exacerbation of itch, and is spread by close contact. A family history of similar complaints is usually present.

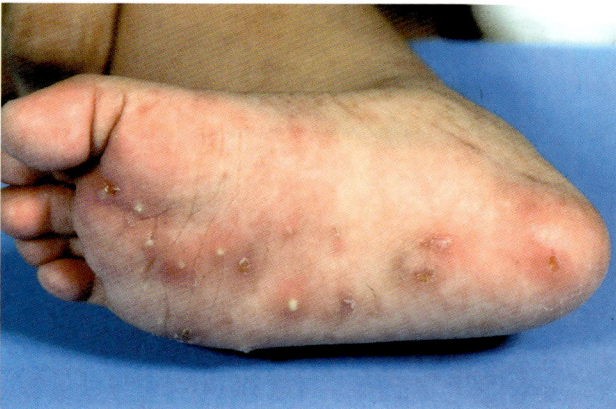

Figure 5–101 □ **Scabies.** Numerous pustules and vesicles and erythematous papules are seen on the sole of this infant. Scabies is usually treated with malathion or emulsion benzyl benzoate, but these are not suitable for infants, who should be treated with permethrin.

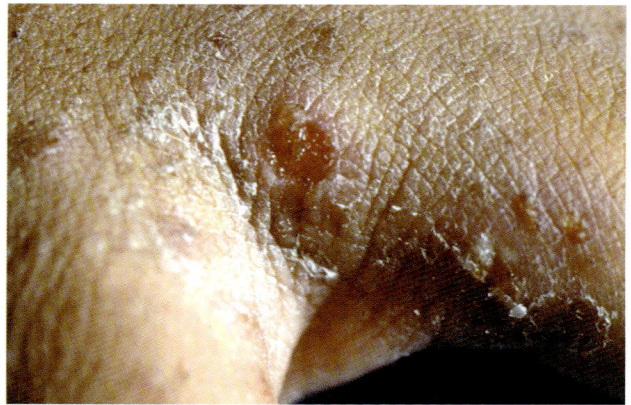

Figure 5–102 □ **Scabies.** Excoriation and a scabies burrow are seen on the finger. These thread-like structures are not commonly seen in scabies patients in the tropics, but are pathognomonic of the infestation. Microscopic examination is diagnostic if the mite, eggs, or feces (scybala) are seen.

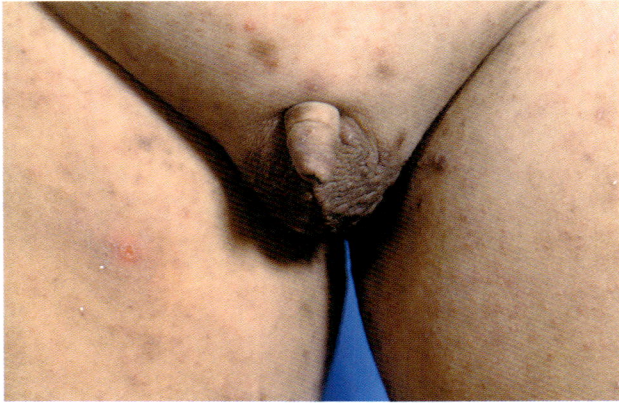

Figure 5–103 □ **Scabies.** Intensely itchy erythematous and excoriated papules and nodules in the suprapubic region, penis, and scrotum. This clinical presentation is very characteristic. Post-scabetic nodules and itching can sometimes persist for many weeks after the initial infestation has been treated, and may be treated with topical steroid creams.

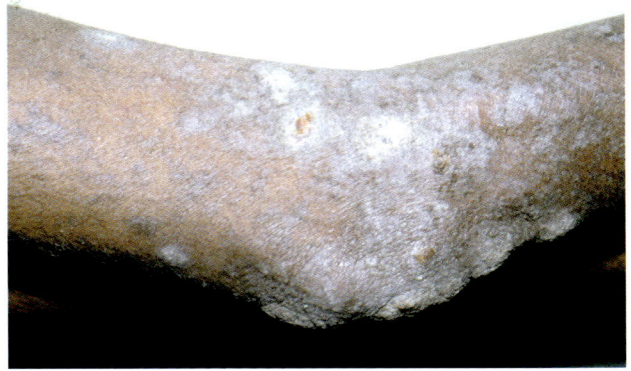

Figure 5–104 □ **Norwegian scabies.** Heavily crusted plaques and keratotic lesions are seen on the elbow. In this condition, thousands of mites have populated the skin, and the patient represents a reservoir from which infestation occurs in those who has close contact with the patient. Paradoxically, despite the high mite load, these patients do not complain of itch. Patients with Norwegian scabies usually have neurological abnormalities (e.g. mental retardation) or are immunosuppressed (e.g. AIDS, malignancy). Ivermectin, given in a single dose (0.2 mg/kg), has been successfully used in treatment.

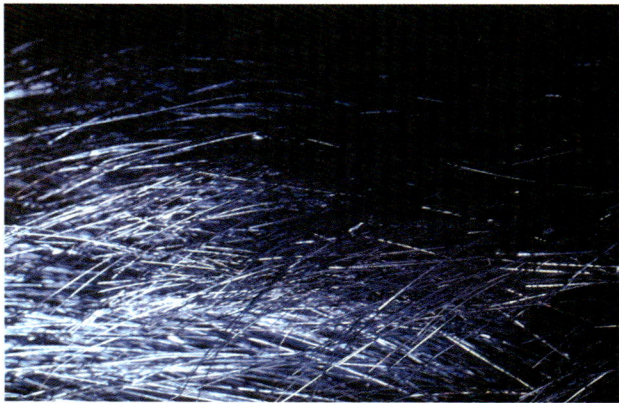

Figure 5–105 □ **Pediculosis capitis.** Nits are attached to the hair shaft. These white particles represent the eggs laid by *Pediculus humanus capitis*, or the head louse. The infection is transmitted through combs, hairbrushes, and caps. It is characterized by itching on the scalp, especially in the occipital and postauricular region. Treatment is with 0.5% malathion, which is rubbed into dry hair and scalp, and allowed to dry naturally. It is washed off after 12 hours.

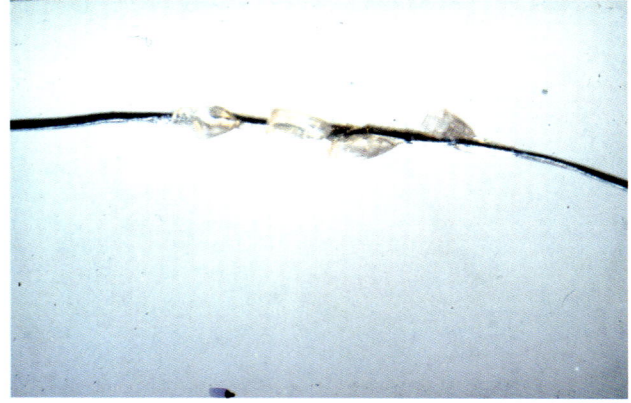

Figure 5–106 □ **Pediculosis pubis.** Pubic lice can be seen as dark black specks that are just visible to the naked eye. Because of intense itching, secondary bacterial infection and eczematization can occur, and bluish-gray macules – maculae caeruleae – are occasionally seen on the thighs. The causative organism is *Phthirus pubis*, and this is often sexually transmitted. The pubic louse can also affect other hair-bearing areas like the axillae and eyebrows. This is a close-up view of a pubic hair showing several nits attached to the hair shaft. These are white, oval, firm particles that cannot be easily detached from the hair.

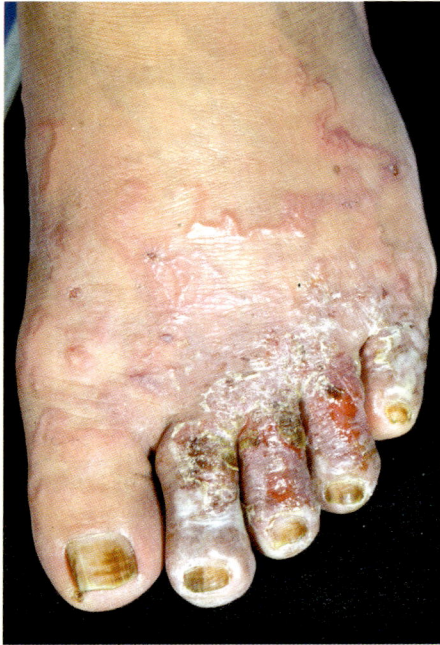

Figure 5–107 □ Cutaneous larva migrans. Erythematous, thread-like, tortuous lesions on the dorsum of the toes, with some areas showing vesiculation. This is also known as a creeping eruption, and is due to the migratory skin lesions caused by movements within the skin of animal hookworm larvae, usually *Ankylostoma braziliense* or *A. caninum*.

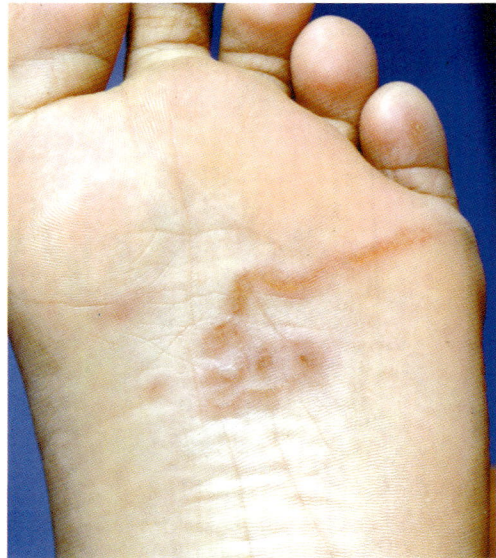

Figure 5–108 □ Cutaneous larva migrans. Tortuous cord-like lesions on the sole of a patient who acquired the infection by walking barefoot on the beach. Man is an accidental host of the hookworm larvae, and the infection is largely self-limiting.

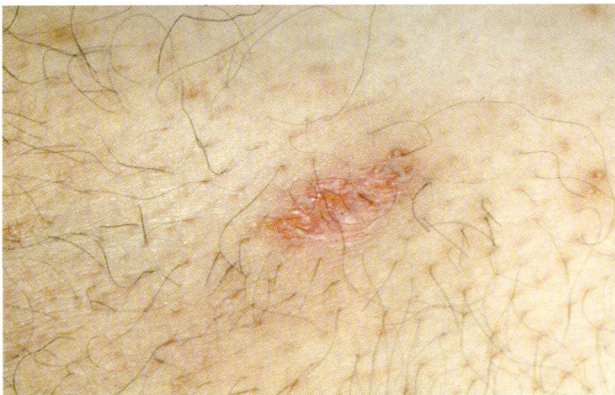

Figure 5–109 □ Cutaneous leishmaniasis. An imported case of cutaneous leishmaniasis presenting as a scaly thin plaque on the axilla of a soldier who was bitten by a sandfly in Belize. Human leishmaniasis is usually classified as cutaneous, mucocutaneous, or visceral. This is a case of "New World" cutaneous leishmaniasis, caused by *Leishmania brasiliensis* and *L. mexicana*, which is endemic in South and Central America.

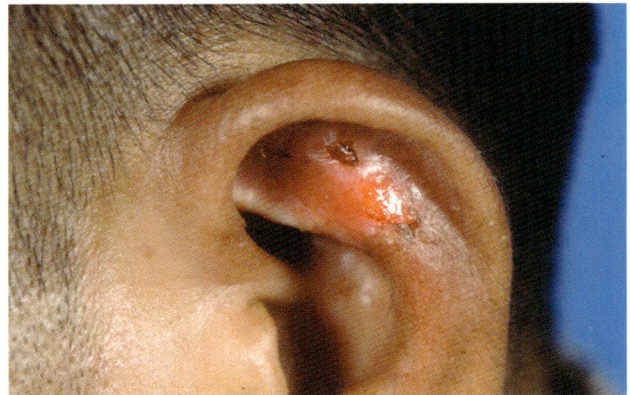

Figure 5–110 □ Cutaneous leishmaniasis. Another imported case presenting with an oozy plaque on the external ear. Cutaneous leishmaniasis can present in various clinical forms, reflecting the different natural histories caused by different organisms as well as variety in host response. This patient had responded well to a ten-day course of sodium stibogluconate.

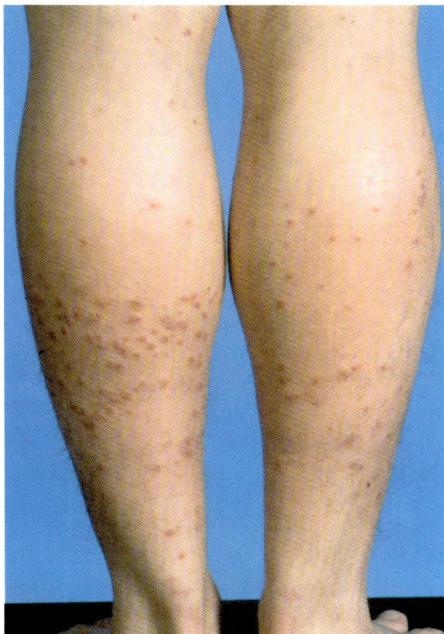

Figure 5–111 □ **Insect bite reaction.** This patient developed numerous grouped, pruritic erythematous papules after multiple insect bites. Mosquitoes, fleas, ants, and other arthropods commonly bite human skin, and the immune reaction to the bites is responsible for the resultant lesions. Often, as in this case, the offending insect is not identified.

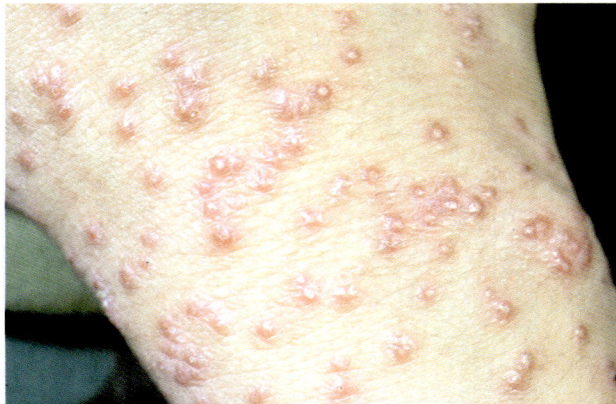

Figure 5–112 □ **Insect bite reaction.** Multiple grouped, erythematous and intensely itchy papules have developed on the dorsum of the hand following ant bites. Topical and short courses of systemic steroids, in severe cases, are useful.

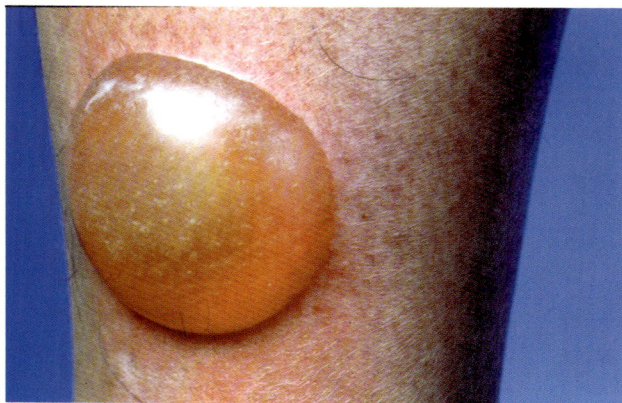

Figure 5–113 □ **Bullous insect bite reaction.** A large tense bulla has developed on the leg of this patient following a probable flea bite. The bullous insect bite reaction occurs because of a severe immune response.

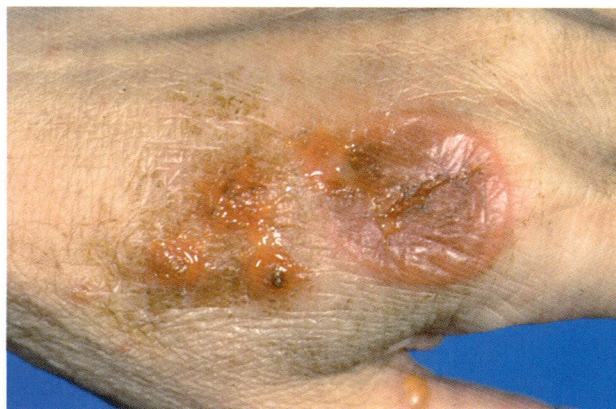

Figure 5–114 □ **Bullous insect bite reaction.** Several intensely erythematous papulovesicles and a large bulla have developed on the dorsum of the hand. They are due to bites from animal mites (*Cheyletiella*) from the patient's pet cat.

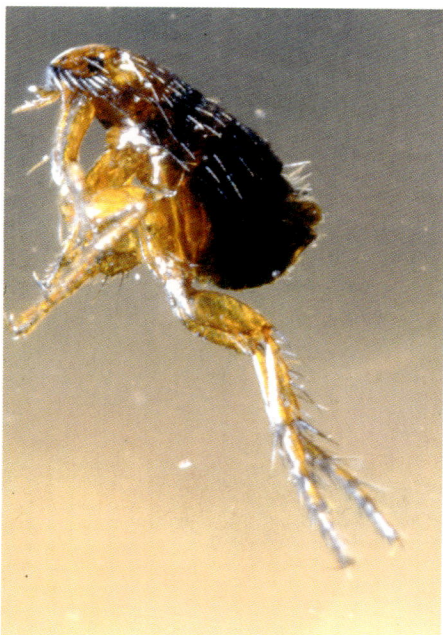

Figure 5–115 □ Flea. The cat flea, *Ctenocephalides felis*, seen under the microscope. Animal fleas are tiny, red-brown insects.

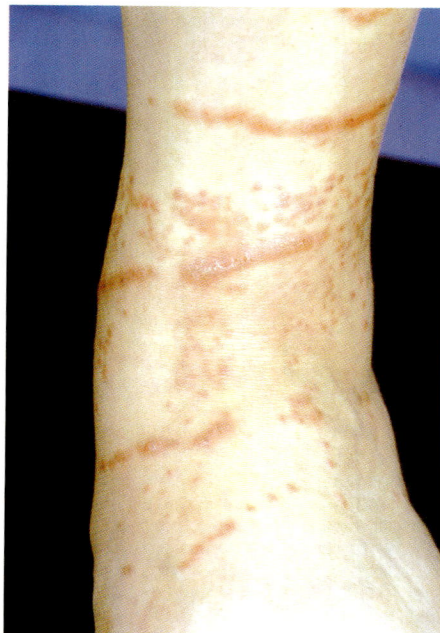

Figure 5–116 □ Jellyfish sting. Stings due to jellyfish are amongst the most common envenomations encountered by humans in marine environments. This patient developed a flagellate or whiplike pattern following jellyfish stings. This immediate reaction is due to toxin-mediated skin changes. The linearly arranged, rounded patterns due to the stinging capsules, or nematocysts, on the tentacles are clearly visible.

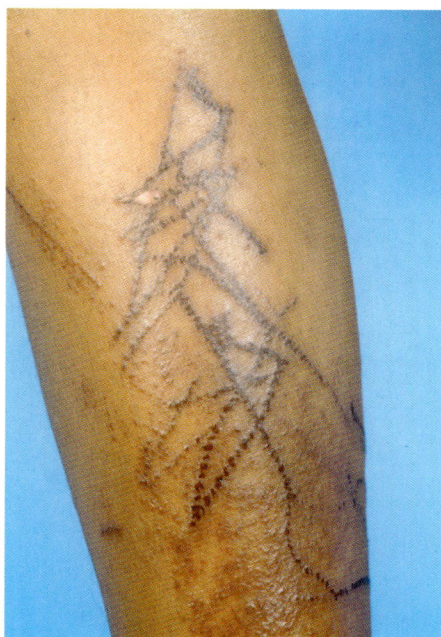

Figure 5–117 □ Jellyfish sting. A bizarre array of whip-like, pigmented streaks is seen here. There is an eczematous plaque on the lower aspect of the leg. For delayed-type hypersensitivity reactions such as these, topical steroids and antihistamines are useful.

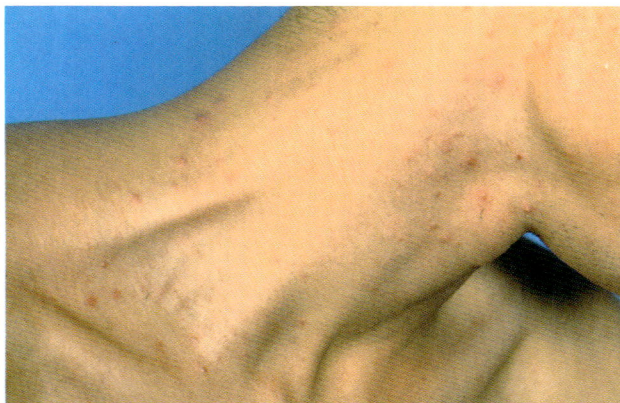

Figure 5–118 □ **Swimmer's itch.** Itchy erythematous papules on the neck of a patient. This is a form of cercarial dermatitis, caused by cercariae of non-human schistosomes, belonging to the group trematoda. It is associated with swimming in freshwater lakes, and is limited to exposed parts of the body. Clinically, the appearance is similar to insect bites. This is in contrast to seabather's itch, which occurs after swimming in salt water and typically affects the parts of the body covered by the swimsuit.

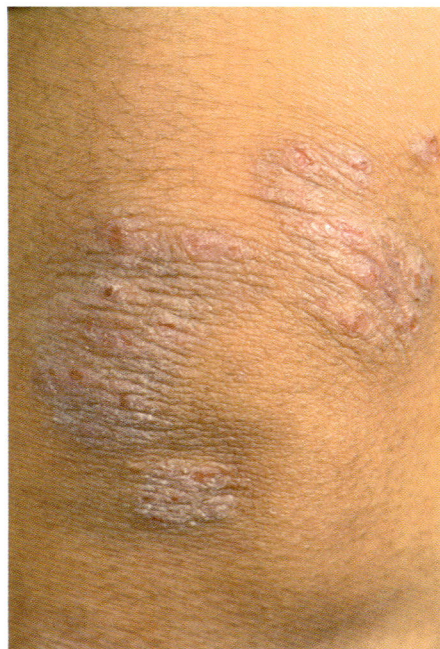

Figure 5–119 □ **Sea urchin thorn foreign body granuloma.** This patient developed erythematous plaques on the knee after being injured by sea urchin thorns whilst diving. The resultant granulomatous response represents a foreign body reaction to the retained spine fragments of the sea urchin.

Skin Tumors

Tan S.H. and Ee M.H.L.

The skin is home to a diverse group of tumors. A skin tumor can be defined as an abnormal mass of tissue arising from tissue or cellular components in the skin. This definition covers most neoplastic proliferations which form discrete lumps. In this chapter, however, we have expanded the term "tumor" to include hamartomas and nevi. A hamartoma is a convenient term for a tumor-like malformation, comprising a single-cell type or mixture of cells in the organ, in this case the skin, in which it occurs. Such lesions, if presenting at birth, are further referred to as nevi. Harmatomas and nevi, although non-neoplastic, clinically present with discrete and localized lesions characteristic of tumors.

CLASSIFICATION

Skin tumors can be broadly classified according to the biological behavior, *viz.* benign and malignant. Within the category of epidermal tumors, there is also a group of pre-malignant tumors. These tumors are cytologically malignant but biologically still benign, and have the potential to develop into invasive carcinomas. This group includes actinic keratoses, arsenical keratoses, and Bowen's disease. The most widely used classification of skin tumors is still histological, according to the tissue or cellular components in which they arise.

CLINICAL APPROACH

A clinical approach to skin tumors can be developed, even from the point of the untrained eye. This is because all skin tumors can be divided into epidermal or dermal and subcutaneous tumors. The presence of surface changes, like scaling or a warty or verrucous appearance, suggests an epidermal tumor, while dermal or subcutaneous tumors generally do not exhibit overlying epidermal changes. The growth pattern of the tumor also contributes to the appearance of the tumor. A diffusely infiltrative tumor within the epidermis will manifest clinically as a plaque, e.g. Bowen's disease, mycosis fungoides, while an expansile tumor spreading centrifugally will result in a tumor nodule, e.g. nodular basal cell carcinoma, melanoma.

By combining the clinical characteristics, such as the color, shape, consistency, site, distribution, and age of the patient, one can often arrive at, or at least narrow down, the clinical diagnosis (Table 6.1). As a broad-based clinical approach, grouping lesions according to the main clinical characteristics is particularly helpful, e.g. clinically pigmented skin tumors include benign tumors such as seborrheic keratoses, melanocytic nevi, dermatofibroma, and malignant tumors such as basal cell carcinoma and melanoma. Lesions which look yellowish, are often sebaceous in origin or xanthomatous (due to lipid deposits). One can also easily recognize vascular tumors which are red or purplish.

HISTOLOGICAL CLASSIFICATION

This chapter is organized according to the histological classification of skin tumors, as this is the most comprehensive approach. In this classification, tumors are grouped under the tissue or cellular components in which they arise:

I. Epidermal tumors
II. Dermal and subcutaneous tumors
III. Adnexal tumors
IV. Tumors of melanocytes
V. Tumors of lymphocytes
VI. Cutaneous metastases

Epidermal Tumors (Figures 6–1 to 6–28)

Within the group of epidermal tumors, seborrheic keratoses are the most common skin tumors, and clinical (and histological) subtypes exist. These are usually removed for cosmesis. However, an irritated seborrheic keratoses can be clinically difficult to differentiate from a viral wart, and sometimes, squamous cell carcinoma. Similarly, an acanthotic seborrheic keratoses is often mistaken for a melanocytic nevus or a pigmented basal cell carcinoma. In these clinical situations, it is imperative that biopsy be done for histological confirmation. Basal cell carcinomas (BCC) in Asians are often of the pigmented type, a distinct difference from those seen in Caucasians, which are non-pigmented and often of the superficial type. Therefore, although both BCC and melanoma are pigmented, the site of presentation is a useful distinguishing feature as melanomas are usually found on acral sites in Asians.

Whilst sun exposure is one of the major factors for cutaneous carcinogenesis, arsenical ingestion through traditional sources of medicine in Singapore or contaminated well water in Malaysia, Bangladesh, and Taiwan, is also a significant predisposing factor. Affected individuals develop arsenic keratoses on non-sun-exposed sites on the trunk, palms, and soles. These patients often develop multiple skin cancers like Bowen's disease and squamous cell carcinomas after a latency period of 30 to 40 years.

Dermal and Subcutaneous Tumors (Figures 6–29 to 6–51)

Dermal or subcutaneous tumors refer to tumors which arise from structures located in the dermis or subcutis, respectively. It should be remembered that adnexal tumors, although often dermal in location, are tumors of epidermal-derived structures. The category of dermal tumors can be subdivided into connective tissue, vascular, neural, smooth muscle, and histiocytic tumors. Although, as a rule, dermal-centered tumors do not have epidermal changes, exceptions are seen in dermatofibroma which is often hyperkeratotic with surface scaling, and vascular tumors like strawberry nevus and pyogenic granuloma show a lobulated surface and surface crusting respectively. The soft gelatinous consistency is characteristic of lipomas and neurofibromas, whilst a firm consistency is present in tumors or reactive hyperplasia of fibrous tissue or muscular tissue.

Adnexal Tumors (Figures 6–52 to 6–68)

Adnexal tumors constitute a category of tumors which are often located on the head or scalp as can be appreciated from the abundance of hair follicles and sebaceous glands in these locations. Sebaceous tumors have a yellowish color whilst others may be skin-colored, such as trichoepitheliomas and syringomas. The eccrine tumors, in contrast, are commonly found on the limbs.

Tumors of Melanocytes (Figures 6–69 to 6–88)

Tumors of melanocytes, which are the pigment-forming cells in the basal layer of the epidermis, constitute the next most common group after epidermal tumors, when one considers acquired melanocytic nevi. Dysplastic nevus, whether solitary or the syndrome, and melanoma are extremely uncommon in Asians. The most common type of melanoma in this region is the acral lentiginous melanoma and several typical presentations are illustrated in this chapter. To the primary care physician, it should be remembered that any pigmented lesion on the foot or nail bed must be viewed with suspicion and early referral to the dermatologist is warranted.

Tumors of Lymphocytes and Cutaneous Metastases (Figures 6–89 to 6–114)

One should be mindful of tumors in the skin which can be due to infiltration by non-resident cells. Skin tumors, presenting as multiple lesions, can be due to lymphomas or metastases to the skin. The spectrum of cutaneous lymphomas reflects the heterogeneity of this group of skin tumors, ranging from indolent subtypes like mycosis fungoides to aggressive lymphomas like subcutaneous panniculitis-like T-cell lymphoma and NK/T-cell lymphoma, which often have systemic involvement; both are more prevalent in the Asia-Pacific region.

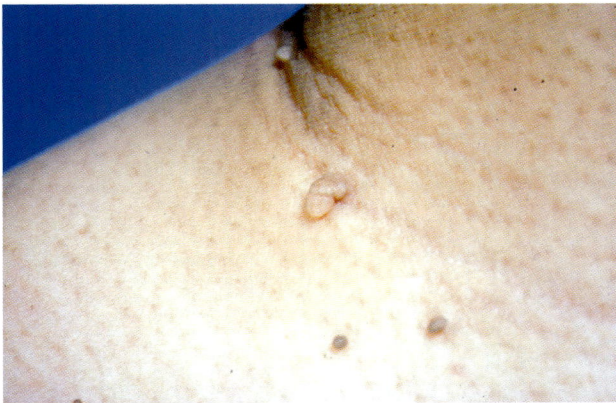

Figure 6–1 □ Skin tags. These common benign epithelial tumors, also referred to as achrochordons or fibroepithelial polyps, are seen in the intertrigious areas, especially on the neck and axillae. The appearance is unmistakable: sessile or pedunculated, soft, skin-colored to pigmented protrusions.

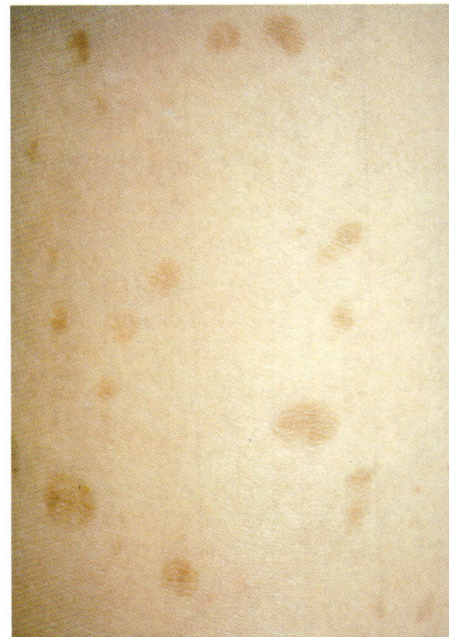

Figure 6–2 □ Seborrheic keratoses – flat. These early seborrheic keratoses are often found in association with solar lentigines on sun-exposed sites such as on the forearms. They are often multiple and appear as just palpable, well-circumscribed, brown lesions with a rough surface.

Table 6–1 Clinical approach to skin tumors

	Benign	Pre-malignant or borderline malignant	Malignant
Pigmented tumors	seborrheic keratoses, acquired melanocytic nevus, dermatofibroma	giant congenital melanocytic nevus, dysplastic nevus	basal cell carcinoma (pigmented), melanoma
Non-pigmented epidermal tumors	keratoacanthoma epidermal nevus	actinic keratoses, arsenic keratoses, Bowen's disease	basal cell carcinoma (superficial, ulcerated, nodular, morphoeic), squamous cell carcinoma, extramammary Paget's disease
Skin-colored lesions	trichoepithelioma, syringoma, fibrous papule (nose), intradermal melanocytic nevus, cyst, connective tissue nevus	–	–
Yellow lesions	sebaceous hyperplasia, sebaceous adenoma, xanthogranuloma	nevus sebaceous, sebaceous epithelioma	sebaceous carcinoma
Red lesions	pyogenic granuloma, hemangioma, eccrine poroma, reactive lymphoid hyperplasia	Kaposi's sarcoma –	angiosarcoma –
Pedunculated lesions	skin tags, dermatosis papulosis nigra, polypoid intradermal melanocytic nevus	–	–
Soft tumors	neurofibroma lipoma	–	neurofibrosarcoma
Firm to hard tumors	leiomyoma, pilomatrixoma	–	dermatofibrosarcoma protuberans
Multiple tumors	dermatofibroma neurofibroma	–	lymphoma metastases

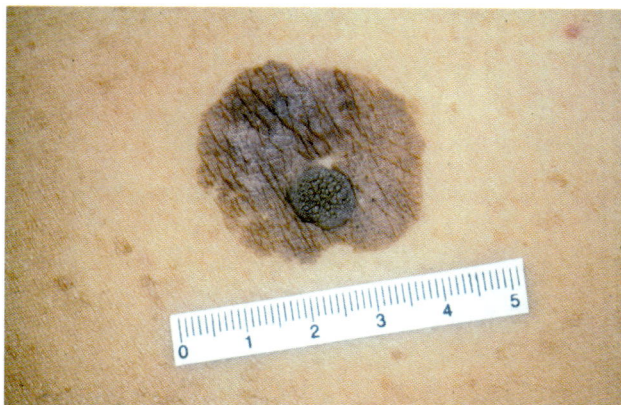

Figure 6–3 □ **Seborrheic keratoses – flat.** In this more developed lesion, warty plaques are seen on an underlying seborrheic keratoses, which is superficial and flat-topped. Note the sharply demarcated margins.

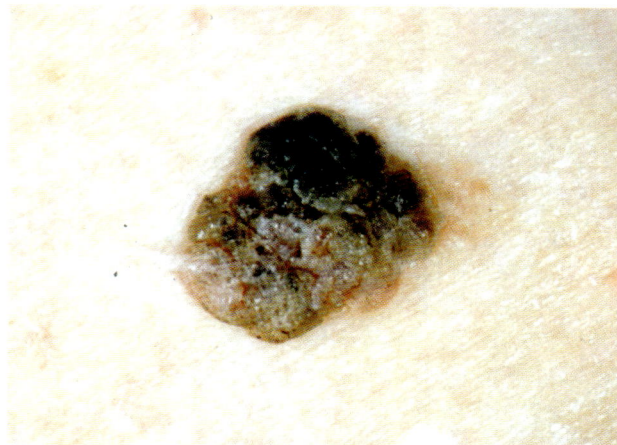

Figure 6–4 □ **Seborrheic keratoses – verrucous.** This established lesion is heavily pigmented and has a warty, mammillated surface. The typical "stuck on" appearance gives the impression that it can be easily picked off.

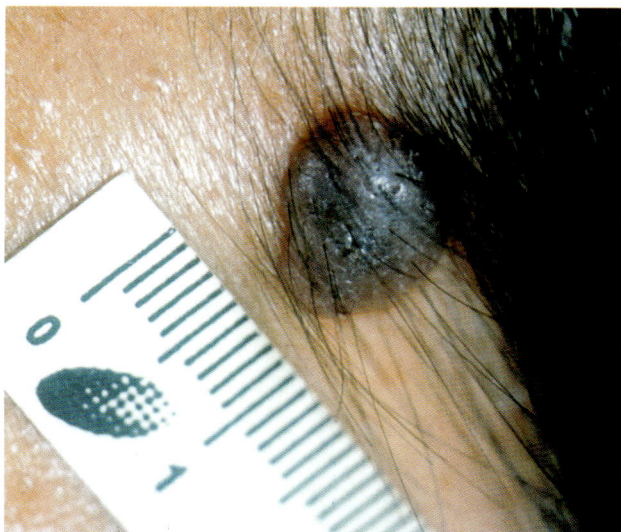

Figure 6–5 □ **Seborrheic keratoses – acanthotic.** This clinical subtype of seborrheic keratoses is often mistaken for a melanocytic nevus or basal cell carcinoma. The dark brown to black lesion is dome-shaped and sharply demarcated. It is characterized by a lack luster appearance and plugged follicular orifices are often seen on the surface.

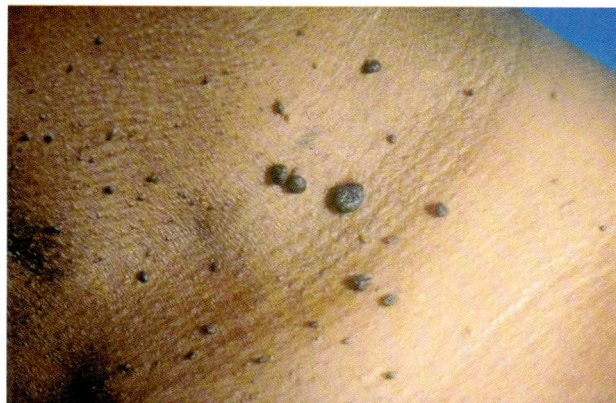

Figure 6–6 □ **Seborrheic keratoses – dermatosis papulosa nigra.** These are variants of seborrheic keratoses in pigmented races. They are often multiple and seen in the intertriginous areas and on the upper parts of the face. Although these pedunculated papules resemble skin tags, they are more heavily pigmented.

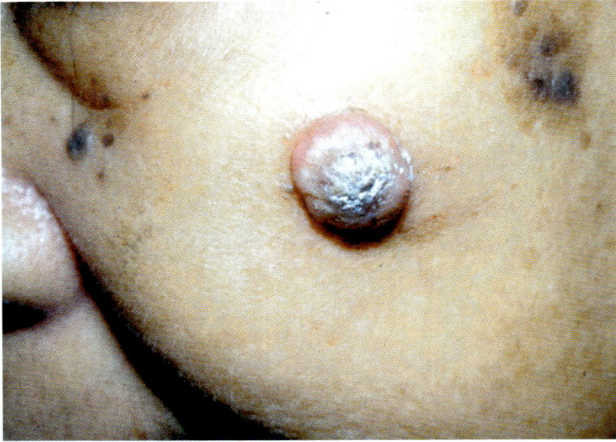

Figure 6–7 □ Keratoacanthoma. This benign epidermal tumor has a distinctive clinical appearance, presenting as a cup-shaped, flesh-colored to erythematous nodule with a keratin-filled central crater. The feature distinguishing it from a squamous cell carcinoma is its rapid evolution, becoming relatively large within weeks to a few months.

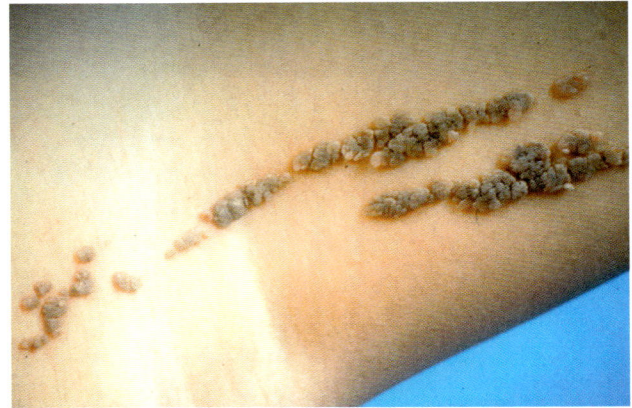

Figure 6–8 □ Epidermal nevus – linear. This nevus is present at birth or in early childhood. Here, the typical features of warty, closely-set, pigmented papules are seen on the arm. The distribution is linear, following the lines of Blashko.

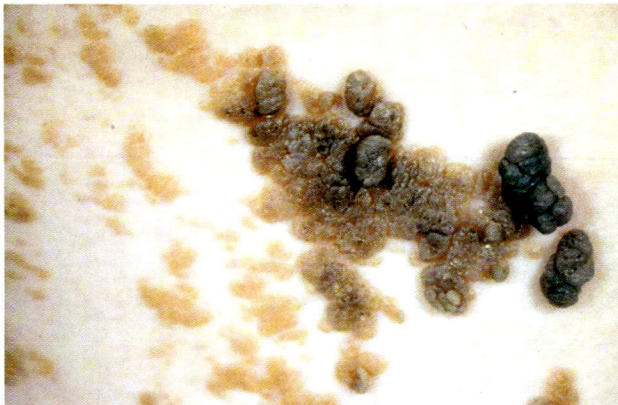

Figure 6–9 □ Epidermal nevus – localized. Epidermal nevus can take the form of a localized or zosteriform plaque with polypoid protrusions. When more extensive, they can be part of the epidermal nevus syndrome, in which there is involvement of the skeletal, ocular, and central nervous systems.

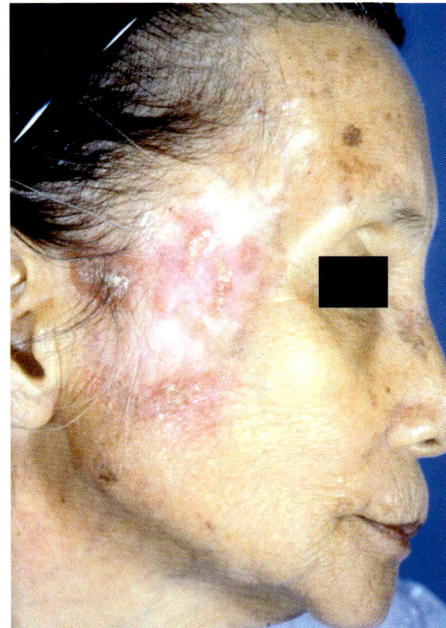

Figure 6–10 □ Actinic keratoses. These erythematous keratotic papules and plaques are actinic keratoses arising from a background of photodamaged skin in an elderly woman. The areas of hypopigmentation are due to post-cryotherapy pigmentary changes.

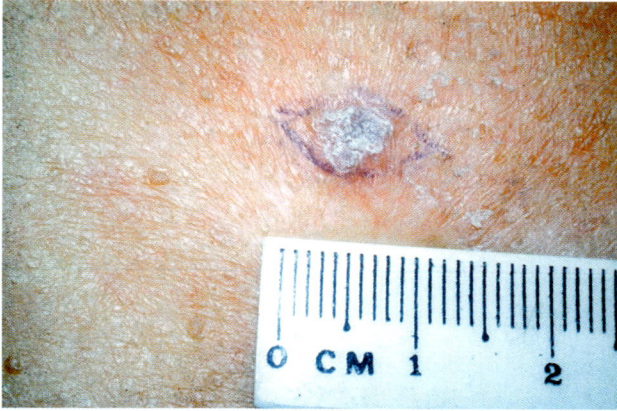

Figure 6–11 □ Actinic keratoses. A close-up of an actinic keratoses showing an elevated, indurated base, suspicious of malignancy change. Actinic keratoses can develop into a squamous cell carcinoma.

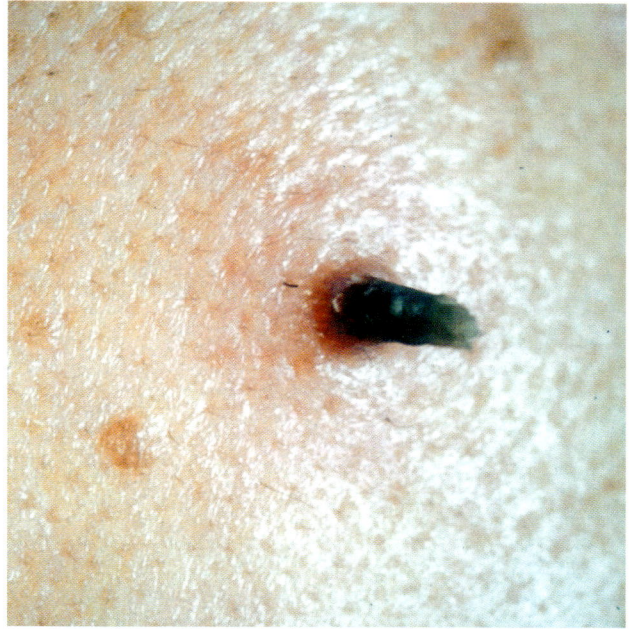

Figure 6–12 □ Cutaneous horn. A conical, markedly hyperkeratotic protrusion may be a harbinger of an underlying viral wart, seborrheic keratoses, or a squamous cell carcinoma. In this 87-year-old patient, histology reveals a squamous cell carcinoma-in-situ. A cutaneous horn warrants an excision biopsy.

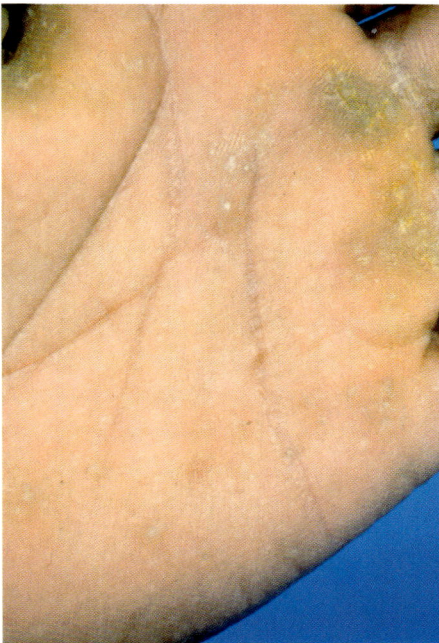

Figure 6–13 □ Arsenical keratoses – palm. These punctate keratoses are due to arsenic, characteristically affecting the palms and soles (see Figures 6–14 and 6–15). They develop as pits and small areas of hyperkeratoses, which may be at the sites of friction. In this locality, arsenic exposure is mostly through consumption of traditional Chinese medicine.

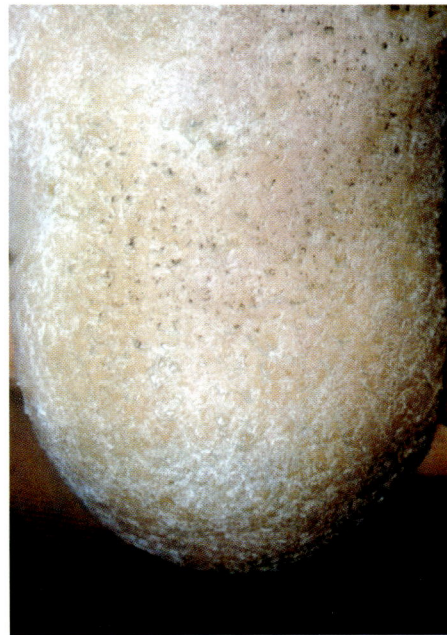

Figure 6–14 □ Arsenical keratoses – sole. The extent, multiplicity and bilateral involvement of these corn-like keratoses on the soles make this clearly distinguishable from plantar warts. Arsenical keratoses may progress to squamous cell carcinoma.

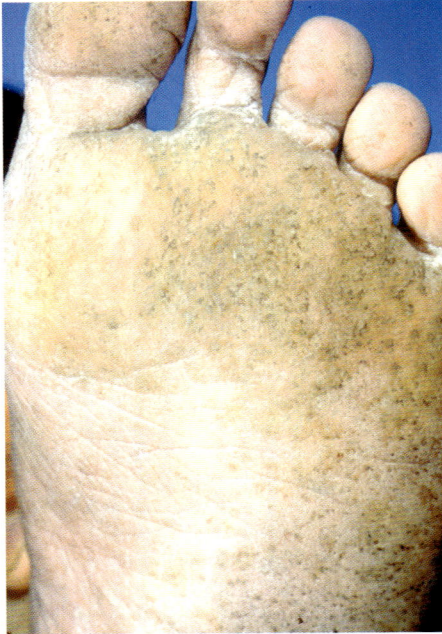

Figure 6–15 □ Arsenical keratoses – sole. These keratoses often impart a dirty look on the soles. Other causes of punctate keratoses, such as punctate keratoderma, appear in early life. The clinical recognition of arsenical keratoses helps to prompt the clinician in eliciting the relevant history. In this Bangladeshi patient, the source of arsenic is likely contaminated well water.

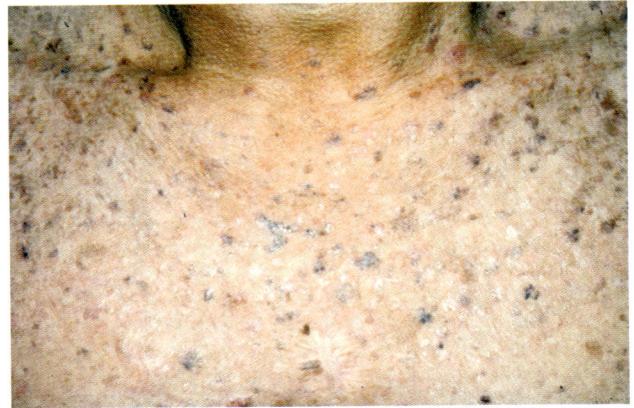

Figure 6–16 □ Arsenical keratoses – chest. Arsenic keratoses appearing as brown keratotic lesions on the upper trunk may resemble seborrheic keratoses or actinic keratoses. However, the guttate hypopigmented macules in the background are stigmata of previous arsenic exposure.

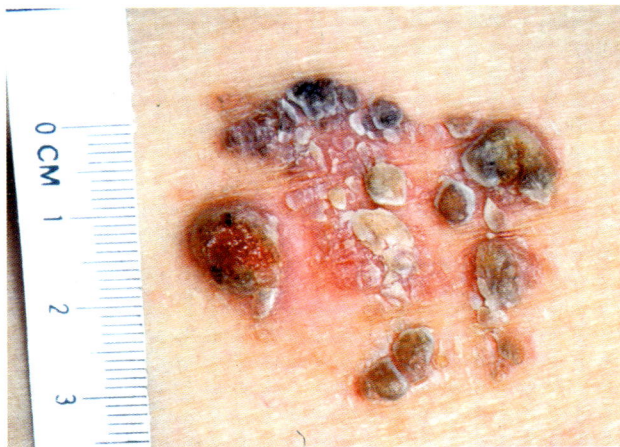

Figure 6–17 □ Bowen's disease. This is squamous cell carcinoma-in-situ, often on sun-exposed sites in Caucasians. Here, a close-up view of a lesion shows an erythematous lesion with an irregular border and little infiltration. Within the patch are areas of scaling and crusting. A persistent eczematous or psoriasiform patch not responding to treatment should raise suspicion of Bowen's disease.

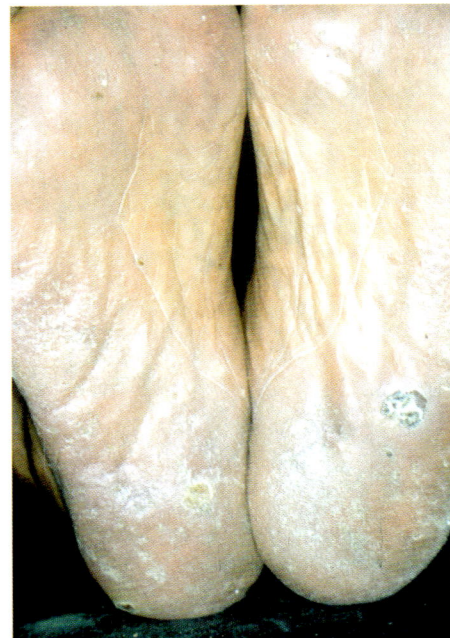

Figure 6–18 □ Bowen's disease – multiple. Multiple lesions of Bowen's disease on the left sole, occurring in a patient with previous arsenic ingestion. Note the plantar pits and keratoses. This 65-year-old patient who had asthma more than 20 years ago, was treated with Chinese herbal medicine, a well-known source of arsenic at that time.

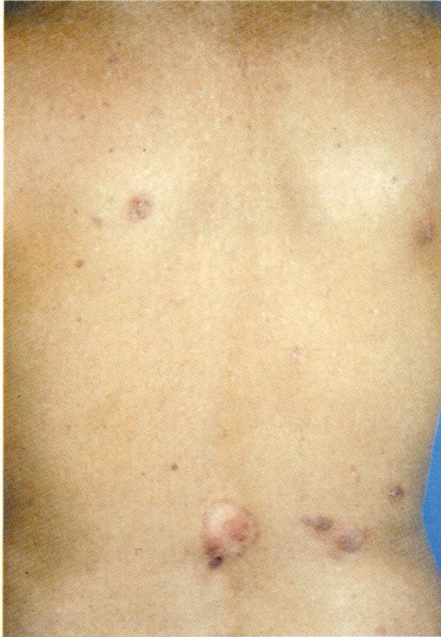

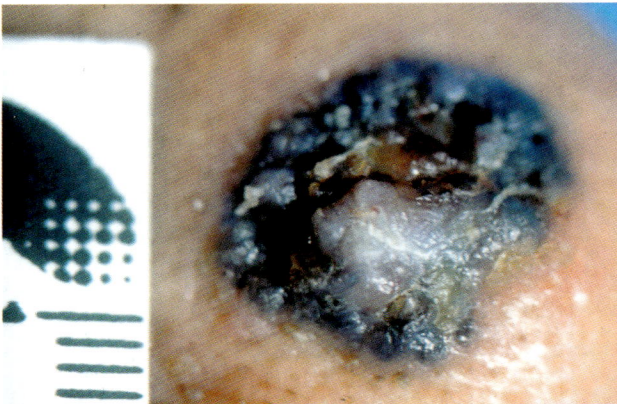

Figure 6–20 □ Basal cell carcinoma – pigmented. Basal cell carcinomas in Asians are typically pigmented and occur principally in the upper central part of the face. This lesion on the left cheek shows a raised translucent pearly border. Although it may resemble a melanoma, the face is an extremely uncommon site for melanomas in Asians.

Figure 6–19 □ Bowen's disease – multiple. Multiple plaques of Bowen's disease occurring on non-exposed skin caused by the ingestion of arsenic. Note the classical raindrop or guttate hypomelanosis in the background. These patients often develop multiple skin cancers over many years.

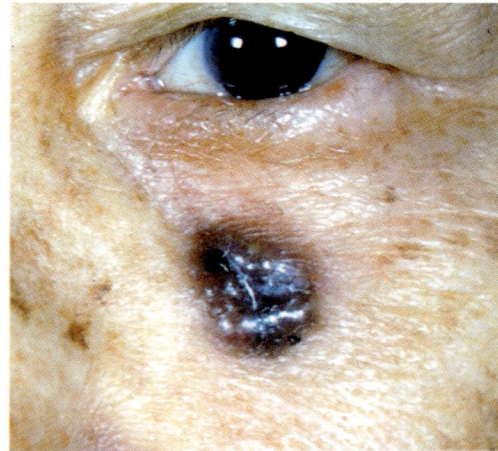

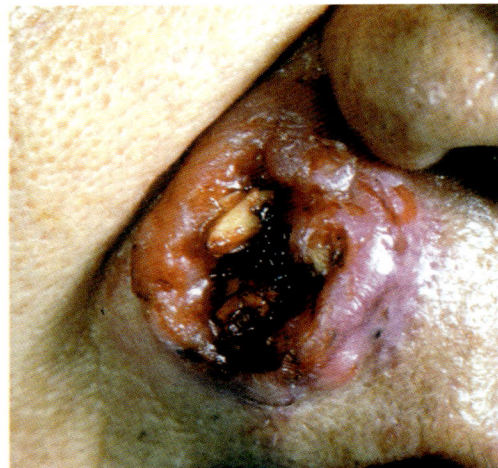

Figure 6–21 □ Basal cell carcinoma – pigmented. This pigmented basal cell carcinoma on the nose shows a pearly center that has partially ulcerated, resulting in a raised papular border.

Figure 6–22 □ Basal cell carcinoma – ulcerative. This large neglected rodent ulcer has been present for ten years. The enlarging basal cell carcinoma ulcerates in the center, leaving the characteristic rolled borders. Although basal cell carcinomas rarely metastasise, they can be locally invasive and destructive.

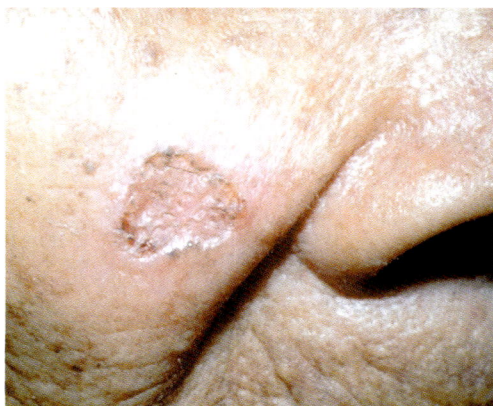

Figure 6–23 □ Basal cell carcinoma – morphoeic. A depressed atrophic plaque may be a rare presentation of basal cell carcinoma. Unlike the other forms, this variety lacks the translucency although a lightly pigmented border can be appreciated here. The extensive infiltrative nature of this subtype of basal cell carcinoma makes it notoriously difficult to treat as pathological extent is difficult to delineate.

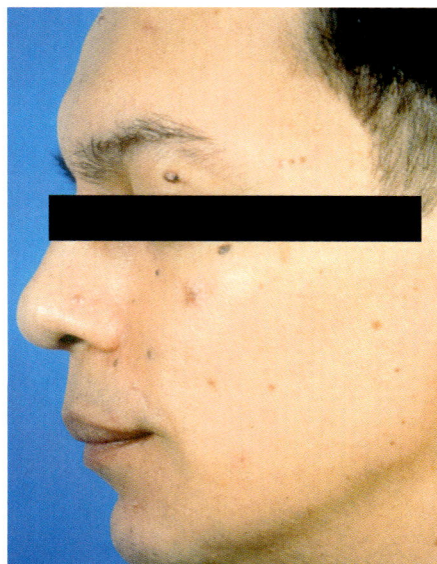

Figure 6–24 □ Nevoid basal cell carcinoma syndrome (Gorlin's syndrome). Multiple basal cell carcinomas are present on the face of this young man. The appearance of tumors can be varied, ranging from brown, dome-shaped papules to soft and nodular lesions, occurring on both exposed and covered areas. This condition is autosomal dominant and is associated with multiple birth defects and tumors especially central nervous system tumors.

Figure 6–25 □ Nevoid basal cell carcinoma syndrome. Varying in numbers, small, symmetrical, shallow pits are seen over the palms and soles and are virtually pathognomonic. Basal cell carcinomas can develop in these pits. This syndrome has been mapped to chromosome 9q22, and mutation of *patched* gene, a developmental gene important in cell growth regulation, has been identified.

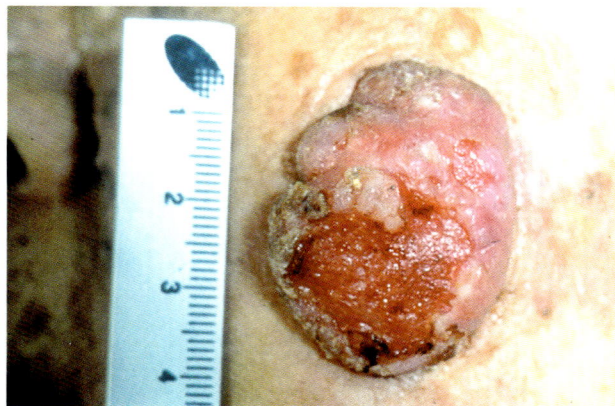

Figure 6–26 □ Squamous cell carcinoma. Squamous cell carcinomas are most commonly seen on sun-exposed sites. Here, a large fleshy and fungating tumor is seen on the cheek of an elderly man. Adjacent skin shows actinic damage. A large neglected tumor is at high risk for regional and distant spread, and has a poorer prognosis.

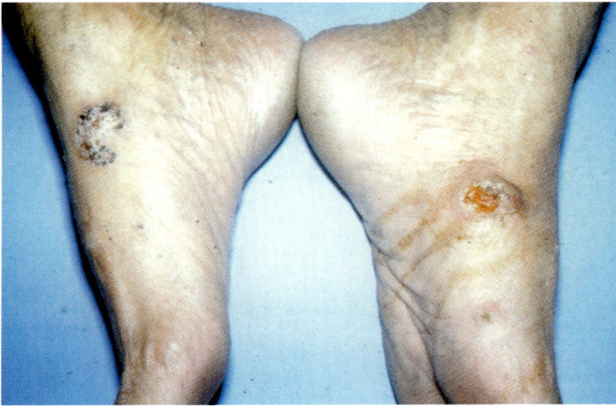

Figure 6–27 □ Squamous cell carcinoma. An indurated, elevated, ulcerated tumor of squamous cell carcinoma is seen on the left foot of this patient whilst on the right, Bowen's disease is present in the form of an annular, pigmented, hyperkeratotic lesion. This patient had previous arsenic exposure.

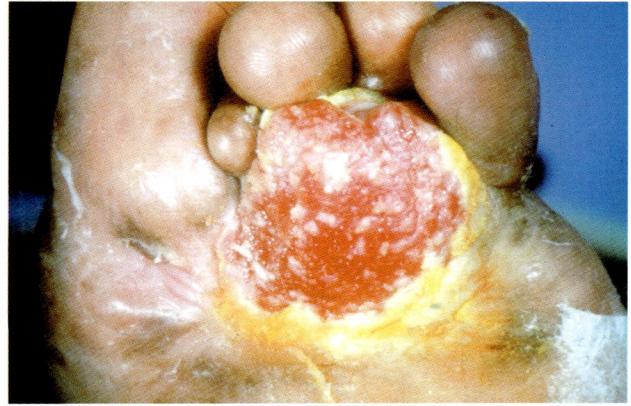

Figure 6–28 □ Squamous cell carcinoma. An old scar or ulcer can be the site for the development of squamous cell carcinoma. This beefy erythematous tumor arises from a chronic neuropathic ulcer on the foot of a patient suffering from Hansen's disease. Any non-healing ulcer should be biopsied to exclude malignant transformation.

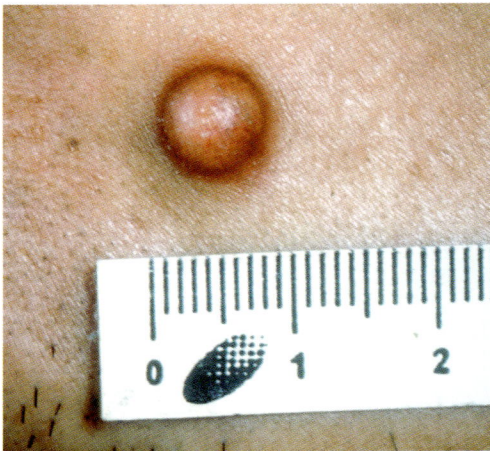

Figure 6–29 □ Dermatofibroma. This is a common fibrous tumor, typically found on the extremities of young adults. The lesion is clinically diagnosable: a round or oval firm dermal papule or nodule, which is pigmented. The color can be reddish-brown because of epidermal hyperpigmentation or blue-black because of hemosiderin deposits.

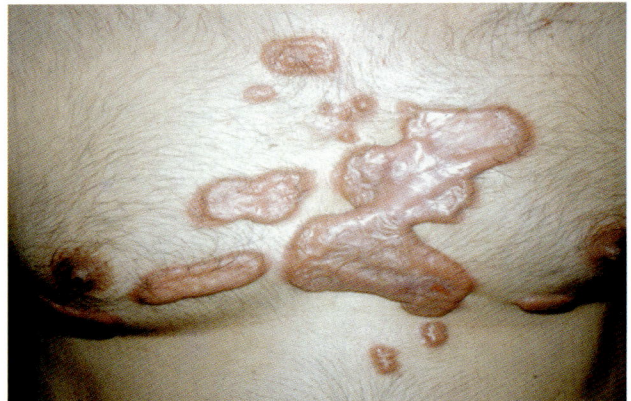

Figure 6–30 □ Keloid. These firm plaques on the pre-sternal region are keloids, a condition affecting individuals who are constitutionally predisposed. Early lesions are erythematous while older ones are usually skin-colored. They occur at sites of injury, such as acne, or may be spontaneous. They can sometimes cause itch, pain, or a burning sensation.

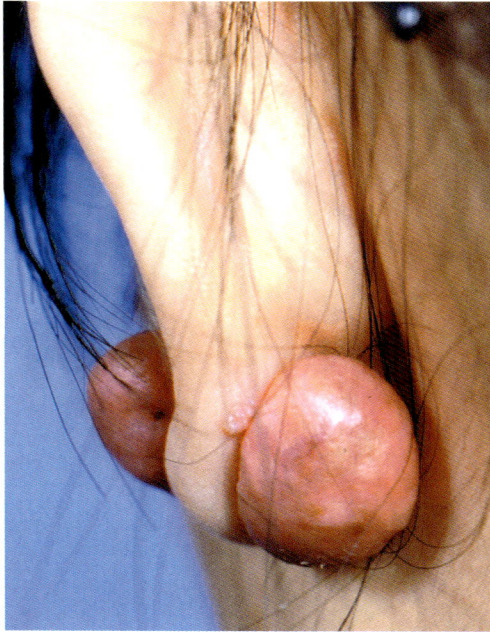

Figure 6–31 □ Keloid. Another site of predilection for keloids is the ear lobe, following ear piercing. This shows a large dumb-bell keloid, which can be cosmetically disfiguring. It can be debulked by laser surgery, with post-operative, intra-lesional steroid injections to prevent recurrences.

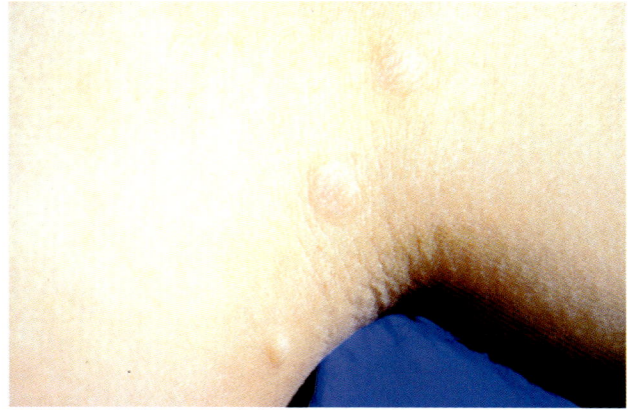

Figure 6–32 □ Connective tissue nevus. This can occur as solitary or multiple lesions and appear as asymptomatic, flesh-colored plaques or nodules on the trunk and upper part of the arms during childhood. It is a hamartoma of the skin in which there is increased dermal collagen or elastic tissue. Some cases may be familial and associated with bony lesions (Buschke-Ollendorff syndrome).

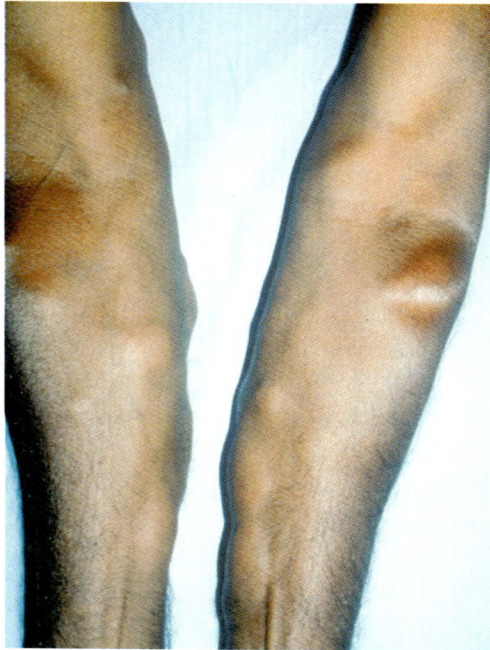

Figure 6–33 □ Lipoma. This is easily diagnosed clinically by its soft consistency, as a round or lobulated subcutaneous nodule that is movable against the skin. Multiple lipomas can occur in the setting of Dercum's disease and benign symmetric lipomatosis. There is no systemic association and neither is there a malignant potential.

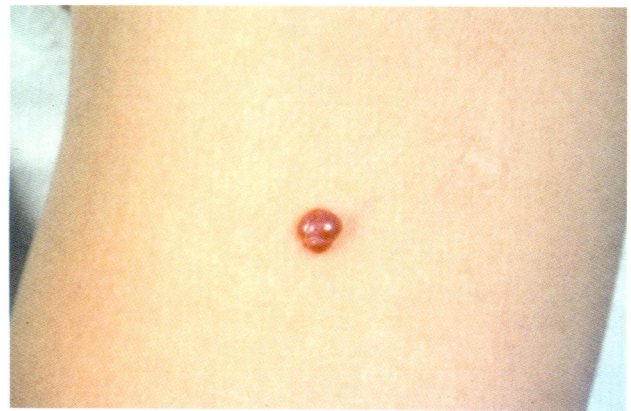

Figure 6–34 □ Pyogenic granuloma. A common benign vascular tumor, pyogenic granuloma, is easily recognized as a polypoid, cherry-red lesion occurring at sites of minor trauma. The lips and fingers are favored sites. It can bleed easily and older lesions show an eroded or crusted surface.

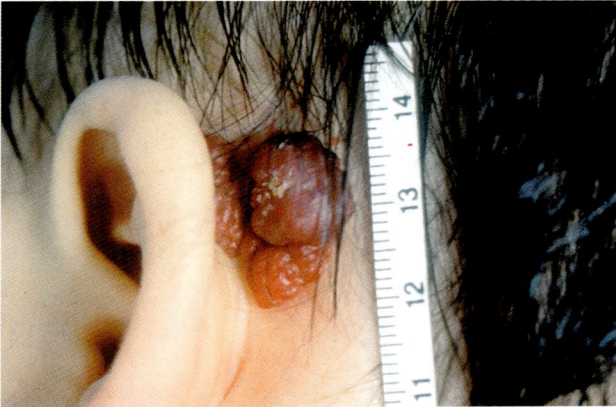

Figure 6–35 □ Capillary hemangioma. This is also referred to as a strawberry nevus as can be appreciated by the appearance of this tumor in the retroauricular region of a one-year-old child. The onset is in the first few weeks of life and the lesion grows to its maximum size by the sixth month. Complete spontaneous resolution occurs in the majority of cases.

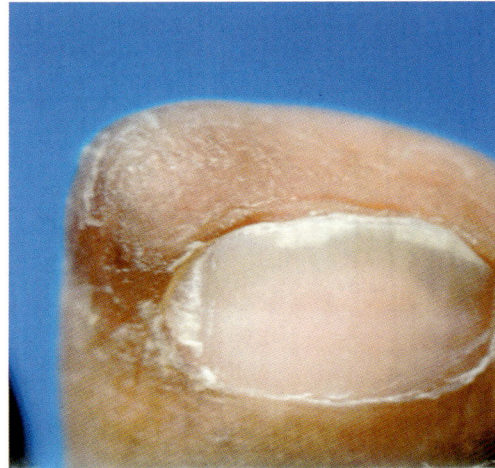

Figure 6–36 □ Glomus tumor. This tumor is almost always a solitary purplish dermal nodule on the finger or toe. Pain is a characteristic feature. It is a benign neoplasm derived from the glomus bodies, arteriovenous anastomosing shunts found primarily in the dermis of fingertips, which serve as thermoregulatory receptors.

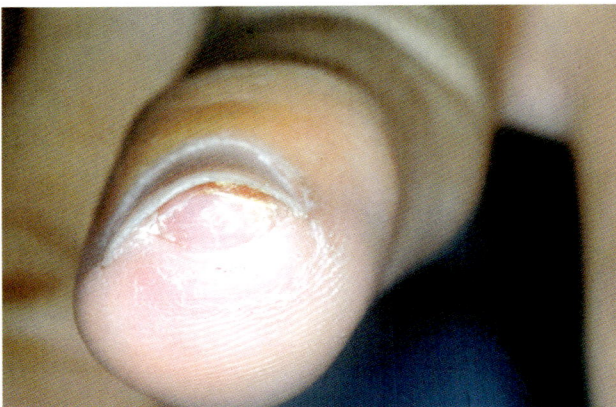

Figure 6–37 □ Glomus tumor. A glomus tumor located in the subungal area of the finger. The absence of trauma and the presence of pain are helpful clues. The diagnosis can be confirmed by ultrasound pre-operatively.

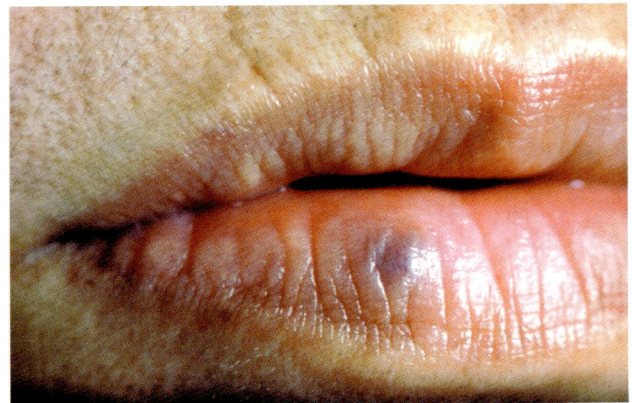

Figure 6–38 □ Venous lake. This vascular malformation is commonly located on the vermilion border of the lips. It appears as a dark-bluish papule and can be mistaken for a melanocytic lesion. The compressible nature of this lesion is a useful distinguishable feature.

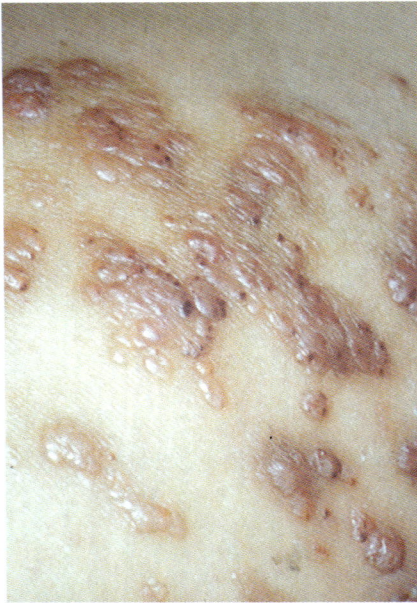

Figure 6–39 □ Lymphangioma circumscriptum. A developmental anomaly of lymphatic vessels; this is a superficial lymphangioma which typically presents with multiple clusters of clear vesicles on the trunk, buttocks, or limbs. The appearance has been likened to frog spawn. Superficial as it looks, there is often a deeper feeding vessel which explains the tendency to recur after superficial ablation.

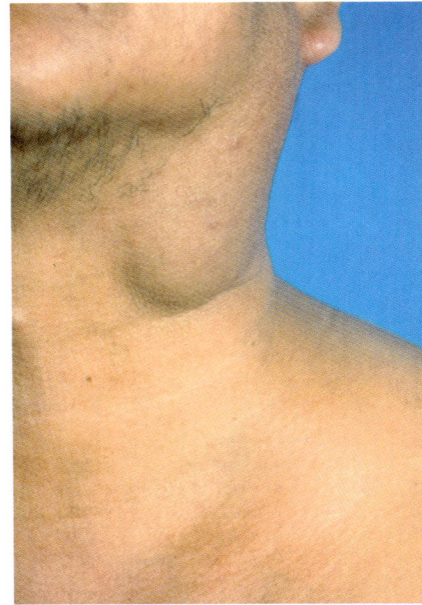

Figure 6–40 □ Kimura's disease. This is an allergic, inflammatory disorder of unknown etiology, predominantly seen in Asia, particularly the Far East. The typical presentation is illustrated here: a middle-aged Chinese man with a subcutaneous mass in the head and neck region. There is often associated lymphadenopathy, peripheral eosinophilia and elevated serum IgE. This disease should be distinguished from a malignancy.

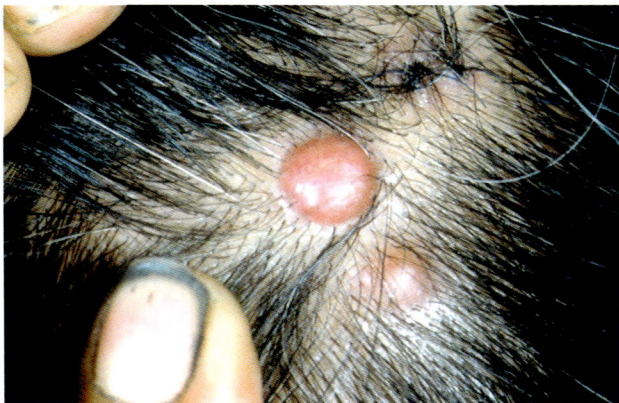

Figure 6–41 □ Angiolymphoid hyperplasia with eosinophilia (AHLE). Whether AHLE, which is mostly reported in the West, is the same entity as Kimura's disease is still debatable. However, there are distinguishable clinical and histological features. The lesions of AHLE are smaller and more superficial. Lesions are common on the scalp and periauricular regions, appearing as red or plum-colored nodules.

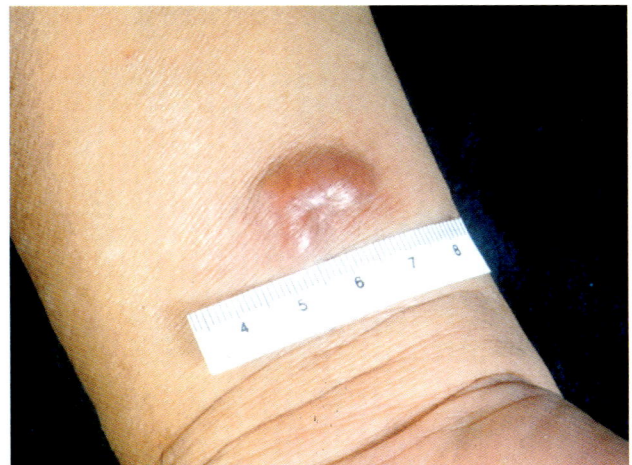

Figure 6–42 □ Angiolymphoid hyperplasia with eosinophilia (AHLE). A solitary plum-colored lesion of AHLE on the wrist of a 69-year-old Chinese man. There is no associated lymphadenopathy or peripheral eosinophilia. Histologically, the epithelioid or histiocytic appearance of endothelial cells, and an inflammatory component including infiltration by eosinophils, are characteristic.

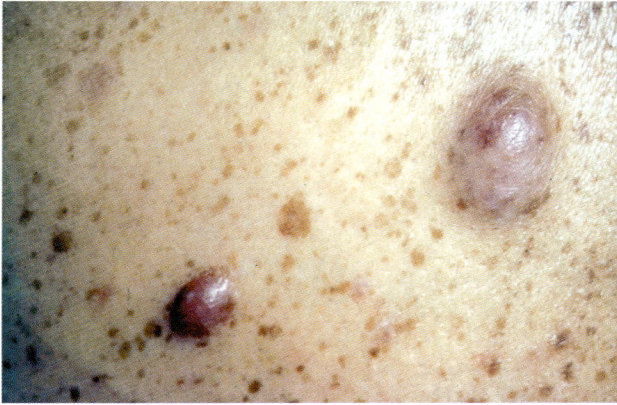

Figure 6–43 □ Neurofibroma. Neurofibromas can occur as a solitary lesion or multiple widespread lesions in the setting of von Recklinghausen's disease. Note the café au lait macules in the background. Neurofibromas, even when solitary, can be diagnosed clinically by its soft consistency and tendency to invaginate on pressure.

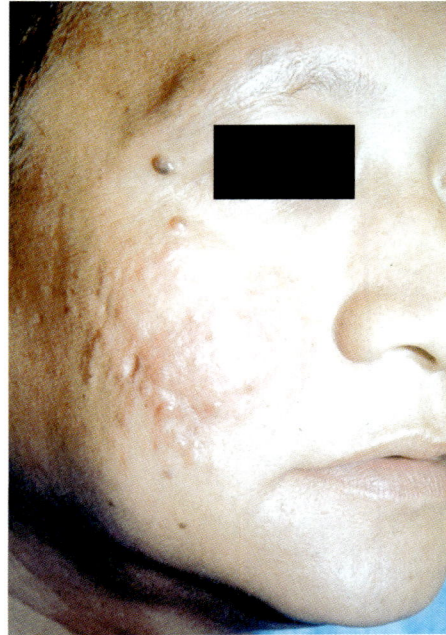

Figure 6–44 □ Leiomyoma. This is a tumor derived from the arrector pili muscle. In this patient, skin-colored clustered papulonodules coalesce to form a plaque on the right cheek. The face is a site of predilection and solitary lesions larger than 2 cm are not uncommon. Pain can be a feature.

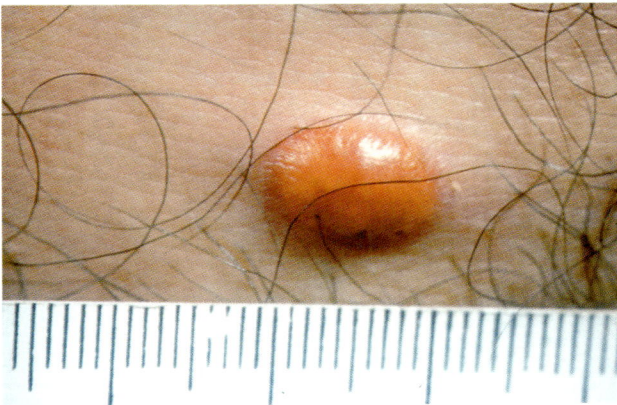

Figure 6–45 □ Juvenile xanthogranuloma. This is classified as non-X (non-Langerhans cell) histiocytosis, most commonly seen in the paediatric age group. It usually presents as solitary or multiple reddish-brown papules or nodules on the head and neck region, upper trunk, or proximal limbs. There is a tendency for lesions to involute spontaneously.

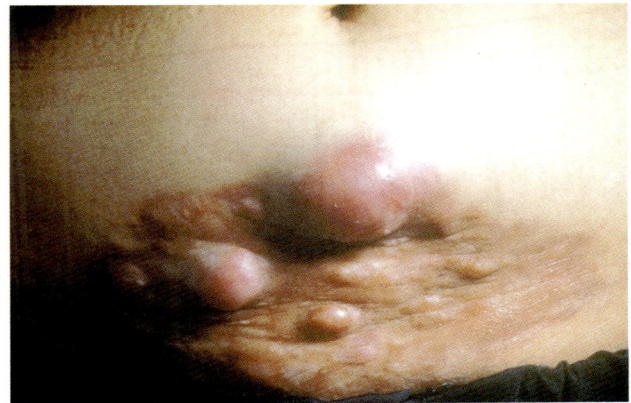

Figure 6–46 □ Dermatofibrosarcoma protuberans. Typical appearance of multiple reddish-brown nodules arising in an indurated plaque on the lower abdomen of this female patient. Dermatofibrosarcoma protuberans is a slow-growing fibrohistiocytic tumor which is locally aggressive, often seen on the trunk. This tumor can be mistaken for keloids and suspicious lesions should be biopsied for diagnosis.

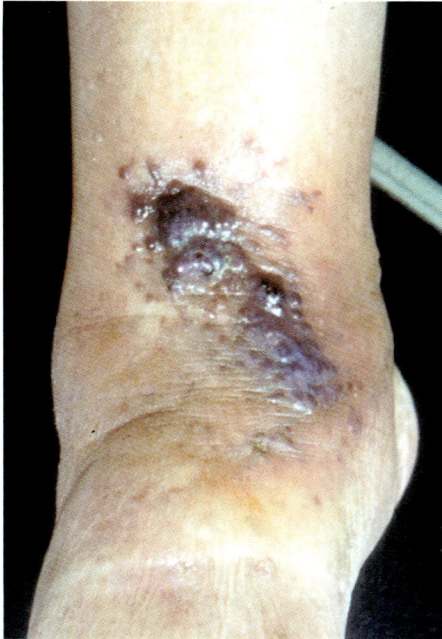

Figure 6–47 □ Kaposi's sarcoma – classic type. This affects predominantly men in their 50s to 70s and is non-AIDS-related. The lesions are common on the lower legs and feet. Multiple purplish papulonodular lesions with accompanying edema are evident over the dorsum of the right foot of this patient.

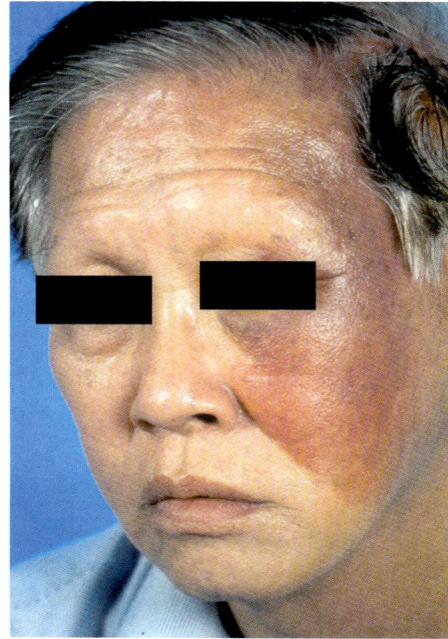

Figure 6–48 □ Angiosarcoma. This presents most commonly with lesions on the face or scalp of elderly individuals. Appearance can vary, ranging from red to purplish nodules or plaques. Here, a flat infiltrating dusky red area affecting the left side of the face is seen, resembling a port wine stain. An onset in later life should raise the suspicion of an angiosarcoma.

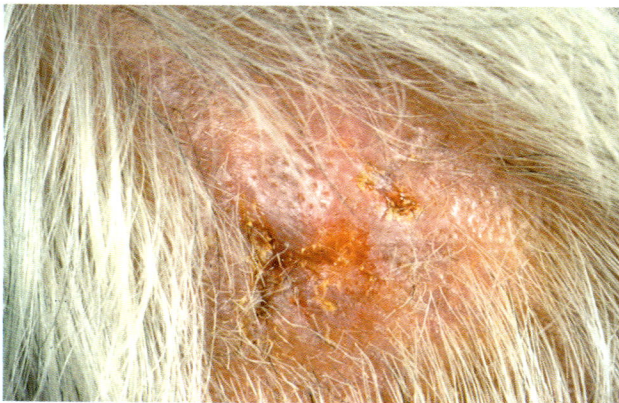

Figure 6–49 □ Angiosarcoma. In this elderly patient, an erythematous, indurated plaque is seen on the frontal scalp. Along with angiosarcoma, other diseases which may enter into the differential diagnosis are cutaneous lymphoma and metastasis.

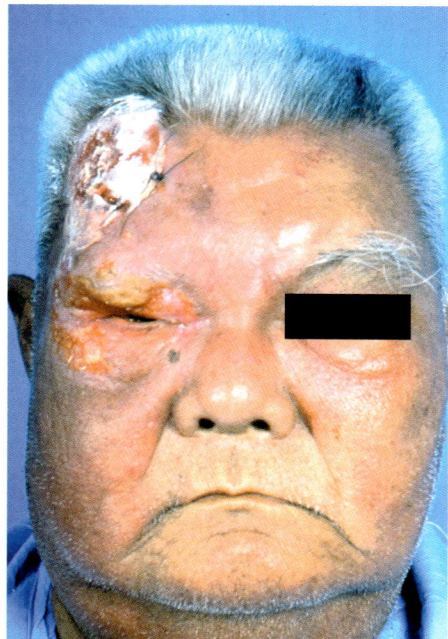

Figure 6–50 □ Angiosarcoma. Very rarely, the presentation of an angiosarcoma may be atypical, as in this patient who presented with bilateral erythema and swelling of the face, mimicking a cellulitis. The lesions eventually ulcerated.

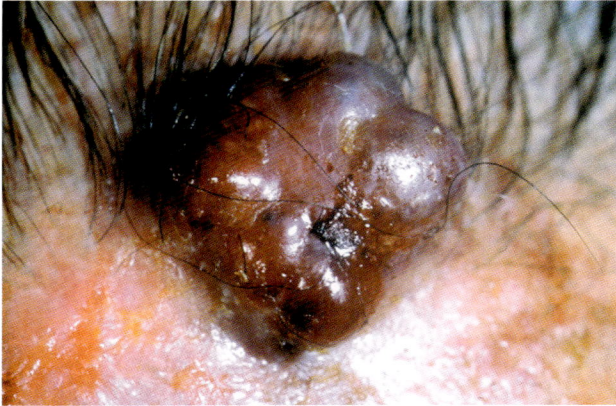

Figure 6–51 □ Merkel cell carcinoma. Also known as neuro-endocrine carcinoma, this tumor usually arises on the sun-exposed skin on the head and neck region of elderly patients. It may have a reddish nodular appearance, averaging 2 cm in diameter which sometimes resemble an angiosarcoma. This is an aggressive tumor with tendency to recurrences and has a metastatic potential.

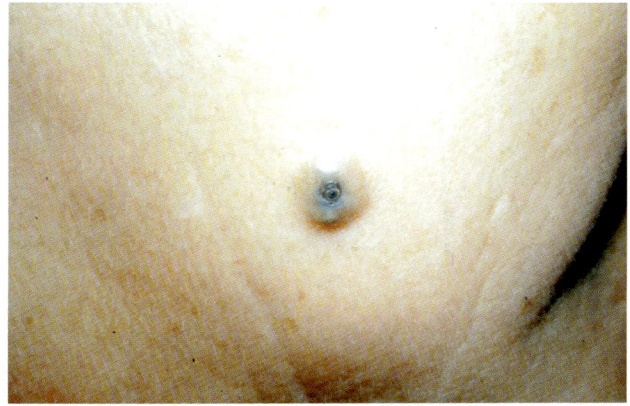

Figure 6–52 □ Epidermal cyst. A cyst with a characteristic central punctum on the cheek. Occasionally, it can discharge creamy, yellow, foul-smelling contents. The much popularized name of sebaceous cyst is a misnomer as this is derived from the infundibular portion of the hair follicle.

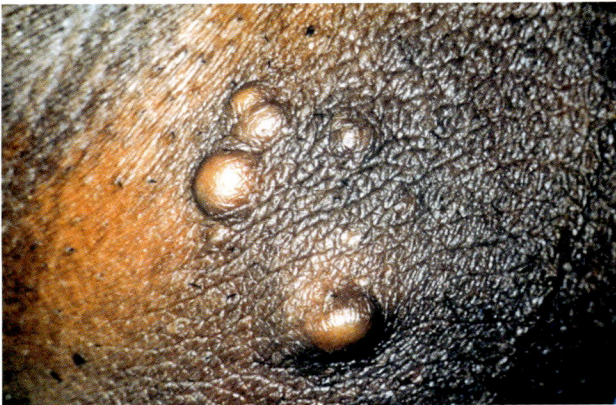

Figure 6–53 □ Epidermal cyst. Multiple epidermal cysts on the scrotum. Dystrophic calcification can result in hard chalky nodules, which may prompt a differential diagnosis of calcinosis cutis.

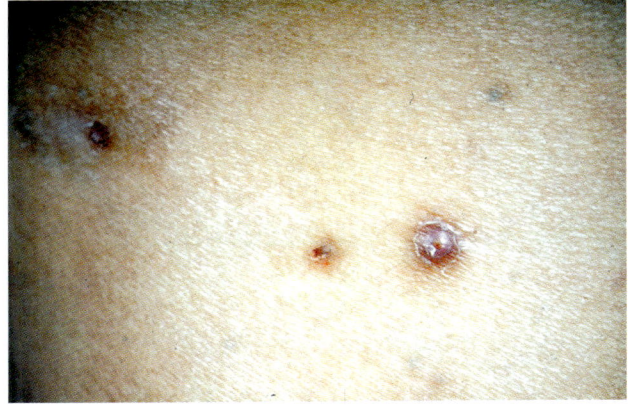

Figure 6–54 □ Vellus hair cyst. This can occur in an eruptive form, as multiple small often bluish papules with a predilection for the chest in young adults. They are thought to develop from an abnormality of vellus hair follicles and may have an autosomal dominant inheritance.

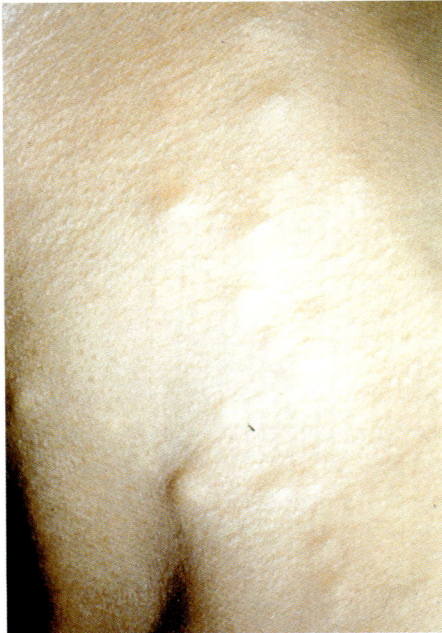

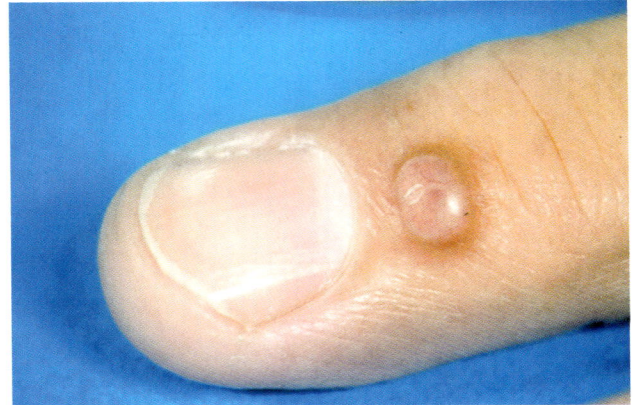

Figure 6–56 □ Mucous cyst – digital. This occurs as a shiny, tense cystic, dome-shaped nodule on the dorsum of the fingers and toes, usually overlying the distal interphalangeal joint. Recurrences after excision is a common problem due to its connection with the underlying joint cavity.

Figure 6–55 □ Steatocystoma multiplex. This condition presents with multiple scattered, smooth, flesh-colored, mobile cysts, commonly on the chest and forearms. It is thought to represent a nevoid malformation of the sebaceous duct and may be of autosomal dominant inheritance, as with vellus hair cysts.

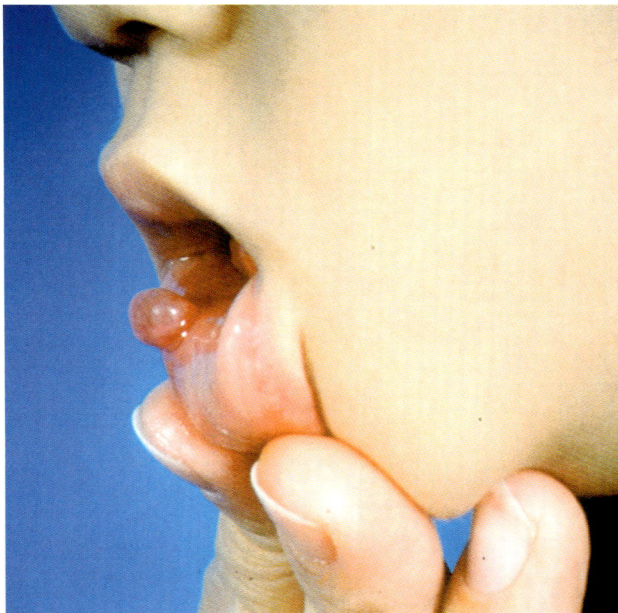

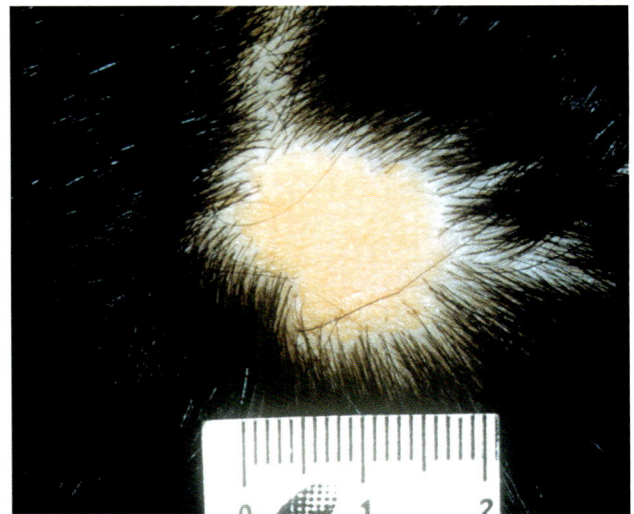

Figure 6–58 □ Nevus sebaceous. Nevus sebaceous is an organoid nevus presenting at birth as a slightly raised hairless plaque on the scalp or, less commonly, on the face. Note the yellowish color, which is often a useful clue to its sebaceous origin. This nevoid malformation involves sebaceous glands, hair follicles, and the epidermis.

Figure 6–57 □ Mucocele (mucous cyst). This lesion is usually found on the lower lip or buccal mucosa, and results from the rupture of the duct of salivary glands with extravasation of mucus into the submucosal tissues. The lesion feels firm and cystic, and has a translucent appearance, ranging from a whitish to reddish color. The nodule can be up to 1 cm in size.

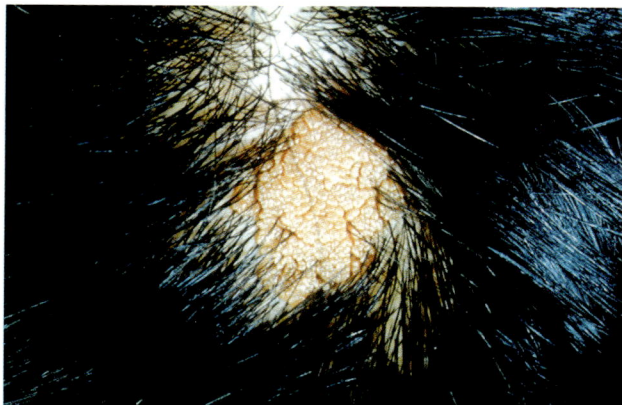

Figure 6–59 □ Nevus sebaceous. Lesion assumes a more verrucous appearance at puberty due to maturation of sebaceous glands and papillomatous epidermal hyperplasia. Development of a new papulonodular lesion on a pre-existing nevus sebaceous should raise the suspicion of an associated basal cell carcinoma, or other adnexal tumors such as syringo-cystadenoma papilliferum.

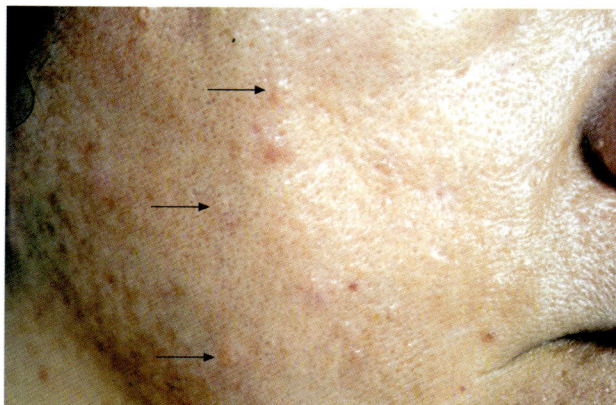

Figure 6–60 □ Sebaceous hyperplasia. This presents commonly as multiple yellowish papules on the face in middle-aged or elderly individuals. The lesions are about 1 to 3 mm in diameter and have an umbilicated center. These lesions have no clinical significance apart from cosmetic concern.

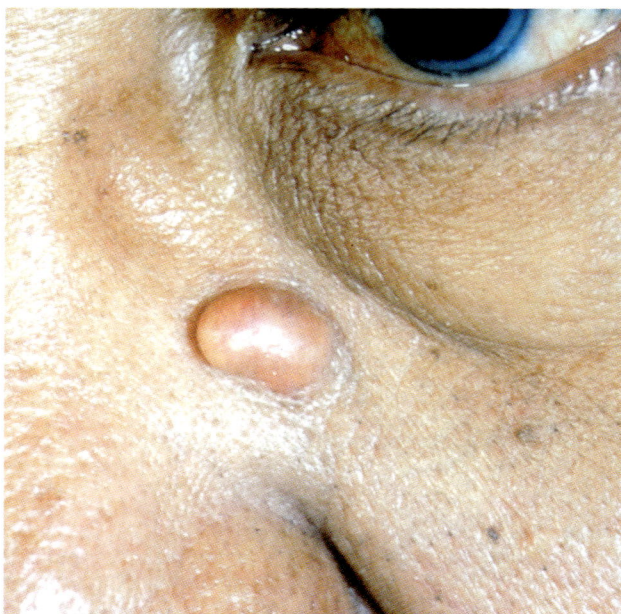

Figure 6–61 □ Sebaceous adenoma. This is an uncommon benign tumor, occurring as a yellowish or flesh-colored tumor on the face or scalp in elderly patients. Sebaceous adenoma, either solitary or multiple, may be associated with a systemic cancer, usually of the gastrointestinal tract, as part of the Muir-Torre syndrome.

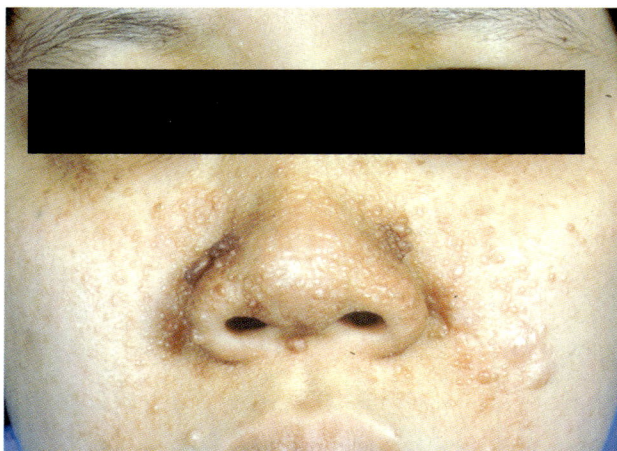

FIGURE 6–62 □ Adenoma sebaceum. These are cutaneous markers of tuberous sclerosis and occur typically around the nasolabial folds. They are angiofibromas histologically. The clinical context of epilepsy and mental retardation helps to differentiate this from multiple trichoepitheliomas (see Figure 6–63).

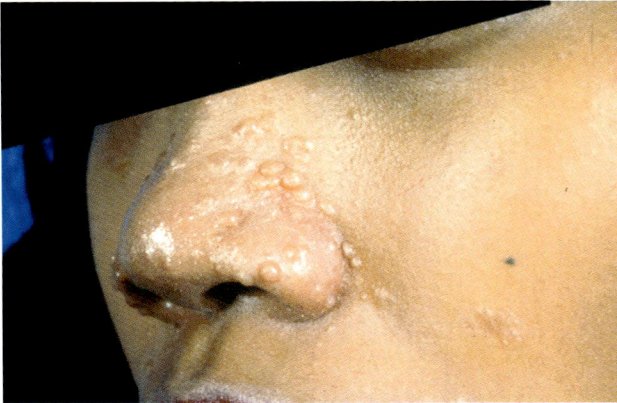

Figure 6–63 □ Trichoepithelioma. This is regarded as a hair-follicle hamartoma, and may present as solitary or multiple lesions. When multiple, they usually appear at puberty as smooth, dome-shaped, and translucent papules on the face, on and around the nose. It is an autosomal dominant condition (epithelioma adenoids cysticum).

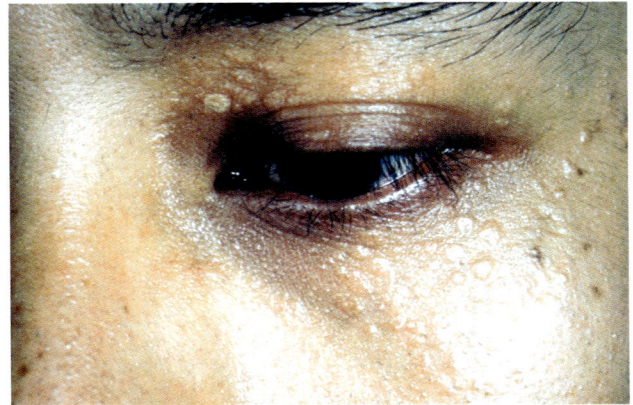

Figure 6–64 □ Syringoma. This is a relatively common eccrine tumor presenting commonly in young women and is not familial. The presentation is often with multiple skin-colored, flat-topped papules on the lower and upper eyelids. Eruptive forms occurring on other sites, e.g. the trunk, are rare presentations.

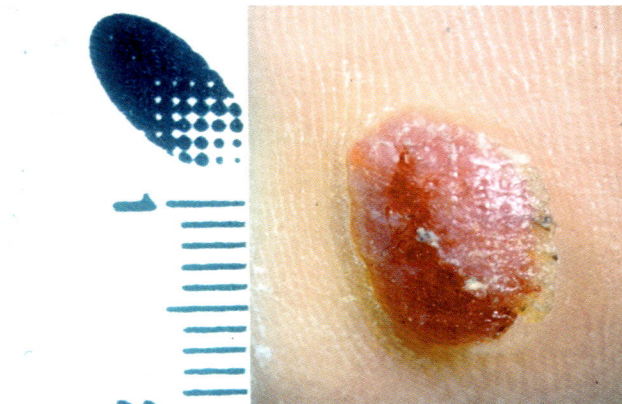

Figure 6–65 □ Eccrine poroma. This is one of the easiest adnexal tumor that can be diagnosed clinically. Most of these lesions are found on the soles and palms, appearing as an exophytic, pink, or red lesion. It is sharply demarcated, and an epidermal collarette can be appreciated, as seen in this lesion. This tumor arises from the intraepidermal portion of the eccrine duct.

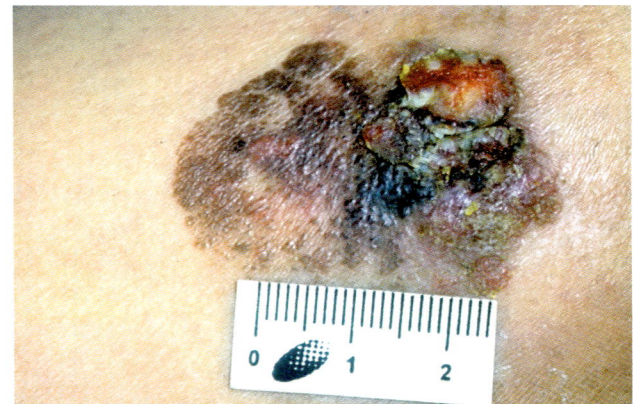

Figure 6–66 □ Porocarcinoma (malignant eccrine poroma). Malignant transformation can arise from a pre-existing eccrine poroma or it can be denovo. This has a predilection for older individuals and for acral sites. It presents usually as a verrucous plaque or polypoid growth. In this instance, the pigmentation and appearance resemble pigmented Bowen's disease clinically. Metastases can occur in porocarcinoma.

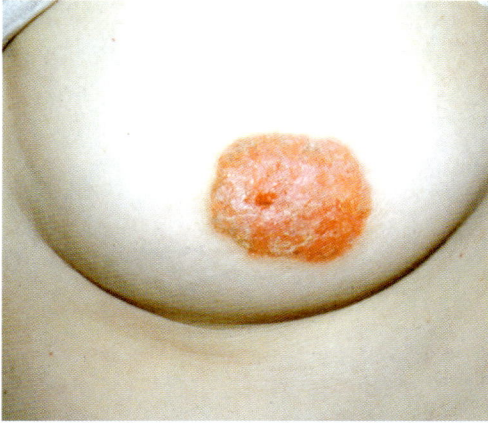

Figure 6–67 □ Paget's disease – nipple. This is intraductal breast carcinoma, occurring mainly in women in their 50s and 60s. It presents typically as marginated scaling and crusting due to epidermal invasion of the nipple and areola by malignant cells. This needs to be differentiated from eczema of the nipples which is often bilateral, runs a relapsing course and responds to treatment with topical steroids.

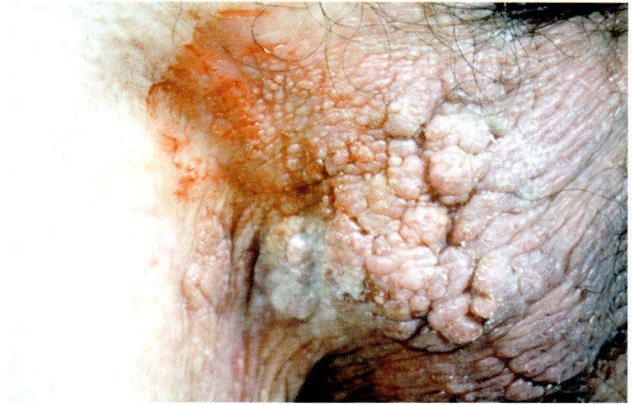

Figure 6–68 □ Extramammary Paget's disease. This lesion is the counterpart of Paget's disease in extramammary sites, frequently occurring in the anogenital region in elderly individuals. It presents as an indurated, sometimes verrucous plaque or as a weepy, eczematized area on the groin. It is important to recognize this tumor, as a primary carcinoma can be found in the urogenital tract or colorectum in a number of cases.

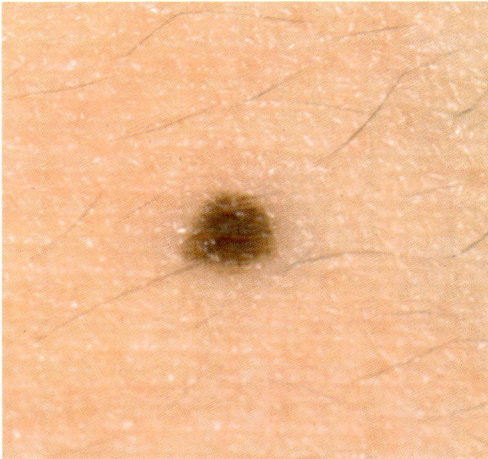

Figure 6–69 □ Junctional melanocytic nevus. This most commonly arises in childhood and adolescence and presents as a small symmetrical pigmented macule which is just palpable. It is often more darkly pigmented than a simple lentigo.

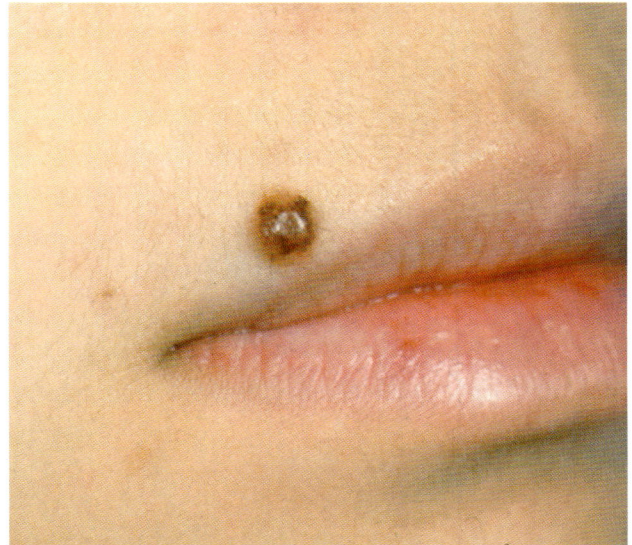

Figure 6–70 □ Compound melanocytic nevus. This represents the next stage of melanocytic nevi where lesions often become raised and more pigmented in late childhood and adolescence. The surface may be smooth or slightly papillated, and the center may be more pigmented than in the periphery.

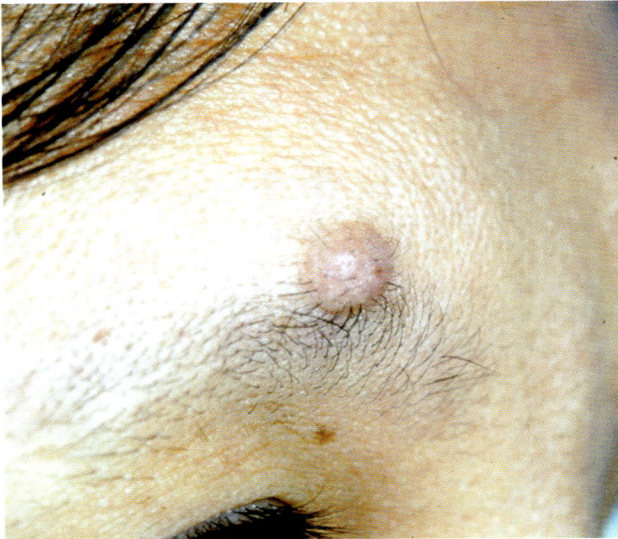

Figure 6–71 □ Intradermal melanocytic nevus. As the lesion ages, it becomes less pigmented and may be skin-colored while maintaining a dome-shaped, hemispherical appearance. This represents a histological change from compound to predominantly intradermal pattern of nevus cell nests.

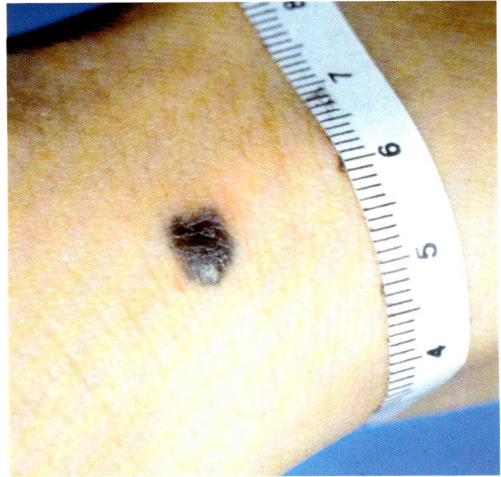

Figure 6–72 □ Blue nevus. This lesion presents as a rounded papule of dark-blue or blue-black pigmentation, often on the extremities, buttocks, and face. It is produced by the developmental arrest of migration of melanocytes to the dermoepidermal junction. However, its appearance in later life is not uncommon. The blue color is a result of reflective qualities of light by the heavily pigmented dermal lesion (Tyndall phenomenon).

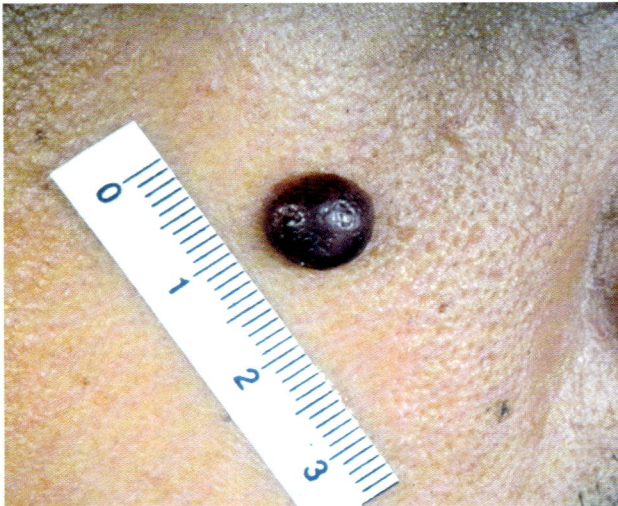

Figure 6–73 □ Spitz nevus. A benign melanocytic lesion occurring mainly in childhood and early adulthood, the Spitz nevus has a predilection for the face, especially the cheeks, and lower extremities. Although pigmented, it often has a reddish hue due to dilated capillaries and measures less than 1 cm. The circumscription, symmetry, and often the age of the patient set it apart from a melanoma.

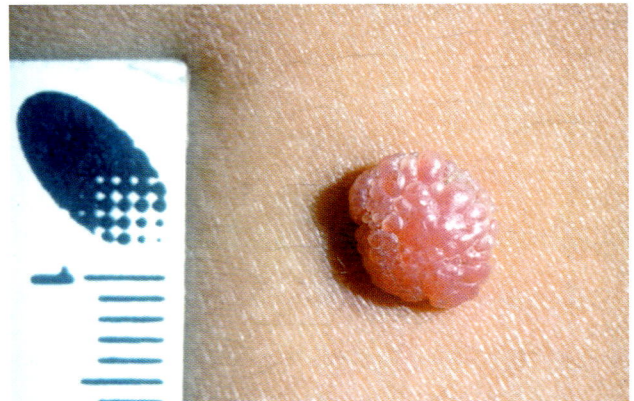

Figure 6–74 □ Spitz nevus. This lesion, in a child, is more pink. In some cases, there is a resemblance to a pyogenic granuloma. However, ulceration and bleeding are uncommon.

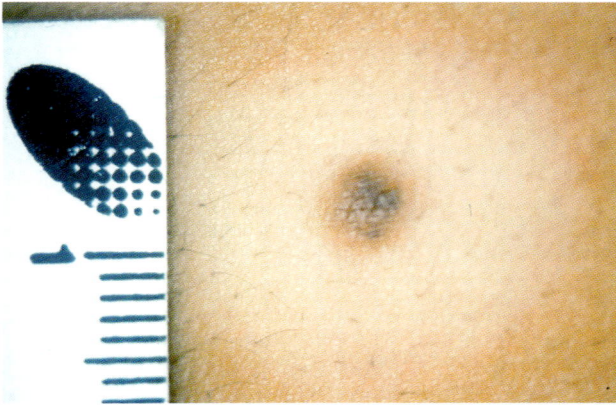

Figure 6–75 □ Halo nevus. This clinically distinctive phenomenon is caused by a lymphocytic immune response against the nevus, causing a rim of depigmentation around a nevus, which has often been present for many years. It may subsequently lead to a complete disappearance of the nevus. The surrounding depigmentation is symmetrical, contrasting with that seen in regressing melanomas, which is often irregularly distributed.

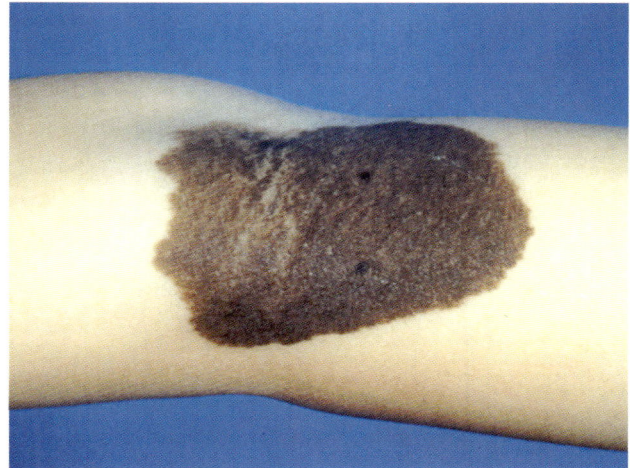

Figure 6–76 □ Congenital melanocytic nevus. Compared to acquired melanocytic nevi, congenital melanocytic nevi are usually larger in size but are commonly smaller than 1.5 cm. The usual location is on the trunk or extremity. At puberty, the nevus often becomes raised, more darkly pigmented, and may be covered with hairs. Large or giant congenital melanocytic nevi (defined as larger than 20 cm) have a distinct malignant potential.

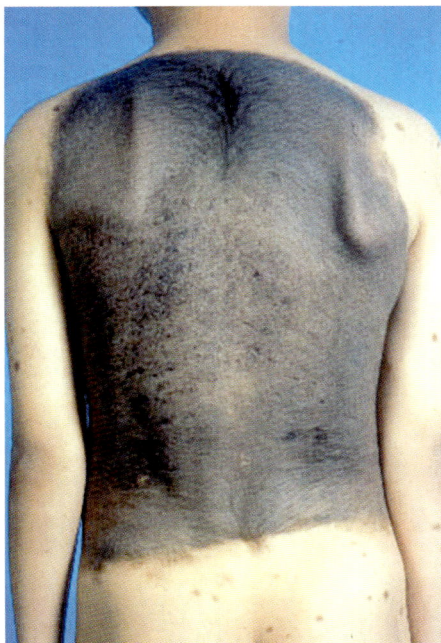

Figure 6–77 □ Giant congenital melanocytic nevus. This usually covers a major part of the trunk, head, or extremity, giving rise to terms such as garment nevus, bathing trunk nevus, or giant hairy nevus. There may also be melanocytic involvement of the central nervous system. The emergence of a nodule or satellite lesion in congenital melanocytic nevus should raise the suspicion of a malignancy.

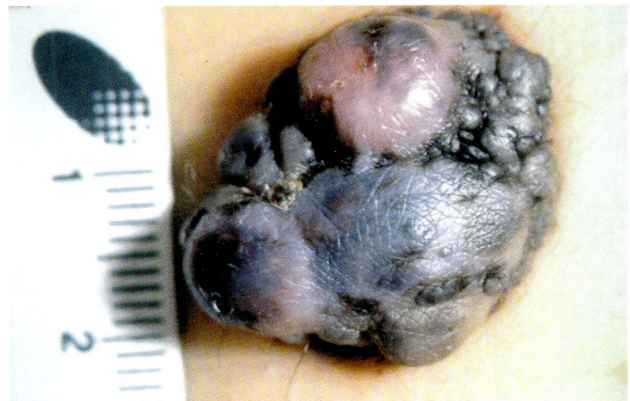

Figure 6–78 □ Melanoma arising in a congenital melanocytic nevus. This multinodular lesion with varying pigmentation developed in a pre-existing congenital melanocytic nevus in a 22-year-old woman. It turned out to be a nodular melanoma.

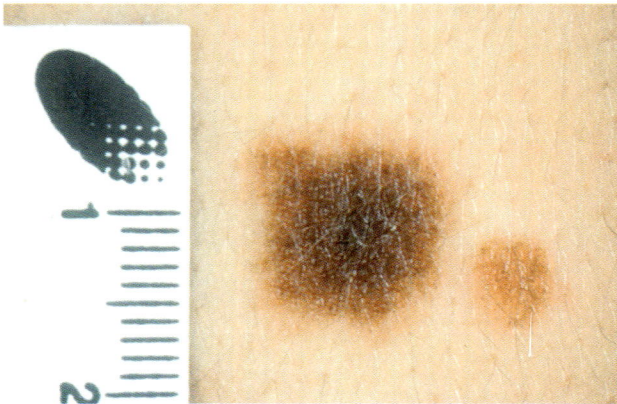

Figure 6–79 □ Dysplastic nevus. Dysplastic nevi are a rarity in Asians. The dysplastic nevus is often larger than 0.5 cm in diameter, has an irregular border, and may be surrounded by a reddish hue. The lesion is usually slightly raised or flat and may have uneven pigmentation. Such a lesion may be a precursor to a melanoma and should be excised for histological diagnosis.

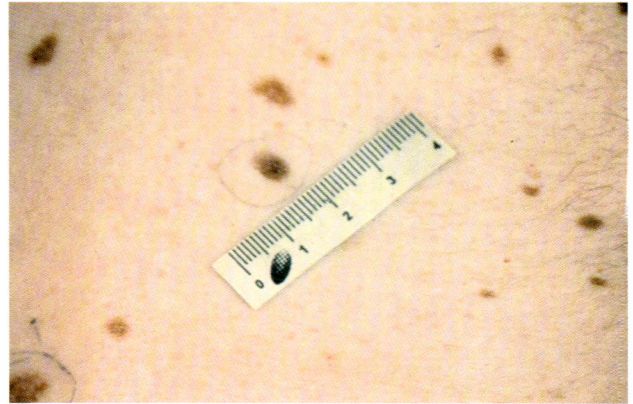

Figure 6–80 □ Dysplastic nevi. Multiple dysplastic nevi can occur in large numbers in Caucasians. These nevi, particularly in the context of the familial dysplastic nevus syndrome, identify a subset of patients who are at high risk cf developing melanoma. Close follow-up for early clinical detection of melanoma is essential to clinical management.

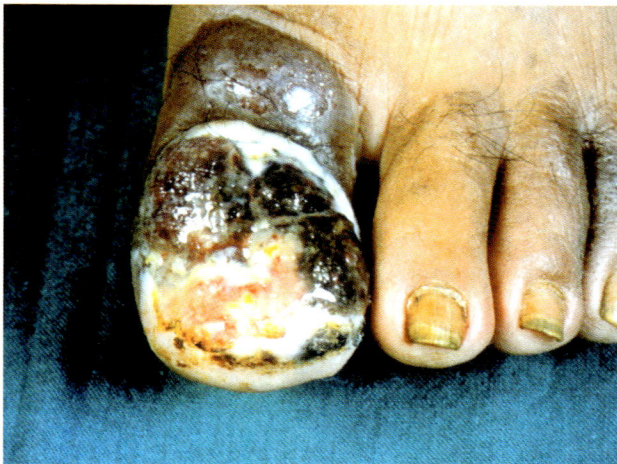

Figure 6–81 □ Acral lentiginous melanoma. Melanomas in Asians are almost exclusively of the acral lentiginous type. The mean age of presentation is the 70s. The sites of predilection are the feet, followed by the hands, with the big toes and thumbs being most commonly affected. Here, it appears as an ulcerated melanotic tumor.

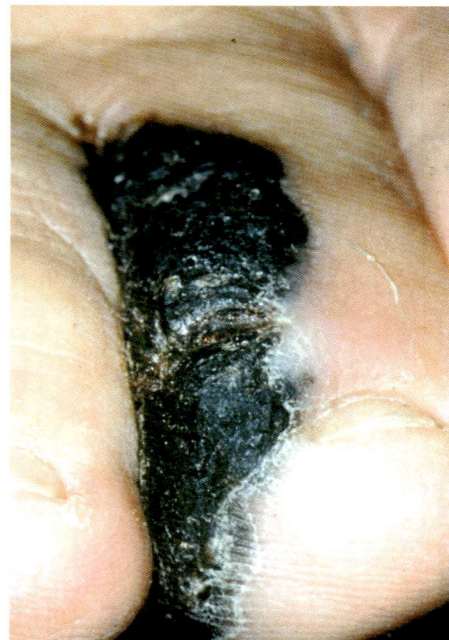

Figure 6–82 □ Acral lentiginous melanoma. This melanoma presents as an irregular, heavily pigmented plaque, involving the toe cleft.

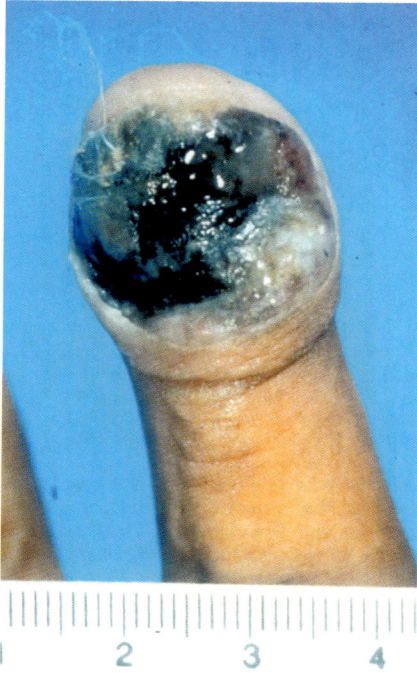

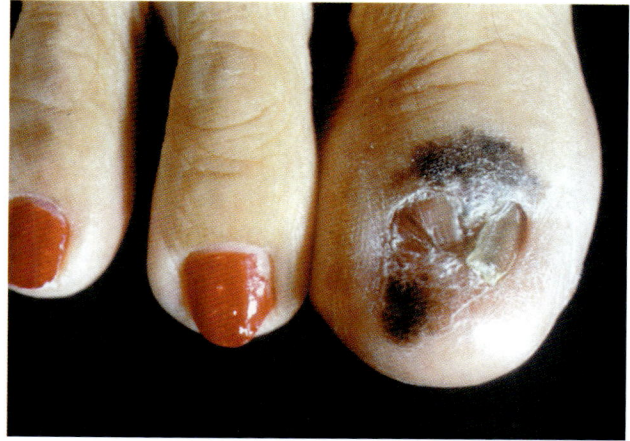

Figure 6–84 □ Acral lentiginous melanoma. In this lesion, the nail is not only destroyed but there is obvious periungual pigmentation on the nail fold proximal and distal to the nail, indicative of periungual or subungual melanoma.

Figure 6–83 □ Acral lentiginous melanoma. Subungual location of acral melanomas occurs with almost equal frequency on the hands and the feet. There is complete destruction of the nail bed by this invasive, raised tumor.

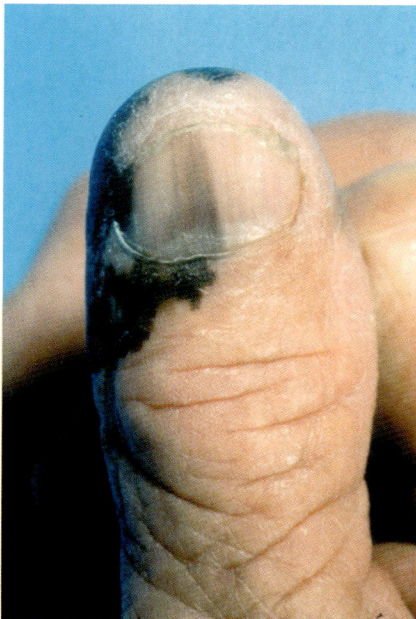

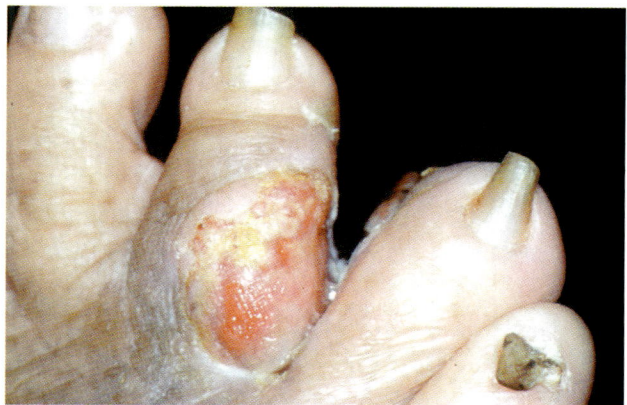

Figure 6–86 □ Acral lentiginous melanoma. This amelanotic variant is an atypical presentation of acral lentiginous melanoma, appearing as a flesh-colored, ulcerated nodule. A high index of suspicion is required to avoid delayed diagnosis.

Figure 6–85 □ Acral lentiginous melanoma. Acral melanoma may present in the early phase as a black longitudinal streak of the nail. The extension of the pigmentation on the nail fold and distally is an extremely useful diagnostic sign of a melanoma (Hutchinson's sign), differentiating it from benign pigmentation involving the nail.

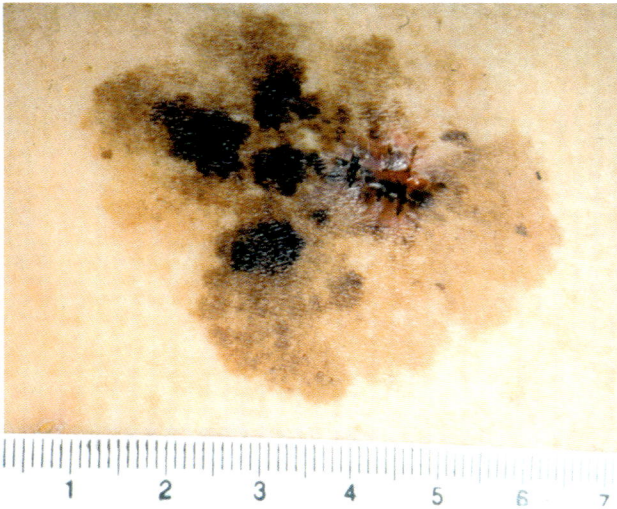

Figure 6–87 □ Superficial spreading melanoma. This type of melanoma is characterized by its radial (pagetoid) growth pattern clinically and histologically, and is rare in Asians. The trunk appears to be a site of predilection and the lesion shows variegated pigmentation with an expanding irregular border.

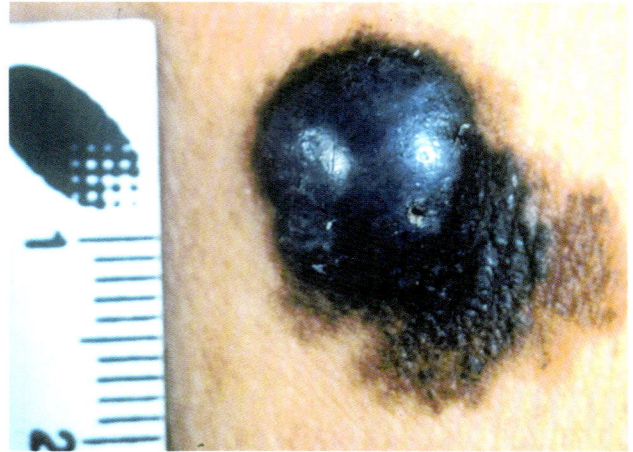

Figure 6–88 □ Superficial spreading melanoma with invasive dermal component. This melanoma is located on the back of a 78-year-old woman. It has a flat component with an irregular border, corresponding to a pagetoid pattern of growth. Dermal invasion and tumor progression result in a tumor nodule.

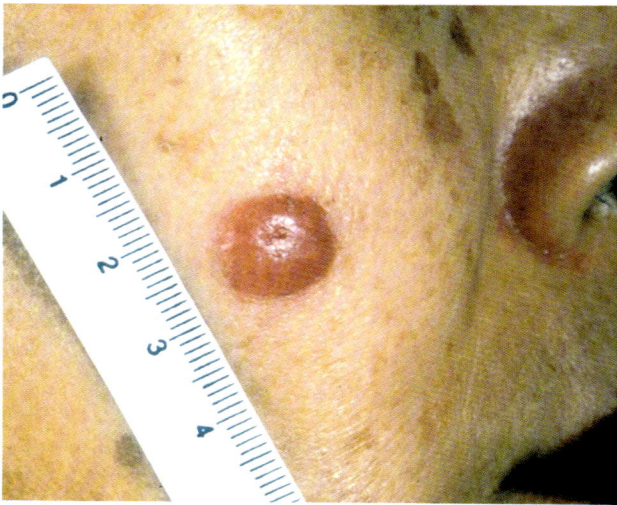

Figure 6–89 □ Lymphocytoma cutis. This refers to benign lymphoid hyperplasia mimicking a cutaneous lymphoma clinically and histologically (pseudolymphoma). The face is a common site of involvement. Lesions can be solitary, as illustrated, or multiple. They are usually papulonodular, and red-brown or violaceous in color. Known antigenic stimuli include tick and arthropod bites, drugs, gold, and tattoos.

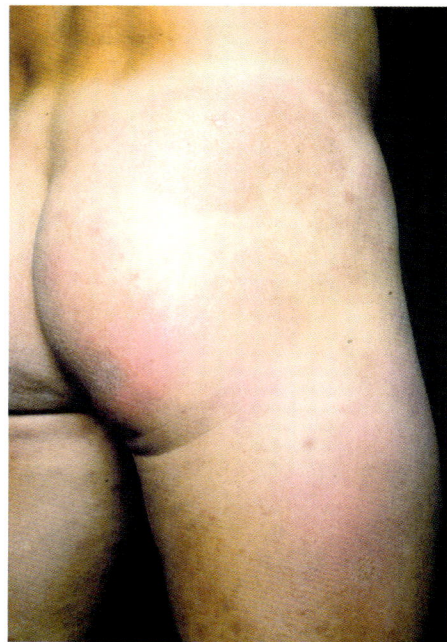

Figure 6–90 □ Mycosis fungoides – patch stage. An indolent cutaneous T-cell lymphoma, this is also the most common form of cutaneous lymphoma. In the early stages of the disease, lesions appear as erythematous to brown, slightly scaly patches in a bathing trunk distribution, typically involving the buttocks.

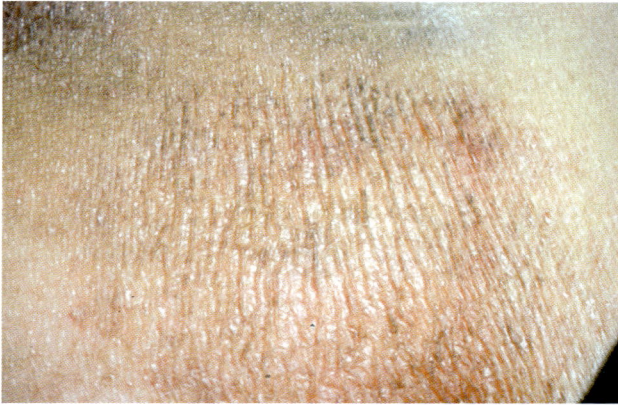

Figure 6–91 □ Mycosis fungoides – patch stage. Early patch stage mycosis fungoides is often a source of diagnostic difficulty. Although it presents like an eczema, the patches are usually thin and atrophied and have a wrinkled, papery-thin appearance.

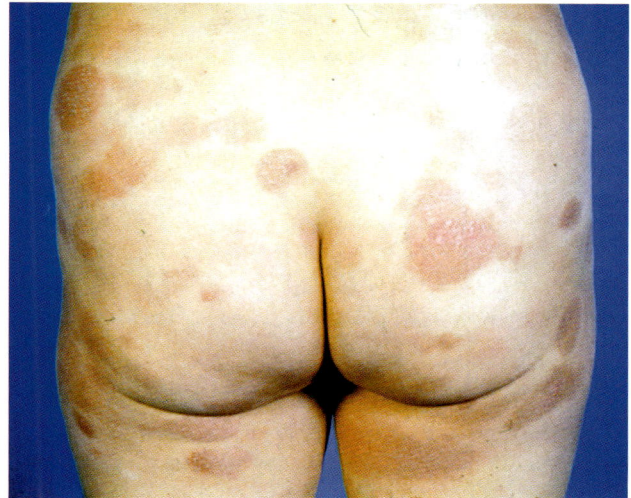

Figure 6–92 □ Mycosis fungoides – plaque stage. In this patient, progression of patch stage of mycosis fungoides leads to the development of infiltrated erythematous plaques in a typical distribution. Lesions are of varying sizes and have irregular borders.

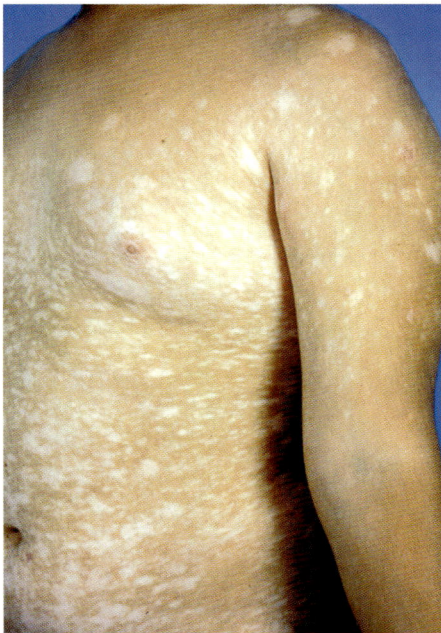

Figure 6–93 □ Mycosis fungoides – hypopigmented. This variant of mycosis fungoides is well-recognized in Asian and black patients. It is predominantly seen in children and young adults, presenting with hypopigmented, mildly scaly macules and patches. Lesions can be widespread as in this 13-year-old patient. Unlike vitiligo, the margins of lesions are less well-defined.

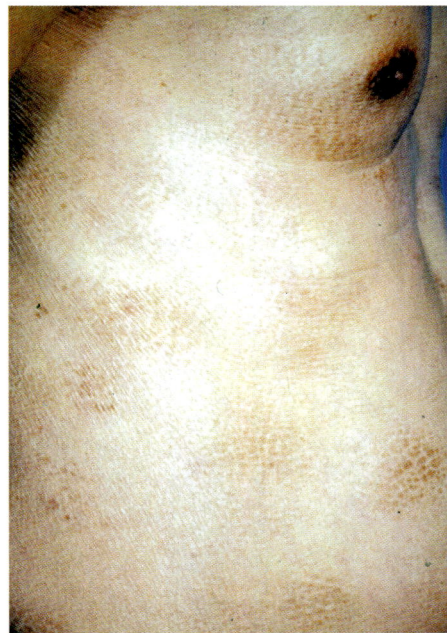

Figure 6–94 □ Mycosis fungoides – ichthyosiform. Besides being a manifestation of an internal malignancy, acquired ichthyosis can be the presenting features of mycosis fungoides. Note the predominantly truncal distribution, brown patches with fine fish-like scales.

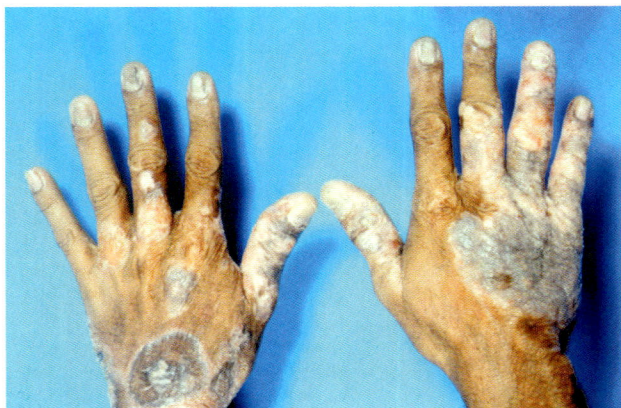

Figure 6–95 □ Mycosis fungoides – acral. Mycosis fungoides can present predominantly on acral sites, as in this patient who had chronic hyperpigmented and hypopigmented plaques on the dorsa of his hands and fingers for 16 years at the time of diagnosis. The lesions are persistent and progressive, and steroid-unresponsive.

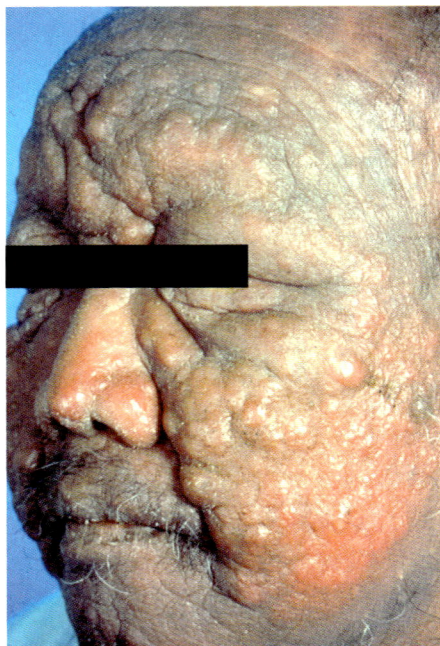

Figure 6–96 □ Mycosis fungoides – follicular. Infiltrated follicular papulonodular lesions on the face are a rare manifestation of mycosis fungoides, which runs a more aggressive course. On histology, the hair follicles are infiltrated by neoplastic lymphocytes. This patient also has classical lesions of mycosis fungoides on the trunk.

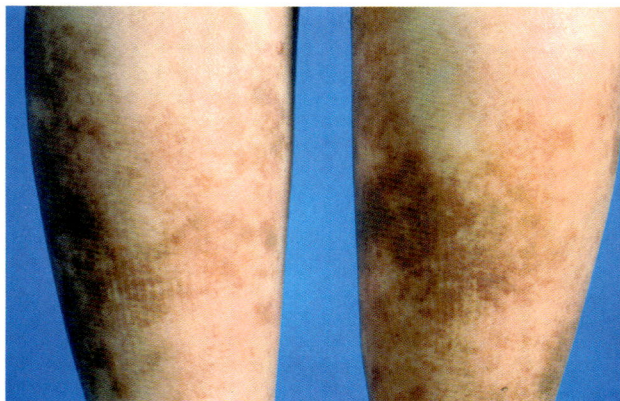

Figure 6–97 □ Mycosis fungoides – pigmented purpura-like. This variant of mycosis fungoides presents with purpuric patches and plaques on the legs, closely resembling pigmented purpuric dermatosis. In this patient, there was extensive involvement up to the lower trunk and histology clinched the diagnosis.

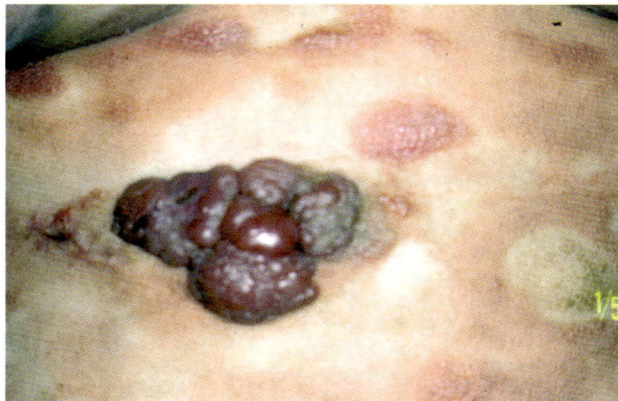

Figure 6–98 □ Mycosis fungoides – tumor stage. This patient shows advanced disease with a tumor arising from pre-existing plaque stage. Multiple infiltrated plaques, some of which are annular in appearance, are seen in the background. Tumor-stage mycosis fungoides is associated with a less favorable, long-term outcome than that at the patch or plaque stage.

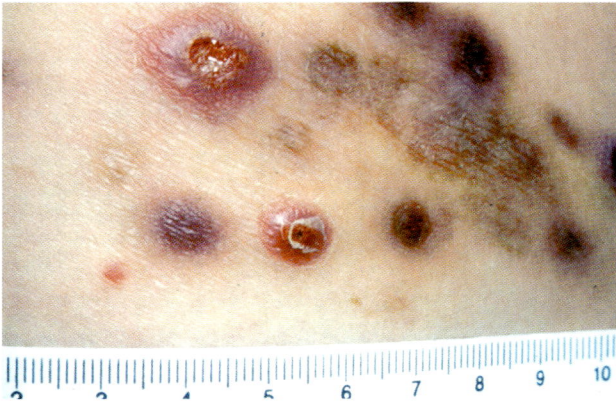

Figure 6–99 □ Lymphomatoid papulosis. Now regarded as a low-grade T-cell lymphoma, lymphomatoid papulosis presents with ulcerated and crusted lesions, which are less than 1 cm in diameter. The papulonecrotic lesions can occur in crops or as scattered lesions, typically running a relapsing course.

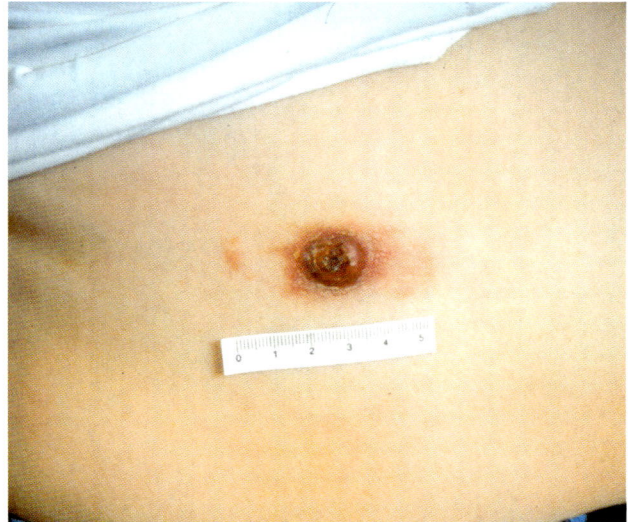

Figure 6–100 □ Primary cutaneous CD30+ large cell T-cell lymphoma. This noduloulcerative lesion is solitary and occurs in a patient with lymphomatoid papulosis. It is larger than the lesions of lymphomatoid papulosis (more than 1 cm) and histology showed a majority of CD30+ infiltrating neoplastic T-cells. This form of lymphoma carries an excellent prognosis.

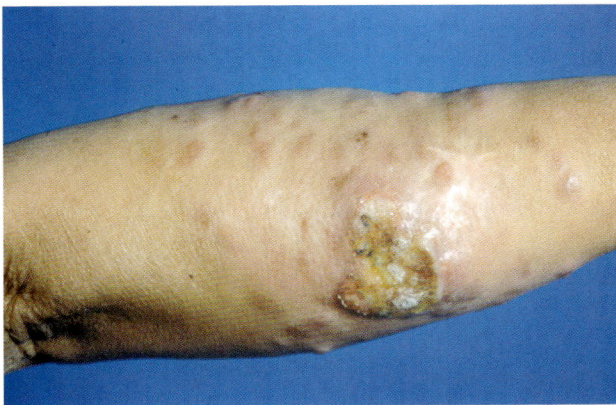

Figure 6–101 □ Secondary cutaneous CD30+ large cell T-cell lymphoma. Ulceration is characteristic of CD30+ cutaneous T-cell lymphoma, often resulting in the initial consideration of an infective lesion. A group of tumors can present in a localized distribution as illustrated here: a fungating, ulcerated tumor with smaller papulonodular lesions developing at the periphery.

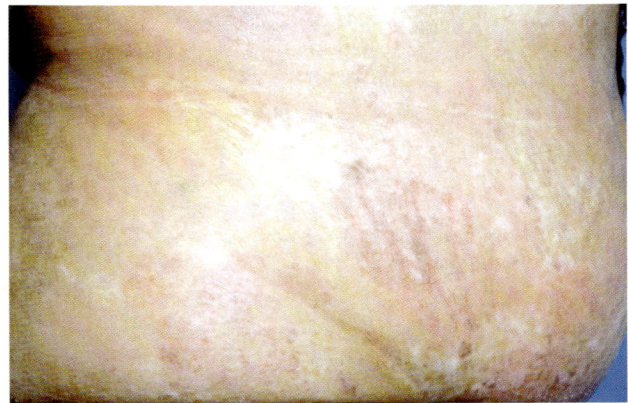

Figure 6–102 □ Cutaneous CD30+ large cell T-cell lymphoma secondary to mycosis fungoides. The patient in Figure 6–101 shows widespread involvement by mycosis fungoides. Note the large erythematous patches and thin plaques with hypopigmented areas.

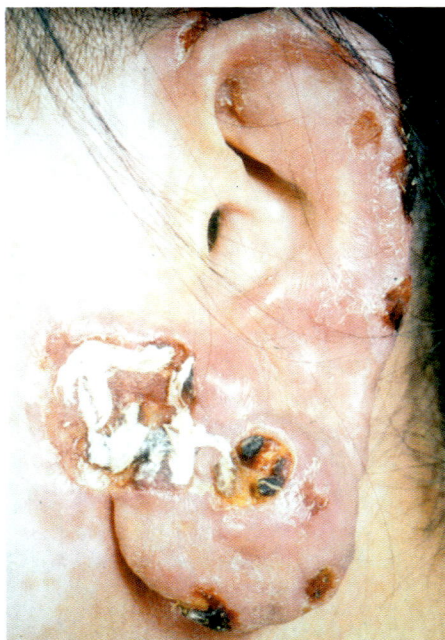

Figure 6–103 □ Cutaneous CD30+ large cell T-cell lymphoma secondary to systemic lymphoma. Infiltrative ulcerative lesions on the ear lobes and pinna, as in this patient, may prompt an initial diagnosis of lepromatous leprosy. However, this patient had extensive ulcerative lesions elsewhere (see Figure 6–104).

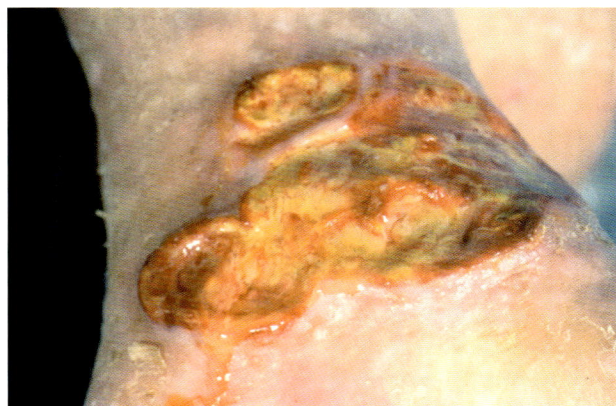

Figure 6–104 □ Cutaneous CD30+ large cell T-cell lymphoma secondary to systemic lymphoma. Ulcerative lesions on the lower left leg of the patient in Figure 6–103. The patient had lung involvement and died of advanced disease two years after presentation.

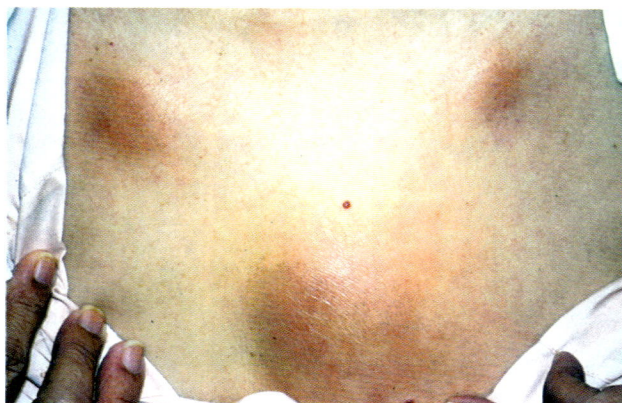

Figure 6–105 □ Subcutaneous panniculitis-like T-cell lymphoma. This unique subtype of T-cell lymphoma is more commonly seen in this part of the world than in the West. Here, one sees multiple subcutaneous nodules on the chest. The entity is so-named as the lymphoma is often misinterpreted as a panniculitis in its early phases.

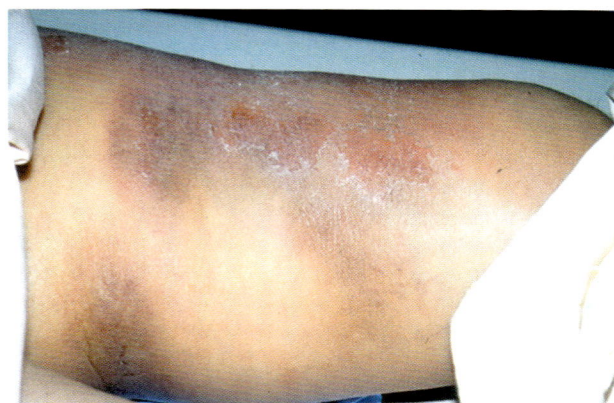

Figure 6–106 □ Subcutaneous panniculitis-like T-cell lymphoma. The other sites of predilection are the extremities. In this patient, the affected thigh is swollen with multiple dusky-looking subcutaneous plaques. Systemic involvement was present in the lymph nodes, bone marrow, and pelvis.

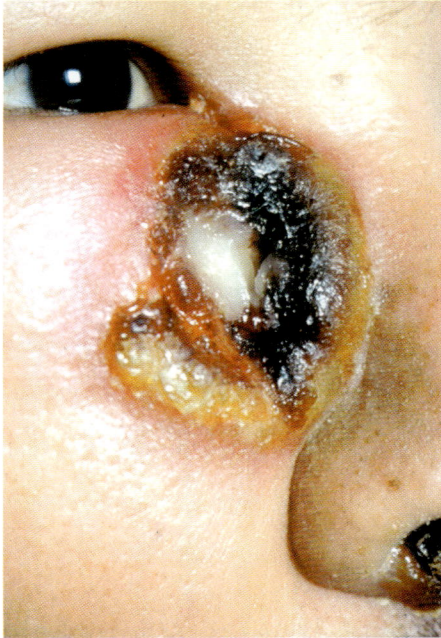

Figure 6–107 □ NK/T-cell lymphoma – nasal type. This Epstein-Barr virus (EBV)-associated lymphoma is more common in the Asia-Pacific region. The lymphoma is derived from natural killer (NK) or T-cells with NK-like features. Midline nasal or facial structures are the typical sites of involvement. Ulceration of lymphoma results from vascular destruction and tumor necrosis which are characteristic histological features.

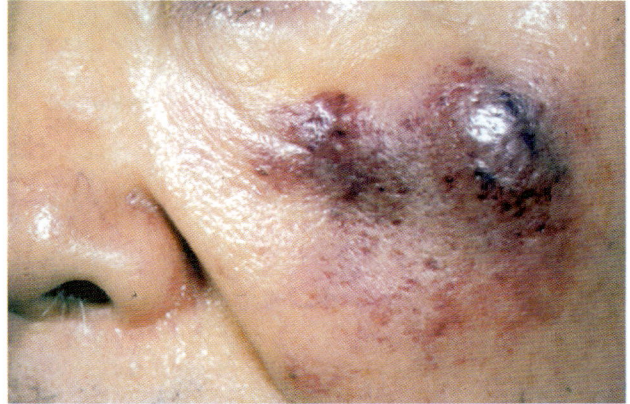

Figure 6–108 □ NK/T-cell lymphoma – disseminated. This tumor can present in sites other than the nasal region. In this patient, there are tumid dusky lesions on the cheeks and disseminated lesions elsewhere (see Figure 6–109). The patient did not have nasal or extracutaneous involvement at the time of presentation.

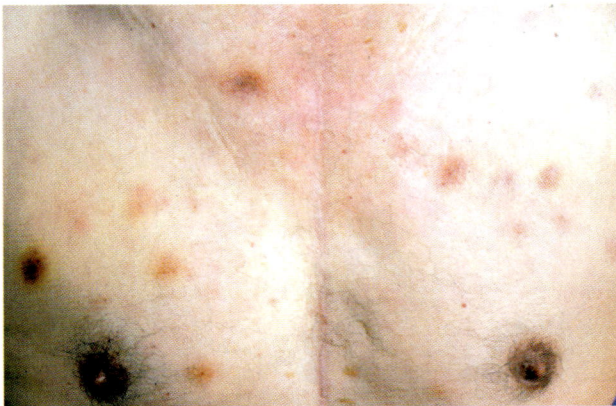

Figure 6–109 □ NK/T-cell lymphoma – disseminated. This patient had widespread multiple lesions on the trunk. The presence of disseminated disease carries an even poorer prognosis of this aggressive lymphoma. The patient eventually died of metastatic disease four years later.

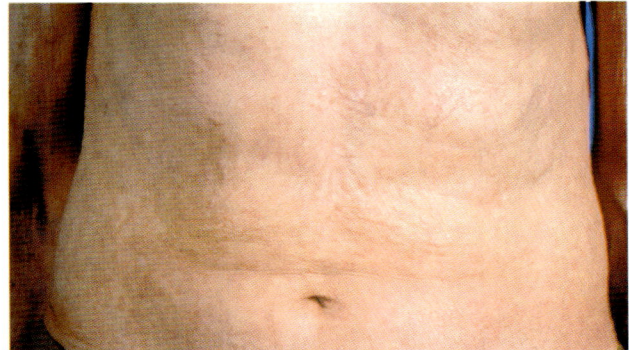

Figure 6–110 □ Adult T-cell lymphoma/leukaemia. This subset of T-cell lymphoma, related to HTLV-1 infection, is most frequently reported in the Carribbean region and Japan. This 71-year-old patient presented with smoldering papulonodular lesions for six years before he developed leukemia with multi-organ involvement.

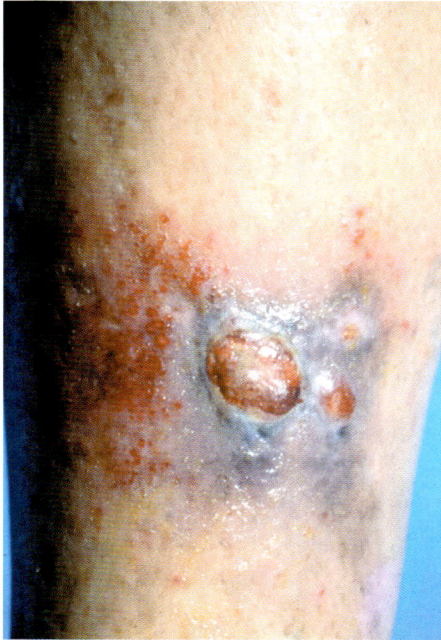

Figure 6–111 □ Large B-cell lymphoma of the leg. This nodular fleshy plaque on the leg of an 83-year-old man is histologically diagnosed as diffuse large B-cell lymphoma. This appears to be a distinctive subset of cutaneous B-cell lymphomas, presenting on the legs of elderly patients and carries a less favorable prognosis than other forms of primary cutaneous B-cell lymphoma.

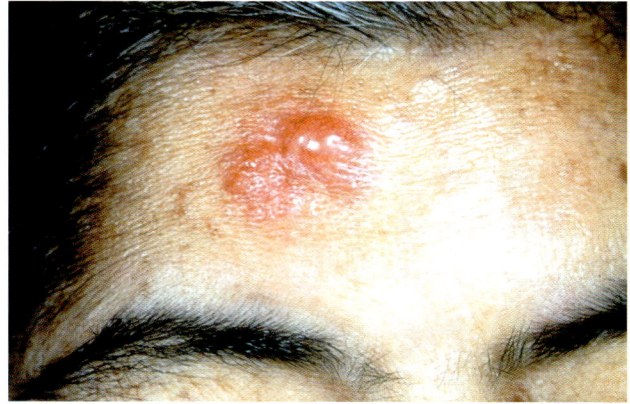

Figure 6–112 □ Cutaneous follicular center cell lymphoma. This middle-aged lady presents with erythematous nodules on the face, some of which have been self-healing for over a year. One such lesion is illustrated here: an irregular nodular plaque which is enlarging. This is a low-grade, primary, cutaneous B-cell lymphoma, which typically presents in the head and neck region.

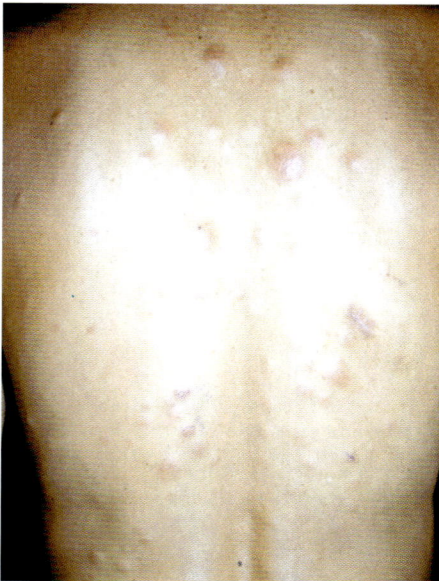

Figure 6–113 □ Cutaneous metastases. Multiple dermal nodules of sudden onset can be a manifestation of metastatic disease, following lymphatic or hematogenous spread. In this case, the patient has nasopharyngeal carcinoma.

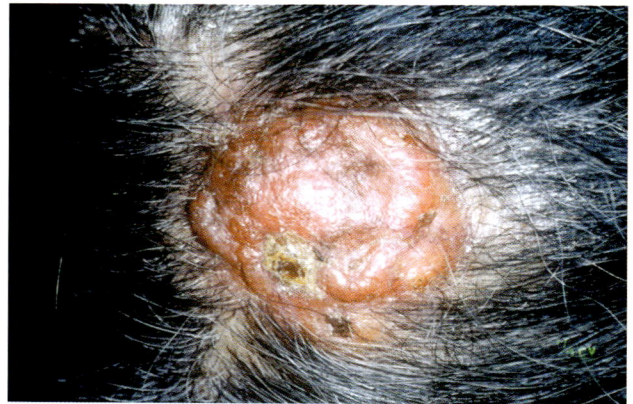

Figure 6–114 □ Cutaneous metastasis. The scalp is one of the favored sites for metastases because of its vascularity. This erythematous fleshy nodule is secondary to an adenocarcinoma in the colon. In some cases, the cutaneous metastasis may be the first indication of visceral cancer.

Pediatric Dermatology

Loh H.T.H. and Theng C.T.S.

Pediatric dermatology has emerged over the years as an important subspecialty of dermatology. Children, be they neonate, infant, toddler, or adolescent, are very dynamic beings, developing and changing constantly. New skin diseases will appear at different stages of development, and similarly, a skin disease will change in clinical features as the child grows older. Some skin diseases are unique in childhood whilst others overlap with those in adults. This chapter aims to highlight the common as well as some unique skin conditions seen in children.

VASCULAR TUMORS AND MALFORMATIONS (Figures 7–1 to 7–12)

Hemangioma typically appears not at birth but shortly afterward. There is a period of rapid growth within the first year that plateaus, with subsequent involution over the next several years. Treatments, such as intralesional and systemic steroids, surgical excision, or pulsed dye laser, are normally reserved for those lesions on critical anatomical sites, such as the periorbital and nasal areas, or if complicated by ulceration which is healing poorly. Unlike hemangiomas, vascular malformations are always present at birth and remain stable in size with no tendency to involute spontaneously. The malformation may affect capillaries, venules, or larger veins. Superficial lesions such as those affecting the capillaries, for example, port wine stains, respond well to the pulsed dye laser. Tufted angioma is a rare vascular tumor presenting at an older age and is associated with Kasabach-Merritt syndrome (thrombocytopenia, microangiopathic hemolytic anemia and consumption coagulopathy).

NEVI (Figures 7–13 to 7–17)

Nevi are harmatomas of skin cells. Those derived from melanocytes are termed melanocytic nevi. Melanocytic nevi can be divided into congenital and acquired types which have different clinical and histological features. Congenital melanocytic nevi are present at birth or appear within the first year of life. They are commonly larger than acquired melanocytic nevi with occasional giant lesions covering large areas of the body. A giant congenital melanocytic nevus is associated with significant risk of melanoma transformation and long-term follow-up with photographic documentation is necessary.

Epidermal nevi are derived from embryonic ectodermal cells that can differentiate into keratinocytes and other epidermal appendages. Keratinocyte nevi and sebaceous nevi are the more commonly seen epidermal nevi. Keratinocyte nevi are a cosmetic concern mainly and the risk of a secondary tumor developing is very low. They may be treated by carbon dioxide laser ablation or electrocautery, although recurrence often occurs following treatment. Sebaceous nevi, on the other hand, are associated with the development of secondary tumors usually after puberty; hence surgical removal is often advocated.

ACUTE EXANTHEMS (Figures 7–18 to 7–25)

An acute exanthem describes a rash of acute onset due to a bacterial or viral infection and drugs. Of these, viral exanthems are the most common exanthems encountered in clinical practice. With the implementation of compulsory MMR immunization in most Asian countries, classic viral exanthems, such as measles, rubella, and mumps, are now rarely encountered. Newer exanthems, such as erythema infectiosum, Giannotti-Crosti syndrome, and unilateral laterothoracic exanthem, are increasingly being described and recognized.

The morphology of a viral exanthem can be rather non-specific and similar to a drug exanthem. Differentiation of the two often relies on the distribution and evolution of the rash, and the temporal relationship to any drug ingested. Useful differential features include the association of a febrile illness in viral exanthem and the presence of significant pruritus in drug exanthem. Careful history-taking and subsequent drug allergy evaluation (including an oral drug provocation test) are essential approaches in evaluating such patients.

Whilst most exanthems are relatively benign and can be left on its own to resolve spontaneously, notable exceptions include Kawasaki disease and meningoccocemia which must be diagnosed early to start specific medical treatment to minimize subsequent morbidity or mortality.

INFECTIONS (Figures 7–39 to 7–42)

Bacterial and viral infections are common in children. Impetigo, viral wart, and molluscum contagiosum are the most common skin infections seen. *Staphylococcus* and *streptococcus* are the most common causative agents in impetigo, the bullous variety being caused by *Staphylococcus*. Mild bacterial infections can be treated effectively with topical antibiotics such as topical fucidin or mupirocin. More severe and extensive bacterial infections require the administration of systemic antibiotics either orally or parenterally. Viral wart and molluscum contagiosum in children can be difficult to treat. Locally destructive methods commonly used in adults, such as cryotherapy and electrocautery, cause pain and are poorly tolerated by most young children. In Asians with pigmented skin, post-inflammatory pigmentary changes secondary to such destructive treatment can be long lasting and disfiguring. As these viral skin infections often clear eventually when the body's acquired immunity develops, reassurance to parents regarding the benign and self-resolving nature of the disease is often enough to convince them to opt for expectant management. Should active treatment be opted for, all attempts must be made to minimize the discomfort of treatment, for example, applying a topical anesthetic to the area prior to destructive treatment.

INFLAMMATORY DERMATOSES
(Figures 7–54 to 7–57, 7–61 to 7–63)

Atopic dermatitis is common in most developed Asian cities as in the West. The onset is often within the first year of life. Differentiation from infantile seborrheic dermatitis can be difficult, with less pruritus and involvement of the groin area suggesting seborrheic dermatitis. In tropical countries, hot weather and sweating are common aggravating factors, and they make the application of oily ointments uncomfortable. Diaper dermatitis is an irritant contact dermatitis due to urine and feces retained within the diaper. It is very common with the increasing use of diapers in preference to napkins. Psoriasis is relatively uncommon in children but earlier onset may signify more severe disease and familial involvement. Lichen striatus is not uncommon; it invariably resolves spontaneously though the initial extension of lesions along Blaschko's lines often causes much concern to parents.

PIGMENTARY DISORDERS
(Figures 7–26 to 7–34)

Pigmentary birthmark is a frequent reason for referral to the dermatology clinic. Often, the pigmentary birthmark poses no problem other than cosmetic concerns (e.g. nevus depigmentosus, Mongolian blue spot, nevus of Ota). However, some of them reflect an underlying genetic mosaicism and are associated with systemic anomalies (e.g. linear and whorled hyperpigmentation, incontinentia pigmenti, hypomelanosis of Ito). Some pigmentary birthmarks act as an early marker for an underlying syndrome (e.g. café au lait macule, ash leaf macule). An accurate diagnosis is essential before advising parents on the implications and prognosis. Acquired hypopigmentary disorders, such as pityriasis alba or post-inflammatory hypopigmentation, are more obvious in pigmented Asian patients. Depigmentary disorders, such as vitiligo, are particularly disfiguring and carry a significant social stigma in certain cultures such as in the Asian-Indians.

MASTOCYTOSIS (Figures 7–43 to 7–45)

Mastocytosis is a term used to describe a wide spectrum of conditions characterized by local or diffuse increase of mast cells in the skin or other organs. The severity and prognosis are related to total increase in mast cells load as reflected in the extent of systemic involvement. Localized cutaneous lesions without systemic involvement, for example in mastocytoma and urticaria pigmentosa, carry a good prognosis, whilst the rare mast cell leukemia has a very poor prognosis. At presentation, a detailed physical examination is necessary, and long-term follow-up is required to monitor the evolution.

HISTIOCYTOSIS (Figures 7–50 to 7–53)

Histiocytosis is a term used to describe all proliferative disorders of monocytes, macrophages (non-Langerhans cell histiocytosis), and dendritic cells (Langerhans cell histiocytosis). The proliferation can involve a local cutaneous site or multiple internal organs or as leukemia. Some examples are given in this chapter.

NEONATAL CONDITIONS
(Figures 7–35 to 7–37)

A group of common transient disorders seen in neonates deserves special mention. Erythema toxicum neonatorum is the most common eruption seen in neonates. Reassurance is all that is required for anxious parents. Stork mark or nevus flammeus neonatorum may at times be confused with port wine stain but it becomes lighter and resolves with time. Milia are multiple small epidermal cysts seen commonly in neonates. Also commonly seen are sebaceous hyperplasias on the nose, as well as acneiform eruptions often termed as neonatal acnes. Both are due to the relative hyperandrogenic state of neonates immediately after birth. The cutaneous features of neonatal lupus erythematosus (Figure 7–58) are transient but the associated complete heart block must not be missed. Genodermatoses, such as the congenital ichthyoses and epidermolysis bullosa, may present during the neonatal period; this group of disorders are covered in Chapter 8 on genodermatoses.

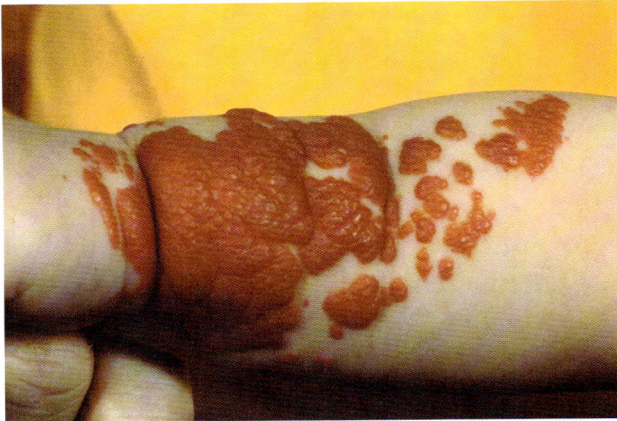

Figure 7–1 □ Hemangioma. Hemangioma of infancy is the most common benign tumor in childhood. It exhibits a proliferation and involution phase. This picture shows a typical "strawberry nevus", which presents clinically as bright red lobulated nodules or plaques. A hemangioma grows rapidly for up to one year of life. Shortly afterwards, it begins to involute. Full involution may take up to ten years.

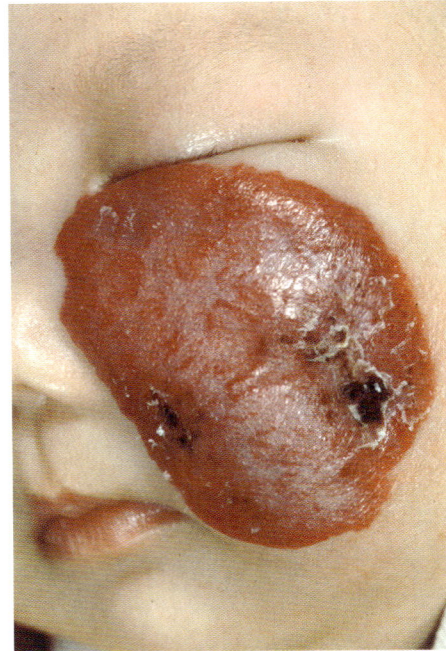

Figure 7–2 □ Hemangioma. Ulceration is a complication of hemangioma which necessitates medical intervention. Amblyopia is another complication where active treatment is indicated. Hemangiomas occurring in the periorbital region may obstruct the visual axis causing subsequent maldevelopment of normal binocular vision. A referral for ophthalmologic assessment is warranted in such cases.

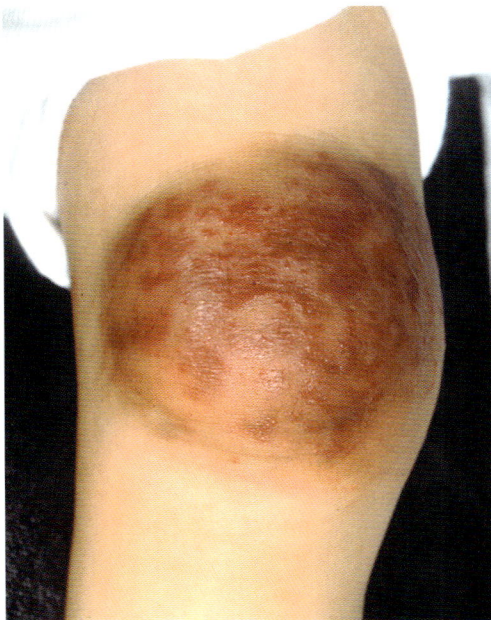

Figure 7–3 □ Tufted angioma. This slow-growing, reddish-brown vascular plaque on the lower limb is a tufted angioma, a rare vascular tumor. Tufted angiomas usually appear in childhood. The typical sites of involvement are the neck, upper trunk, and shoulders. They may grow slowly for several years before stopping and generally do not regress spontaneously. Kasabach-Merritt syndrome can occur with a large tufted angioma.

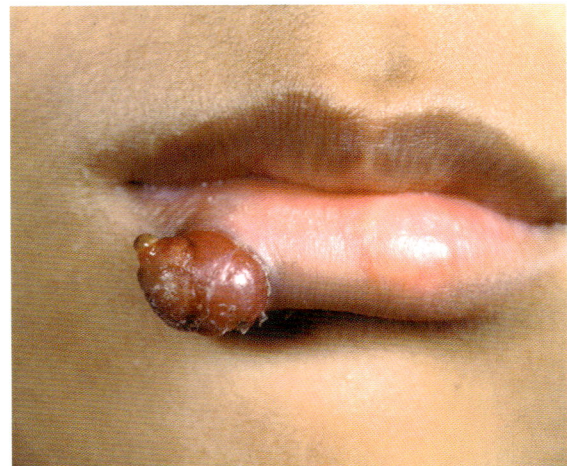

Figure 7–4 □ Pyogenic granuloma. This fleshy red nodule on the lower lip is a classical example of a pyogenic granuloma. Pyogenic granuloma is a relatively common benign vascular lesion that presents clinically as a bright red, polypoid, friable papule, or nodule which often bleeds after minor trauma. There may be a history of preceding trauma.

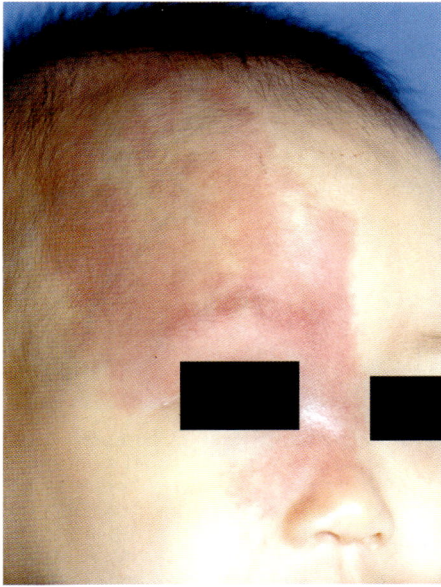

Figure 7–5 □ Port wine stain. This young child presented at birth with a unilateral erythematous vascular patch over the face. Port wine stain is a capillary malformation that persists throughout life. It frequently occurs on the face and is usually unilateral. It presents as a vascular macular patch at birth, which may gradually darken and become hypertrophic with time. The presence of port wine stain in the distribution of the ophthalmic branch of trigeminal nerve may indicate an underlying Sturge-Weber syndrome.

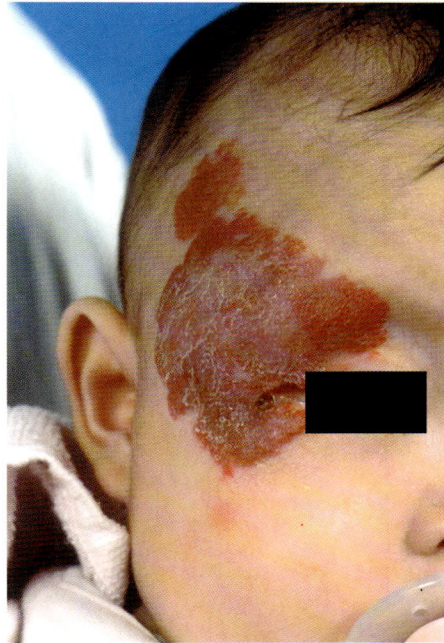

Figure 7–6 □ Venous malformation. This young boy has a vascular malformation not only affecting the capillary (as in port wine stain) but also the deeper venous vessels. The lesion appears as a raised erythematous plaque rather than a flat lesion as in port wine stain.

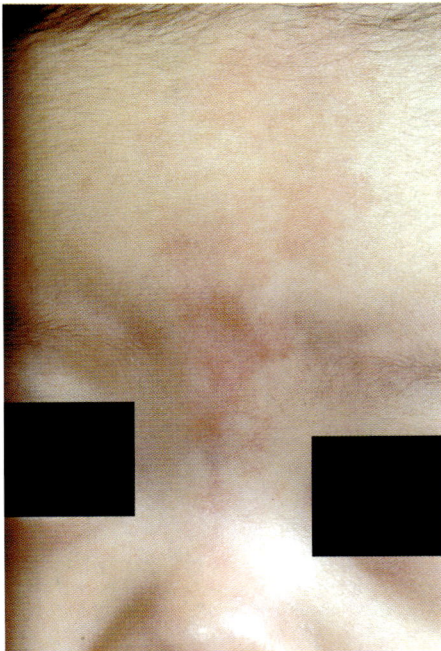

Figure 7–7 □ Nevus flammeus neonatorum. Commonly known as stork mark, nevus flammeus neonatorum is much more common than port wine stain. Generally lighter than port wine stain, it is commonly found on the midline glabella, eyelids, and occipital scalp. The facial lesions are usually transient and lighten or resolve within the first year of life. The occipital lesions tend to persist.

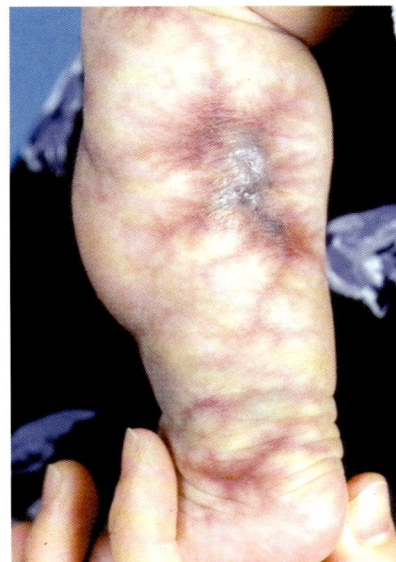

Figure 7–8 □ Cutis marmorata telangiectatica congenita. Cutis marmorata telangiectatica congenita is a vascular disorder that presents as an erythematous reticulate macule or patch giving a mottling appearance. In severe cases, there may be atrophy or ulceration as seen in this baby girl. It may be localized or generalized. The lower limbs are the most commonly affected sites. They usually resolve over time but ulcerated lesions often leave scars and persistent pigmentation. Vascular malformation, skeletal and neurological anomalies are known associations.

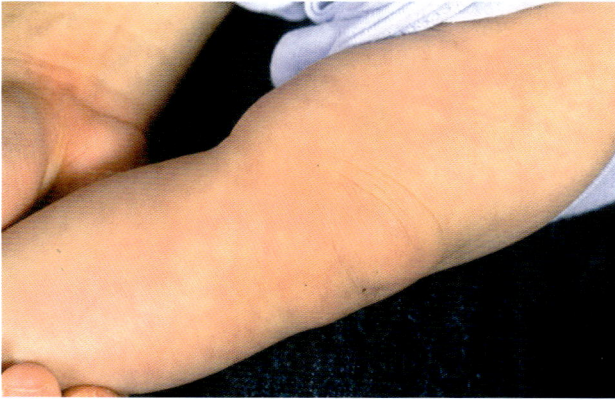

Figure 7–9 □ Cutis marmorata. This picture shows cutis marmorata in a baby. This is a physiological phenomenon commonly seen in infants upon exposure to cold. It appears as diffuse, reticulate, erythematous macules on the exposed limbs. The transient nature of the lesion distinguishes it from cutis marmorata telangiectatica congenital. No atrophy and ulceration are seen in this condition.

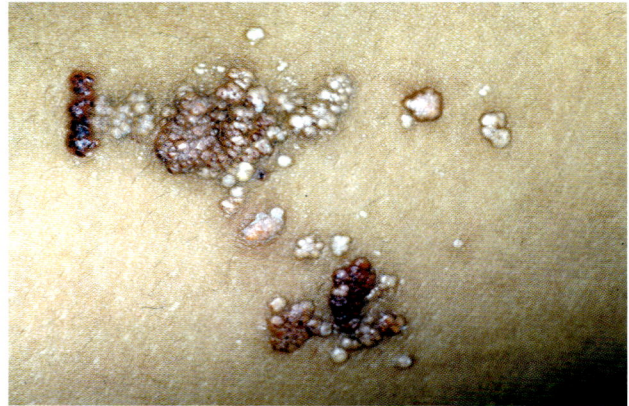

Figure 7–10 □ Lymphangioma circumscriptum. Lymphangioma circumscriptum is the most common form of cutaneous lymphatic malformations. It presents clinically as translucent or hemorrhagic vesicles occurring in clusters, classically described as "frog-spawn" as illustrated in this picture. It may occur at birth or appear later in life. It commonly occurs on the shoulders, axillae, and proximal extremities. Recurrences following surgical excision are common.

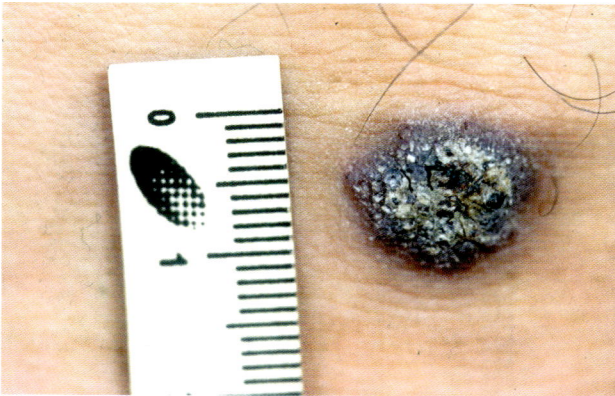

Figure 7–11 □ Angiokeratoma of Mibelli. Angiokeratomas are composed of dilated vessels in the capillary dermis associated with epidermal hyperkeratosis. There are several subtypes of angiokeratomas. Angiokeratoma of Mibelli usually appears during childhood to adolescence; it appears as a verrucous, hyperkeratotic purplish nodule or plaque as seen on the left heel of this boy. It commonly occurs on the dorsum of the hands and feet.

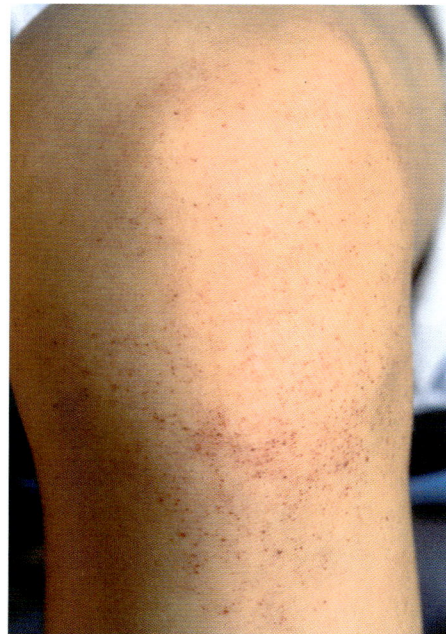

Figure 7–12 □ Angiokeratoma corporis diffusum. Angiokeratoma corporis diffusum presents with eruption of multiple scattered small, red, non-blanchable papules as seen on the knee of this boy. Sites of predilection include the buttocks, abdomen, flanks, and thighs. The condition may be associated with lysosomal hydrolase α-galactosidase deficiency (Fabry's disease). Fabry's disease is an autosomal recessive condition associated with renal, cardiac, and ocular abnormalities.

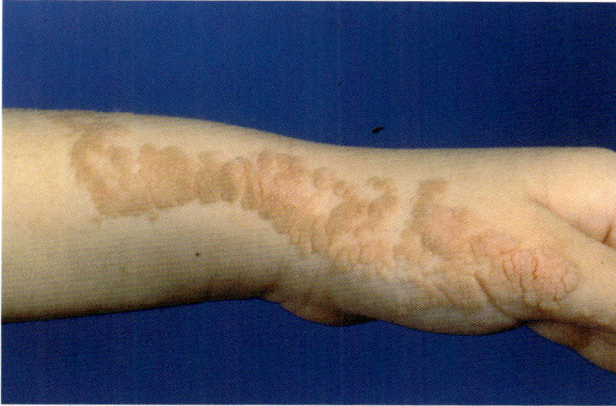

Figure 7–13 □ Epidermal nevus. This lesion on the forearm of this child is a linear verrucous epidermal nevus. An epidermal nevus is a harmatoma of the epidermal structures of the skin. It usually presents at birth or infancy and gradually enlarges during childhood and plateaus in the adolescent years. On the limbs, it tends to follow the lines of Blaschko. It often presents initially as closely grouped papules that subsequently coalesce to form a verrucous plaque.

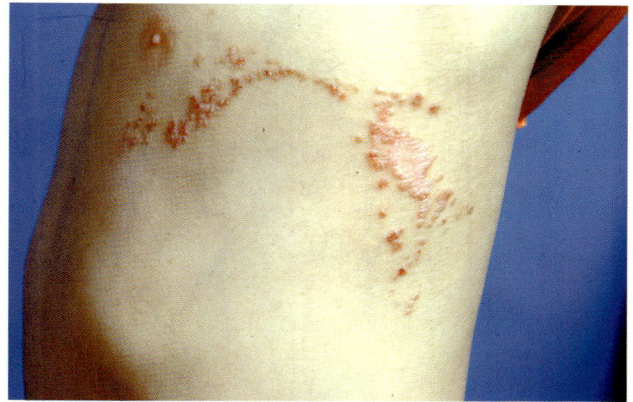

Figure 7–14 □ Inflammatory linear verrucous epidermal nevus. This adolescent girl has an inflammatory linear verrucous epidermal nevus on her trunk, seen here as unilateral, erythematous, coalescing papules and plaques in a linear distribution on the trunk. The lesions are inflamed and pruritic. Inflammatory linear verrucous epidermal nevus is usually localized and unilateral although bilateral widespread lesions may occur.

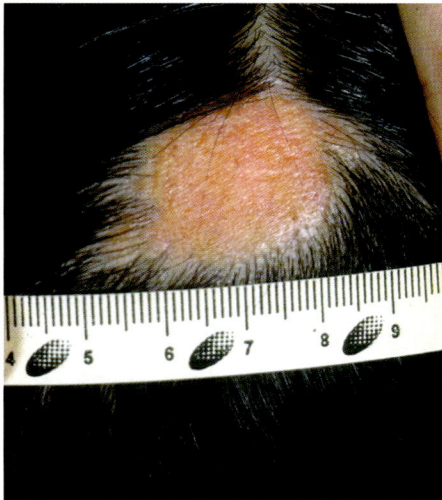

Figure 7–15 □ Nevus sebaceous. This yellowish verrucous plaque on the scalp of this four-year-old child is a nevus sebaceous. It often presents at birth as a relatively flat lesion on the face or scalp. After puberty, it becomes thicker and more verrucous. There is an increased risk of developing tumors such as syringocystadenoma papilliferum and basal cell carcinoma later in life (usually after puberty). Treatment by surgical excision is therefore recommended.

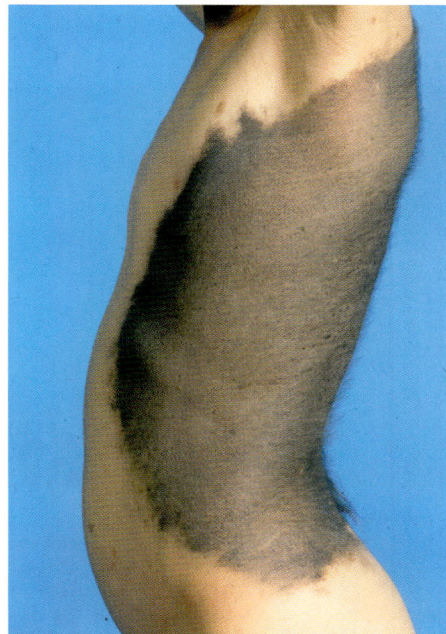

Figure 7–16 □ Congenital melanocytic nevus. This child presented at birth with a large pigmented hairy plaque on the trunk. This is a giant congenital melanocytic nevus or bathing trunk nevus. Satellite nevi are seen near the main lesion. A giant congenital melanocytic nevus has a significant risk of malignant change. Such lesions should be closely followed up for life. Involvement over the head, neck, and spine may be associated with leptomeningeal melanocytosis.

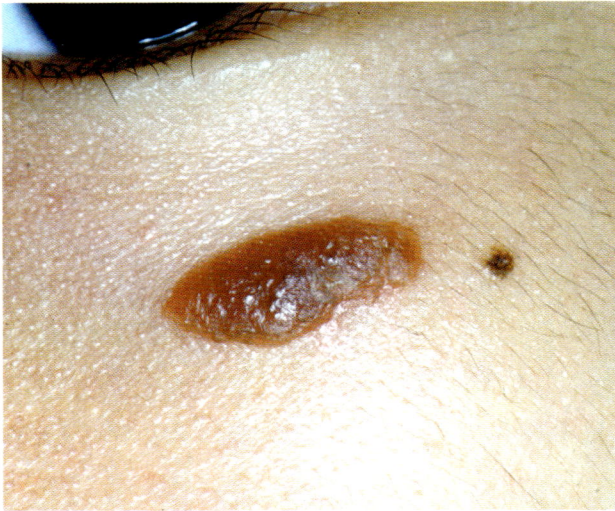

Figure 7–17 □ Spitz nevus. This reddish-brown nodule on this child is typical of a Spitz nevus. This uncommon nevi of melanocytic origin occurs mainly on the face, neck, and lower extremities. It is a benign lesion although the histological features may resemble malignant melanoma. Treatment is by surgical excision.

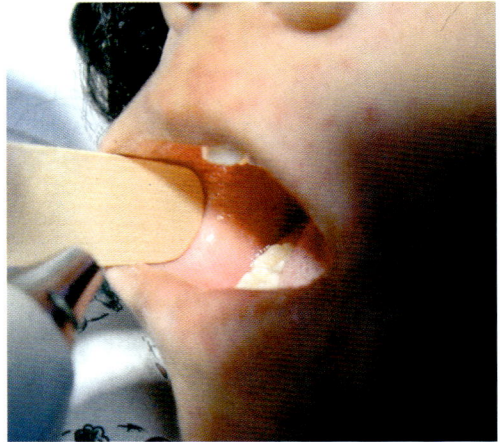

Photograph courtesy of Professor Quak Seng Hock, The Children's Medical Institute, National University Hospital, Singapore.

Figure 7–18 □ Measles. The exanthem is preceded by a prodrome of high fever, coryza, cough, conjunctivitis, and Koplik's spots for two to four days. It appears initially as an erythematous maculo-papular rash along the hairline and retroauricular skin with a subsequent downward spread. It is asymptomatic and fades with fine skin peeling from head down by day 5. Koplik's spots appear as white papules on red bases on the lateral buccal mucosae.

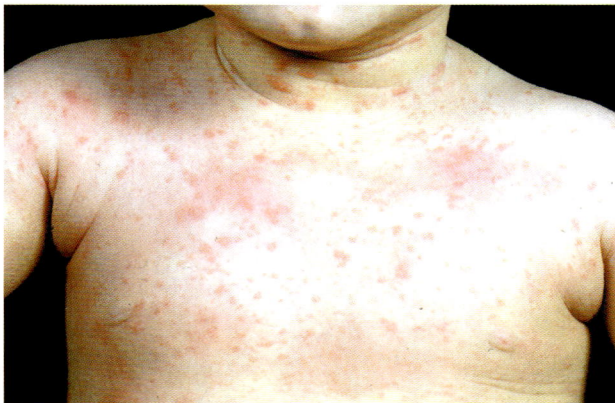

Figure 7–19 □ Roseola. After having a high fever for three days, this child has developed an erythematous maculo-papular rash on his trunk on the fourth day coinciding with resolution of the fever. This is typical of roseola infantum (exanthema subitum). The exanthem usually fades within 48 hours. Roseola is a common cause of febrile convulsions in an infant and is caused by human herpesvirus 6.

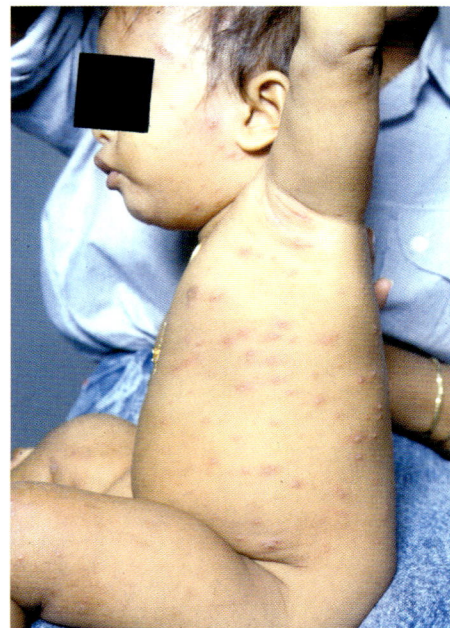

Figure 7–20 □ Varicella (chicken pox). Multiple erythematous macules, vesicles, and crusted erosions are present on the trunk and face of this boy. The exanthem of varicella is typically polymorphic with different lesions at different stages of development. Significant pruritus may be present. The eruption lasts seven to 14 days and appears in crops.

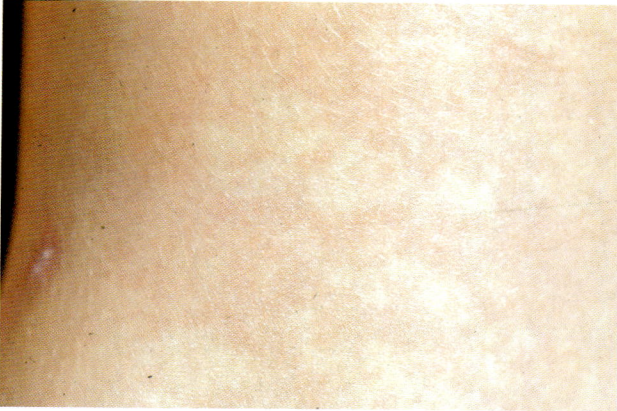

Figure 7–21 □ Erythema infectiosum. Erythema infectiosum or "Fifth disease" is caused by parvovirus B19. It typically presents with a "slapped cheek" appearance of the face, which is followed by a reticulated maculo-papular rash developing on the lower limbs as seen in this child. Mild constitutional symptoms precede the development of skin manifestations. The disease is self-limiting and resolves spontaneously over several days.

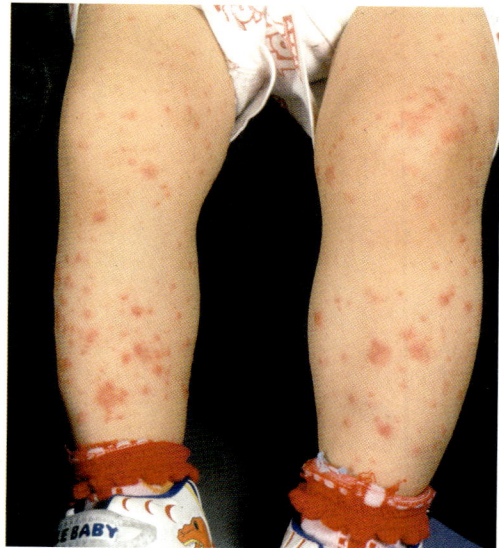

Figure 7–22 □ Giannotti-Crosti syndrome. This child has monomorphic, erythematous papules which are symmetrically distributed over the lower limbs. This is Giannotti-Crosti syndrome. The eruption occurs mainly in pre-school children. It is associated mainly with viral infections such as the Epstein-Barr and hepatitis B virus. It usually resolves within several weeks and does not normally recur.

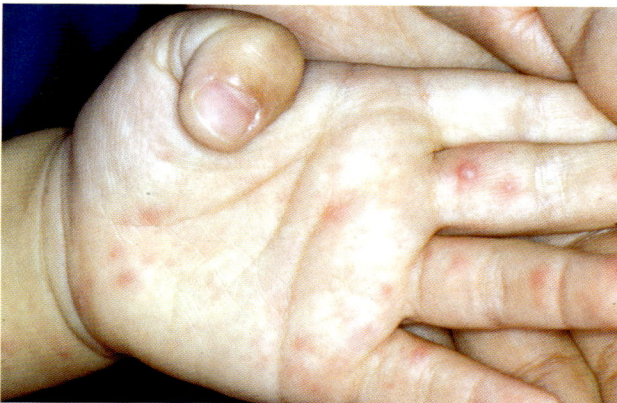

Figure 7–23 □ Hand, foot and mouth disease. There are multiple vesicles on erythematous bases on the palm of this young child with hand, foot, and mouth disease. Similar vesicles on the soles and painful oral ulcers are present as well. He is febrile with mild constitutional symptoms. This is usually a benign self-limiting infection, commonly caused by the coxsackie virus and enterovirus. Recent outbreaks in Southeast Asia and Taiwan due to enterovirus 71 resulted in some mortality in pre-school children.

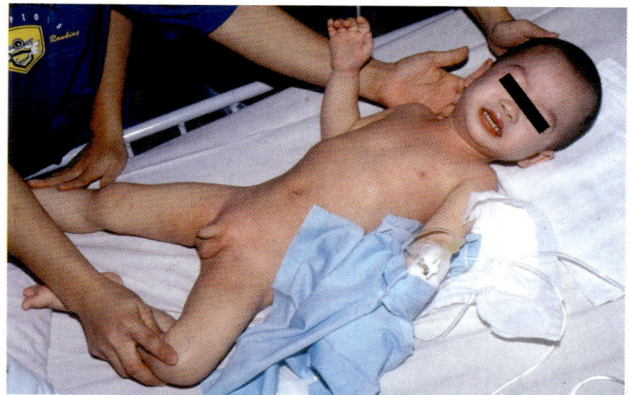

Photograph courtesy of Professor Quak Seng Hock, The Children's Medical Institute, National University Hospital, Singapore.

Figure 7–24 □ Kawasaki's disease. This young child has high fever, irritability, conjunctivitis, stomatitis, a strawberry tongue, cervical lymphadenopathy, intense erythema of hands and feet, and an erythematous maculo-papular rash. He fulfills the diagnostic criteria for Kawasaki's disease. Early recognition of this disease is important for timely administration of intravenous immunoglobulins, which has been shown to prevent the complication of myocarditis and the formation of coronary artery aneurysm.

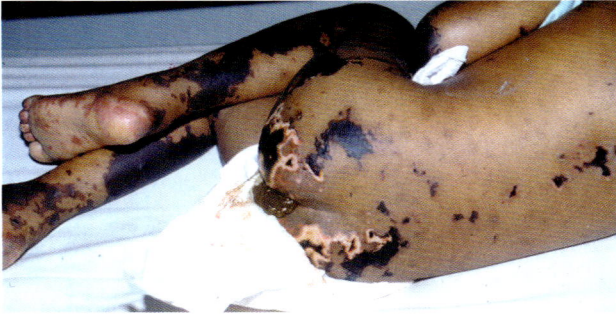

Photograph courtesy of Professor Quak Seng Hock, The Children's Medical Institute, National University Hospital, Singapore.

Figure 7–25 □ Meningococcal septicemia. This is a rapidly progressing fatal complication of meningococcal infection. The rash often appears early when other clinical features are non-specific, and thus recognition is important for early intervention to avert mortality. The rash appears initially as petechiae or purpuric macules which coalesce to form large, irregular, hemorrhagic, and necrotic lesions. Skin lesions may be generalized affecting both trunk and limbs extensively.

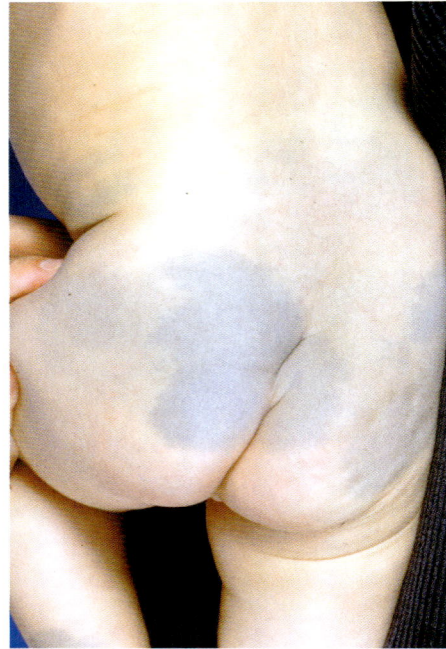

Figure 7–26 □ Mongolian blue spot. This is a very common birthmark found in Asian babies. It usually presents at birth as a bluish-gray patch over the lumbar-sacral area. The pigmentation comes from melanocytes entrapped deep in the dermis during their embryonic migration from the neural crest to the epidermis. The pigmentation usually resolves spontaneously by early childhood.

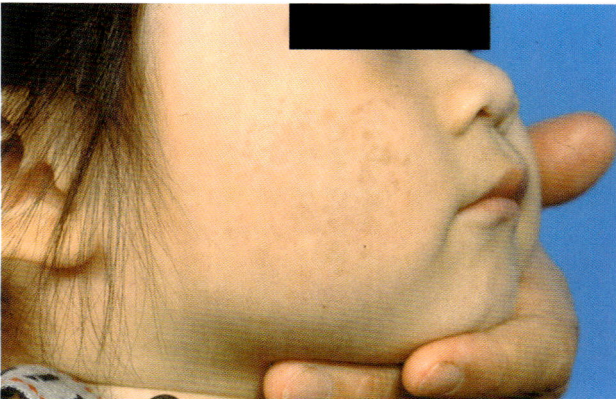

Figure 7–27 □ Nevus of Ota. This is a condition of dermal melanocytosis seen predominantly in Asian-Orientals. It is usually unilateral and presents as a blue-gray speckled confluent macule or patch over the forehead, temple, zygomatic, or periorbital areas. It may be associated with scleral and retinal hypermelanosis as well as glaucoma. This condition responds well to the Q-switched Alexandrite and Q-switched Nd-YAG lasers although multiple treatment sessions are required.

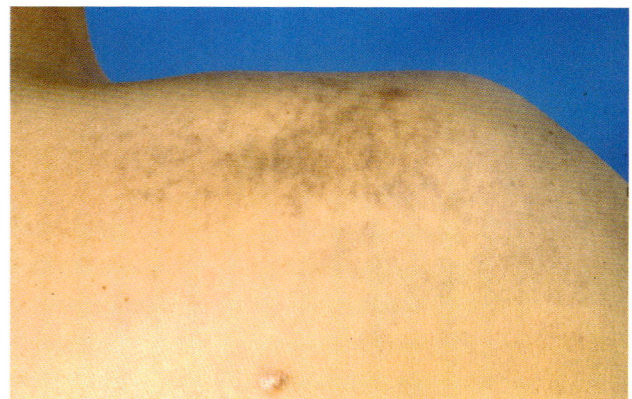

Figure 7–28 □ Nevus of Ito. This dermal melanocytosis is the counterpart of nevus of Ota that occurs on the upper arm or shoulder instead of on the face. Nevus of Ota and nevus of Ito typically appear at birth or shortly afterwards, or during early adolescence.

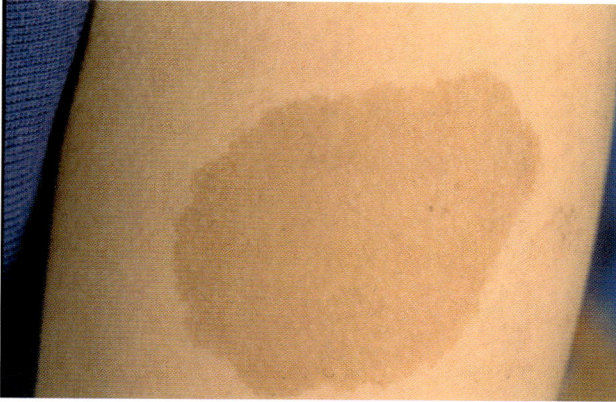

Figure 7–29 □ Café au lait macule. This often appears at birth or early infancy as a well-circumscribed, tanned, brown macule varying in size from a few millimeters to more than 10 cm. The number varies from being solitary to multiple. The border may be regular or irregular. Presence of multiple lesions is a marker for neurofibromatosis.

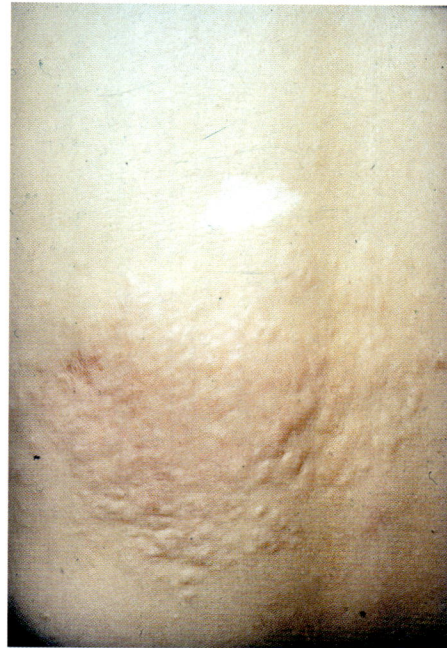

Figure 7–30 □ Ash leaf macule. This is often the first manifestation of tuberous sclerosis especially if multiple. It presents at birth or early infancy as a well-circumscribed, hypopigmented macule with irregular borders. This patient with tuberous sclerosis also has a large confluent shagreen patch (a connective tissue nevus) on the lower back below the ash leaf macule.

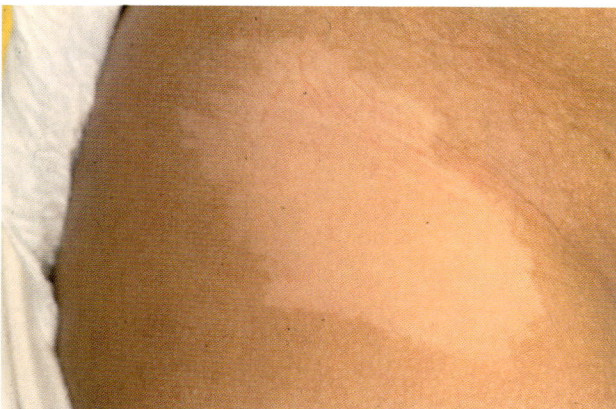

Figure 7–31 □ Nevus depigmentosus. This nevoid lesion presents at birth as a solitary, well-circumscribed patch of hypopigmentation with irregular outline on the face, trunk, or limbs. The lesion is usually a few centimeters in size. The lesion often persists with no effective treatment available. Multiple lesions can occur, and may pose a diagnostic difficulty from ash leaf macules of tuberous sclerosis.

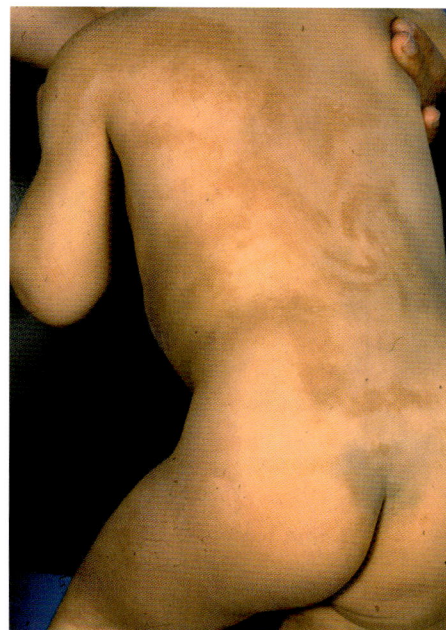

Figure 7–32 □ Linear and whorled hypermelanosis. This is the term used to describe a sporadic disorder of hyperpigmentation seen at birth or that develops within first two years of life. The pigmentation is distributed along lines of Blaschko in a linear and whorled pattern. Co-existing cardiac and neurological anomalies have been reported.

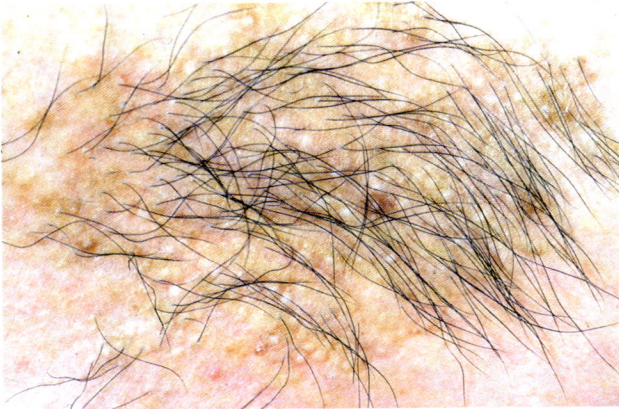

Figure 7–33 □ Becker's nevus. This sporadic condition appears around puberty with an area of hyperpigmentation and hypertrichosis. The pigmentation is light to dark brown, irregular, and often geographical. It appears most commonly on the trunk and upper shoulder.

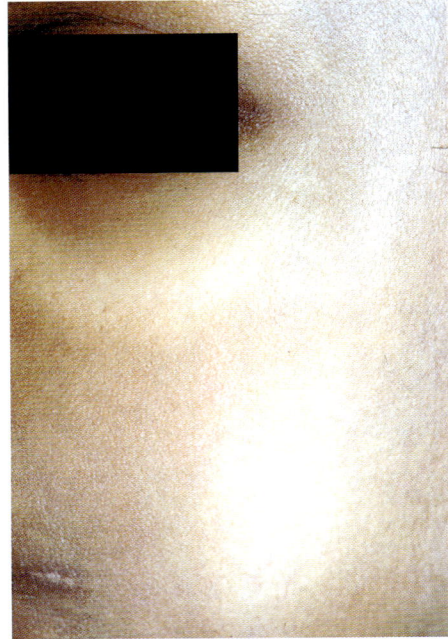

Figure 7–34 □ Pityriasis alba. This benign inflammatory dermatosis primarily affects young children aged six to 12 years. It appears on the face and arms as single or multiple patches of hypopigmentation with indistinct edges. The lesions measure one to several centimeters in size. Fine scaling may be present. The condition is asymptomatic and often persists for several months to years. It is more obvious in pigmented Asians or after sun tanning.

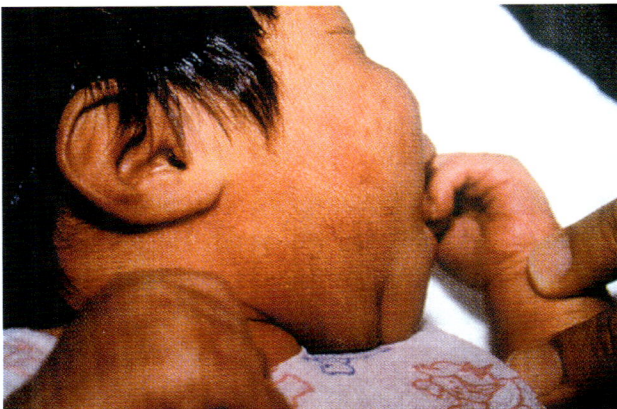

Photograph courtesy of Professor Quak Seng Hock, The Children's Medical Institute, National University Hospital, Singapore.

Figure 7–35 □ Erythema toxicum neonatorum. This is the most common transient rash seen in neonates. This idiopathic rash usually appears during the first week of life as multiple erythematous macules or patches with or without a central papule or pustule. The eruption is found mainly on the trunk but involvement of the face and limbs have been seen as well. It is asymptomatic and resolves spontaneously after a few days.

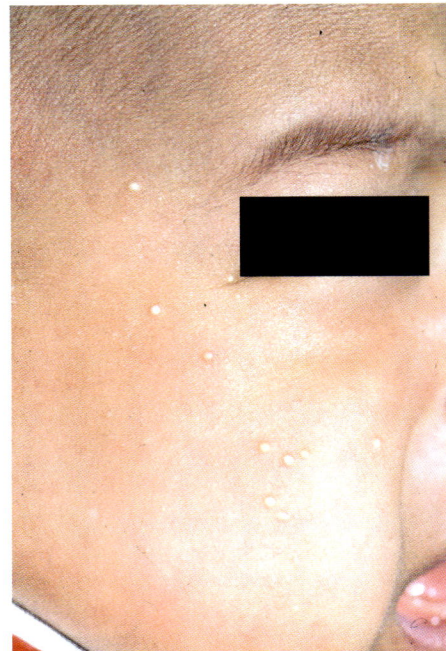

Figure 7–36 □ Milia. This is a very common transient skin finding in neonates. Multiple white or yellow small papules are found on the nose, cheeks, chin, and forehead. They often resolve spontaneously within a few weeks. Epstein's pearls are essentially milia found on the hard palate in newborns.

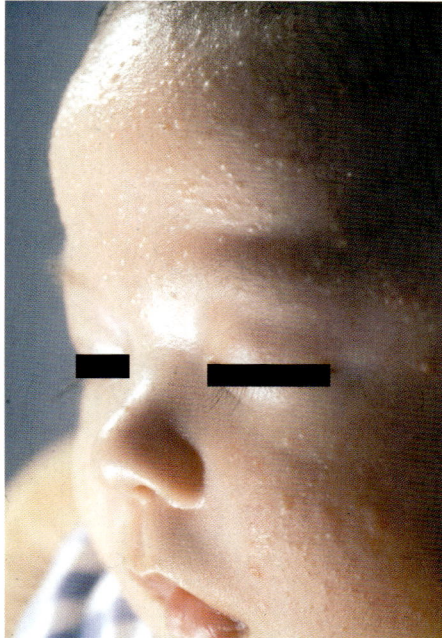

Figure 7–37 □ Miliaria. Miliaria is thought to be eccrine disorders secondary to occlusion of the sweat ducts. Heat and humidity leading to increased sweating are the primary stimuli. Depending on the level of occlusion, papules, vesicles, or pustules may result. This baby has miliaria pustulosa and rubra appearing as multiple small, red papules and pustules on the face.

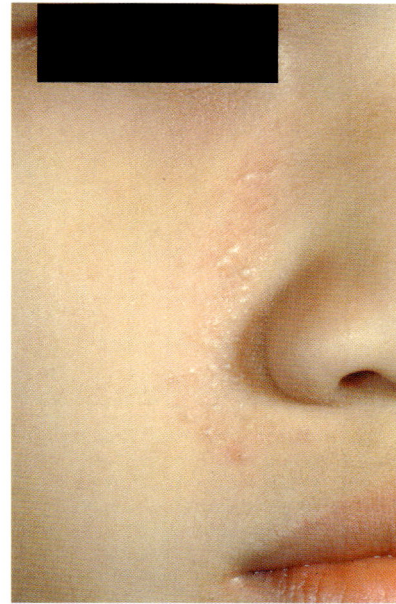

Figure 7–38 □ Milia en plaque. This young girl presents with multiple milia overlying an erythematous, linear plaque on the right medial cheek along the right nasolabial fold. Previously reported cases have involved predominantly the ears and the eyelids.

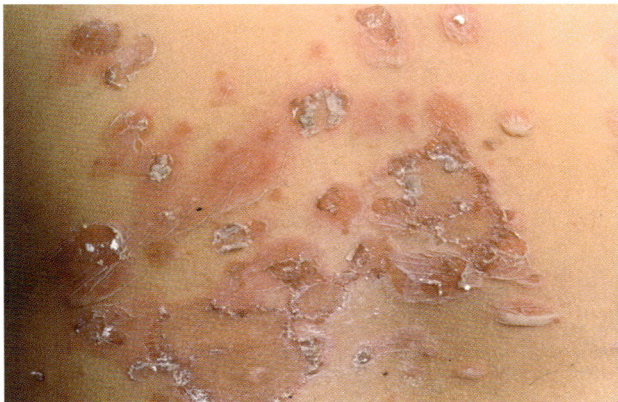

Figure 7–39 □ Bullous impetigo. Impetigo is a common childhood bacterial skin infection. Multiple thin-roofed bullae occur in the bullous variety of impetigo. These would rupture easily, leaving behind weeping denuded areas. Pus can sometimes be present within the bullae. *Staphylococcus aureus* producing epidermolytic toxin is responsible. This condition should be treated with a course of systemic antibiotics such as cloxacillin or cephalexin.

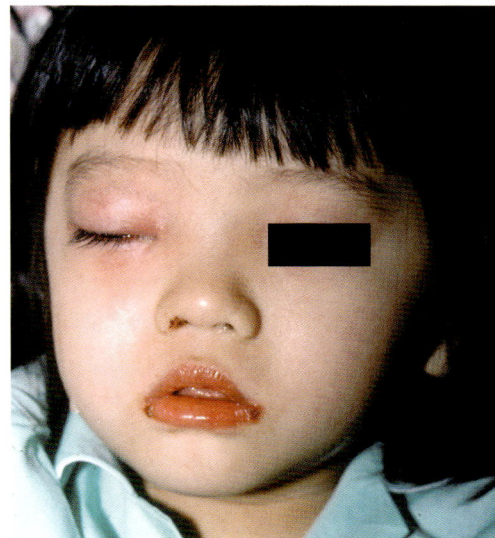

Photograph courtesy of Professor Quak Seng Hock, The Children's Medical Institute, National University Hospital, Singapore.

Figure 7–40 □ Periorbital cellulitis. Cellulitis is skin infection involving the deep dermis and subcutaneous tissue. It presents as erythematous swelling with indistinct and spreading borders. Involvement of the periorbital area and face of young children is often due to *Hemophilus influenzae* rather than *Staphylococcus aureus* or *Streptococcus pyogenes* which are the most common organisms causing cellulitis elsewhere. Urgent ophthalmologic referral is needed if there is evidence of orbital extension.

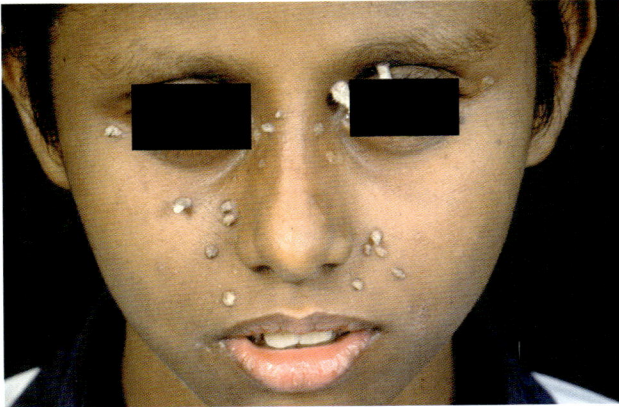

Figure 7–41 □ Viral wart. Viral wart is caused by the human papilloma virus. This boy has multiple filiform-type warts on his face. The lesions appear as papilliferous projections on fleshy bases. Psychological distress associated with these unsightly lesions often necessitates treatment. Light electrocautery and cryotherapy are common therapies used, although post-inflammatory pigmentary changes are common in pigmented Asians.

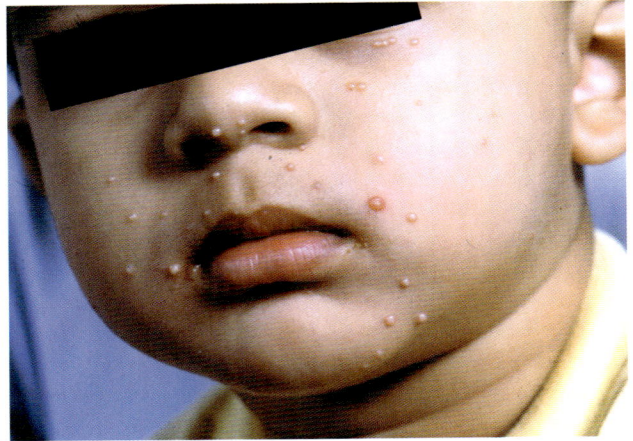

Figure 7–42 □ Molluscum contagiosum. This common childhood infection is caused by a pox virus. The typical morphology is that of a dome-shaped, flesh-colored, or pearly papule with an umbilicated center. The papule is usually less than 1 cm in size. Lesions occur commonly on the axillae, neck, and trunk. Ano-genital lesions do not necessarily signify sexual abuse in children.

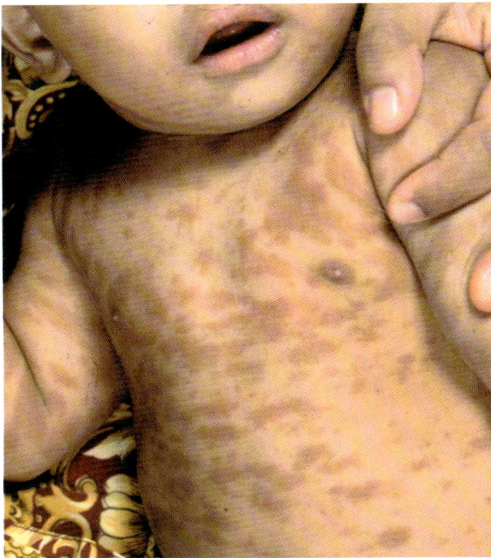

Figure 7–43 □ Urticaria pigmentosa. This is the most common mastocytosis in children. This child presents with multiple reddish-brown macules and plaques on the trunk and limbs. Systemic involvement is uncommon in children as compared to adults.

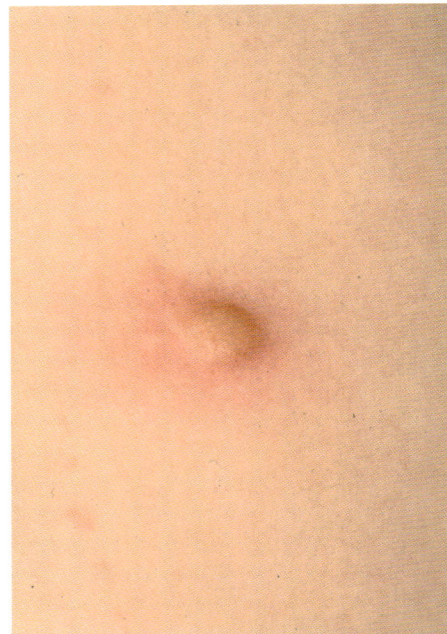

Figure 7–44 □ Urticaria pigmentosa – Darier's sign. An urticarial reaction comprising a weal and erythema forms soon after rubbing the lesion of urticaria pigmentosa. This reflects degranulation of the mast cells. Patients with urticaria pigmentosa should avoid ingestion of mast cells degranulators such as opiates, polymyxin, and non-steroidal anti-inflammatory drugs.

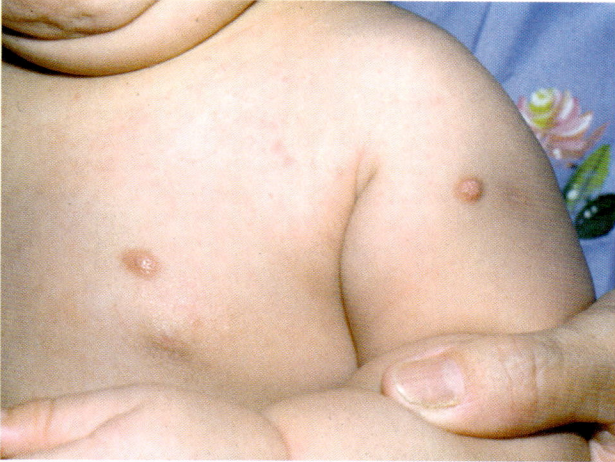

Figure 7–45 □ Mastocytoma. This is the second most common mastocytosis in children after urticaria pigmentosa. The lesion appears as a reddish-brown macule, papule, or nodule. Onset is usually during the first two years of life. Darier's sign may be positive. Multiple lesions may be present as seen in this baby. Systemic involvement is uncommon.

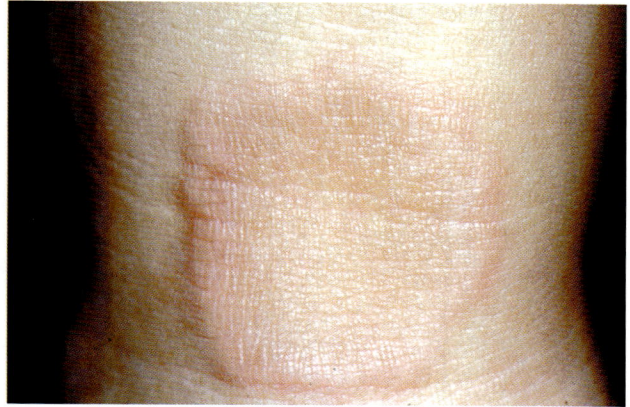

Figure 7–46 □ Granuloma annulare. This self-limiting, benign, inflammatory condition affects children and young adults. Histologically, there is degeneration of dermal collagen and the presence of a lympho-histiocytic infiltrate within the dermis. The most common form in children is the localized variant which consists of multiple smooth, firm, skin-colored papules forming an annular plaque as shown in this picture.

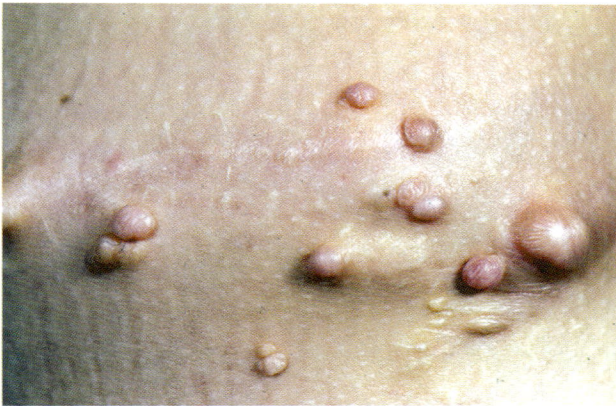

Figure 7–47 □ Connective tissue nevi. These are hamartomas of collagen and elastin. They present at birth or during the first few years of life as multiple, smooth, irregular papules, nodules, and plaques on the trunk and extremities. The lesion may be skin-colored or yellowish. They may occur as part of a syndrome such as Buschke-Ollendorf syndrome and tuberous sclerosis.

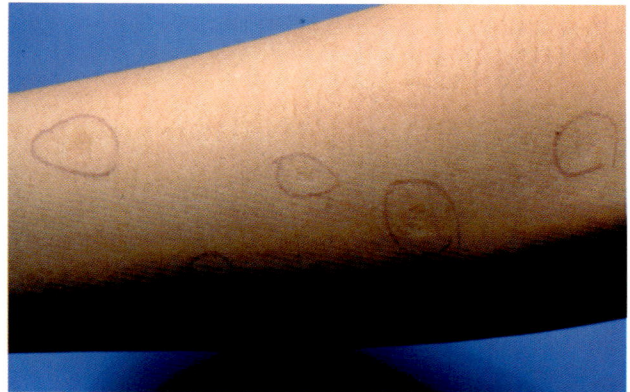

Figure 7–48 □ Primary anetoderma. This is an idiopathic disorder characterized by focal loss of elastic tissue leading to depressed lesions with an atrophic, wrinkled appearance. On palpation, an indentation into the dermis can be felt. The lesions may be preceded by erythematous inflammatory phase. Anetoderma can also be secondary to infections such as syphilis and chicken pox.

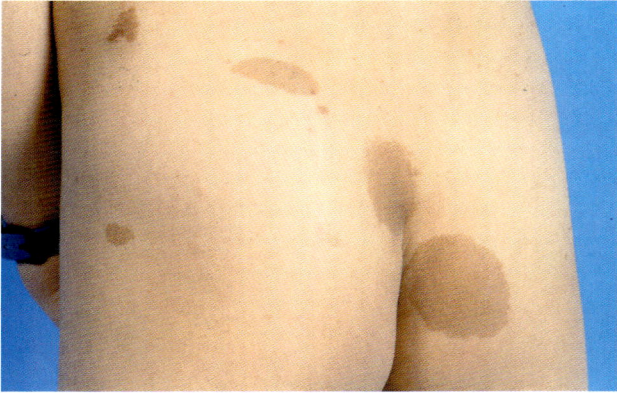

Figure 7–49 □ Neurofibromatosis. Multiple café au lait macules (more than six) is a major defining criteria for neurofibromatosis. As cutaneous neurofibromas do not appear until adulthood in most cases, the presence of multiple café au lait macules allows the diagnosis of neurofibromatosis to be made at an early age.

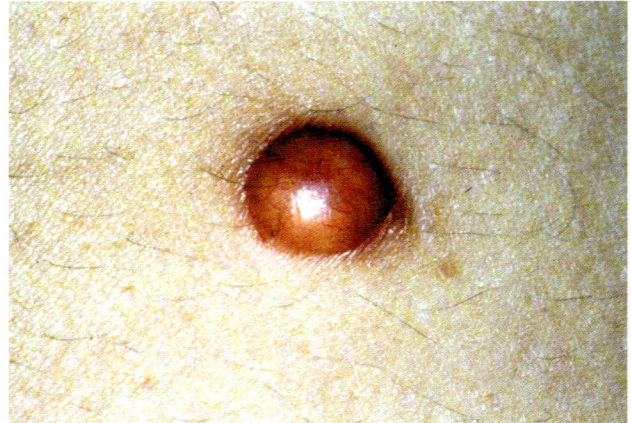

Figure 7–50 □ Juvenile xanthogranuloma. Juvenile xanthogranuloma is a non-Langerhans cell histiocytosis affecting mostly children within the first year of life. The lesion appears as a smooth, firm, dome-shaped papule or nodule. Early lesions appear reddish-brown whilst late lesions take on a yellowish-orange color. Juvenile xantho-granulomas often regress spontaneously after several years.

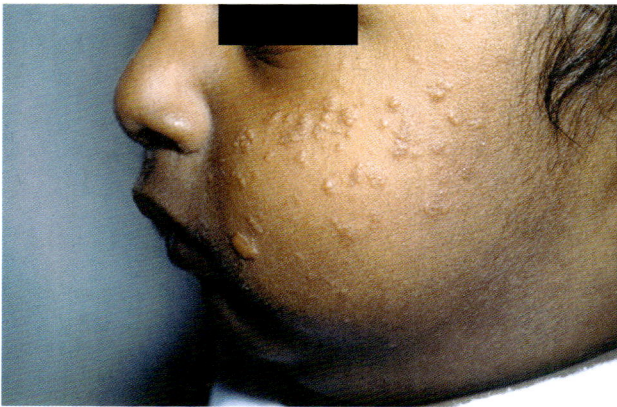

Figure 7–51 □ Eruptive xanthoma. This baby has multiple reddish-yellow papules on his face which have erupted in crops. Blood lipid and lipoprotein profile need to be evaluated to exclude any familial hyperlipoproteinemia.

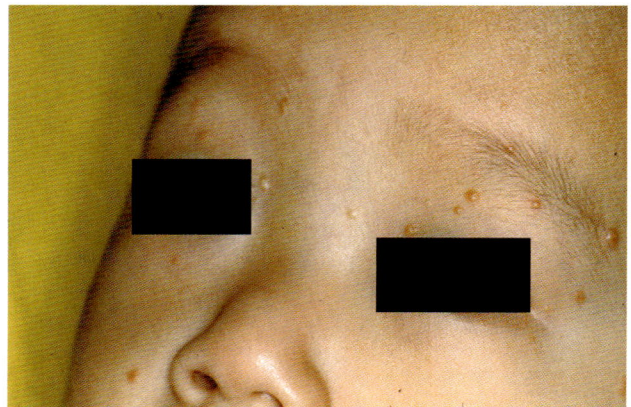

Figure 7–52 □ Benign cephalic histiocytosis. This is a benign non-Langerhans cell histiocytosis. It presents in an infant as multiple yellowish-brown papules on the face, neck, and shoulders. This condition is asymptomatic and usually resolves spontaneously over several years.

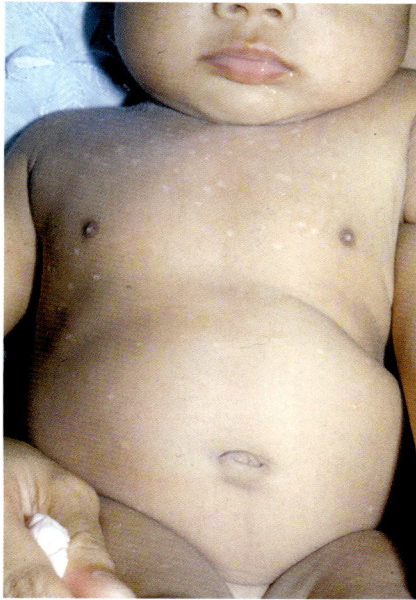

Figure 7–53 □ Letterer-Siwe disease. This is the disseminated form of Langerhans cell histiocytosis affecting young children. The cutaneous lesions comprise generalized erythematous papules which may become confluent, crusted, ulcerated, or purpuric. The areas of predilection are the scalp, groin, and intertriginous areas. The disease may involve the bones, central nervous system, lungs, and internal organs.

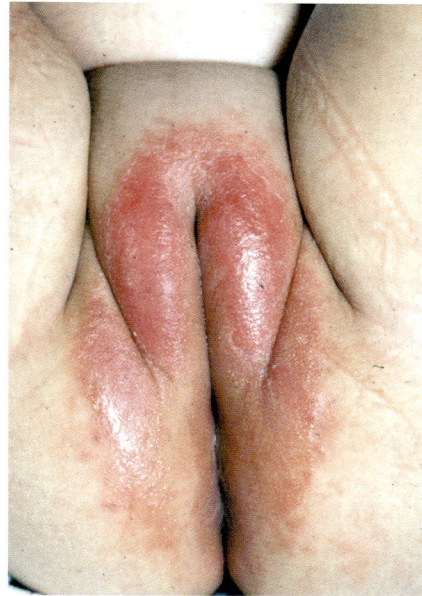

Figure 7–54 □ Diaper dermatitis. This results from irritant contact dermatitis due to prolonged contact with feces and urine and is associated with diaper use. The rash appears as shiny, erythematous patches and plaques affecting the nappy areas, often sparing the skin folds. Co-existing candidal infection is common. The key to prevention is frequent changes of diapers. Mild topical steroids help to quickly reduce the inflammation in severe cases.

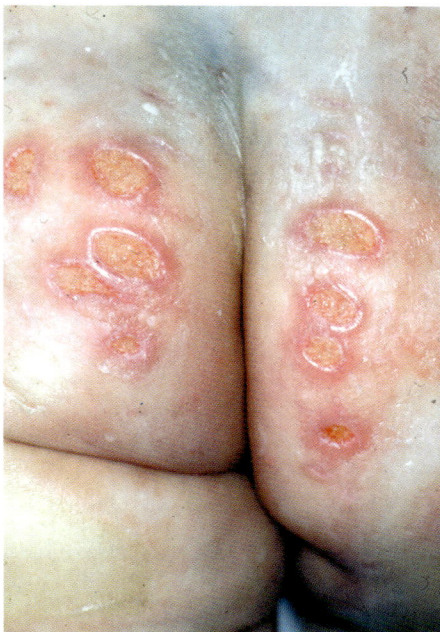

Figure 7–55 □ Jacquet's dermatitis. This is a less common morphological subtype of diaper dermatitis. It presents as papuloulcerative lesions. The ulcers have a punched-out appearance.

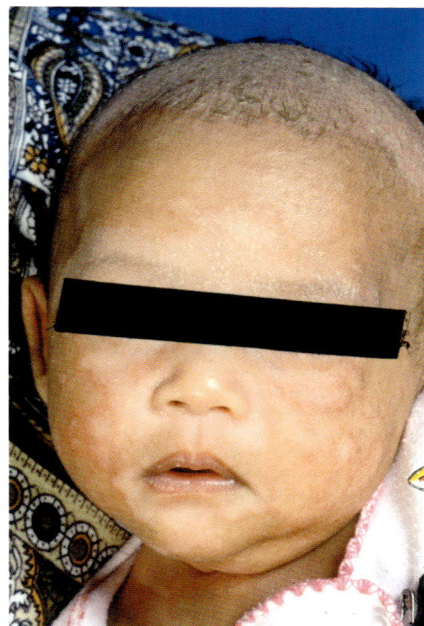

Figure 7–56 □ Infantile seborrheic dermatitis. This condition typically presents at two to six weeks of age with yellowish, greasy scales on the scalp (cradle cap). The scales tend to be adherent and confluent. Scaly, erythematous papules on the face and groin are often seen at the same time or shortly afterwards. Itch is not a prominent symptom as compared to atopic dermatitis.

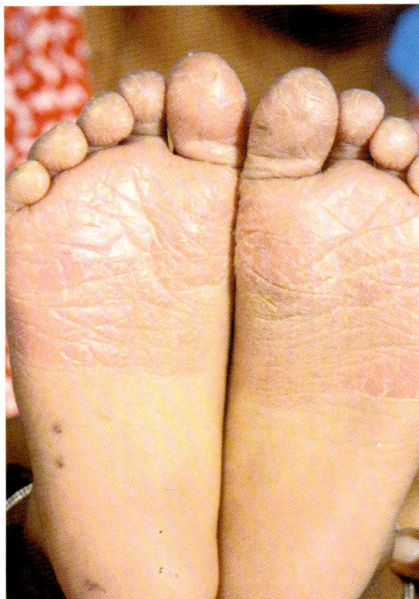

Figure 7–57 □ Juvenile plantar dermatosis. This condition affects pre-pubertal children. The characteristic appearance comprises shiny erythema hyperkeratosis and fissuring of skin affecting the soles of both feet symmetrically. The dorsums of the feet are spared. The plantar side of the big toe and forefoot is usually affected. Response to topical steroids is variable and the condition tends to remit spontaneously after puberty.

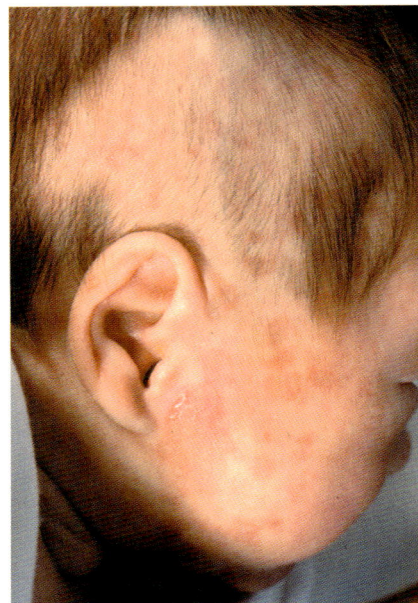

Figure 7–58 □ Neonatal lupus erythematosus. This is a rare disorder due to transplacental transfer of IgG autoantibodies (anti-Ro, anti-La, anti-U1-RNP). The rash appears at birth or shortly after as well-demarcated, scaly, erythematous patches and plaques affecting the face, neck, and scalp. There may be associated congenital heart block and hematological abnormalities. Often, the mother is healthy but serologically positive.

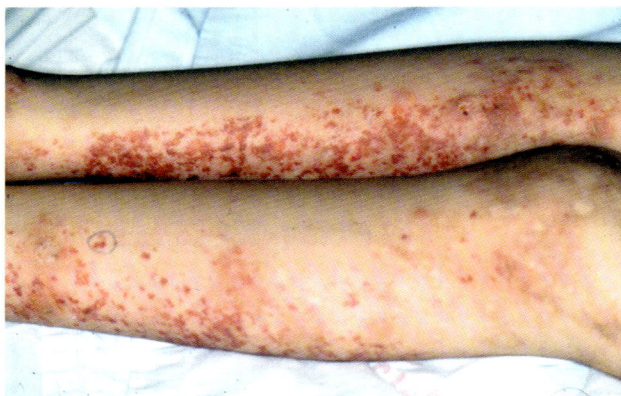

Figure 7–59 □ Henoch-Schönlein purpura. This is a small vessel vasculitis with IgA deposition, predominantly but not exclusively seen in children. It occurs as an acute eruption of purpuric papules on the lower legs extending to the buttocks. The eruption often occurs in crops. There are associated joint, renal, and gastro-intestinal complications which must be evaluated.

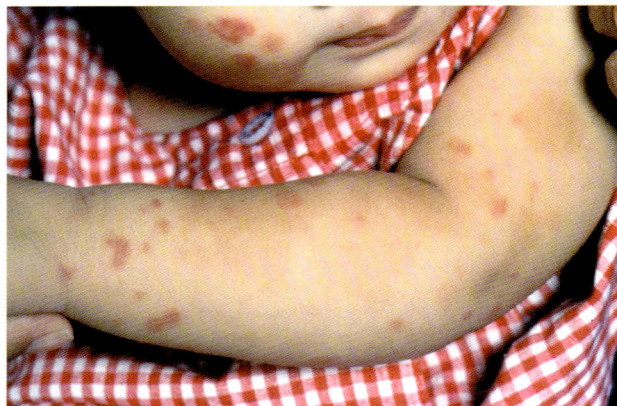

Figure 7–60 □ Acute hemorrhagic edema of infancy (Finkelstein's disease). This is a leukocytoclastic vasculitis typically affecting young infants less than three years old. Often preceded by a history of upper respiratory illness, it appears abruptly in a non-toxic child as targetoid purpura affecting mainly the face and extremities. The lesions often resolve over a few weeks. Recurrences have been reported but long-term complications are uncommon.

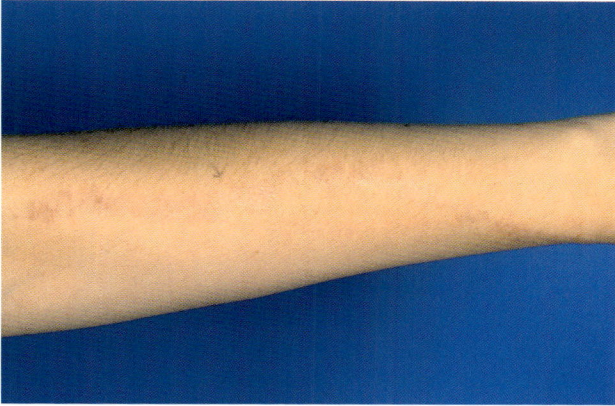

Figure 7–61 □ Lichen striatus. This is an idiopathic dermatosis affecting mainly young children. It appears as red or flesh-colored lichenoid papules often coalescing into linear plaques on the limbs or trunk following Blaschko's lines. Itch is often minimal. Spontaneously resolution over several months to years is to be expected.

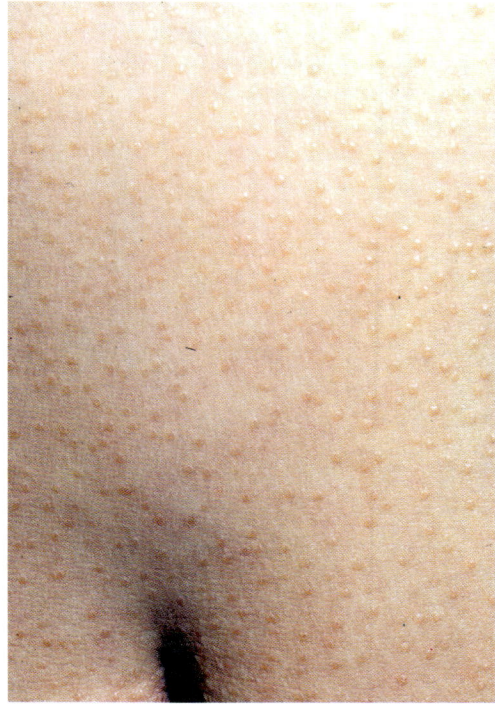

Figure 7–62 □ Lichen nitidus. An idiopathic disorder predominantly affecting children and adolescents, it presents as an acute eruption of small, flat-topped, skin-colored shiny papules on the upper limbs and trunk. Itch is usually minimal. Köebnerization can occur. Spontaneous resolution normally occurs but this may take several years.

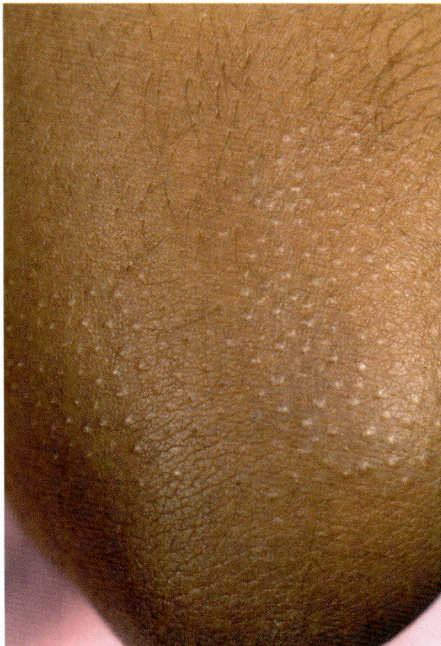

Figure 7–63 □ Lichen spinulosus. This presents most commonly during adolescence as circumscribed areas of grouped follicular papules with horny spines. It is asymptomatic and usually resolves within one to two years. Topical keratolytics such as salicylic acid may be used if treatment is desired.

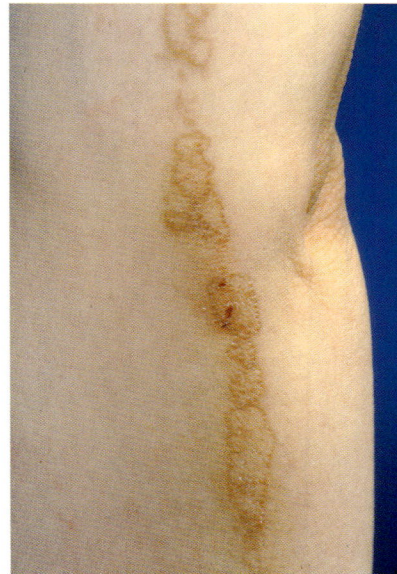

Figure 7–64 □ Linear porokeratosis. Linear porokeratosis is one of the clinical subtypes of porokeratosis, a disorder of epidermal differentiation involving a mutant clone of keratinocyte. It usually presents at birth or during childhood as linear, keratotic plaques rimmed by a prominent double-edge border. The lesions are distributed along the lines of Blaschko. The lesions are usually asymptomatic but carry a risk of malignant transformation.

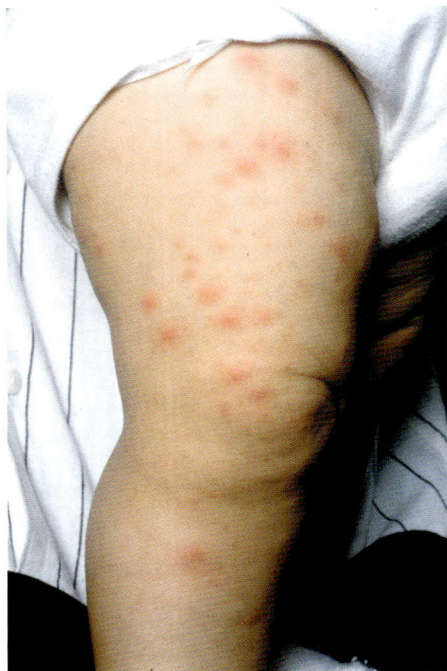

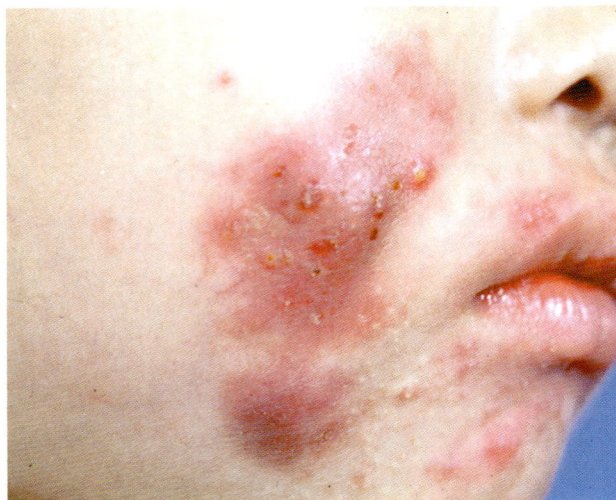

Figure 7–66 □ Infantile acne vulgaris. This 20-month-old boy has severe inflammatory acne on both cheeks. Erythematous papules, pustules, nodules, and comedones are present. Infantile acne is rare, predominantly affecting boys and in most cases without an underlying endocrine abnormality. Treatment with systemic antibiotics may be needed to reduce the risk of scarring in severe cases.

Figure 7–65 □ Papular urticaria. This is a hypersensitivity reaction to insect bites occurring in young children. It presents as groups of urticarial papules and nodules, often on exposed parts of the body. The lesions are pruritic and may become secondarily infected following self-excoriations.

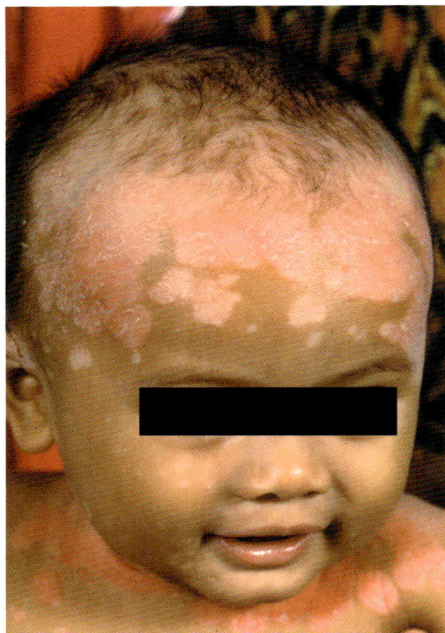

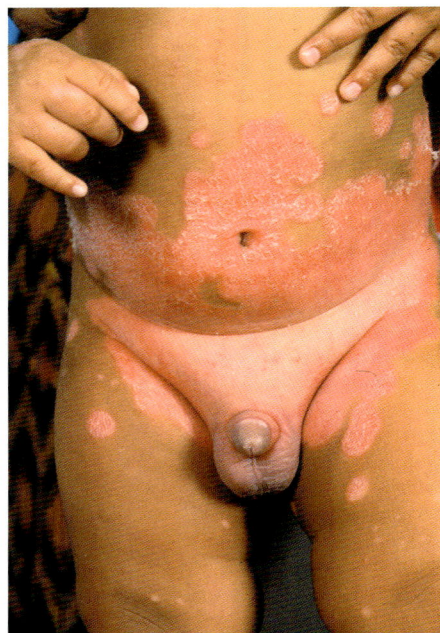

Figure 7–67 □ Infantile psoriasis. Psoriasis can present during early infancy. Often, there is a family history of psoriasis. The morphology is similar to that in adults with well-demarcated, scaly, erythematous plaques as seen in this 10-month-old baby. The scalp, extensor surfaces, groin, and trunk are commonly affected sites.

Figure 7–68 □ Infantile psoriasis. The groin is often involved in infantile psoriasis and may be misdiagnosed as diaper dermatitis. Scaling is often not prominent in occluded areas but the sharp borders, the involvement of skin folds, and the presence of psoriatic lesions elsewhere help point to the diagnosis.

Genodermatoses

Chan Y.C., Goh B.K., and Giam Y.C.

The genetic origin of such dermatoses results in the hereditary nature of the disorder, which means that families and generations may be similarly afflicted. A detailed family history and pedigree tree are therefore a prerequisite in the evaluation of any suspected genodermatosis. It must also be noted that the genetic defect may result from a new mutation or deletion which occurs sporadically; as such, a negative family history does not preclude the diagnosis of genodermatosis. Polygenic disorders, like atopic dermatitis and psoriasis, are excluded from this category.

In the overall management of genodermatoses, the diagnostic evaluation and therapeutic management must be complemented by comprehensive and compassionate genetic counseling on the spectrum of phenotypic expression, prognosis, and potential transmission risk of the disease.

Currently, there are no good population-based epidemiological data on genodermatoses in the Asian population. Thus, this is a potential area for further research. However, personal communications with pediatric dermatologists from Thailand, the Philippines, Indonesia, Sri Lanka, and Malaysia suggest that the following genodermatoses are more commonly seen in Southeast Asia: (a) autosomal dominant conditions like ichthyosis vulgaris, neurofibromatosis type 1, Darier's disease, Hailey-Hailey disease, steatocystoma multiplex, epidermolysis bullosa simplex, tuberous sclerosis, porokeratosis of Mibelli, autosomal dominant palmoplantar keratoderma; (b) autosomal recessive conditions like lamellar ichthyosis, Netherton syndrome, pretibial epidermolysis bullosa dystrophica; (c) X-linked dominant conditions like incontinentia pigmenti; and (d) heterogeneous conditions like pseudoxanthoma elasticum (which exhibits both autosomal dominant and autosomal recessive inheritance).

INHERITANCE PATTERNS

The following patterns of inheritance can be seen:

Autosomal Dominant Inheritance

Genetic traits are called dominant when they are expressed in a heterozygous state. Dominant traits usually involve defects of structural proteins. For instance, the gene mutation in neurofibromatosis type 1 causes a defect in neurofibromin. However, exceptions to the rule exist and some autosomal dominant genodermatoses are metabolic disorders. For example, porphyria cutanea tarda is characterized by a deficiency of the enzyme uroporphyrinogen decarboxylase. Interestingly, molecular genetics has shown that benign hamartomas or malignant tumors of the skin or viscera in some classical autosomal dominant disorders like neurofibromatosis, tuberous sclerosis, and nevoid basal cell carcinoma syndrome demonstrate homozygosity for the underlying gene. This suggests that these tumors are localized "recessive" manifestations that arise after a spontaneous mutation of the normal allele in a person with a pre-existing inherited mutant allele ("double hit" phenomenon).

The expression of an autosomal dominant trait may be highly variable, even amongst family members. Such variable expression is well-demonstrated in neurofibromatosis type 1, where one family member may be severely disfigured with multiple neurofibromas but another may only have café au lait macules and axillary freckling. "Incomplete penetrance" means that the trait is present but not detectable in some individuals. An autosomal dominant disorder with a variable expression or incomplete penetrance can pose a challenge in genetic counseling.

For the children of an affected individual, the recurrence risk is 50% (one out of two children is expected to be affected).

Autosomal Recessive Inheritance

Genetic traits are called recessive when they are only expressed in a homozygous state. This means that two identical alleles have to be present in a given gene locus before manifestations of the disease are evident.

As a general rule, autosomal recessive traits are due to enzyme deficiency. For example, transglutaminase 1 is deficient in lamellar ichthyosis. Autosomal recessive traits are generally more severe and often have a poorer prognosis compared to autosomal dominant traits.

Individuals with autosomal recessive disorders show relatively constant involvement and resemble one another like siblings. For children of two heterozygous parents, the risk of recurrence is 25% (one out of four children is expected to be affected; two out of four are expected to be carriers).

X-linked Inheritance

Males have only one X chromosome and hence most of the X-linked genes are present in a hemizygous state, i.e. they do not have a corresponding loci on the Y chromosome. X-linked gene defects are expressed to a more severe degree in hemizygous males than in heterozygous females. In females, one of the two X chromosomes present in each cell is inactivated at an early stage of embryogenesis – a mechanism known as lyonization. The inactivated X chromosome can be either the maternal or paternal one in different cells of the same person, but the inactivated X chromosome remains the same in all daughter cells of a given cell line. This functional X chromosome may give rise to a characteristic pattern of skin lesions which follow the lines of Blaschko.

X-linked recessive traits like X-linked recessive ichthyosis occur almost exclusively in male individuals. Characteristically, one generation is skipped as the disease is transmitted by healthy female carriers. X-linked dominant, non-lethal traits occur in both sexes and can be difficult to differentiate from autosomal dominant traits. An indication of autosomal dominant inheritance is the transmission of the disorder from father to son, as fathers do not give their X chromosome to their sons.

X-linked dominant, male-lethal traits like incontinentia pigmenti occur almost exclusively in females as the mutation has a lethal effect on hemizygous male embryos. The exceptional male survivors may have an XXY constitution, an early post-zygotic mutation or a gametic half-chromatid mutation.

Gonadal Mosaicism

An autosomal dominant trait may occur in several siblings although both parents are healthy. This phenomenon has been proven to be due to gonadal mosaicism. This means that some of the germ cells in the father or the mother carry the genetic mutation, but his or her somatic cells are unaffected. This situation is caused by a late post-zygotic mutation affecting some of the germ cells. This concept of gonadal mosaicism is important for genetic counseling. The risk of recurrence for such apparently normal parents who have one child with an autosomal dominant disorder, is very low, but not zero.

DIAGNOSTIC APPROACH

The diagnostic approach to a patient with a possible genodermatosis begins with the consolidation of essential information. The history of a proband's presenting signs and symptoms as well as a detailed family history, including a pedigree diagram, are crucial to the diagnosis. The proband is often a child and the history should be taken from the parents or a knowledgeable caregiver. A thorough physical examination is then carried out to detect anomalies, both cutaneous and extracutaneous. The examination includes growth parameters like height, weight, and head circumference as well as a developmental assessment. Photography should be done, especially for documentation of difficult cases. Relevant investigations, including blood tests, skin biopsies, chromosome analysis, genetic testing, and radiology, are then performed. Referral to the appropriate specialty should be considered for evaluation of any extracutaneous anomalies found.

Rare genodermatoses pose additional diagnostic challenges. However, the clinician who is faced with such a situation may turn to several avenues for assistance: (1) Ask the world experts. With electronic mail and digital photography, one can consult many experts around the world simultaneously for advice; (2) Do a database search. Genetic databases like POSSUM®, the London Dysmorphology Database or the Online Mendelian Inheritance in Man (OMIM) database are available for use by the clinician; or (3) Wait and see. With time, more features of the disease may manifest and facilitate the establishment of a clear diagnosis.

GENETIC COUNSELING

The management of a genodermatosis is facilitated by a firm diagnosis, which would then allow the physician and the family to anticipate complications associated with the disease. Counseling of patients and family takes centerstage in the overall management of the disease and must include discussion on prognosis, genetic counseling, and advice on the availability and feasibility of prenatal diagnosis.

A special genetics clinic, if available, will help with the evaluation of transmission risk and in the genetic counseling of patients and their family. Verbal communication by the physician is best supplemented by educational materials and introducing the family to relevant websites and support groups.

Finally, there exists a fairly large group of patients who have diseases which do not yet fit into any known diagnosis. Despite this handicap, the physician can still help the patient by treating any complication as it arises. Genetic counseling is hindered by lack of a firm diagnosis. The usual scenario is an affected child born to normal parents and the family history reveals no features of the disease. In such a case, the physician can inform the parents that the recurrence risk is at most 25%, assuming that in the worst case scenario, the mutation is an autosomal recessive one.

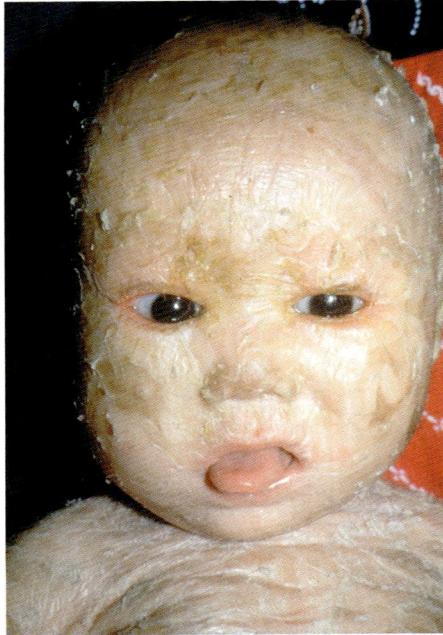

Figure 8–1 □ Lamellar ichthyosis. This child is born a collodion baby. The collodion membrane is beginning to slough off, leaving generalized hyperkeratotic and large brown scales. Ectropion and eclabium pose problems. This is usually an autosomal recessive condition and mutations in the transglutaminase 1 gene have been found in some families.

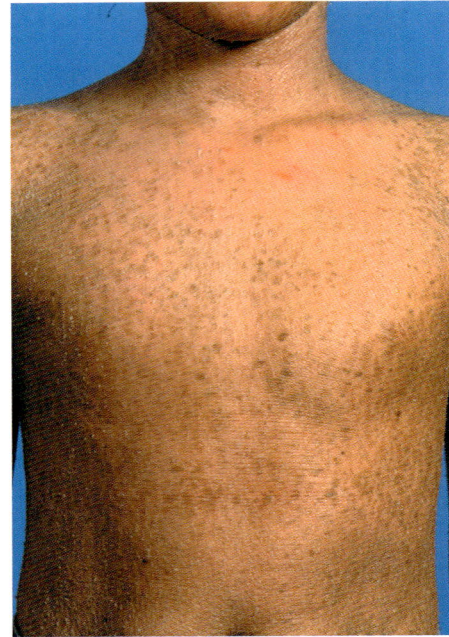

Figure 8–2 □ Lamellar ichthyosis. After the disappearance of the collodion membrane, a mosaic pattern of scaling gradually becomes established, as shown on the chest of this 12-year-old Malay boy with lamellar ichthyosis.

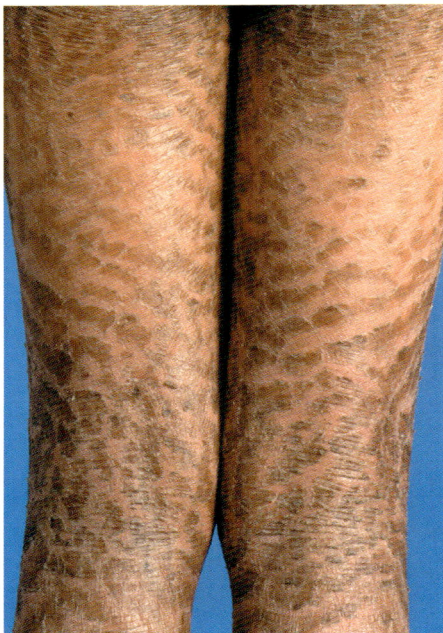

Figure 8–3 □ Lamellar ichthyosis. The scales are large, brown, and plate-like, with the borders having the tendency to curl up. Flexural involvement tends to be more severe, as in the child's popliteal fossae.

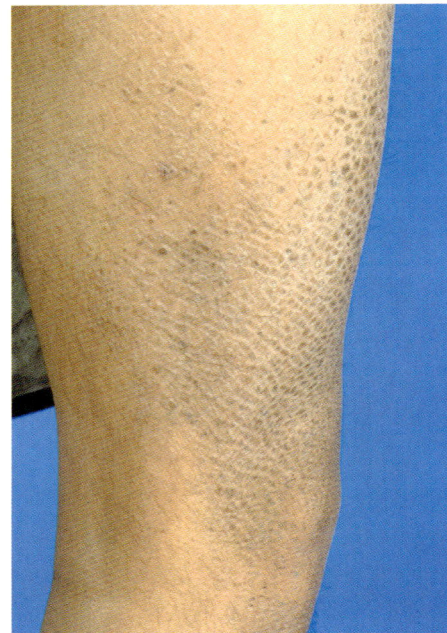

Figure 8–4 □ Ichthyosis vulgaris. This is the most common form of ichthyosis, with the incidence ranging from 1:250 to 1:2,000. It is inherited as an autosomal dominant trait, and often presents in infancy. Fine, bran-like scaling with accentuation on the extensor extremities of this boy and sparing of the flexures are characteristic.

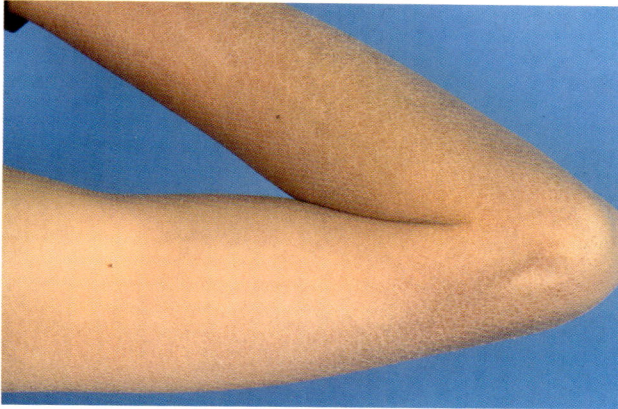

Figure 8–5 □ X-linked recessive ichthyosis. This 18-year-old Chinese male has ichthyosis involving almost all the body surfaces, with the exception of his face, palms, and soles. The scales are large and yellow-brown. Involvement of the neck has given rise to the description "dirty neck disease". This X-linked recessive condition is due to deficiency of steroid sulphatase. Absence of placental steroid sulphatase activity may lead to prolonged labor. Cryptorchidism occurs in about 20% of affected males.

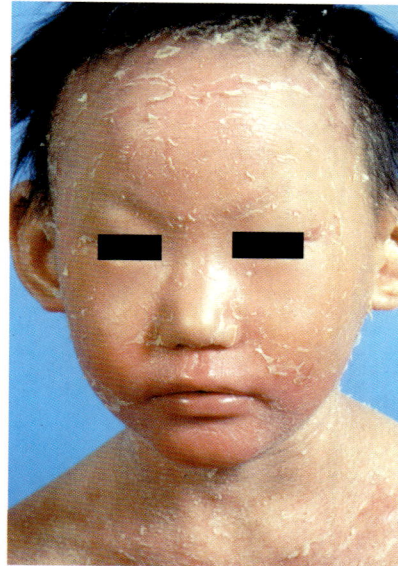

Figure 8–6 □ Non-bullous congenital ichthyosiform erythroderma. Children with this autosomal recessive condition may present at birth as a collodion baby, similar to lamellar ichthyosis. After infancy, generalized erythroderma with white scales, as shown in this picture of a nine-year-old Chinese boy, is characteristic. Complications include heat intolerance (due to decreased ability to sweat) and secondary fungal infection. Some patients' condition may improve at puberty.

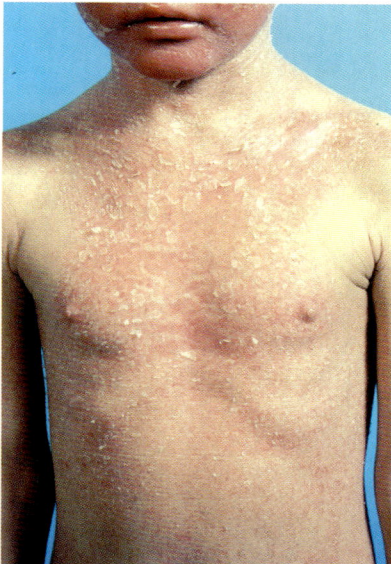

Figure 8–7 □ Non-bullous congenital ichthyosiform erythroderma. Erythema and whitish scales are typical of this condition. In contrast, patients with lamellar ichthyosis exhibit darker scales and less erythema.

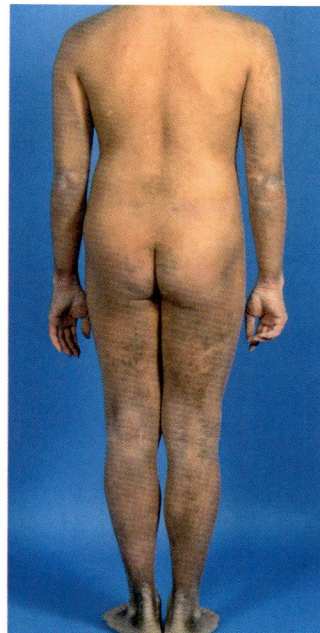

Figure 8–8 □ Epidermolytic hyperkeratosis. This is an autosomal dominant genodermatosis linked to mutation of genes encoding K1 and K10. Typically, erythroderma with widespread bullae and denuded skin occurs in the newborn. Over time, the blistering eruption resolves and is followed by areas of hyperkeratosis with thick spiny scales. Patients with epidermal nevi may be at risk of having children with generalized epidermolytic hyperkeratosis.

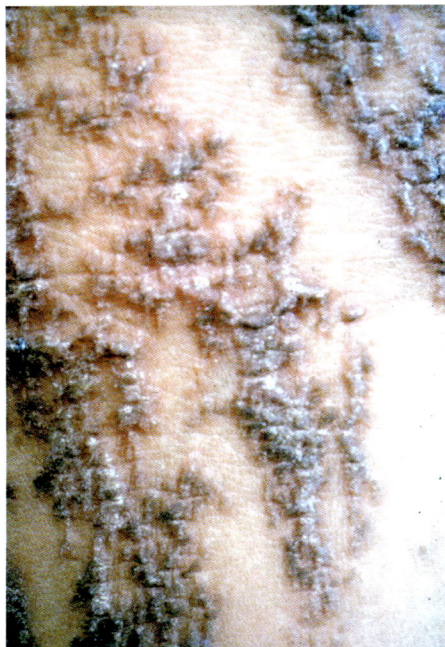

Figure 8–9 □ **Epidermolytic hyperkeratosis.** A close-up view of the lesion showing the hyperkeratosis with thick spiny scales. Flexural areas tend to be more severely affected. Bacterial colonization of the skin may result in malodor.

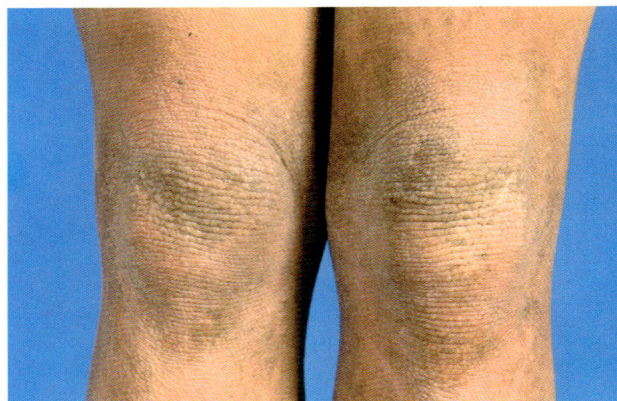

Figure 8–10 □ **Epidermolytic hyperkeratosis.** With time, the erythroderma lessens, but the hyperkeratosis persists to some degree throughout the afflicted person's life.

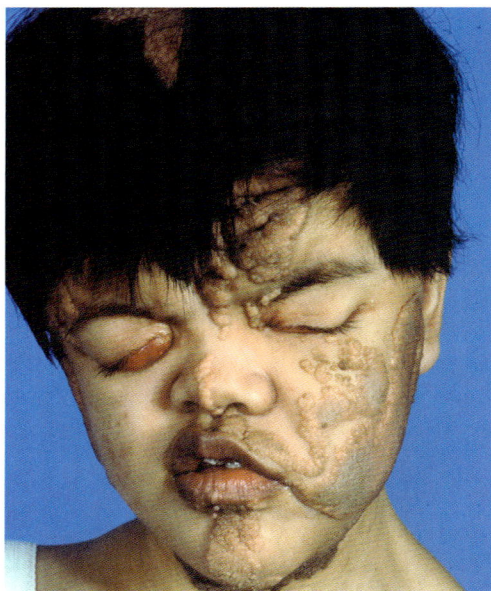

Figure 8–11 □ **Epidermal nevus syndrome.** This syndrome consists of epidermal nevi associated with neurological, skeletal, ocular, and other organ system abnormalities. This 15-year-old Chinese female has mental retardation, nevus sebaceous on her scalp and face, and a lipodermoid tumor over her right eye.

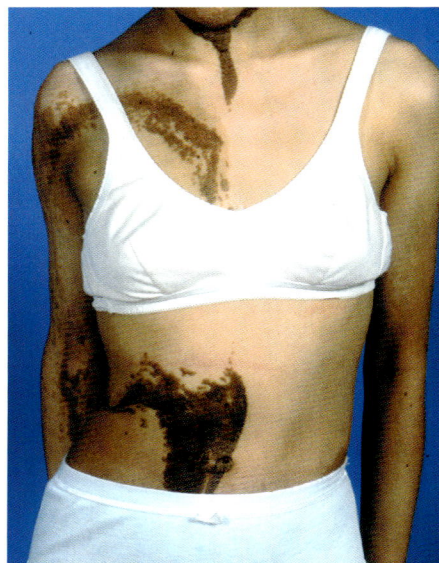

Figure 8–12 □ **Epidermal nevus syndrome.** The patient in Figure 8–11 showing the epidermal nevi, presenting as hyperpigmented verrucous plaques, distributed along the lines of Blaschko on her limbs, neck, chest, and abdomen.

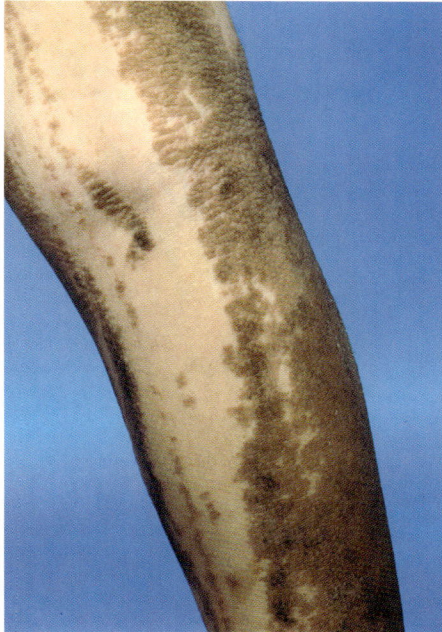

Figure 8–13 □ Epidermal nevus syndrome. The patient in Figure 8–11 has epidermal nevi distributed in a linear fashion, along the lines of Blaschko, on her lower limbs. A sporadic genetic mutation is believed to be the cause. This disorder has been associated with an increased risk of malignancy, particularly Wilm's tumor.

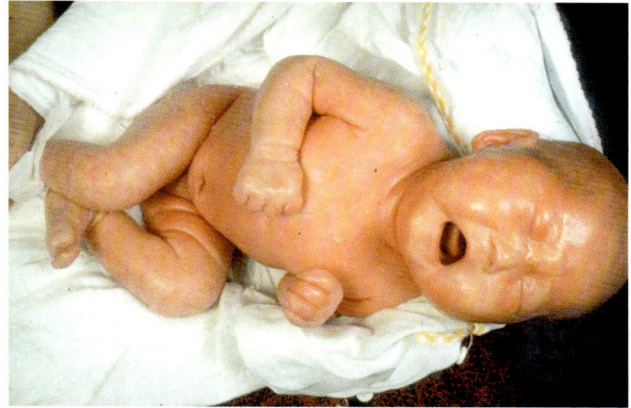

Figure 8–14 □ Netherton syndrome. This is an autosomal recessive condition that is characterized by a unique ichthyosis, "bamboo-hair shaft" abnormalities, atopic diathesis, and erythroderma. At birth, a generalized ichthyosiform erythroderma is the most common presentation, as seen in this newborn Chinese female. Hypernatraemic dehydration and failure to thrive are possible complications. Mutation in the gene encoding a novel serine protease inhibitor of Kazal type (SPINK5) on chromosome 5q32 has been implicated in the pathogenesis of this condition.

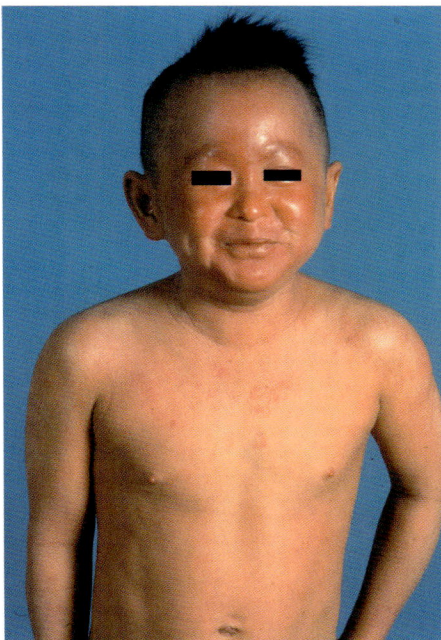

Figure 8–15 □ Netherton syndrome. The associated hair-shaft abnormalities including trichorrhexis invaginata, trichorrhexis nodosa, and pili torti are usually evident after two years of age. This 11-year-old Malay boy is erythrodermic and has short, spiky, brittle hair due to trichorrhexis invaginata.

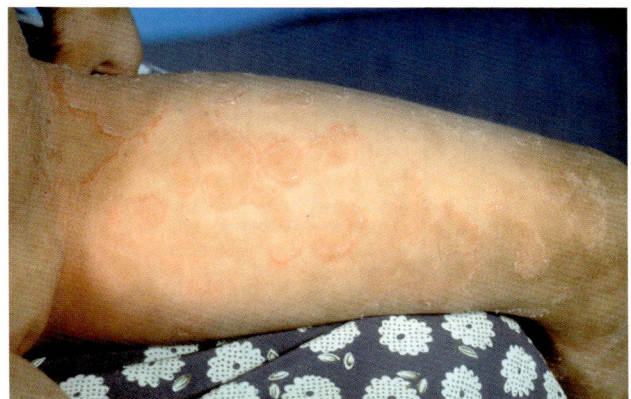

Figure 8–16 □ Netherton syndrome. A unique and less common cutaneous feature of this disorder is ichthyosis linearis circumflexa as seen in this six-year-old Chinese female. This lesion is characterized by circinate or polycyclic erythematous keratotic plaques lined by double-edged scales. This rash may last several weeks to several years.

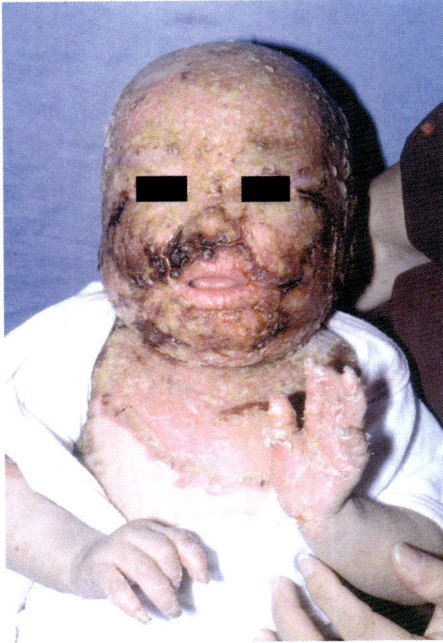

Figure 8–17 □ Erythrokeratoderma variabilis. This autosomal dominant condition is characterized by fixed localized hyperkeratosis and migratory erythema. The latter may be induced by changes in temperature and emotional stress. It usually presents during infancy, progresses through childhood, and stabilises at puberty. The face, extensor surfaces of the extremities, trunk, and buttocks are usually involved.

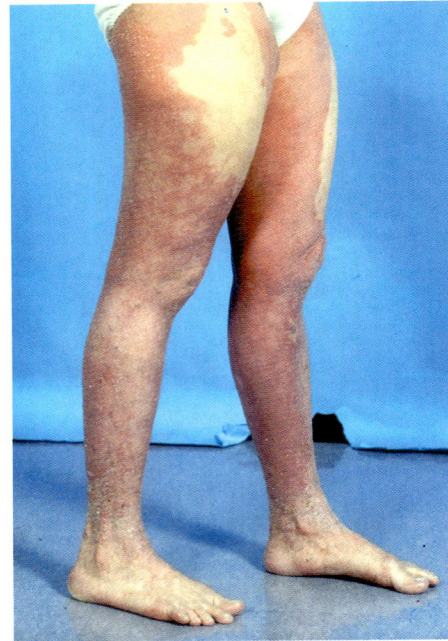

Figure 8–18 □ Erythrokeratoderma variabilis. This 24-year-old Chinese female has fixed erythematous hyperkeratotic plaques on her lower limbs as well as a history of geographic patches of migratory erythema. The gene locus of this disorder has been linked to chromosome 1p36.2-34.

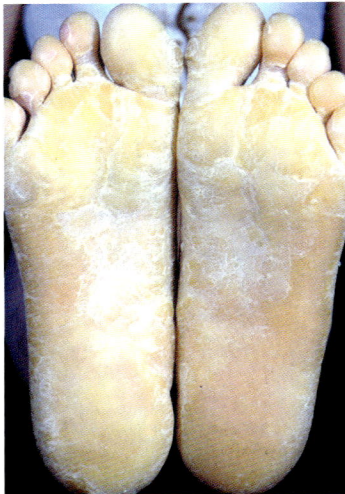

Figure 8–19 □ Palmoplantar keratoderma. The hereditary palmoplantar keratodermas are a heterogeneous group of conditions characterized by abnormal thickening of the palms and soles. They are differentiated by severity (mutilating versus non-mutilating), distribution (punctate versus generalized, limited to palms and soles or extending beyond, i.e. transgrediens), associated abnormalities, histopathology (epidermolytic versus non-epidermolytic), and mode of inheritance. This patient has diffuse yellowish hyperkeratotic thickening of her soles. This is a vertically transmitted trait in her family, likely autosomal dominant.

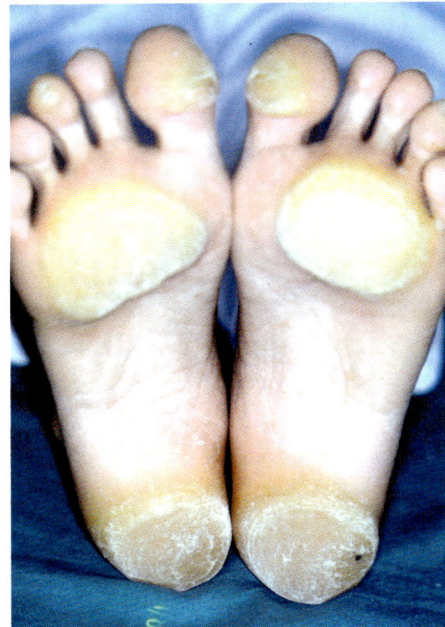

Figure 8–20 □ Palmoplantar keratoderma. In some cases, the plantar keratoderma is not diffuse but localized to the areas of pressure on the sole.

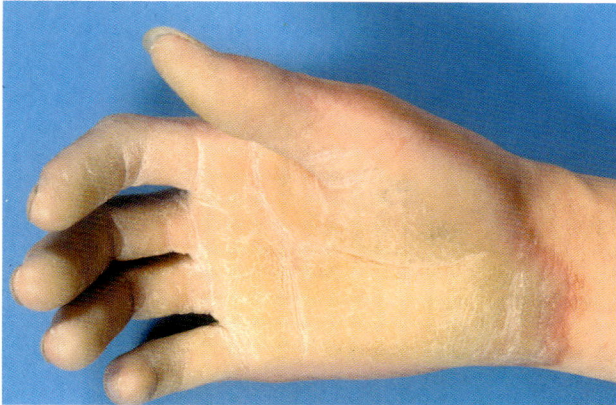

Figure 8–21 □ **Palmoplantar keratoderma.** This patient has diffuse yellowish hyperkeratotic thickening of her palms with a surrounding erythematous rim and no transgrediens, i.e. the dorsum of her hand and forearm are not involved.

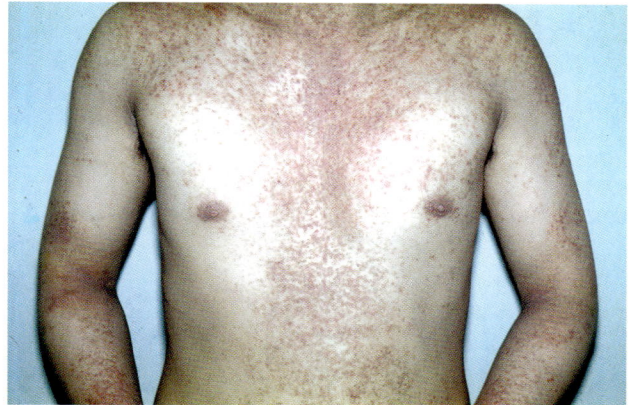

Figure 8–22 □ **Darier's disease.** This is an autosomal dominant genodermatosis with variable penetrance. It is characterized by greasy keratotic papules, commonly distributed in the seborrheic areas of the body (as shown in this 30-year-old Chinese male), palmoplantar pitting, and nail abnormalities. Mutations in the ATP2A2 gene which encodes the sarcoendoplasmic reticulum calcium-ATPase isoform 2 (SERCA2) have been found.

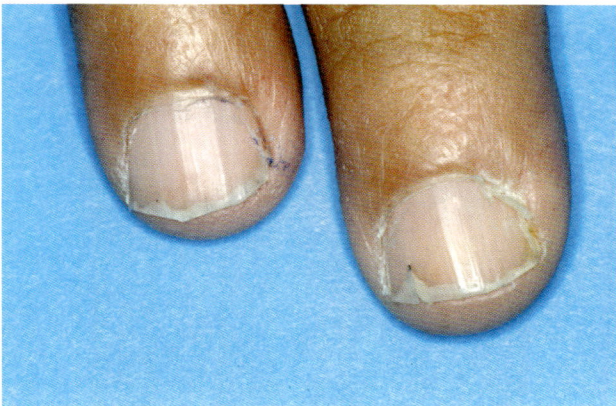

Figure 8–23 □ **Darier's disease.** Red and white striations on the nail plate associated with lamellar V-shaped splitting on the distal nail margin are characteristic.

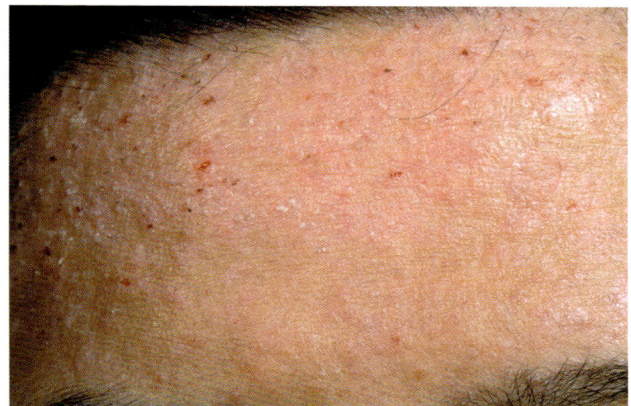

Figure 8–24 □ **Darier's disease.** These greasy and erythematous keratotic papules on the forehead of this 18-year-old Malay male may be mistaken for the lesions of seborrheic dermatitis. The family history and skin biopsy are often diagnostic.

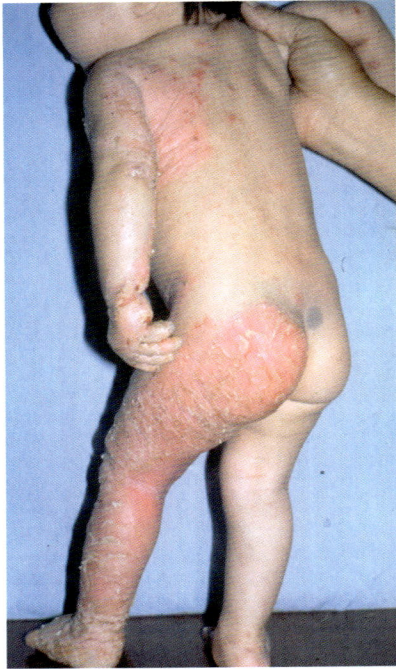

Figure 8–25 □ CHILD syndrome. The acronym stands for **C**ongenital **H**emidysplasia with **I**chthyosiform erythroderma and **L**imbs **D**efects. The mode of inheritance may be sporadic or X-linked dominant, usually lethal to males. It is characterized by unilateral ichthyosiform erythroderma with a clear midline demarcation as shown in this 18-month-old Chinese female. Skeletal, neurological, and visceral abnormalities may be found ipsilateral to the skin lesions.

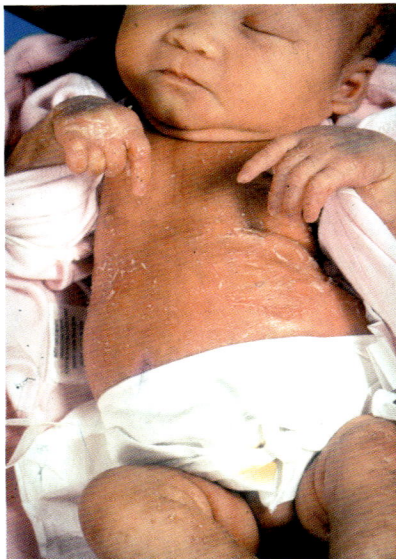

Figure 8–26 □ Conradi-Hünermann syndrome. This child has erythrodermic ichthyosis distributed along the lines of Blaschko, a typical feature in this syndrome, also known as X-linked dominant chondrodysplasia punctata. Other cutaneous features are thick and spiky hyperkeratosis in newborn babies, patchy cicatricial alopecia and, in the older child, follicular atrophoderma.

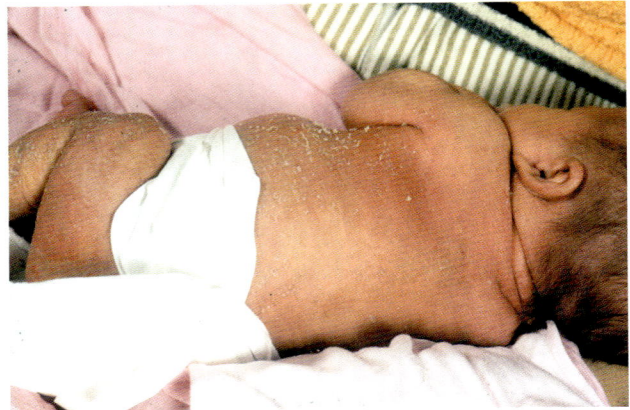

Figure 8–27 □ Conradi-Hünermann syndrome. Non-cutaneous findings include frontal bossing, focal cataracts, and stippled calcifications in areas of enchondral bone formation, short stature, and shortening of legs. Inheritance is X-linked dominant.

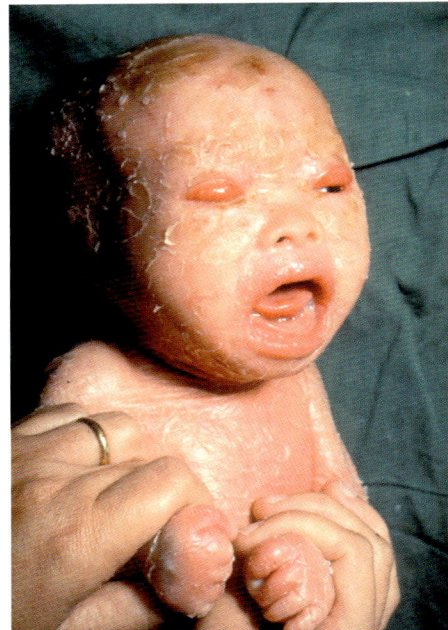

Figure 8–28 □ Harlequin ichthyosis. In this rare autosomal recessive congenital ichthyosis, this newborn is covered with thick, armor-like plates of scale that fissure. Ectropion (eyelid eversion) and eclabium (lip eversion) are typical. Scalp hair, eyebrows, and eyelashes are often absent or sparse. Death from complications of prematurity, respiratory compromise due to limitation of thoracic expansion, sepsis, hypothermia, and dehydration used to be very common.

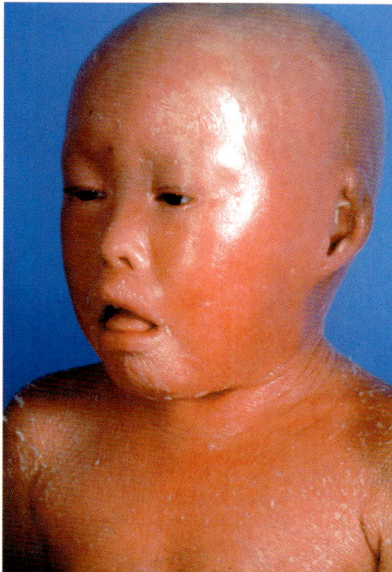

Figure 8–29 □ Harlequin ichthyosis. With modern medical support equipment and meticulous intensive nursing, the chances of survival have improved significantly. Systemic retinoid therapy results in an improvement of the ichthyosis but the child is often left with a persistent erythroderma (as seen here) resembling congenital ichthyosiform erythroderma.

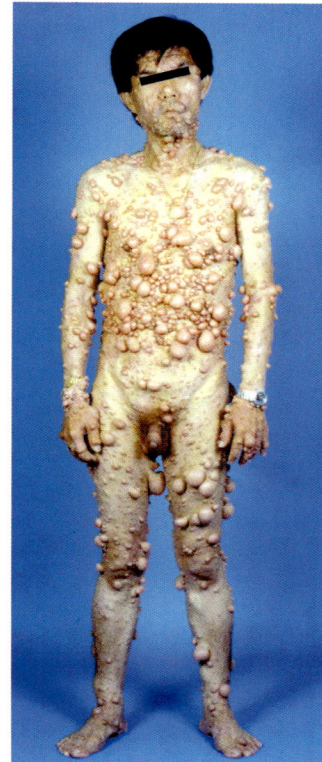

Figure 8–30 □ Neurofibromatosis Type 1. This is an autosomal dominant disorder with variable expressivity. About 50% of the cases are due to spontaneous mutations. Clinical manifestation of the disease is highly variable and runs the full spectrum from very mild to severe, even amongst family members. This patient has florid neurofibromata which has resulted in severe cosmetic disfigurement. Other cutaneous signs of this disease include café au lait macules, inguinal, and axillary freckling. Of concern are malignant degeneration and development of neurofibrosarcomas and malignant schwannomas. Extracutaneous manifestations include learning difficulties, scoliosis, and hypertension. The gene responsible for this disorder is localized to chromosome 17q11.2 and encodes neurofibromin. This protein acts as a tumor suppressor that modulates the products of the ras proto-oncogene.

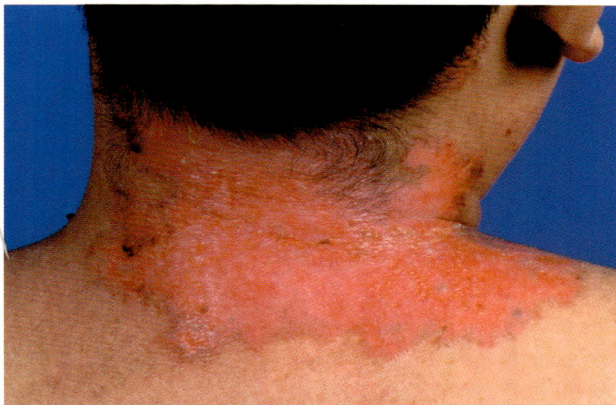

Figure 8–31 □ Hailey-Hailey disease. This is an autosomal dominant disease with onset during the third and fourth decades of life. Vesicles and erosions develop on the neck, axillae, and groin. Crusted and erosive plaques, as shown here, are indicative of the long-standing disease. Histopathology showed suprabasal acantholysis of epidermal cells.

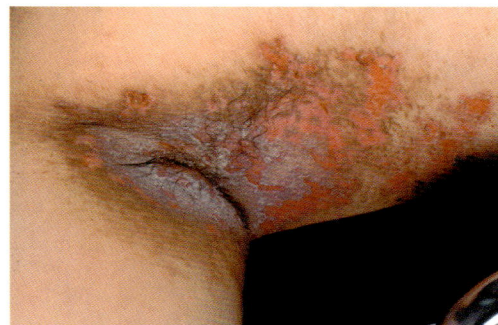

Figure 8–32 □ Hailey-Hailey disease. Chronically affected areas may show maceration and erosive plaques. Secondary bacterial and candidal infections are common, giving rise to symptoms of pain, itch, and malodor. Recent studies have revealed that the Hailey-Hailey disease is caused by mutations in the ATP2C1 gene encoding the secretory-pathway Ca(2+)-ATPase (SPCA1) Ca(2+) pump. This gene has been mapped to 3q21-24.

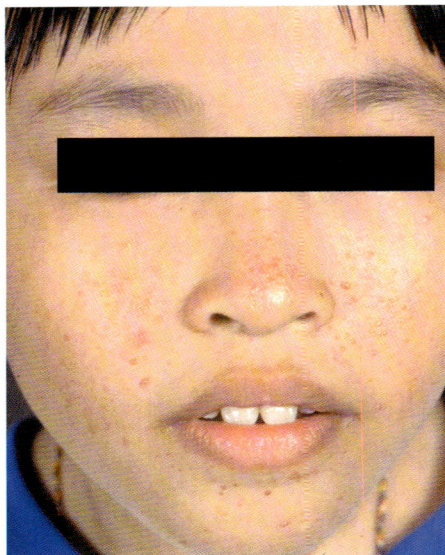

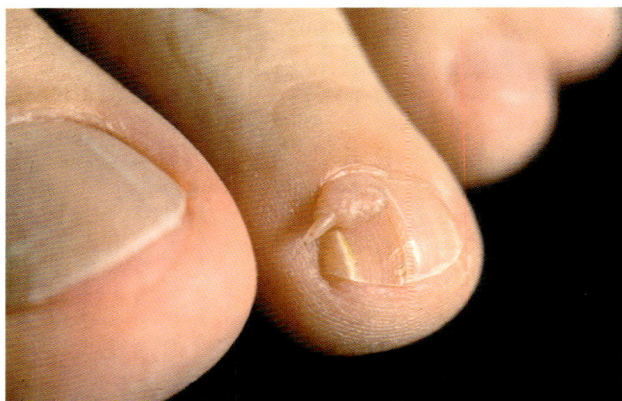

Figure 8–34 □ Tuberose sclerosis. Ash leaf macules or patches are the earliest cutaneous manifestation of this condition. They can present at birth or during infancy. The hypopigmented lesions are typically "ash-leaf" and polygonal in shape although confetti-like macules can be found especially on the pretibial areas.

Figure 8–33 □ Tuberose sclerosis. This is an autosomal dominant condition with variable penetrance. Spontaneous mutation can account for as high as 75% of the cases. Adenoma sebaceum is one of the most common cutaneous manifestations of this disorder. The lesions are red and dome-shaped, and are predominantly clustered around the perinasal areas and cheeks. Histologically, these lesions are angiofibromas.

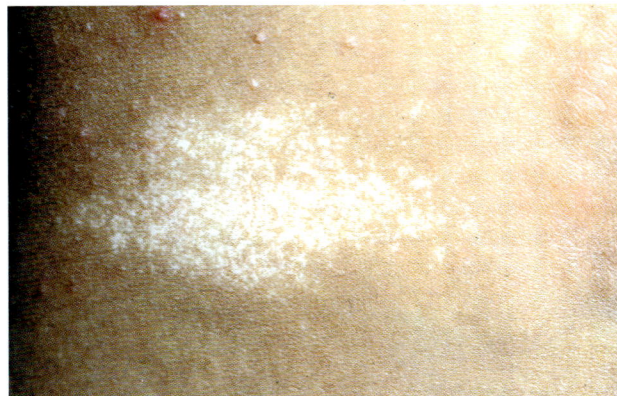

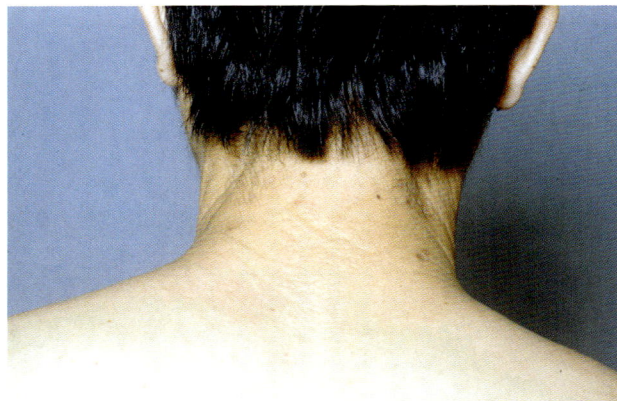

Figure 8–35 □ Tuberose sclerosis. Periungual fibromas (Konen tumors) are found in about 20% of affected individuals. They occur around or under the nail plate and may distort the nail. These fleshy growths may be reddish or flesh-colored and are more commonly found on the toes. The presence of normal epidermal skin lines helps to differentiate them from viral warts. They are pathognomonic of this condition.

Figure 8–36 □ Pseudoxanthoma elasticum. This 30-year-old Chinese male has yellowish papules and plaques on his neck. Other commonly involved sites are the axillae and flexural skin.

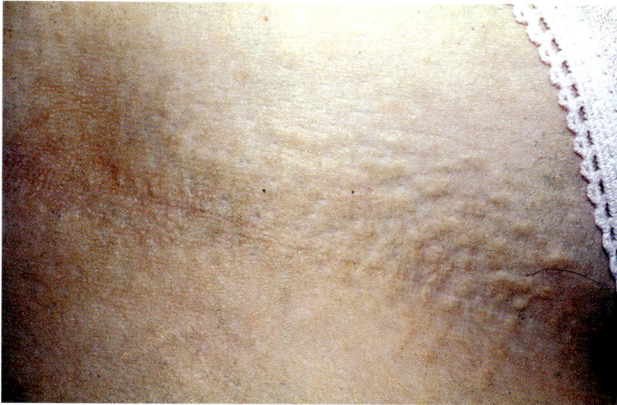

Figure 8–37 □ Pseudoxanthoma elasticum. Typical "xanthoma-like" papules with a cobblestone appearance are seen in this woman. This genetic abnormality of elastic tissue may be autosomal recessively or dominantly inherited. Noncutaneous manifestations include ocular (angioid streaks, retinal hemorrhage), cardiovascular (arterial calcification, intermittent claudication, coronary artery disease, valvular heart disease), and gastrointestinal bleeding.

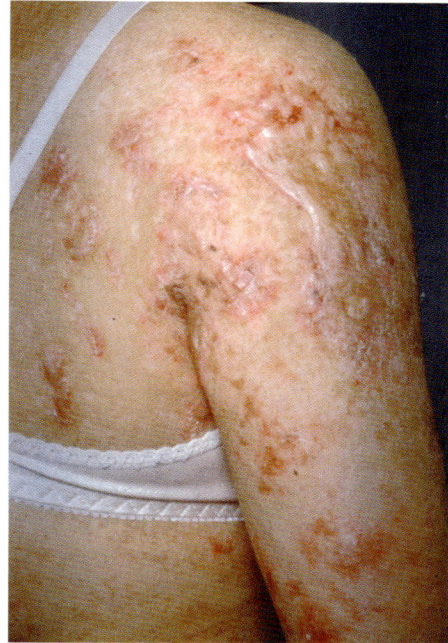

Figure 8–38 □ Focal dermal hypoplasia. This X-linked dominant condition is also known as Goltz syndrome. This girl has linear, streaky, cribriform atrophy with multiple depressions in the skin. Telangiectasia and hyperpigmentation are also present. Patchy thinning to absence of the dermis results in herniation of the subcutaneous fat up into the epidermis, causing small and yellow out-pouchings that are soft and easily depressed.

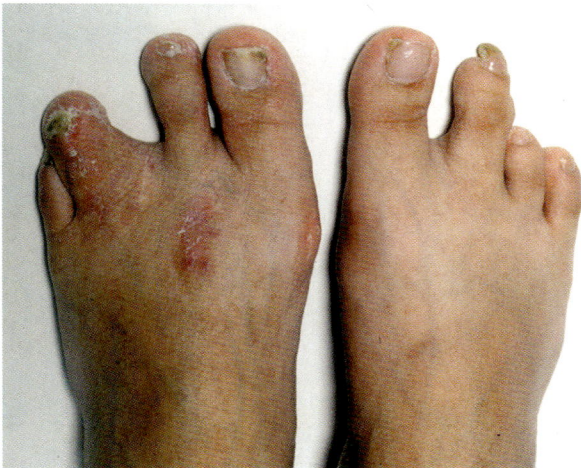

Figure 8–39 □ Focal dermal hypoplasia. Cutaneous or bony syndactyly is relatively common. Hypoplasia or aplasia of the digits can occur. Nail dystrophy is common.

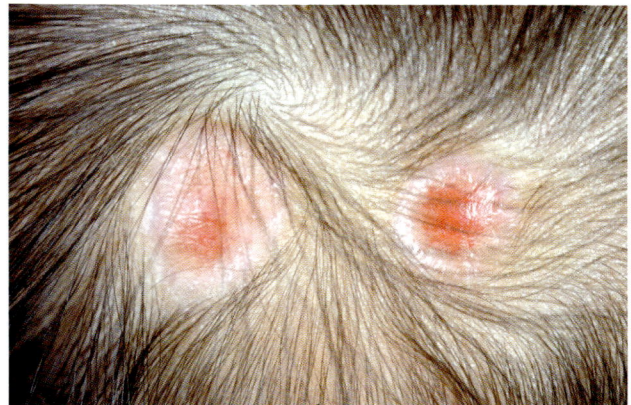

Figure 8–40 □ Aplasia cutis congenita. This is a heterogeneous group of conditions that share in common focal absence of the skin. The defect may be limited to the epidermis, involve full thickness of the skin, or bony defects. The most common site of involvement is the vertex of the scalp. These two scalp defects have healed with scars.

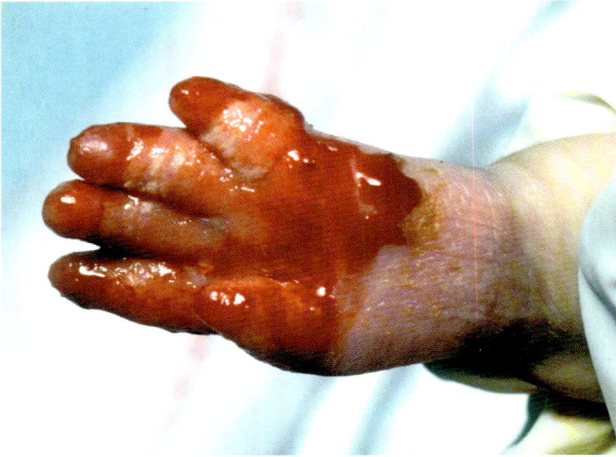

Figure 8–41 □ Aplasia cutis congenita. This shiny, red, glistening defect on the hand may be mistakenly attributed to an injury. The differential diagnosis of epidermolysis bullosa should be considered. Many cases of aplasia cutis congenita are sporadic and some demonstrate autosomal dominant inheritance.

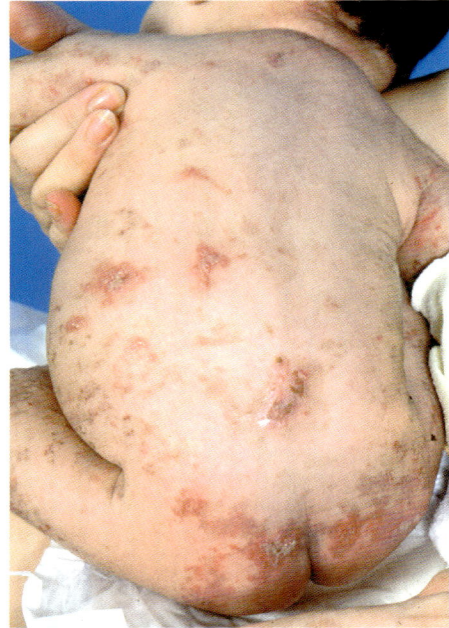

Figure 8–42 □ Incontinentia pigmenti. This X-linked dominant condition, also known as Bloch-Sulzberger syndrome, is often lethal in males. It is due to NF-kappaB essential modulator mutation, the locus of which has been mapped to Xq28. The cutaneous manifestations have four stages: inflammatory (vesicular), proliferative (papular), pigmentary, and atrophic hypopigmented lesions. These lesions are distributed along the lines of Blaschko. Vesicles, erosions, papules, and hyperpigmentation are present on the back of this child.

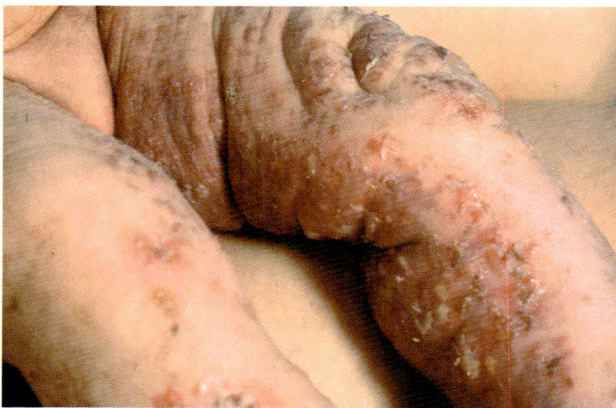

Figure 8–43 □ Incontinentia pigmenti. This is a multisystemic disorder with cutaneous, ocular, dental, cerebral, and skeletal manifestations. Vesicles and verrucous papules are distributed in a linear fashion on the limb, along the lines of Blaschko.

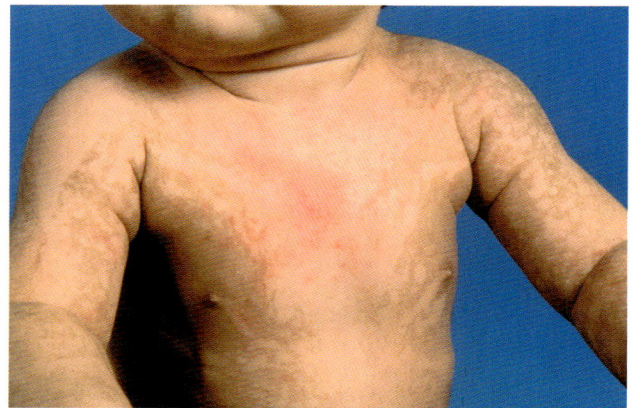

Figure 8–44 □ Incontinentia pigmenti. The vesicles often resolve by the age of six months, and the papules by the first two years of life. The hyperpigmented lesions, shown here on the chest and arms, often fade with age, but may persist into adulthood or become replaced by hypopigmented, slightly atrophic skin.

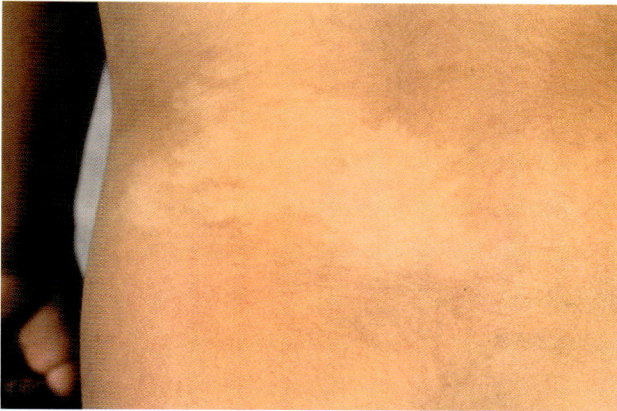

Figure 8–45 □ Hypomelanosis of Ito. Hypopigmentation is distributed in swirls and patches along the lines of Blaschko in this four-year-old Malay girl. The pigmentary disturbance is often noticed soon after birth and is non-progressive.

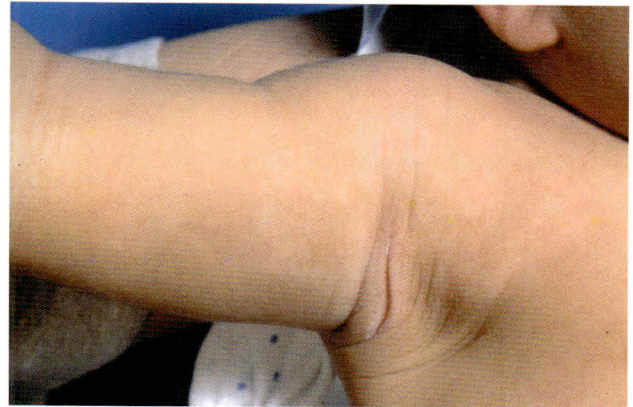

Figure 8–46 □ Hypomelanosis of Ito. The phenotype appears to be non-specific for chromosomal mosaicism, and has been reported in a number of distinct karyotype alterations, some of which are associated with mental retardation, seizures, or structural brain defects. However, it should be emphasized that most patients are otherwise normal and do not have karyotype alterations.

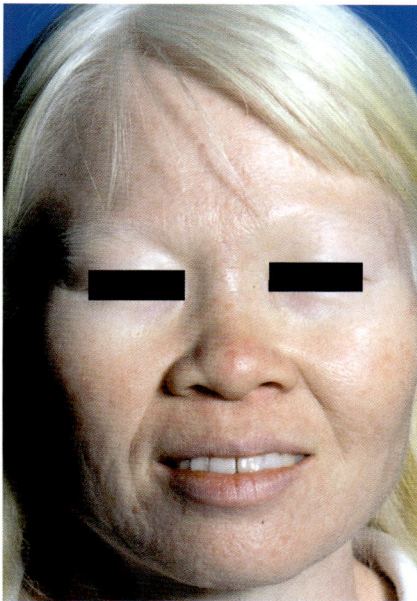

Figure 8–47 □ Albinism. This heterogeneous group of genetic disorders are characterized by congenitally absent or reduced melanin production, in the presence of the normal number, structure, and distribution of melanocytes. The skin, hair and irides may be affected to varying degrees, depending on the molecular defect. This woman of Chinese descent has white hair, hypopigmented skin, and pale irides. Sun protection, including the use of sunblock and protective clothing, monitoring for photo-related complications, like skin cancers, and ophthalmologic evaluation on diagnosis should be advised.

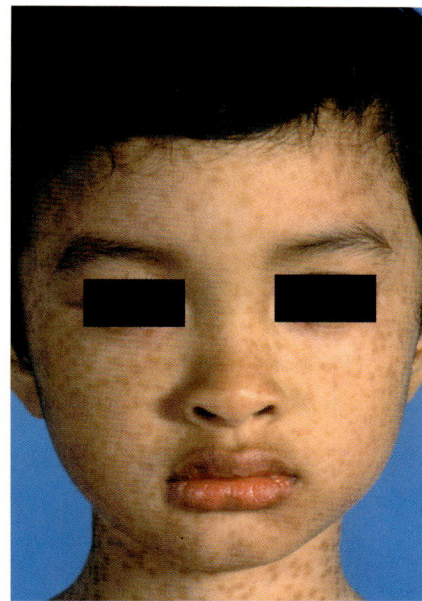

Figure 8–48 □ Multiple lentiginosis syndrome. Multiple lentigines may be presenting feature of genetic disorders like LEOPARD syndrome, Carney complex (including NAME and LAMB syndromes), Peutz-Jeghers syndrome, and Bannayan-Riley-Ruvalcaba syndrome.

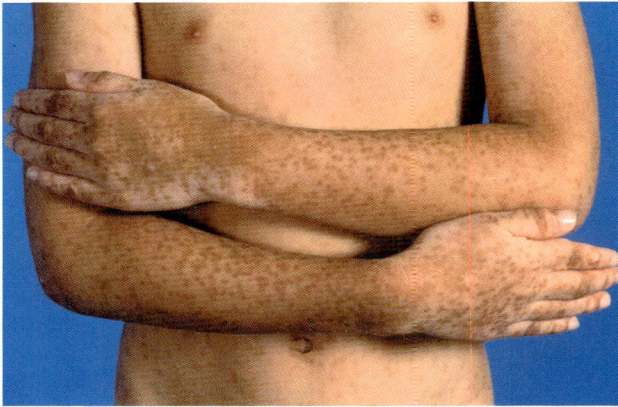

Figure 8–49 □ Multiple lentiginosis syndrome. A family history, complete physical examination (looking particularly for deafness, cardiac, ocular, genital, and growth abnormalities) and electrocardiogram should be done. This boy has multiple lentigines, especially on his face, neck, and limbs but is otherwise normal. His family history is non-contributory.

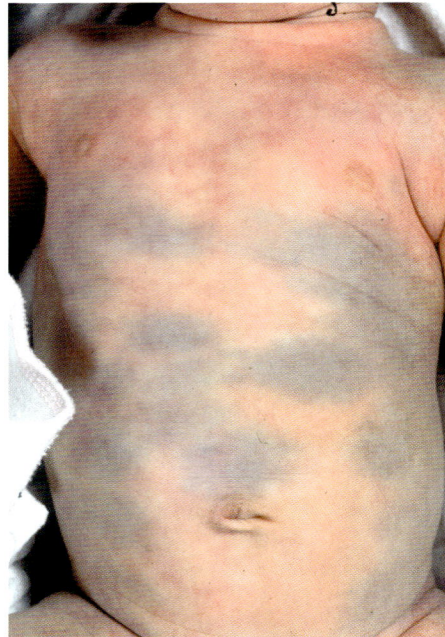

Figure 8–50 □ Phakomatosis pigmentovascularis. This girl has dermal melanocytosis and port wine stains on her trunk. The genetic concept of "twin spots" has been hypothesized to explain this sporadic association of cutaneous vascular malformation with pigmented nevi.

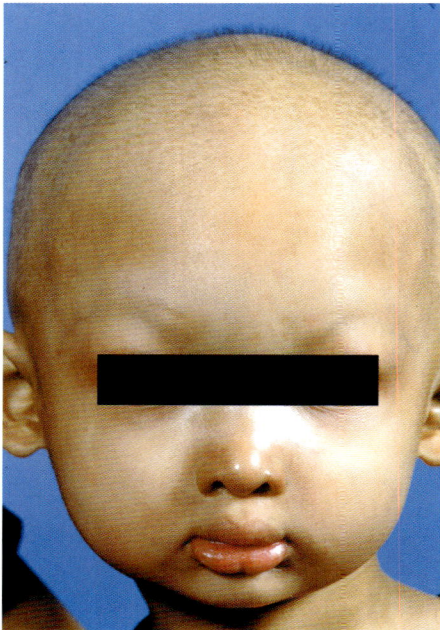

Figure 8–51 □ Hypohidrotic ectodermal dysplasia. This group of inherited disorders share common developmental defects of two or more of the following: hair, teeth, nails, and sweat glands. Hypohidrotic ectodermal dysplasia is an X-linked recessive disorder. This Chinese boy has typical features of sparse and fine hair on the scalp, eyebrow, eyelash, frontal bossing, a concave midface, and full, everted lips due to hypoplastic alveolar ridges as well as markedly reduced sweating. Bouts of fever due to the inability to maintain effective body cooling are typical during childhood.

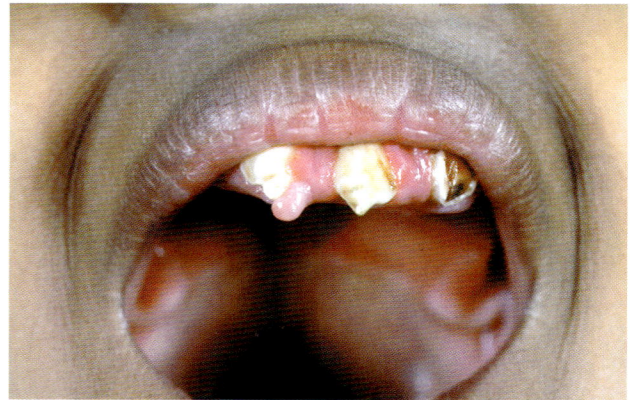

Figure 8–52 □ Hypohidrotic ectodermal dysplasia. Variable hypodontia with peg-shaped teeth is typical. Dental consult should be sought for early restoration with dentures and placement of dental implants.

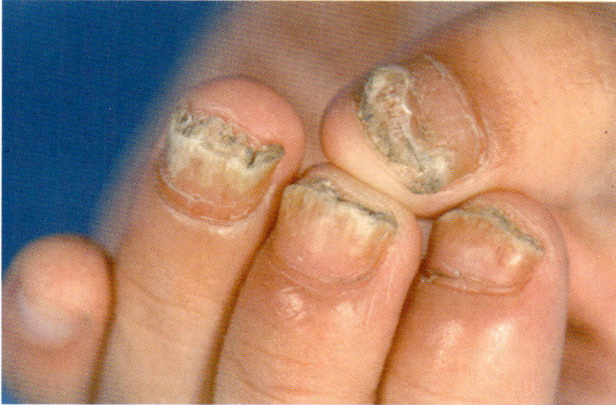

Figure 8–53 □ Pachyonychia congenita. This is a group of autosomal dominant disorders characterized by thickened, friable, and darkened nails, hyperkeratosis of the palms and soles, as well as follicular hyperkeratosis, primarily of the knees and elbows. Nail changes are usually present in infancy; the toe nails and fingernails of the thumbs and index fingers tend to be more severely involved.

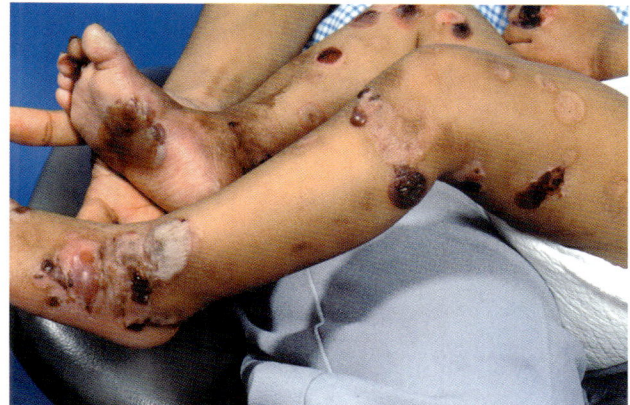

Figure 8–54 □ Epidermolysis bullosa simplex. This autosomal dominant condition is due to mutations in the keratin genes K5 and K14. This boy has developed bullae, most of which are hemorrhagic, over areas of trauma. These bullae heal without scarring, unless infection intervenes.

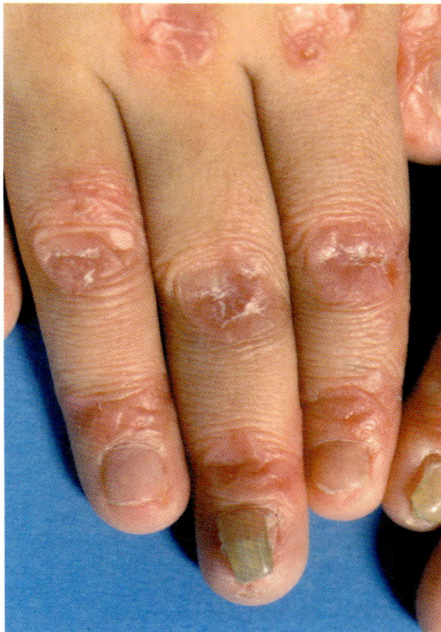

Figure 8–55 □ Epidermolysis bullosa dystrophica. This condition is due to mutations in the collagen VII genes and inheritance may be autosomal dominant or autosomal recessive, the latter having a poorer prognosis. Bullae develop over areas of trauma and heal with scarring. Milia are typically seen.

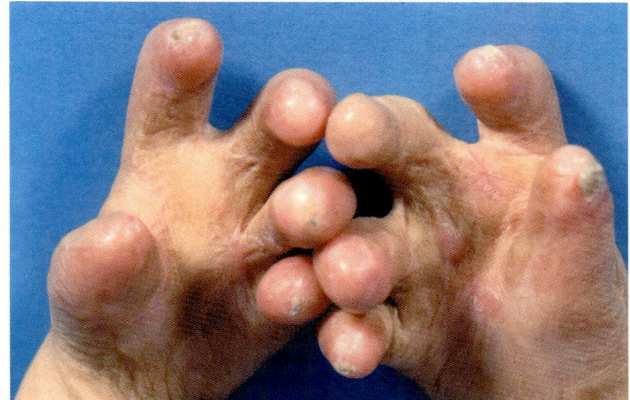

Figure 8–56 □ Epidermolysis bullosa dystrophica. Pseudoamputation of the digits, loss of nails and joint contractures may occur due to scarring. In some patients, fusion of digits leading to a mitten hand deformity may occur. Surgical release of contractures and separation of digits may be required every few years in these patients to preserve hand mobility and function.

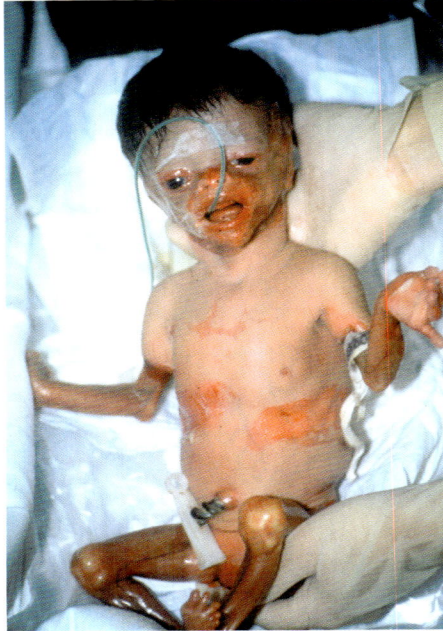

Figure 8–57 □ Junctional epidermolysis bullosa. This child has been feeding poorly due to pain from oropharyngeal erosions, resulting in failure to thrive and malnutrition. Recurrent erosions lead to loss of protein, fluid, and trace minerals like iron and zinc, aggravating his condition. Mutations in the laminin-5, $\alpha6\beta4$ integrin, uncein and BPAG2 genes have been found in this autosomal recessive condition.

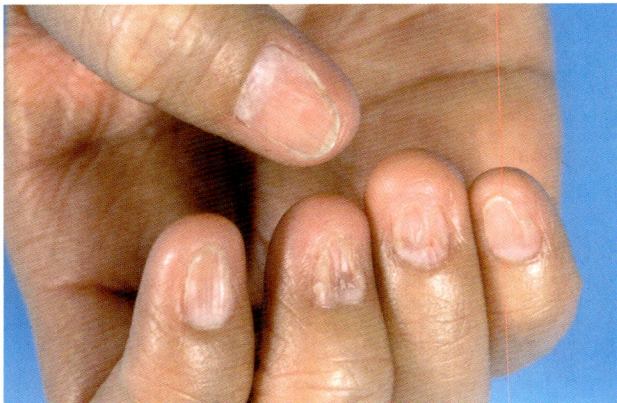

Figure 8–58 □ Dyskeratosis congenita. This X-linked recessive disorder is characterized by reticulate hyperpigmentation, nail dystrophy, oral leukoplakia, and mucocutaneous malignant tumors. Hyperpigmented macules appear on the neck, upper chest, arms, and axillae in childhood. This may progress to involve other skin folds and the lower extremities.

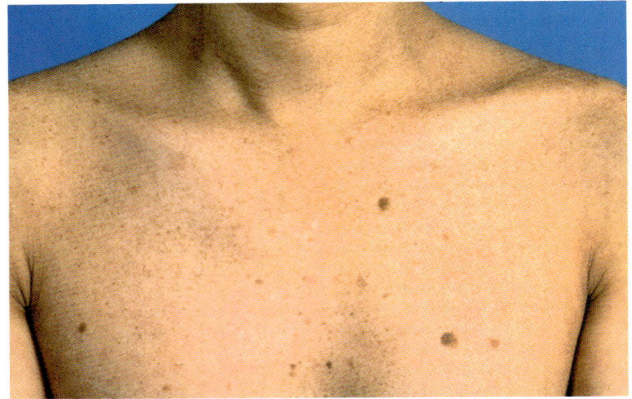

Figure 8–59 □ Dyskeratosis congenita. Nail dystrophy starts as longitudinal ridging and splitting, and progresses to pterygia formation and nail loss. Malignant skin and mucosal tumors, primarily squamous cell carcinoma, develop between the ages of 20 and 50. Bone marrow failure begins in the teenage years in about half of reported patients. Infection, hemorrhage, and malignancy are major causes of death, typically before the age of 40.

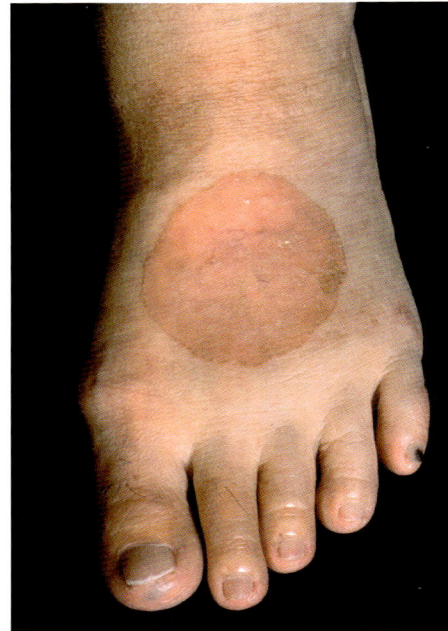

Figure 8–60 □ Porokeratosis of Mibelli. The characteristic lesions are round, erythematous to brown plaques with a surrounding raised and hyperkeratotic rim. There are several variants, including Mibelli (large annular plaques, as shown here), linear, disseminated superficial actinic, and palmoplantar. Inheritance may be autosomal dominant or sporadic.

Photodermatoses

Wong S.N. and Theng C.T.S.

Sunlight. Sun-worshippers embrace it fervently, dermatologists caution against it. We have learnt about the devastating effects of the sun from our fairer counterparts in temperate countries. From skin cancers to photodermatoses to photo-aging, ultraviolet radiation has been implicated as a major etiological factor. Yet, in a climate of unrelenting sunshine punctuated by year-end monsoon showers, skin cancers and the idiopathic photodermatoses are less frequently seen in tropical Asia than in the United States, Europe, or Australia. Some have postulated that skin-hardening consequent to chronic sun exposure during the course of work or daily living could account for the decreased incidence of photosensitive skin conditions. Subtropical Australia, however, with its almost perennial sunshine, is still a brewing pot for photosensitive skin conditions. The common denominating factor in regions with low incidence of photosensitive conditions appears to be pigmentation, whether it be the yellow-brown pigmentation of ethnic Chinese, the medium-brown pigmentation of ethnic Malays or Polynesians, or darker brown pigmentation of ethnic Indians.

Pigmentation, however protective, does have its limitations. Two decades ago, an Asian lady would not dream of going out of the house without an umbrella – for protection against the sun, not the rain, and certainly not when the sun was at its zenith. As the younger generation looked increasingly to the West, the notion of a "beautiful tan" soon set root in the fertile soil of youth. From the poolside to the beach to sidewalk cafés, they deliberately exposed themselves to high levels of ultraviolet radiation in their quest for beauty and acceptance. Apart from photo-aging and pigmentary problems such as solar lentigines and melasma, we have also seen an increase in the incidence of the idiopathic photodermatoses in the past decade.

POLYMORPHOUS LIGHT ERUPTION (Figures 9–1 to 9–8)

As in other parts of the world, polymorphous light eruption is the most commonly seen idiopathic photodermatosis. Papules and eczematous lesions predominate. However, a lichen nitidus-like morphology has also been observed, particularly in darker Asian skin types such as ethnic Indians and Sri Lankans, but also in Malays, Chinese, and Koreans. This morphology has not been described in Caucasian skin but was recently reported in African-Americans.

CHRONIC ACTINIC DERMATITIS (Figures 9–9 to 9–14)

Chronic actinic dermatitis generally affects elderly men. However, in Asia, as in other parts of the world, we are seeing chronic actinic dermatitis in younger adults in association with advanced asymptomatic HIV infection. In such cases, a photodistributed rash may be the initial presenting feature of HIV infection, necessitating a screen for HIV infection in newly diagnosed cases of chronic actinic dermatitis not in the usual age group. We postulate that HIV infection may be predisposed to or hasten the onset of chronic actinic dermatitis.

ACTINIC PRURIGO (Figures 9–15 to 9–17)

In contrast to actinic prurigo in Britain, actinic prurigo in Singapore affects adults rather than pubertal adolescents, and spontaneous resolution does not occur. The similarity to actinic prurigo in American Indians is not limited to age of onset and persistence. Cheilitis, a feature of actinic prurigo in the Americas, was observed in up to 20% of affected patients here. Conjunctivitis, however, has not been observed.

SOLAR URTICARIA (Figure 9–18)

It is often difficult for patients in tropical climates to distinguish between aggravation by heat, by sweating, and by the sun, as all three frequently occur simultaneously. A detailed history may help differentiate between solar urticaria and cholinergic urticaria, but challenge tests, such as exercise challenge test and photoprovocation test, are usually needed to establish the diagnosis.

HYDROA VACCINIFORME (Figures 9–19 to 9–23)

Hydroa vacciniforme, a rare photodermatosis characterized by a vesicular eruption that heals with vacciniforme scarring, occurs typically in children with resolution in adolescence. However, the two cases diagnosed at our center over the last ten years both had a late onset in young adulthood, with no resolution to date.

PHOTOSENSITIVITY SECONDARY TO SYSTEMIC DRUGS (Figures 9–24 to 9–28)

Photosensitivity secondary to systemic drugs is relatively common, comprising about 15% of photodermatoses seen. The main culprits are thiazide diuretics, phenothiazines, and hypo-glycemic agents. The thiazide diuretics, although long known to be associated with photosensitivity and electrolyte disturbances, are still widely prescribed as anti-hypertensive agents as they are inexpensive and efficacious, important factors in Asian countries where healthcare costs are borne largely by the patients. Doxycycline, for similar reasons, is widely used in Asia for treatment of acne vulgaris, and photo-onycholysis occasionally occurs.

PHOTO-ALLERGIC CONTACT DERMATITIS (Figures 9–29 to 9–32)

Photo-allergic contact dermatitis has seen a shift from fragrances as the main photoallergen to sunscreen components in recent years. This has paralleled the increase in sunscreen use and the inclusion of sunscreen components in proprietary cosmetic products to prevent photo-aging and pigmentation. Phototoxic contact dermatitis occurs more in the context of food preparation, such as squeezing lime and grating turnip.

PHOTOSENSITIVITY DUE TO METABOLIC AND GENETIC CAUSES (Figures 9–33 to 9–42)

Photosensitivity due to metabolic and genetic causes such as the porphyrias, pseudoporphyria, and xeroderma pigmentosum is very rarely seen in Asia. Pellagra has become increasingly uncommon with increasing affluence and improved diet.

PHOTO-AGGRAVATED DERMATOSES

A wide range of dermatoses may demonstrate photo-aggravation. These include lupus erythematosus, dermatomyositis, pemphigus foliaceus, herpes simplex, actinic lichen planus, acne vulgaris, atopic dermatitis, and transient acantholytic dermatosis. These conditions are covered elsewhere in this atlas.

UV RADIATION AND SKIN CANCERS

Certain neoplastic diseases, such as squamous cell carcinoma, basal cell carcinoma, actinic keratoses, and malignant melanoma, show a predilection for sun-exposed areas. UVB is thought to be primarily responsible for non-melanoma skin cancers, whilst UVA has been implicated in melanoma. The incidence of these have been low in Asia compared to Western nations, with some of those affected having other predisposing factors such as photo-chemotherapy, or chronic arsenic ingestion, the latter from drinking contaminated well water or consumption of traditional Chinese medicines for asthma.

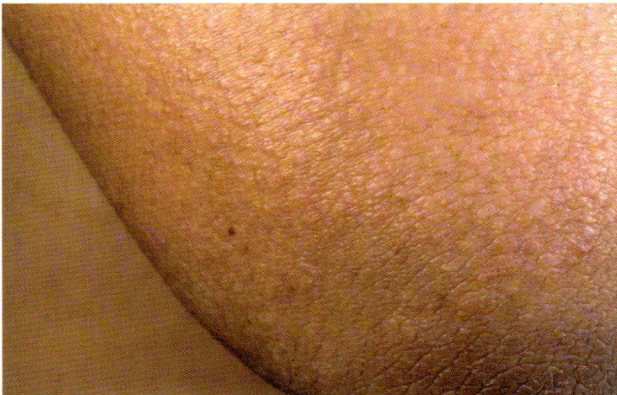

Figure 9–1 □ Polymorphous light eruption – papular variant. Multiple skin-colored to erythematous papules on the extensor aspect of the forearm and elbow. The papular variant is the most common morphology seen, and the distribution is usually patchy. The lesions typically erupt hours after sun exposure and resolve within a few days to two weeks without scarring.

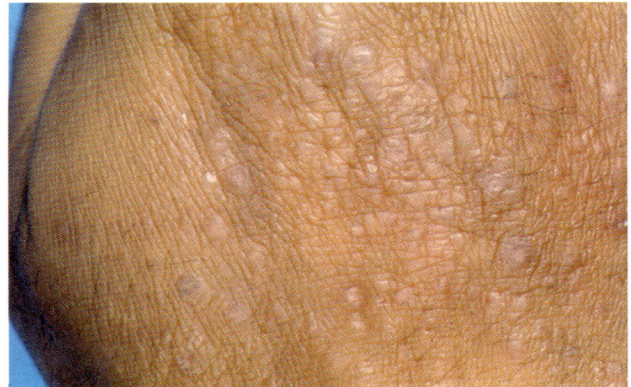

Figure 9–2 □ Polymorphous light eruption – papular variant. Both large and small papules are present. Some are excoriated, a reflection of the pruritus usually experienced. The dorsum of the hands, forearms, and nape of the neck are the most commonly affected sites.

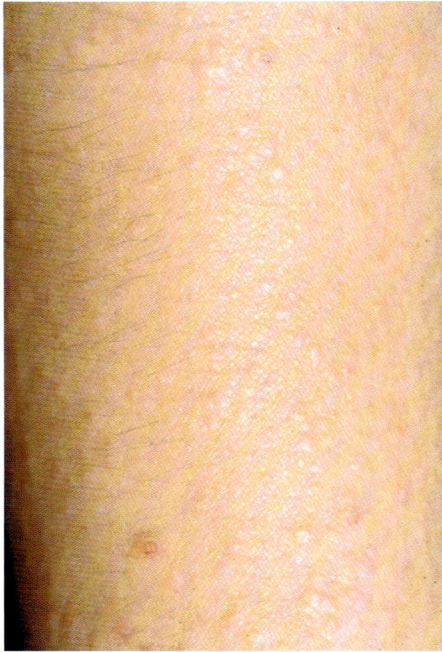

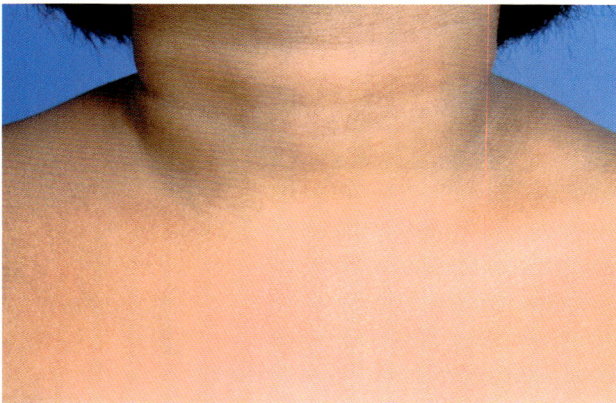

Figure 9–4 □ Polymorphous light eruption – eczema and papules. Eczematous and papular lesions occurring simultaneously in the same patient, hence the term "polymorphous". It is not uncommon to have more than one morphological subtype seen in a patient at any one time. The same patient may also present with a different morphological type at another point in time, although most patients remain "true to type".

Figure 9–3 □ Polymorphous light eruption – papules and plaques. Hypopigmented, slightly pinkish papules coalescing into plaques. In darker-skin types, the lesions may appear hypopigmented and lichenoid in appearance.

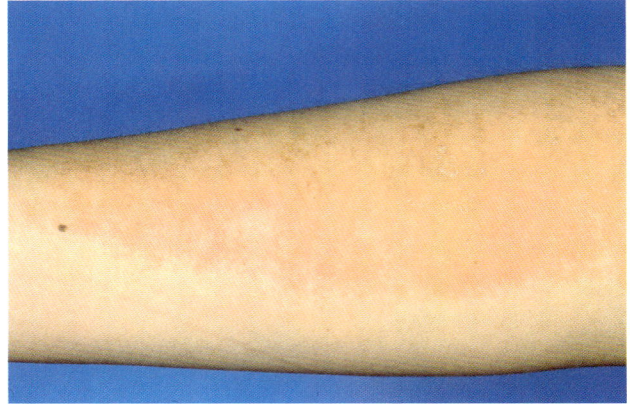

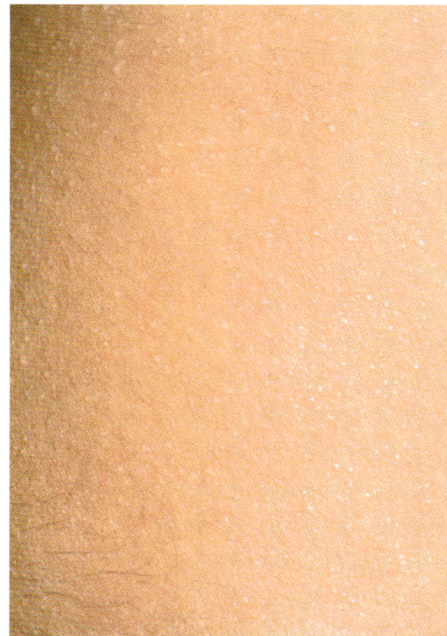

Figure 9–5 □ Polymorphous light eruption – lichen nitidus-like variant. Tiny, shiny, lichen nitidus-like papules over the V of the neck, sparing covered areas. This subtype is not uncommon in Asian skin, and shows a predilection for Indians and darker-skin types. In the West, it has been reported only in African-Americans. Unlike lichen nitidus, it is usually pruritic and confined to photo-exposed areas. It often resolves with post-inflammatory hypopigmentation or hyper-pigmentation.

Figure 9–6 □ Polymorphous light eruption – lichen nitidus-like variant. A close-up view of the forearm of the patient in Figure 9–5 showing the pinpoint, shiny, lichen nitidus-like papules.

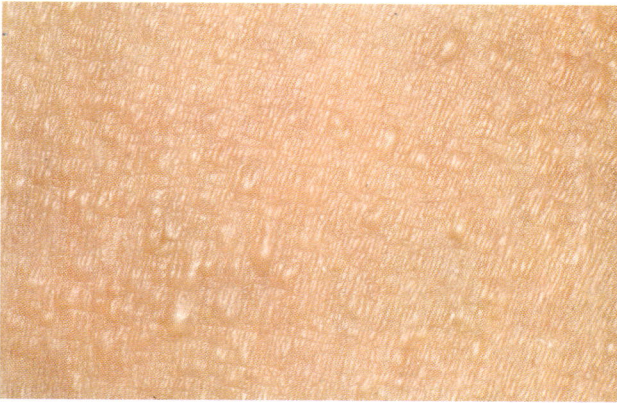

Figure 9–7 □ Polymorphous light eruption – vesicular variant. A close-up showing small vesicles and papulovesicles. Vesicles are a rare presentation of polymorphic light eruption, and are differentiated from hydroa vacciniforme by the lack of scarring on resolution.

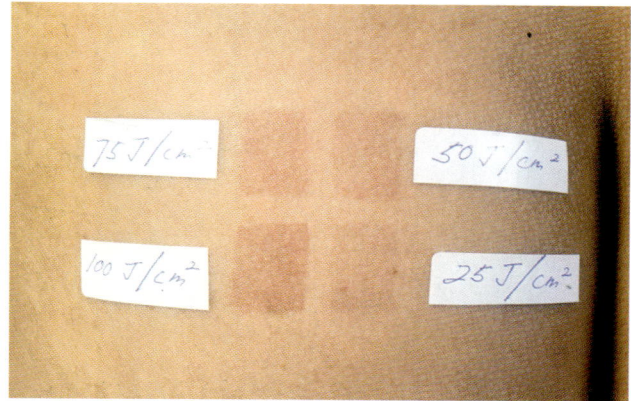

Figure 9–8 □ Polymorphous light eruption – abnormal phototest. This patient has developed erythema to 25 J/cm^2 of UVA with the normal minimal erythema dose (MED) to UVA for his skin type (Fitzpatrick type IV) being more than 80 J/cm^2. About half of patients have abnormal phototests, most commonly decreased MED to UVB, but some to UVA or both. Occasionally, papules typical of the eruption may develop on the irradiated areas.

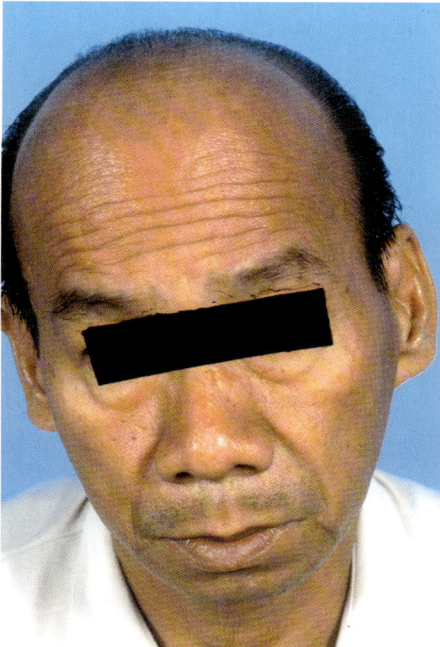

Figure 9–9 □ Chronic actinic dermatitis. Chronic, lichenified, eczematous plaques affecting the convex surfaces of the face and sparing the eyelids, nasolabial folds, and submental region. Chronic actinic dermatitis is an idiopathic primary photodermatosis that preferentially affects elderly males, and presents as chronic eczema affecting predominantly the sun-exposed areas. However, it may also spread to covered areas when severe.

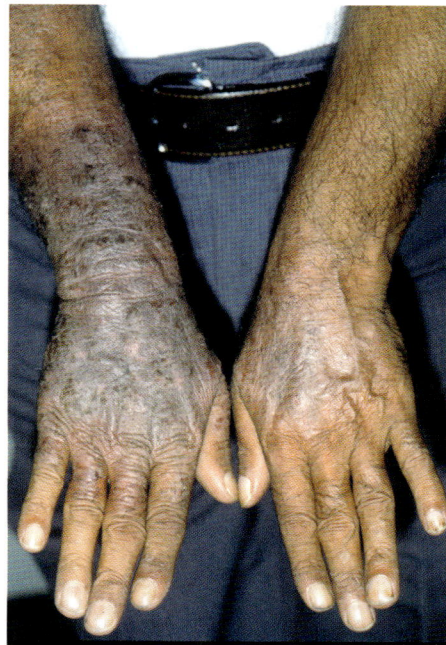

Figure 9–10 □ Chronic actinic dermatitis. Hyperpigmented, eczematous plaques over the dorsum of the hands and wrists. With chronicity, eczema may become hyperpigmented, a phenomenon often seen in pigmented Asians.

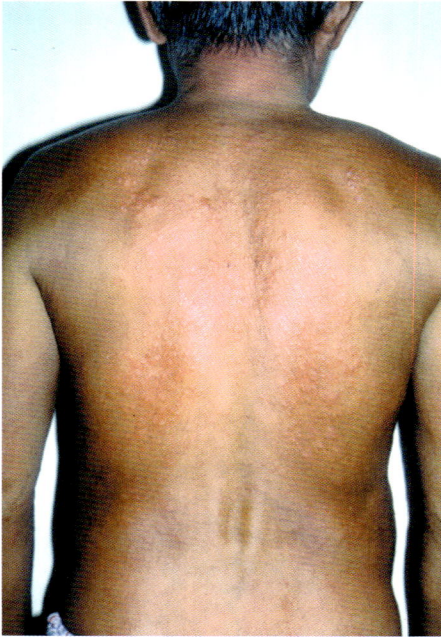

Figure 9–11 □ Chronic actinic dermatitis. Involvement of covered area of the back, with a band of sparing where the collar has conferred protection. Some patients with this distribution have improved with the use of tight-weave, dark-colored clothing and extension of sunscreen use to include covered areas.

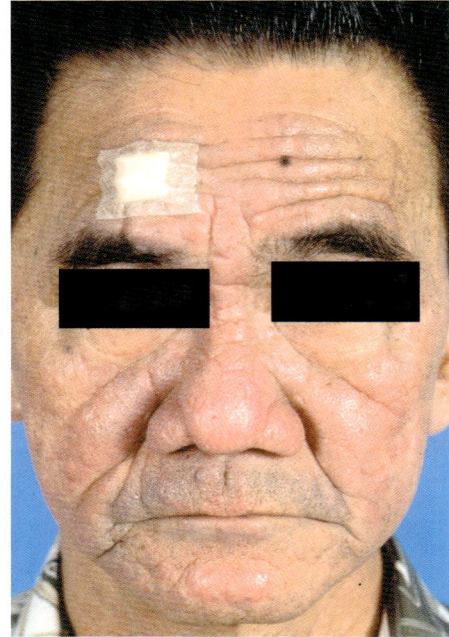

Figure 9–12 □ Pseudolymphomatous chronic actinic dermatitis. Indurated erythematous plaques on the face resembling infiltrated plaques of cutaneous lymphoma, throwing the skin into leonine-like folds. This severe form of chronic actinic dermatitis was previously known as actinic reticuloid. Histologically, dense lymphocytic infiltrates may also resemble lymphoma.

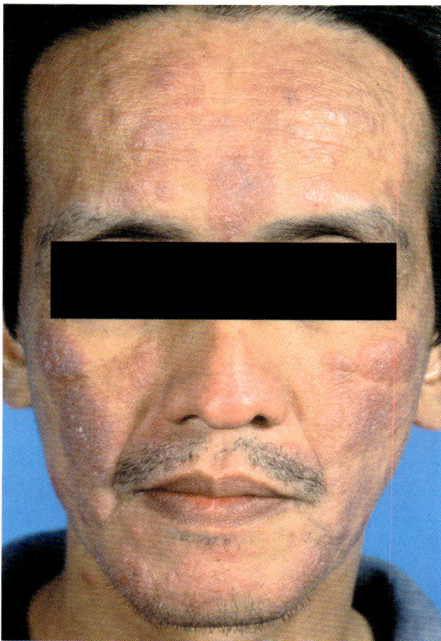

Figure 9–13 □ Chronic actinic dermatitis in HIV. This 40-year-old gentleman is not in the characteristically affected age group. Chronic actinic dermatitis has been reported from our center and in African-Americans to be a presenting feature of advanced asymptomatic HIV infection, where the age of onset is younger than usual. Early age of onset of chronic actinic dermatitis has also been reported in atopic individuals.

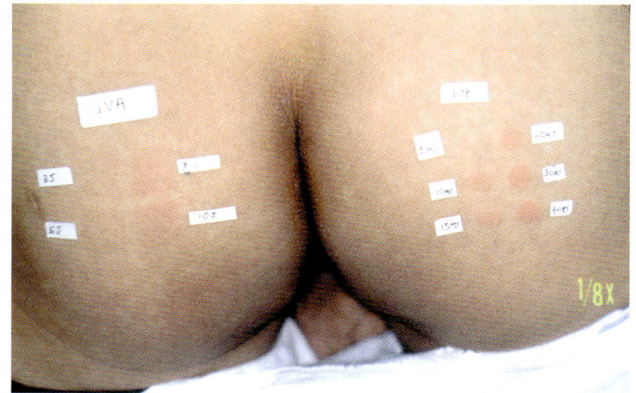

Figure 9–14 □ Chronic actinic dermatitis – phototest. Abnormal phototest demonstrating markedly decreased MED to both UVA and UVB, typical of chronic actinic dermatitis (CAD) seen here. Occasionally, some have reduced MED to UVA or UVB alone.

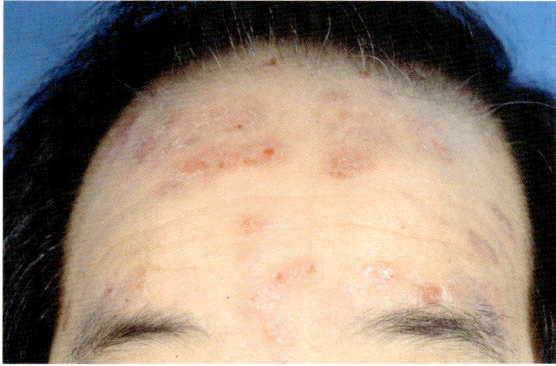

Figure 9–15 □ **Actinic prurigo.** Excoriated erythematous papules and lichenified plaques present symmetrically on the forehead, supraorbital ridge, and dorsum of nose. Some regard this condition as a more severe and persistent form of polymorphous light eruption. Our Asian patients are unusual in that the onset is usually in adulthood, with no spontaneous resolution. Conjunctivitis and cheilitis are other features that are occasionally seen in our tropical variant.

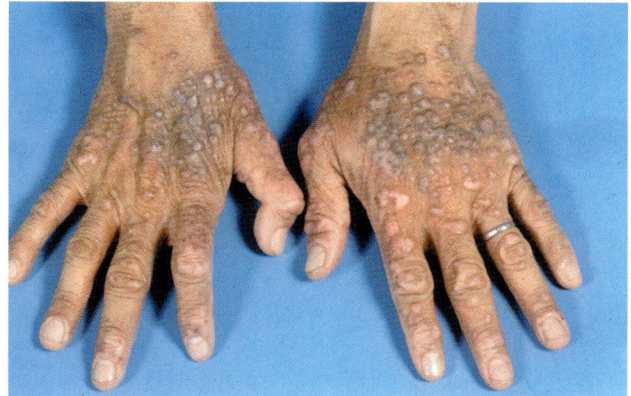

Figure 9–16 □ **Actinic prurigo.** Chronic excoriated prurigo nodules on the dorsum of the hands, a typical site of involvement in actinic prurigo. With chronicity, some nodules have become hyperpigmented with central hypopigmentation, a common observation in pigmented skin types.

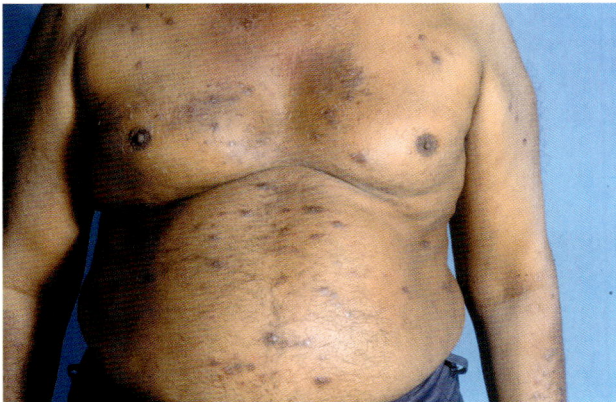

Figure 9–17 □ **Actinic prurigo.** The lesions have spread to the covered areas as well in this Indian patient with severe actinic prurigo. Erythema takes on a more pigmented or purplish hue in such darker-skin types. Phototesting usually reveals reduced MED to both UVA and UVB, and occasionally to UVB only.

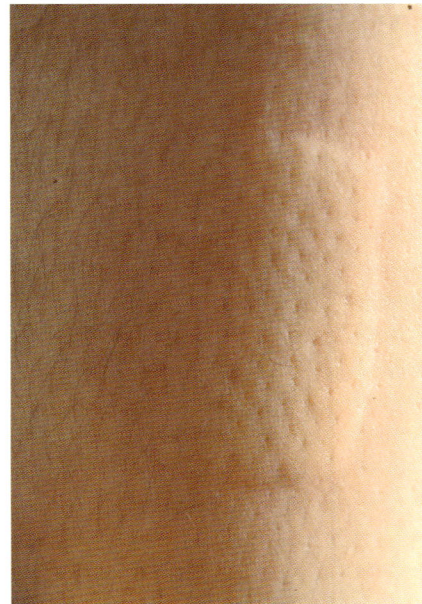

Figure 9–18 □ **Solar urticaria.** Well-demarcated edema induced within 15 minutes following exposure to visible light from a slide projector. Solar urticaria typically develops within minutes of exposure to sunlight, and resolves within a few hours. Patients usually have no visible lesions at the time of consultation, and a phototest is most useful in confirming the diagnosis.

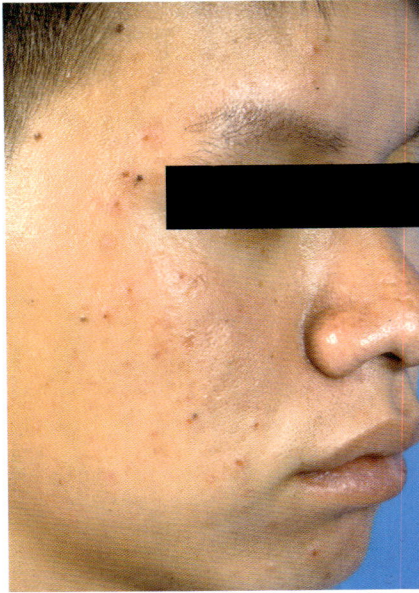

Figure 9–19 □ Hydroa vacciniforme. Necrotic papulo-vesicles in the sun-exposed areas of the face. These lesions are typically distributed over the ears, nose, and cheeks. They start as pruritic erythematous macules within hours of sun exposure, progressing through tender papules to vesicles or bullae that eventually crust and heal with vacciniform scarring. A sharply marginated depressed scar, the final stage of the evolution of lesions, is present at the zygomatic region.

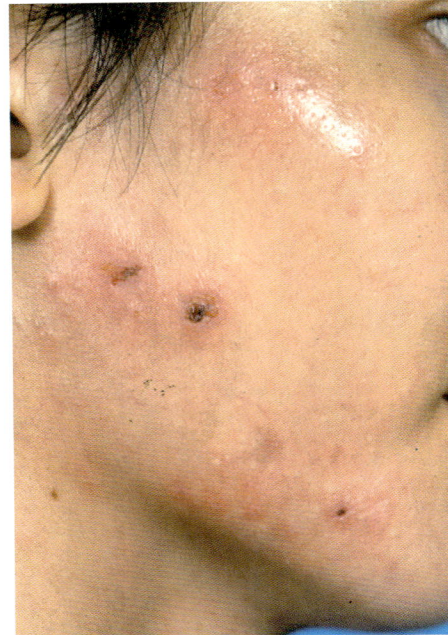

Figure reproduced with permission from *British Journal of Dermatology.*

Figure 9–20 □ Hydroa vacciniforme. A male patient in his early 20s with scattered necrotic papules and papulovesicles on his face. It is unusual for Asians to experience onset in their early 20s, the usual age of onset worldwide being in childhood, with resolution by adolescence or early adulthood.

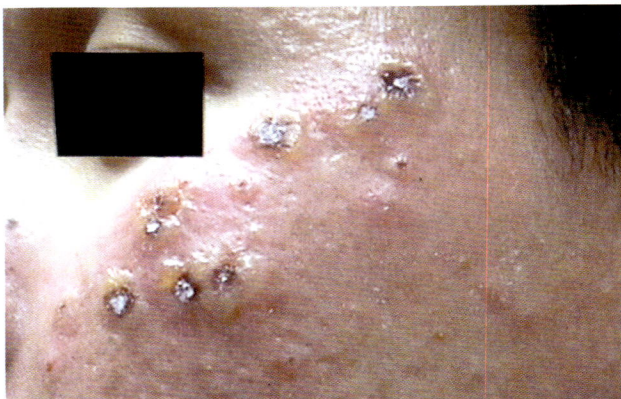

Figure reproduced with permission from *British Journal of Dermatology.*

Figure 9–21 □ Hydroa vacciniforme. Umbilicated vesicles with crusting which typically develop days after the inciting sun exposure.

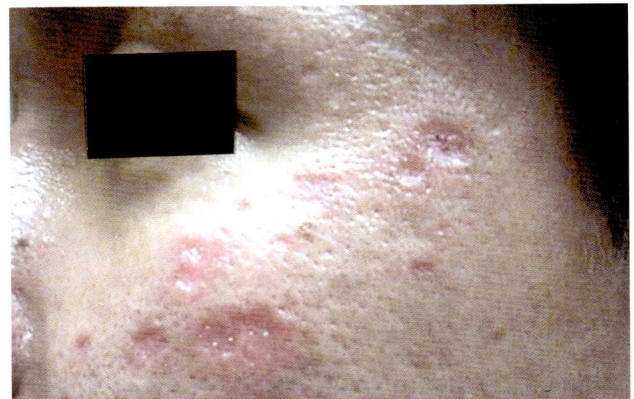

Figure reproduced with permission from *British Journal of Dermatology.*

Figure 9–22 □ Hydroa vacciniforme. The vesicles seen in Figure 9–20 have healed over weeks, leaving vacciniform scars which are characteristic. In contrast, papulovesicular polymorphous light eruption heals without scarring.

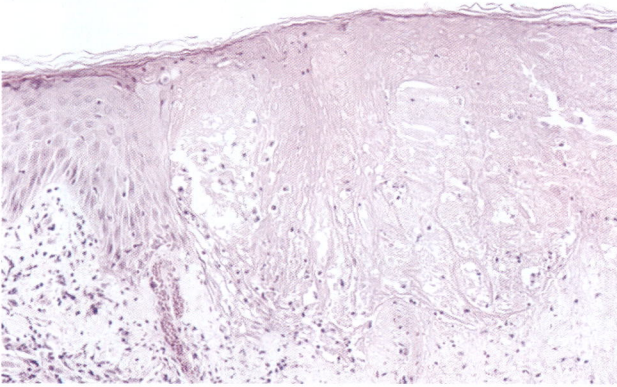

Figure reproduced with permission from *British Journal of Dermatology.*

Figure 9–23 □ Hydroa vacciniforme – histopathology. Vesicle formation with focal epidermal necrosis is characteristic. A superficial dermal perivascular infiltrate of lymphocytes is also seen.

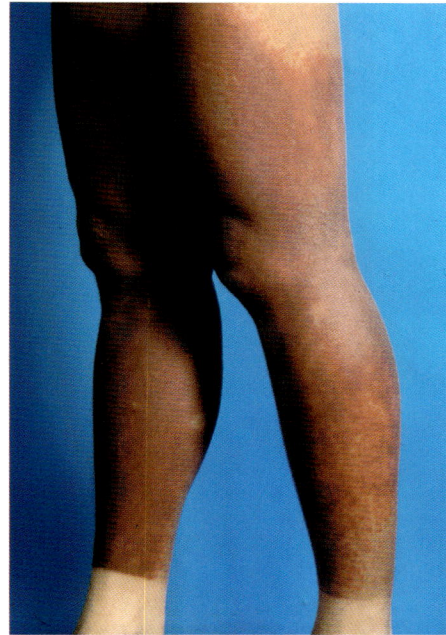

Figure 9–24 □ Phototoxic drug reaction to griseofulvin. Sharply demarcated, sunburn-like, intense erythema, edema, and papules in this patient with phototoxic drug reaction to griseofulvin. Phototoxicity in the acute phase mimicks severe sunburn, and is confined exclusively to areas of skin exposed to light.

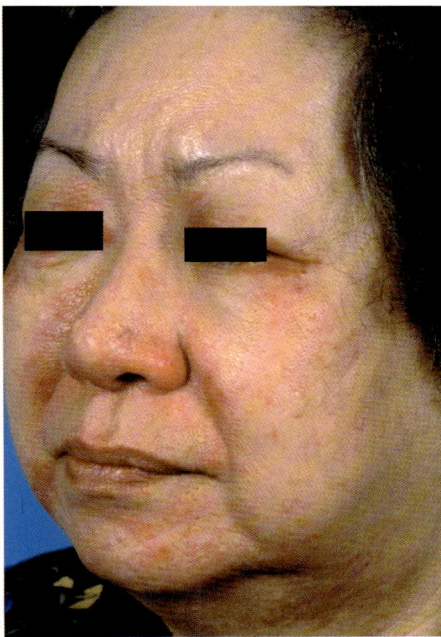

Figure 9–25 □ Phototoxic drug reaction to hydrochlorthiazide. Photodistributed erythema, edema, and erythematous papules on the face of a patient who was on hydrochlorthiazide for control of hypertension. This is the most commonly implicated drug here. Phototesting may reveal decreased MED, usually to UVA.

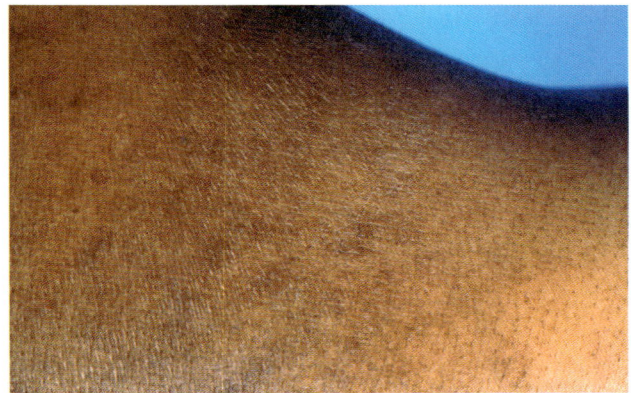

Figure 9–26 □ Phototoxic drug reaction to glibenclamide. Hyperpigmented, eczematous lesions on the extensor aspect of the forearms of this Indian patient on glibenclamide for diabetes mellitus. With repeated exposure, as would occur with chronic medications, chronic changes, such as scaling and lichenification, may occur. The distinction between photo-allergic and phototoxic drug reaction often cannot be made clinically.

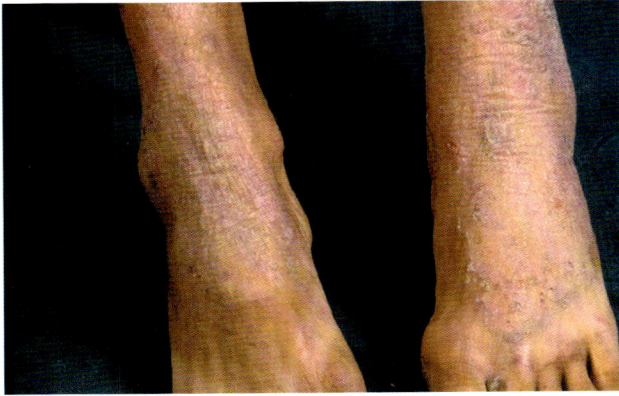

Figure 9–27 □ Chronic phototoxic drug reaction to chlorpromazine. Chronic lichenified, eczematous plaques on the dorsum of the feet of a patient on chlorpromazine for chronic schizophrenia. Although an uncommon site for photodermatitis, this institutionalized patient usually wore long pyjamas with Japanese thongs, leading to this unusual presentation, and a V-shaped zone of sparing on the forefoot.

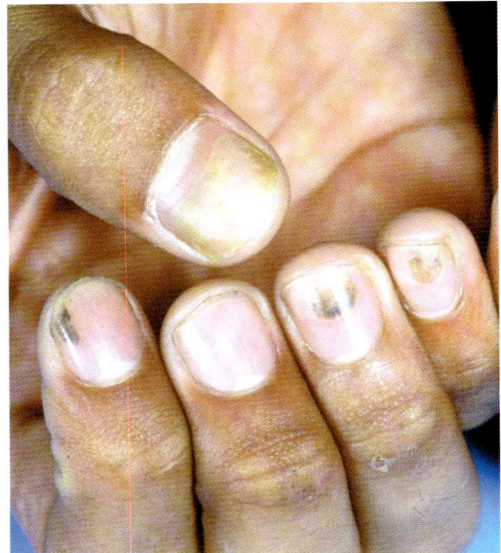

Figure 9–28 □ Phototoxic drug reaction to doxycycline. Separation of the nail from the nail bed has occurred in this patient who developed photo-onycholysis with doxycycline.

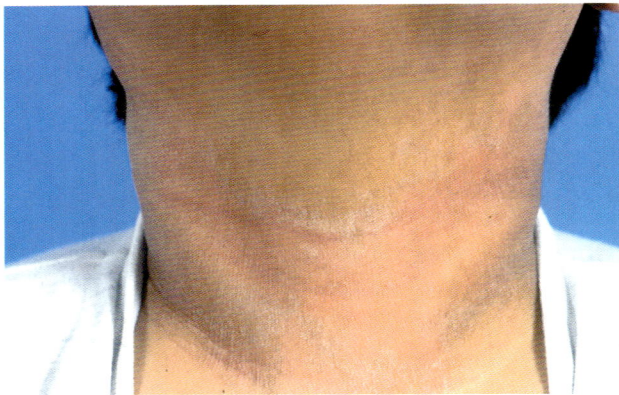

Figure 9–29 □ Photo-allergic contact dermatitis from sunscreen. Erythema and papules affecting the photo-exposed areas of the face and neck, following the use of a sunscreen and subsequent sun exposure. The diagnosis may be confirmed with a photopatch test. Locally, chemical sunscreens are now the most common group of allergens responsible for photo-allergic contact dermatitis. They are found not only in sunscreen lotions but also in lipsticks, lip balms, moisturisers, foundations, face powders, and shampoos.

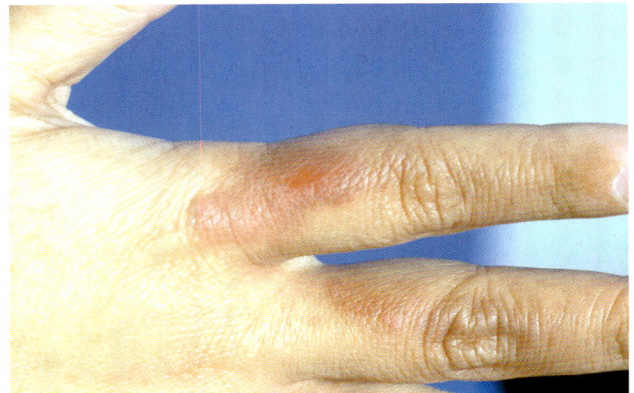

Figure 9–30 □ Phototoxic contact dermatitis from lime juice. Characteristic distribution of phototoxic contact dermatitis from lime juice in the dominant hand occurring after squeezing limes in sunlight. Hyperpigmentation, often not preceded by erythema, occurs and pigmented macules from lime juice droplets may also be seen on the dorsum of the non-dominant hand. These persist for months but eventually resolve.

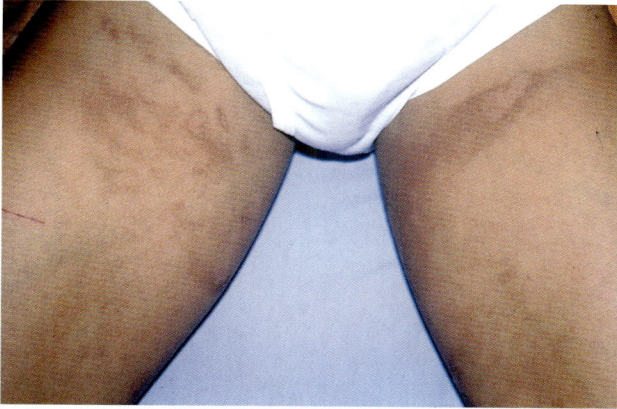

Figure 9–31 □ Phototoxic contact dermatitis from pomelo juice. This man has streaky pigmentation over the thighs, where he had anchored a pomelo (a large citrus fruit) that he had been peeling. Citrus juice contains furocoumarins (plant psoralens), which is phototoxic.

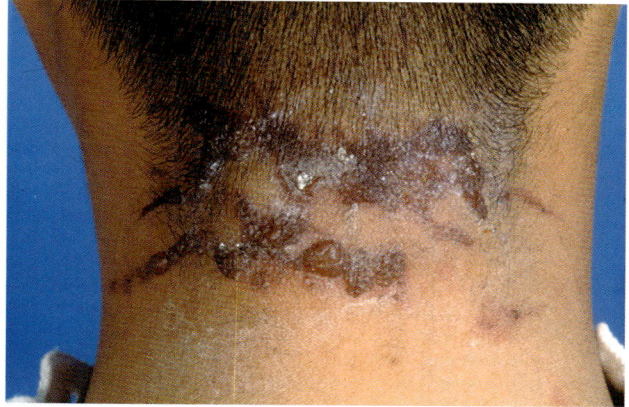

Figure 9–32 □ Phytophotodermatitis. This national serviceman developed acute eczema with linear and confluent areas of erythema and vesiculation at the exposed area of his neck after outfield training. This pattern and distribution are highly suggestive of phytophotodermatitis, possibly to meadow grass.

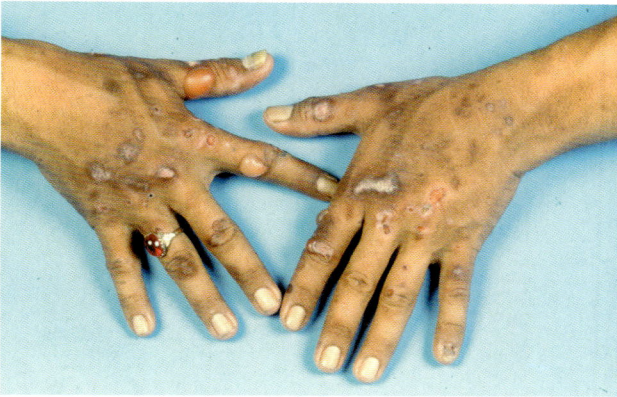

Figure 9–33 □ Porphyria cutanea tarda. Bullae, erosions, scarring, and hyperpigmentation on the hands of a young man with hereditary porphyria cutanea tarda. The most common of the porphyrias seen in dermatological practice, porphyria cutanea tarda is characterized by fragility of the light-exposed skin, most prominently on the hands, but also on other light-exposed areas. The vesicles are characteristically subepidermal with "festooning" of the basement membrane, and little or no inflammatory infiltrate.

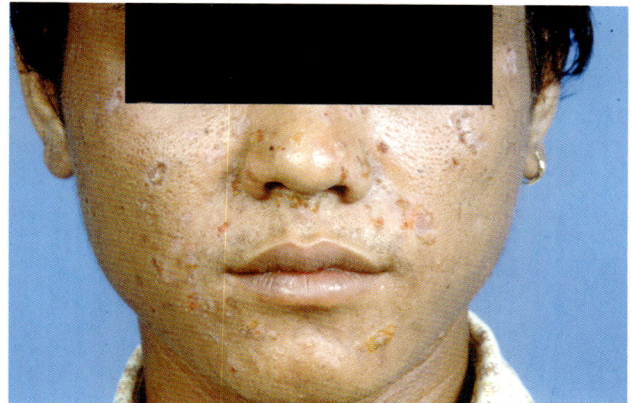

Figure 9–34 □ Porphyria cutanea tarda. Crusted erosions heal slowly with atrophic scarring and milia formation. Additional features such as hypertrichosis, hyperpigmentation, and sclerodermoid plaques will help to differentiate this from hydroa vacciniforme and epidermolysis bullosa acquisita.

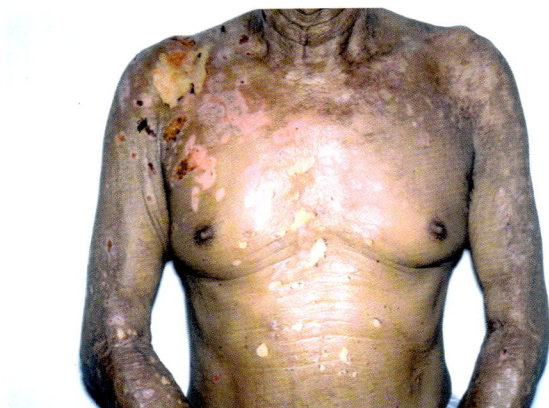

Figure 9–35 □ Porphyria cutanea tarda. Extensive erosions on photo-exposed areas, extending to covered areas of the trunk. The sporadic type is the most common type seen here, usually in the context of middle-aged male alcohol abusers, such as this man with gynecomastia.

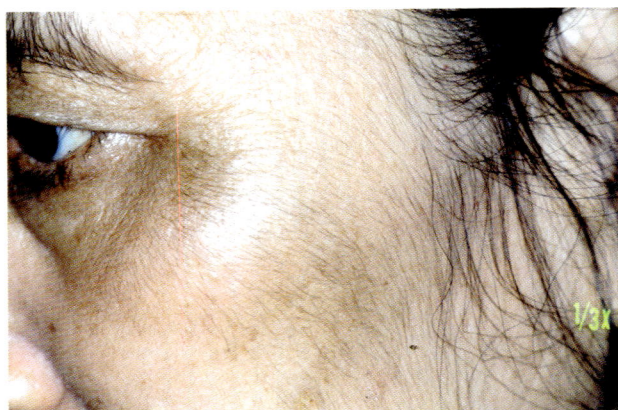

Figure 9–36 □ Porphyria cutanea tarda – hypertrichosis. Hypertrichosis, as seen in this woman, is present in the majority of patients with porphyria cutanea tarda. The malar and temporal regions are the usual areas involved.

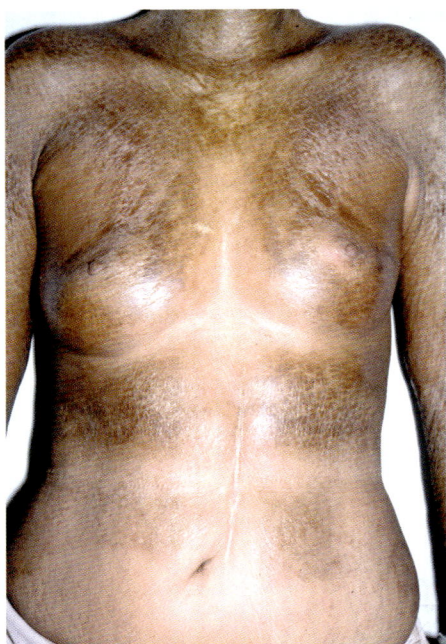

Figure 9–37 □ Porphyria cutanea tarda – sclerodermatous change. Waxy white, sclerodermoid plaques with mottled hyperpigmentation on the chest and abdomen of this elderly woman. These plaques may occur in light-exposed or covered regions, and resemble morphea or scleroderma, both clinically and histologically.

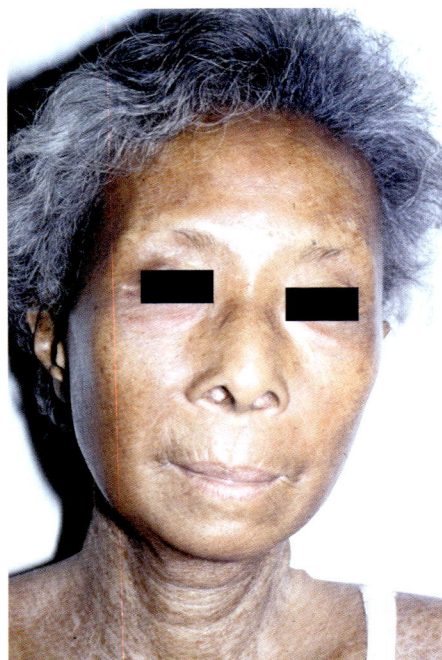

Figure 9–38 □ Porphyria cutanea tarda – sclerodermatous change. The same patient as Figure 9–37 demonstrating scleroderma-like features of beaking of the nose, a youthful taut face despite the graying hairs, and a "purse-string" mouth. Characteristic melasma-like, mottled, hyper- and hypopigmentation is seen on the face and neck.

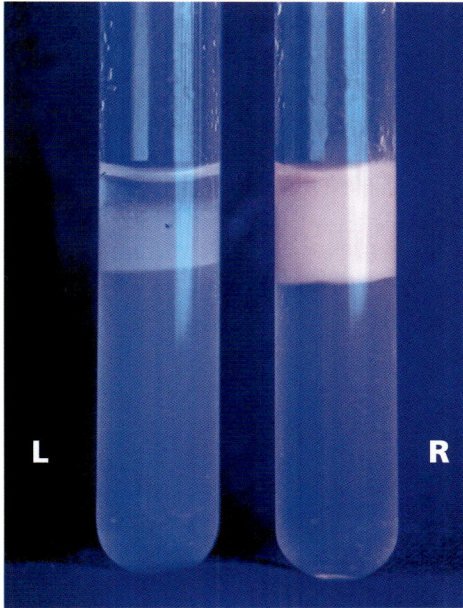

Figure 9–39 □ Porphyria cutanea tarda – urine porphyrin screen. A urine sample (on the right) showing fluorescence with illumination with Wood's lamp. The sample on the left is the negative control. Urine porphyrin excretion is increased in porphyria cutanea tarda, the basis of this test.

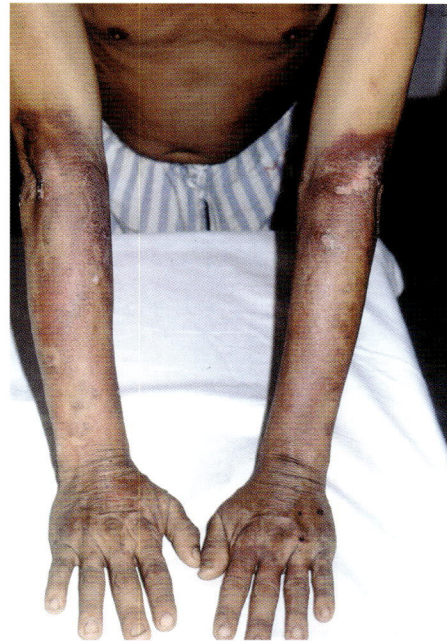

Figure 9–40 □ Pellagra. Sunburn-like erythema and scaling on light-exposed areas, resolving with a dusky, reddish-brown discoloration. Diarrhoea and dementia make up the rest of the classical triad. Pellagra is due to vitamin B3 (niacin) deficiency, and is now rarely seen except in chronic alcoholics or patients with malabsorption due to gastrointestinal disease.

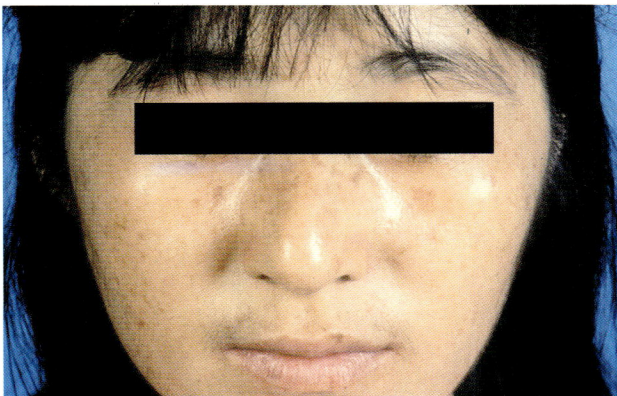

Figure 9–41 □ Xeroderma pigmentosum. Lentigines on the sun-exposed areas of the face and lips in an adolescent. Freckling and increased skin dryness on the exposed parts are the earliest signs of this autosomal recessive syndrome associated with defective DNA repair. Onset is usually in childhood.

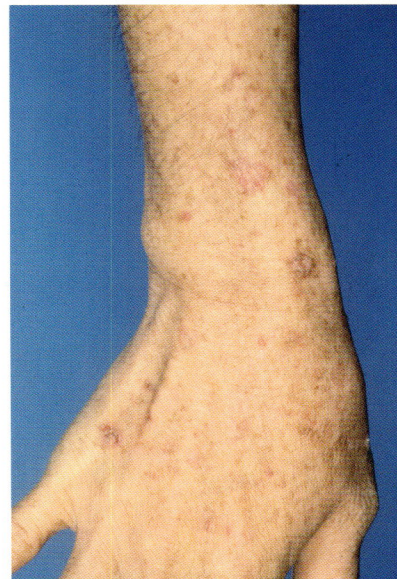

Figure 9–42 □ Xeroderma pigmentosum. Apart from numerous lentigines, the adolescent in Figure 9–41 also has actinic keratoses and scaly red plaques of Bowen's disease (squamous cell carcinoma-in-situ) over the dorsum of her hands and wrists. In this syndrome, malignant tumors, commonly basal cell carcinoma, and squamous cell carcinoma, may first develop as early as the third or fourth year of life. Life expectancy is reduced to less than 20 years in most.

Immunodermatology
Ng P.P.L. and Tang M.B.Y.

IMMUNOBULLOUS DISEASES
(Figures 10–1 to 10–19)

The immune-mediated blistering diseases can be divided into the intraepidermal and subepidermal conditions. Pemphigus (Figures 10–1 to 10–8) is a rare autoimmune intraepidermal blistering condition in which autoantibodies are directed against desmogleins which are responsible for epidermal cell adhesion, resulting in blistering of the skin and mucous membranes. Pemphigus vulgaris and pemphigus foliaceus are the main subtypes. Rarer subtypes include pemphigus vegetans, paraneoplastic pemphigus, IgA pemphigus, and pemphigus herpetiformis.

As the level of the split determines the clinical presentation, pemphigus usually presents with flaccid blisters that are easily eroded, while subepidermal immunobullous diseases (Figures 10–9 to 10–19) tend to present with tense blisters as the autoantibodies are directed against components of the basement membrane zone. Bullous pemphigoid (BP) is the most common of the subepidermal immunobullous diseases. Others include cicatricial pemphigoid (mucous membrane pemphigoid), epidermolysis bullosa acquisita (EBA), linear IgA bullous disease, dermatitis herpetiformis, herpes gestationis, and bullous systemic lupus erythematosus (SLE). Although all present with subepidermal blistering, some clinical and histological features help to differentiate these conditions. Predominance of mucosal involvement suggests mucous membrane pemphigoid, whilst involvement of extensor surfaces and buttocks with intense pruritus and a relatively young age of onset suggests dermatitis herpetiformis.

On histology, bullous pemphigoid tends to have a predominantly eosinophilic infiltrate, whilst a predominance of neutrophils is more commonly seen in EBA, dermatitis herpetiformis, and bullous SLE. Immunofluorescence (IF) is an extremely useful tool in further differentiating these subepidermal immunobullous diseases. Both BP and EBA display linear IgG and C3 deposition on direct immunofluorescence, but on indirect or direct IF using salt split skin, the former displays a "roof" or "roof and floor" pattern, whilst the latter has a "floor" pattern. On direct IF, both linear IgA bullous disease and dermatitis herpetiformis reveal IgA deposits, the former showing a characteristic linear IgA staining at the basement membrane zone, whilst granular IgA deposits are seen in the papillary dermis in the latter.

CONNECTIVE TISSUE DISEASES AND VASCULITIS

Lupus Erythematosus (Figures 10–20 to 10–38)

Skin involvement in lupus erythematosus spans a spectrum from discoid lupus erythematosus (DLE), in which the majority of patients have no systemic complications, acute cutaneous lupus erythematosus (ACLE), which is seen in patients with active SLE, and subacute cutaneous lupus erythematosus (SCLE), which is intermediate in severity. These are considered specific cutaneous lesions as they show characteristic histological changes associated with lupus erythematosus (LE) in contrast to non-specific cutaneous lesions, such as Raynaud's phenomenon, vasculitis, livedo reticularis, and telangiectasia, which may be seen in LE as well as a variety of other autoimmune conditions. There are a few rare variants of cutaneous lupus erythematosus (CLE), namely LE tumidus and LE panniculitis, which are closer to the DLE end of the spectrum and rarely have systemic involvement or positive serological markers.

Dermatomyositis (Figures 10–39 to 10–47)

Dermatomyositis usually presents either to the dermatologist with a skin rash or to the rheumatologist with muscle weakness. At times, the diagnosis may be confused with CLE as they are similar histologically and both are photosensitive conditions. The rash in dermatomyositis, however, has certain characteristic features and should be recognized even in the absence of muscle involvement (amyopathic dermatomyositis or dermatomyositis sine myositis). Early diagnosis is crucial as there is a strong association with an underlying malignancy in both classical as well as amyopathic dermatomyositis. Dermatomyositis may precede the presentation of the malignancy, and therefore, prompt screening

may help to detect the malignancy at an early stage. In addition to the work up for other malignancies, adult Asians of Chinese descent must be screened for nasopharyngeal carcinoma as this is the most common malignancy associated with dermatomyositis in this ethnic group.

Scleroderma (Figures 10–48 to 10–57)

Scleroderma is a term used to describe conditions in which fibrosis of the skin is present. It can be divided into systemic sclerosis and localized scleroderma. Systemic sclerosis can be further divided into diffuse and limited (CREST) forms. Although skin tightness is the usual presenting feature of systemic sclerosis, internal organ involvement, most commonly affecting the esophagus, lungs, heart, and kidney, is the cause of morbidity and mortality associated with the condition. Localized scleroderma does not have systemic involvement and the main variants are morphea, generalized morphea, and linear scleroderma. Lichen sclerosus et atrophicus has also been considered by some to be within the spectrum of localized scleroderma.

Cutaneous Vasculitis (Figures 10–58 to 10–71)

Cutaneous vasculitis can be classified into cutaneous small vessel vasculitis and medium-sized vasculitis although there may be some overlap. Small and medium-sized cutaneous vasculitis have different causes and they can usually be distinguished clinically – the former presenting with purpuric macules, palpable purpura, small ulcers, vesicles, pustules, and hemorrhagic blisters, whilst the latter with ulceration, nodules, livedo reticularis, and digital infarction. Diagnosis of cutaneous vasculitis rests on histology regardless of the size of vessel involvement. Direct IF supplements the information obtained from histology and is the only means of diagnosing

Henoch-Schönlein purpura. The evaluation of the patient with cutaneous vasculitis should be geared toward excluding systemic involvement as well as searching for an underlying cause.

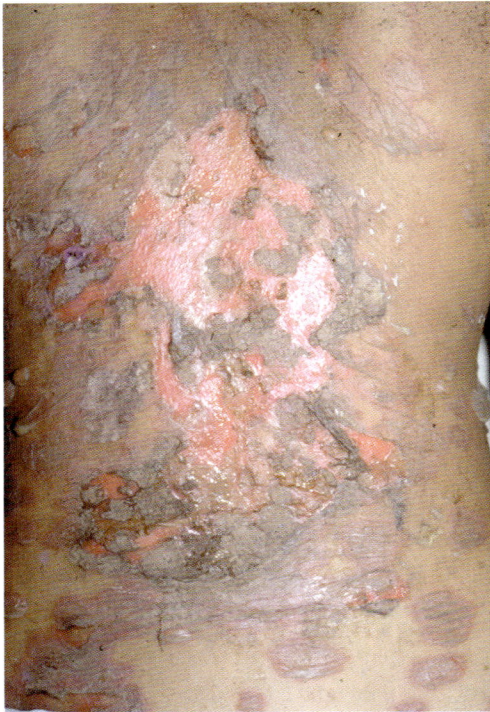

Figure 10–1 □ Pemphigus vulgaris. Confluent areas of painful denuded skin secondary to flaccid blisters that are easily eroded with minimal trauma. Intact flaccid bullae are seen at the lower back and characteristically arise from normal-looking skin. Anti-desmoglein autoantibodies are responsible for the intraepidermal acantholysis of keratinocytes, which can be recognized histologically as suprabasilar cleft formation with an intact basal layer ("tombstone sign"). Lesions heal without scarring although post-inflammatory hyperpigmentation is common in Asians of darker skin.

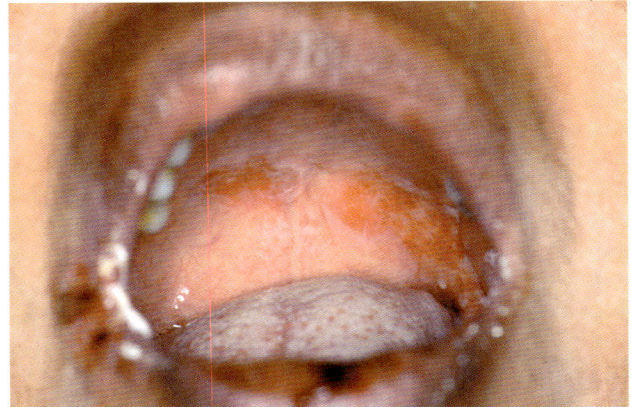

Figure 10–2 □ Pemphigus vulgaris. Painful oral ulcers often precede the development of skin lesions and at times may be the sole manifestation of the disease. They tend to have ill-defined borders and involve the buccal mucosa, gingiva, palate, and tongue. Other mucosal sites, such as the nasal mucosa, vulva, and pharynx, may occasionally be involved. In severe cases of mucosal involvement, paraneoplastic pemphigus and mucous membrane pemphigoid must be excluded.

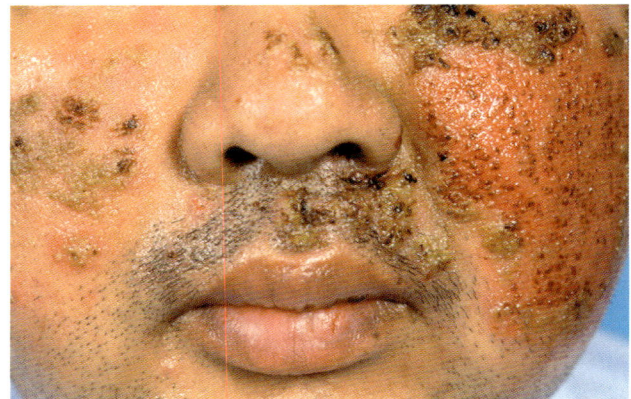

Figure 10–3 □ Pemphigus foliaceus. Also known as "superficial pemphigus", pemphigus foliaceus presents as superficial crusted erosions that resemble impetigo or eroded eczema. There is a predilection for seborrheic areas such as the face, scalp, and chest. Autoantibodies targeting anti-desmoglein 1 are responsible for the acantholysis of keratinocytes in the superficial epidermis usually within the granular layer. In contrast to pemphigus vulgaris, intact blisters are rarely seen and the absence of mucosal lesions is a useful clinical feature to distinguish it from pemphigus vulgaris.

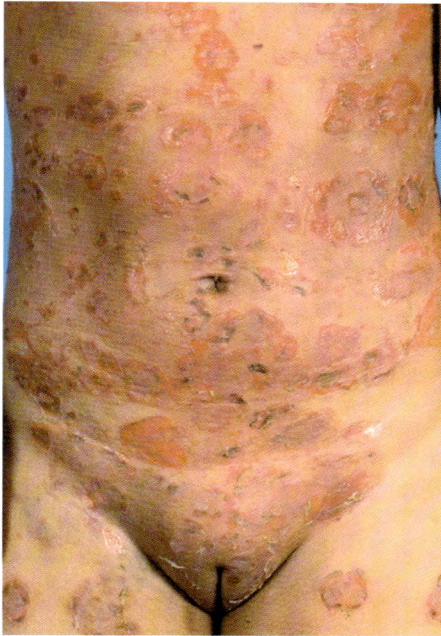

Figure 10–4 □ Pemphigus foliaceus. Multiple superficial crusted erosions on the trunk becoming confluent in some areas. Occasionally, involvement may be very extensive and the clinical presentation may be that of a generalized exfoliative dermatitis. This is more commonly seen in the endemic form of pemphigus foliaceus (Fogo Selvagem) present in South America, in particular Brazil and Columbia.

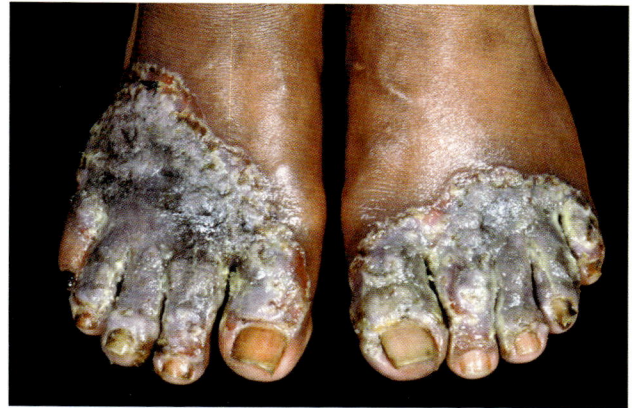

Figure 10–5 □ Pemphigus vegetans. Moist vegetating plaques presenting over the dorsum of both feet with a few peripheral erosions and a prominent edge. Pemphigus vegetans is a rare subset of pemphigus vulgaris and is more commonly seen in intertriginous areas, such as the axillae and groin, although any site may be involved. Small pustules may be seen at the periphery of lesions. Characteristic histological features include hyperkeratosis and papillomatosis of the epidermis with intraepidermal eosinophilic abscesses.

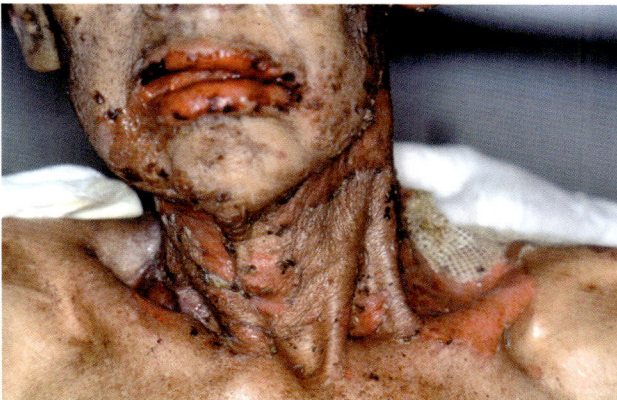

Figure 10–6 □ Paraneoplastic pemphigus. The findings of both crusted mucosal erosions and weepy denuded skin lesions underscore the resemblance of paraneoplastic pemphigus to Stevens-Johnson syndrome. The rash is polymorphic and may present as blisters, erosions, erythema multiforme-like lesions, or lichenoid lesions. Paraneoplastic pemphigus is a rare cutaneous sign of internal malignancy, most frequently a B-cell lymphoproliferative disorder. Non-Hodgkin's lymphoma, chronic lymphocytic leukemia, Castleman's disease, and thymoma are the most commonly associated neoplasms.

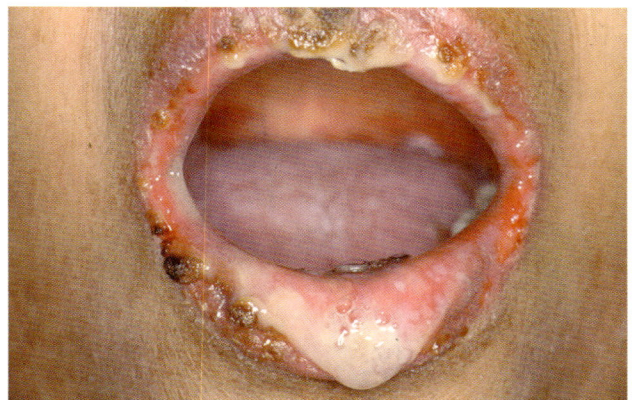

Figure 10–7 □ Paraneoplastic pemphigus. Severe erosive changes affecting the entire surface of the upper and lower lips. Severe mucosal involvement is characteristic of this condition and tends to be very persistent and resistant to therapy unlike the cutaneous manifestations.

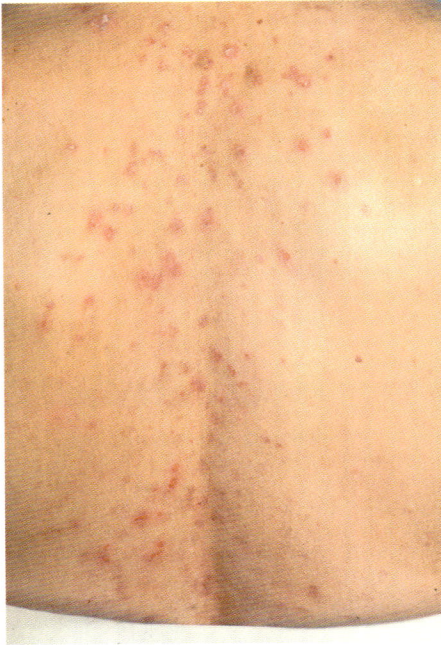

Figure 10–8 □ IgA pemphigus. Superficial healing erosions and a few resolving pustules over the back. This is a rare form of pemphigus presenting with vesiculopustular eruptions in which acantholysis and intraepidermal neutrophil infiltration can be demonstrated on histology and intraepidermal IgA deposition on direct immunofluorescence. Clinically, it may resemble subcorneal pustular dermatosis, pemphigus foliaceus, or even pemphigus vulgaris.

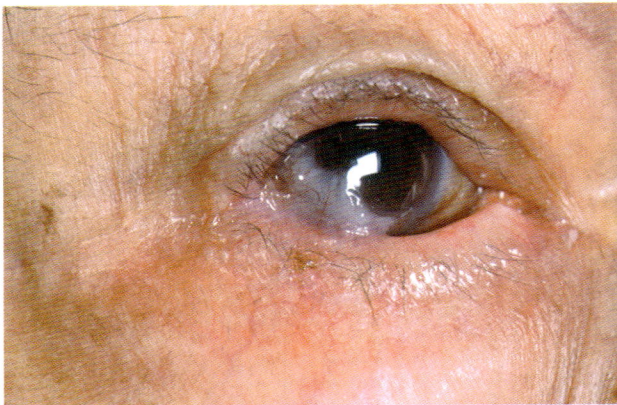

Figure 10–9 □ Bullous pemphigoid. Multiple large tense bullae on the chest of an elderly man. Urticarial-like plaques (as shown in the figure) or occasionally an eczematous rash may precede the development of bullae. Bullae may be hemorrhagic and can arise from erythematous or non-inflamed skin. Rupture of the bullae results in erosions which may leave prominent post-inflammatory hyperpigmentation in darker-skinned Asians. Circulating antibodies against the hemidesmosomal glycoproteins BP180 and BP230 are present but only the former has been shown to induce the subepidermal blistering.

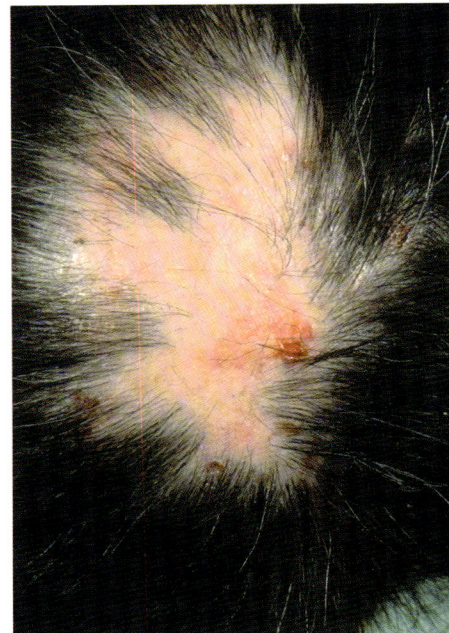

Figure 10–10 □ Mucous membrane pemphigoid. Also known as cicatricial pemphigoid, the severe conjunctival inflammation can lead to symblepharon with partial obliteration and scarring of the conjunctival sulcus as shown. Entropion, corneal scarring, and eventual blindness are serious sequelae. Apart from the eye, other "high risk" sites are the nasopharyngeal, esophageal, laryngeal, and genital mucosa and aggressive therapy is required. Oral mucosa, albeit being the most common site affected, is considered a "low risk" site of involvement.

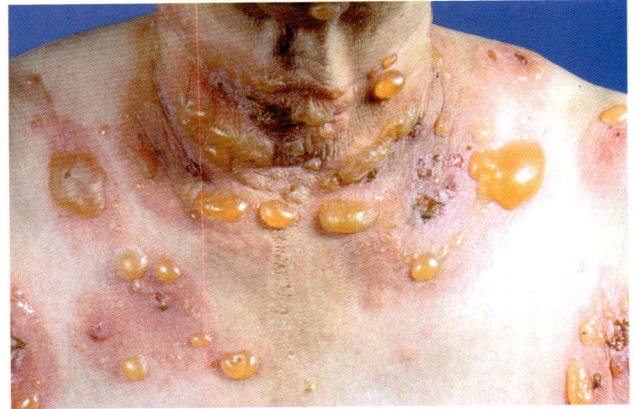

Figure 10–11 □ Localized cicatricial pemphigoid – Brunsting-Perry variant. An area of scarring alopecia with crusted erosions seen at the periphery. A rare variant of cicatricial pemphigoid, it presents with tense bullae affecting predominantly the head and neck region of elderly patients which heal with scarring and atrophy. Mucosal lesions are usually absent.

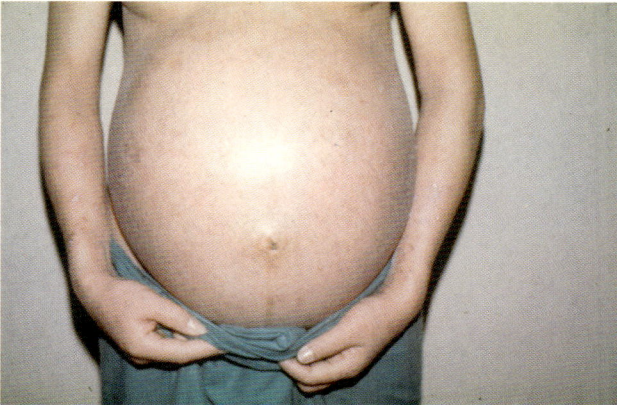

Figure 10–12 □ Pemphigoid gestationis. Resolving urticarial plaques and erosions over the abdomen and arms of a pregnant woman. Initially, the presence of urticarial papules and plaques may resemble polymorphic eruption of pregnancy, however, the subsequent development of vesicles and larger bullae together with a positive direct immunofluorescence will help to clinch the diagnosis. This rare condition often presents in the second trimester, usually beginning around the umbilicus, spreading to involve the abdomen and limbs. It has a tendency to recur and to be more severe in subsequent pregnancies.

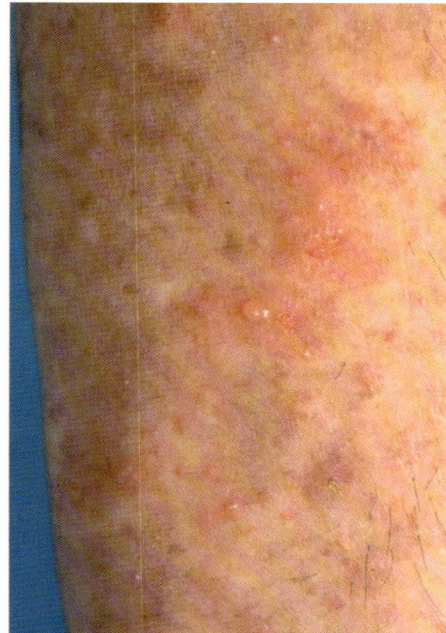

Figure 10–13 □ Epidermolysis bullosa acquisita. Several small tense blisters seen arising from the erythematous skin with a few erosions. The clinical presentation of epidermolysis bullosa acquisita can be diverse. Although classically described as a mechanobullous condition that involves trauma prone sites, patients may present with a bullous pemphigoid-like picture with an inflammatory vesiculo-bullous eruption as seen here. At times, it may present with predominant mucous membrane involvement.

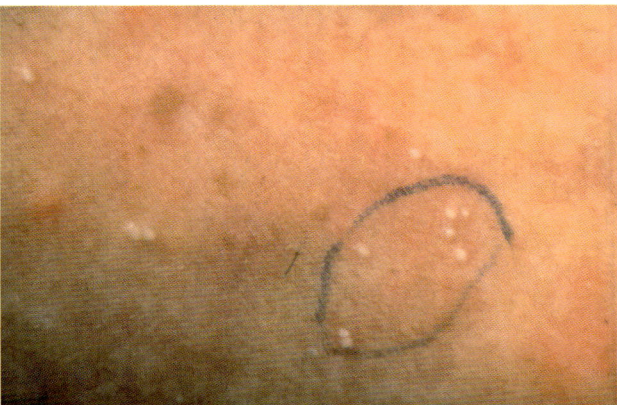

Figure 10–14 □ Epidermolysis bullosa acquisita. Several milia are seen after the resolution of blisters and erosions. Scarring, milia, and hyperpigmentation may be seen in the healing phase of the disease. These features are not, however, invariably present.

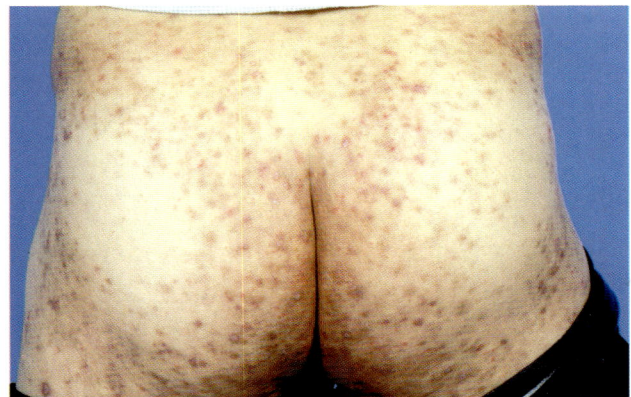

Figure 10–15 □ Dermatitis herpetiformis. Multiple small erosions and excoriated papules seen over the buttocks. Note the marked post-inflammatory pigmentary changes and the presence of a few small intact vesicles. It is an uncommon condition in Asians and a high index of suspicion is needed, especially in patients presenting with unrelenting pruritus and "excoriated eczema" over the extensor surfaces of their limbs and buttocks which are unresponsive to conventional therapy.

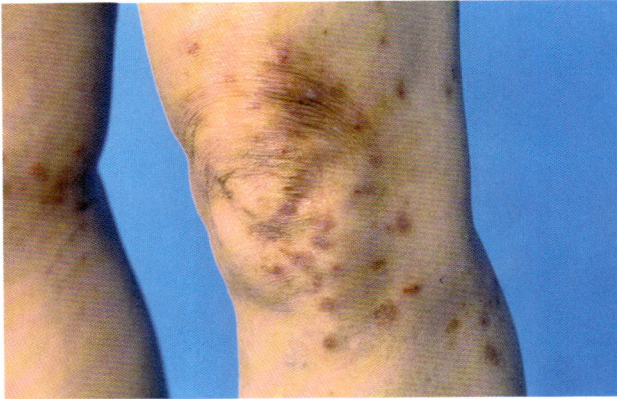

Figure 10–16 □ Dermatitis herpetiformis. Characteristic pruritic erythematous papules and erosions over the extensor surfaces of the knees in the same patient shown in Figure 10–15. Granular IgA deposits in the papillary dermis are pathognomonic. It is associated with gluten-sensitive enteropathy and dapsone is the drug of choice.

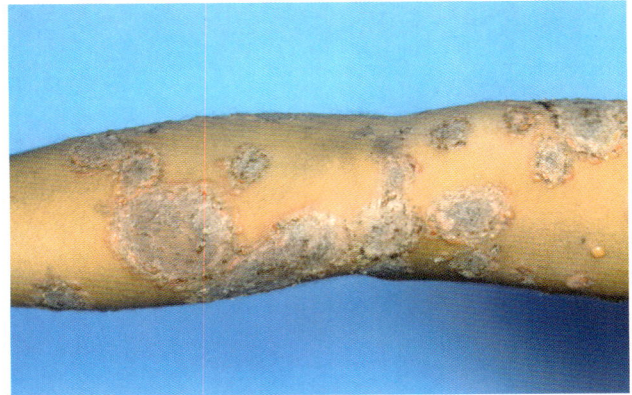

Figure 10–17 □ Linear IgA bullous dermatosis – adult variant. Distinctive annular crusted plaques with a ring of intact vesicles at the periphery. Linear IgA bullous dermatosis can clinically and histologically mimic bullous pemphigoid or, less commonly, dermatitis herpetiformis, but direct immunofluorescence will reveal the diagnostic linear deposition of IgA along the basement membrane zone. This condition has been associated with various malignancies, especially lymphoproliferative types, and drugs, in particular, vancomycin.

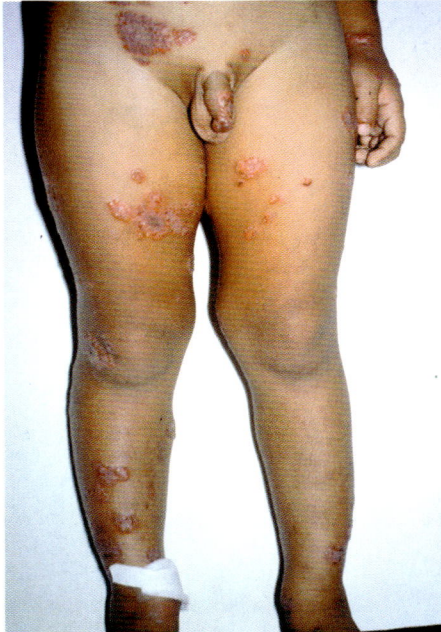

Figure 10–18 □ Linear IgA bullous dermatosis – pediatric variant. Bullae on the limbs and trunk of a child showing the classical "cluster of jewels" configuration. Also known as chronic bullous disease of childhood, the mean age of onset is four to five years, and it commonly affects the face and perineum with secondary generalization. Mucosal involvement is common in both adult and pediatric variants.

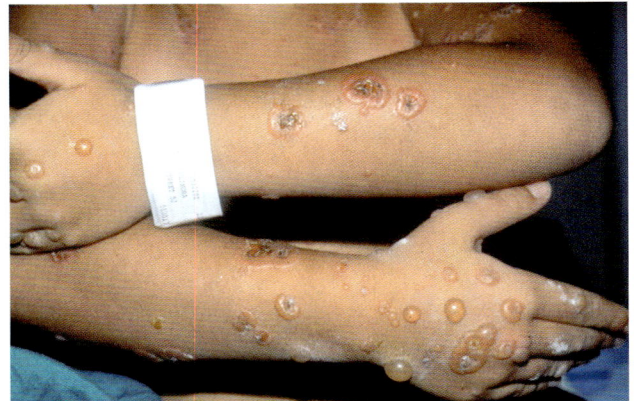

Figure 10–19 □ Linear IgA bullous dermatosis – pediatric variant. Large tense grouped bullae coalescing into a ringed configuration, like a "string of pearls".

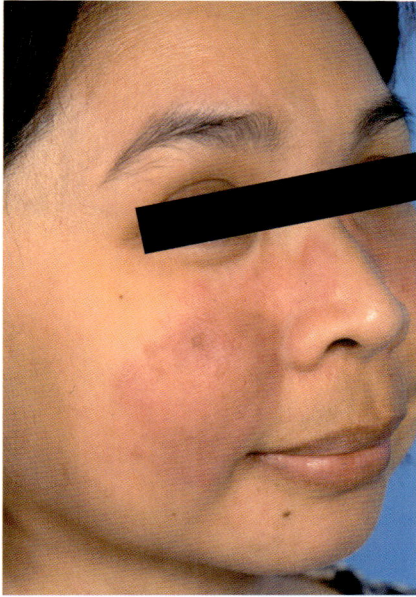

Figure 10–20 □ Acute cutaneous lupus erythematosus.
Erythematous plaque over the malar region characteristic of the "butterfly rash" seen in systemic lupus erythematosus (LE). It is a photosensitive rash and often extends across the bridge of the nose. Acute LE lesions can occur in areas other than the face and present as confluent erythema with a varying degree of edema or, less commonly, as a morbilliform eruption. Further evaluation with anti-nuclear antibodies and anti-double-stranded DNA antibodies is required.

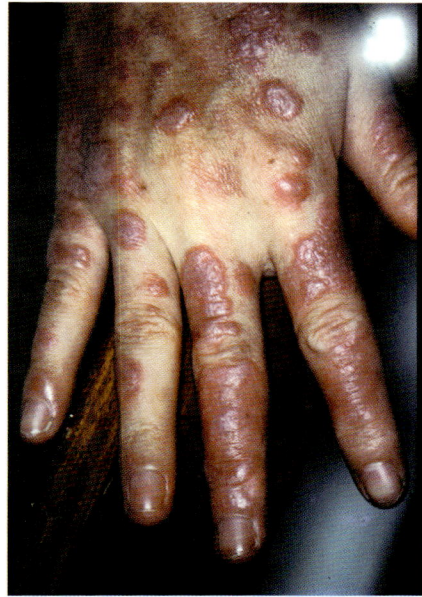

Figure 10–21 □ Acute cutaneous lupus erythematosus.
Erythematous, succulent plaques over the dorsal aspect of the phalanges in a patient with systemic lupus erythematosus, typically sparing the areas overlying the small joints of the hand. The dorsum of the hand is also affected and some periungual erythema can be seen. In contrast, Gottron's sign and papules seen in dermatomyositis occur over the joints.

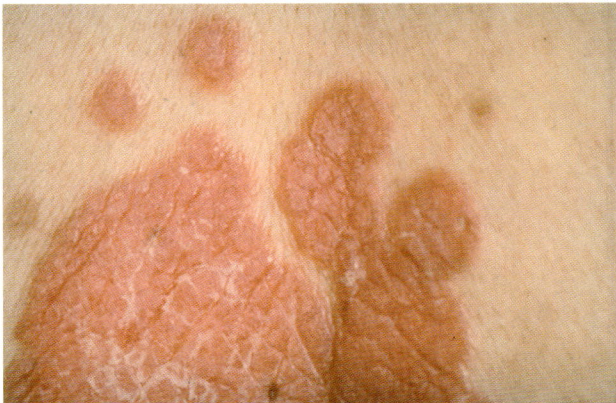

Figure 10–22 □ Subacute cutaneous lupus erythematosus.
Well-demarcated, erythematous, scaly psoriasiform plaques on the trunk of a patient with papulosquamous subacute cutaneous LE (SCLE). SCLE is a subset of cutaneous lupus erythematosus. The majority of patients have anti-Ro antibodies and about half fulfil the ACR criteria for SLE.

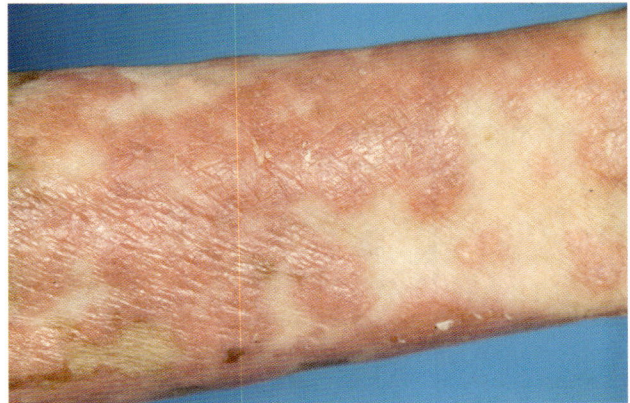

Figure 10–23 □ Subacute cutaneous lupus erythematosus.
Unlike discoid LE, which tends to affect the face and scalp, SCLE tends to affect the limbs and trunk in a photo-distribution and is non-scarring.

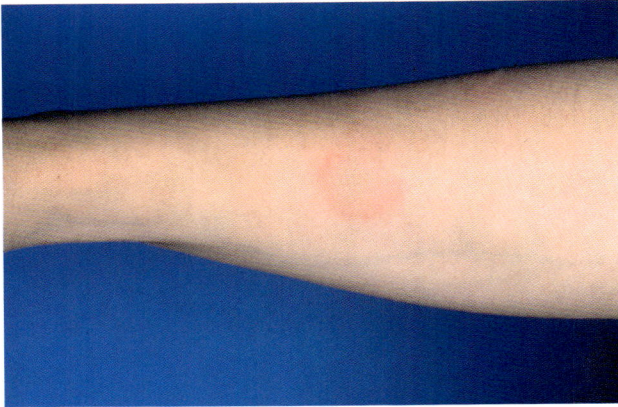

Figure 10–24 □ **Anti-Ro positive annular erythema.** Annular erythematous plaque on the leg of a young Chinese man who is anti-Ro positive. This condition, described mainly in Orientals with either Sjögren's syndrome or SLE, is believed to be the Asian counterpart of annular SCLE. LE-specific histopathologic changes are typically absent, in contrast to annular SCLE.

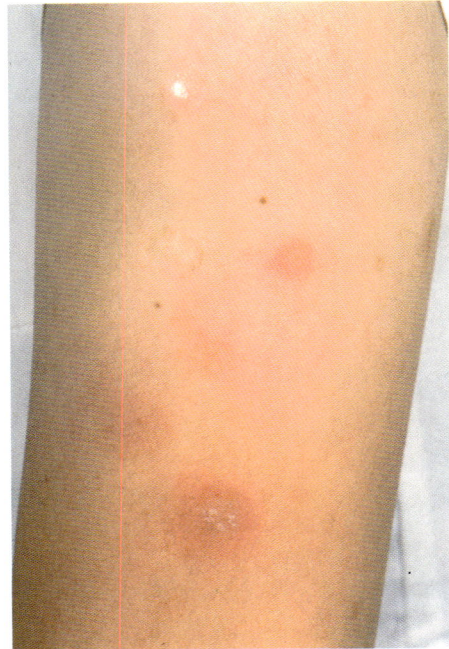

Figure 10–25 □ **Anti-Ro positive annular erythema.** Annular erythematous plaques over the sun-exposed areas of the forearms of a young Chinese female.

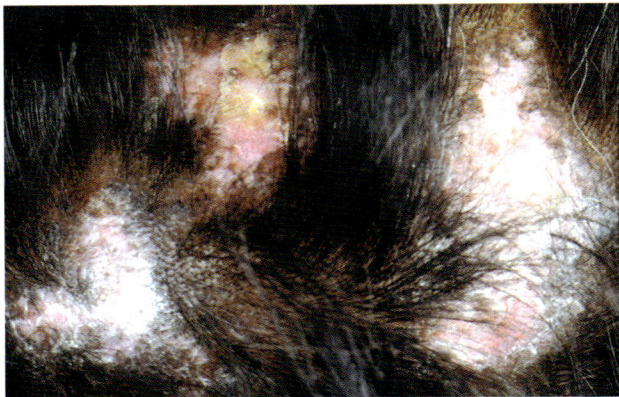

Figure 10–26 □ **Discoid lupus erythematosus (DLE) – scarring alopecia.** Multiple erythematous plaques with active inflammation and adherent scale at the edges associated with scarring alopecia. The centrally scarred areas are devoid of viable follicles and epidermal atrophy and post-inflammatory hypopigmentation are present. Closer inspection may reveal follicular plugging and telangiectasia. DLE is the most common form of cutaneous lupus erythematosus.

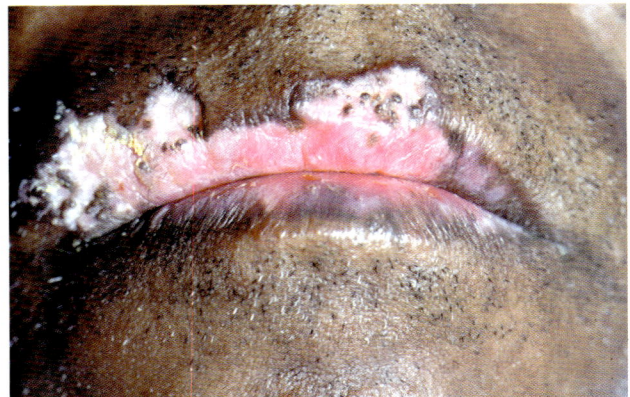

Figure 10–27 □ **Discoid lupus erythematosus.** Typical well-demarcated pink plaques encroaching on the upper lip with marked pigmentary changes seen in an Indian patient. Note the adherent scaling and slightly hypertrophic, pigmented borders. Classical histopathological features of DLE are epidermal atrophy, follicular plugging, and an interface dermatitis with periadnexal and periappendageal lymphocytic infiltrate.

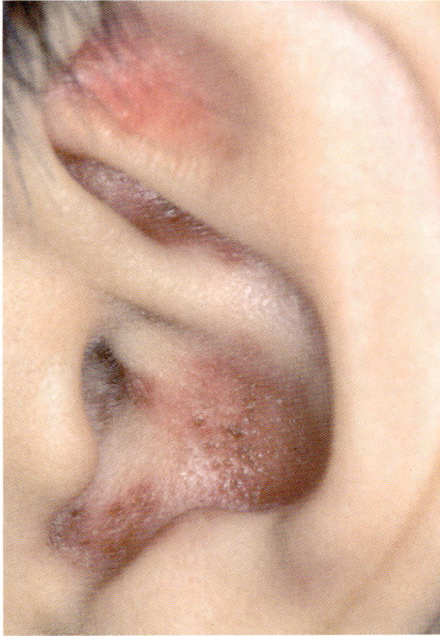

Figure 10–28 □ **Discoid lupus erythematosus.** Erythema with characteristic follicular plugging within the concha of the ear. The ear is a common site of involvement in DLE.

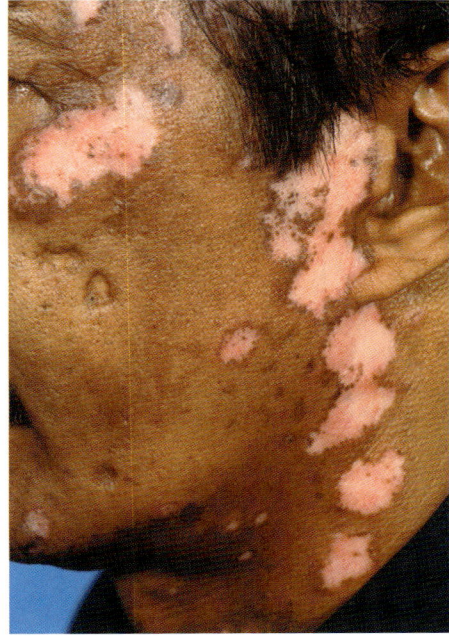

Figure 10–29 □ **Discoid lupus erythematosus.** Multiple atrophic patches with post-inflammatory hypopigmentation seen in the late "burnt-out" stages of DLE. Occasionally, a ring of hyperpigmentation is seen around the areas of hypopigmentation. These severe pigmentary changes are a devastating cosmetic problem for dark-skinned Asian patients and aggressive therapy must be initiated early to prevent such irreversible sequelae.

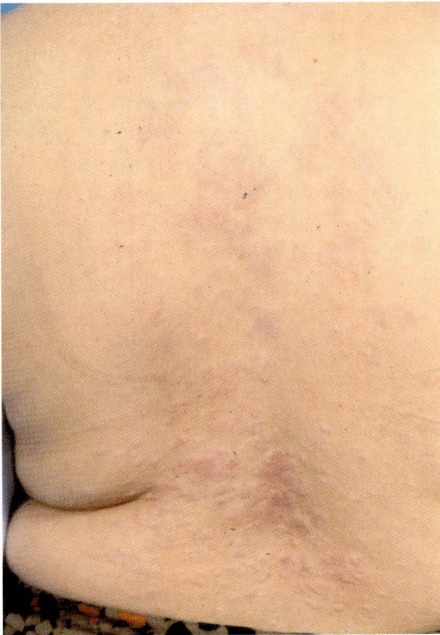

Figure 10–30 □ **Tumid lupus erythematosus.** Multiple erythematous, mildly indurated, urticarial-like plaques on the back. Lesions of tumid LE do not have prominent epidermal changes and resolve with minimal scarring. This is a rare form of cutaneous LE in which there is marked mucin deposition within the dermis, together with a periadnexal and perivascular lymphocytic infiltration. Serological markers of SLE may be negative.

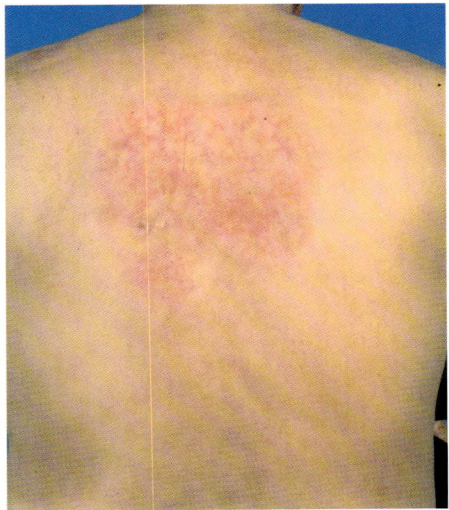

Figure 10–31 □ **Tumid lupus erythematosus.** A large erythematous, succulent plaque on the back with a reticulate appearance in some areas. This lesion responded to intralesional corticosteroid administration.

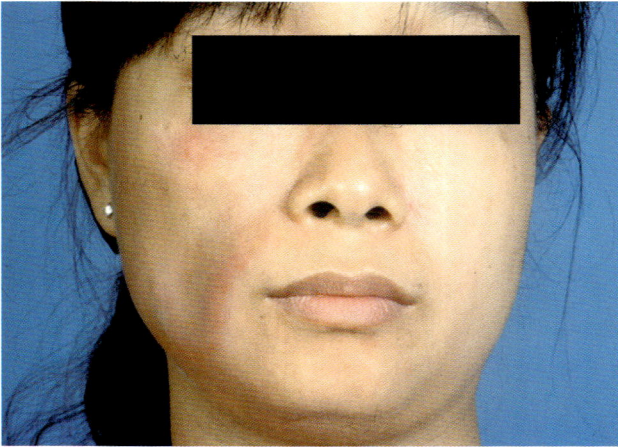

Figure 10–32 □ Lupus erythematosus panniculitis. Disfiguring, asymmetrical loss of subcutaneous fat on the cheek. Note the indurated, erythematous border that connotes disease activity. Histology from this edge will reveal a lobular panniculitis. Although there are no epidermal changes seen clinically in this patient, features of DLE may be seen on histology. LE profundus (or LE panniculitis) is a rare form of cutaneous LE. As in DLE, systemic involvement is uncommon.

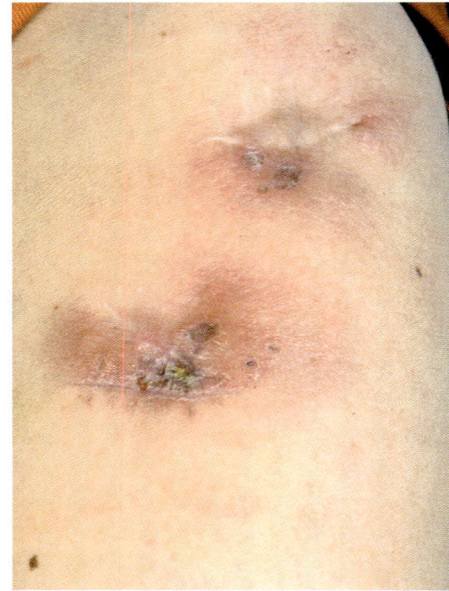

Figure 10–33 □ Lupus erythematosus panniculitis. Erythematous nodules on the upper arm with DLE changes (erythema, atrophy, adherent scale) seen on the overlying skin. Scars from previous incisional biopsies are also seen. The face, trunk, and proximal limbs are commonly affected sites.

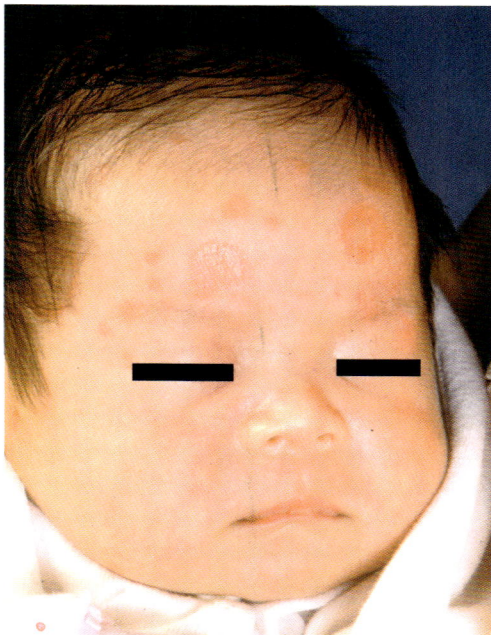

Figure 10–34 □ Neonatal lupus erythematosus. Annular, erythematous papules and plaques over the face of an infant born to a Ro+ mother with systemic LE. Lesions are usually photodistributed and may resemble SCLE. The cutaneous lesions and other systemic manifestations, which include complete congenital heart block, hematological abnormalities, and hepatitis, are due to the transplacental passage of maternal anti-Ro antibodies.

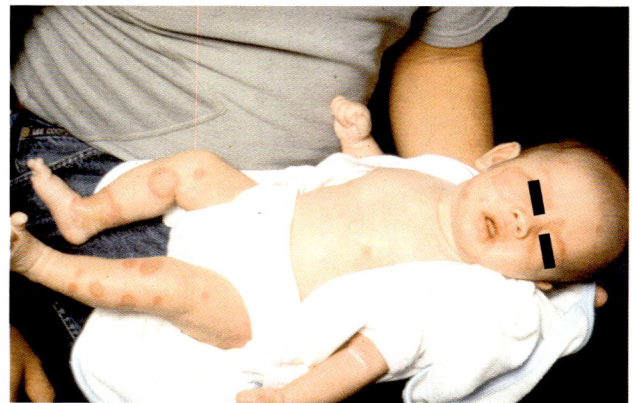

Figure 10–35 □ Neonatal lupus erythematosus. Well-defined, annular, erythematous plaques over the face and legs of an infant. Cutaneous lesions usually appear within the first few weeks of life or, at times, may be present at birth. Spontaneous resolution occurs by the age of six months often with post-inflammatory hyperpigmentation.

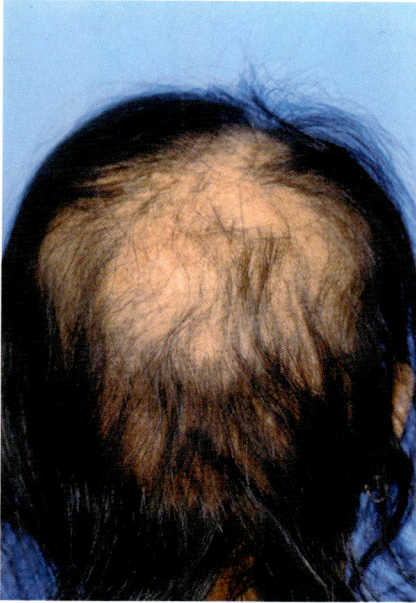

Figure 10–36 □ Diffuse alopecia in systemic lupus erythematosus. Sparse hair density over a large area of the scalp in a patient with active SLE. In contrast to discoid LE, this form of diffuse alopecia is non-scarring. Hair pull is often positive. Possible contributory factors include anemia of chronic disease, renal impairment, nutritional deficiency, chronic telogen effluvium, and medication.

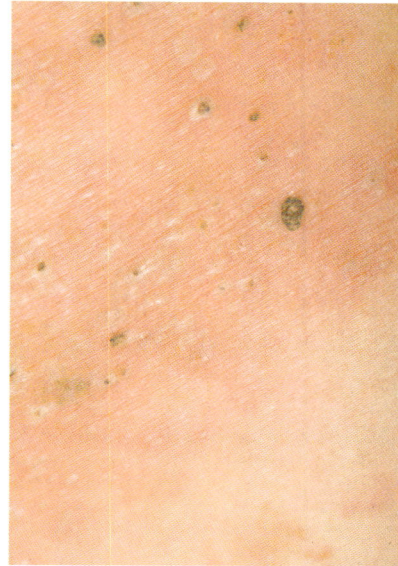

Figure 10–37 □ Bullous systemic lupus erythematosus. Small intact vesicles overlying an area of erythema in a patient with active SLE. Vesiculobullous SLE is a rare cutaneous feature of SLE and occurs predominantly in young females. Blisters are subepidermal with a predominantly neutrophilic infiltrate. Important differential diagnoses include dermatitis herpetiformis, bullous pemphigoid, and epidermolysis bullosa acquisita. Antibodies directed against type VII collagen have been found in bullous LE and the drug of choice is dapsone.

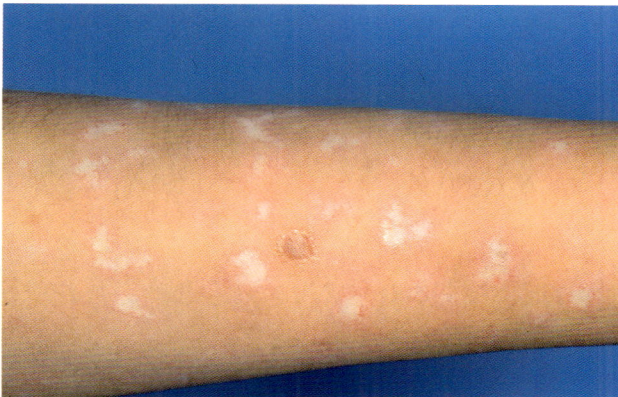

Figure 10–38 □ Anti-phospholipid syndrome. Porcelain-white atrophie blanche lesions on the limb of a patient with SLE and anti-phospholipid syndrome. Anti-phospholipid syndrome is characterized by the presence of anti-phospholipid antibodies causing a hypercoagulable state and presents with vascular thrombosis and recurrent spontaneous abortions. The atrophie blanche lesions are the result of healed ulcerations secondary to thrombosis occurring in the cutaneous vasculature. Other cutaneous manifestations include livedo reticularis, superficial thrombophlebitis, leg ulcers, digital ischemia, and acrocyanosis.

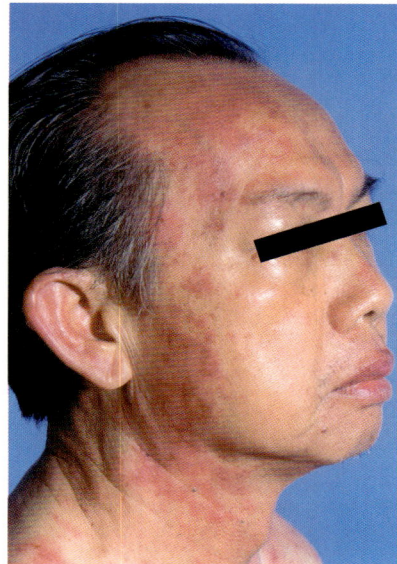

Figure 10–39 □ Dermatomyositis. Violaceous, erythematous, photodistributed rash over the face, ears, and neck. Note the striking characteristic purple-red color of the skin. Skin signs include periorbital heliotrope rash, Gottron's papules, photodistributed, violaceous, poikilodermatous rash, and nail fold telangiectasia. A thorough search for an underlying internal malignancy should be carried out. In Chinese patients, screening for occult nasopharyngeal carcinoma should be performed as it is the most common malignancy associated with both the classical and amyopathic forms of dermatomyositis.

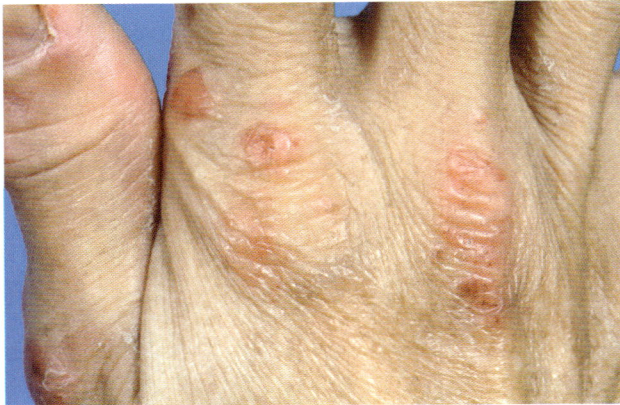

Figure 10–40 □ Dermatomyositis – Gottron's papules. Violaceous, erythematous papules over the metacarpophalangeal joints. Such lesions may also be found over the interphalangeal joints and occasionally over other bony prominences. They may become slightly depressed at the center with an atrophic appearance. Together with Gottron's sign (symmetrical macular violaceous erythema over the same sites), these features are pathognomonic of dermatomyositis.

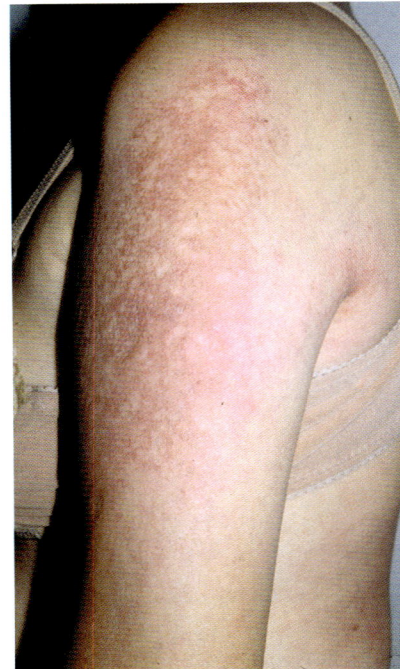

Figure 10–41 □ Dermatomyositis. Poikilodermatous changes are seen over the extensor surfaces of the arm. Other typically affected areas include the upper back and "V" of the neck ("shawl sign"). Skin histology will reveal interface dermatitis with a lymphocytic perivascular infiltrate and mucin deposition.

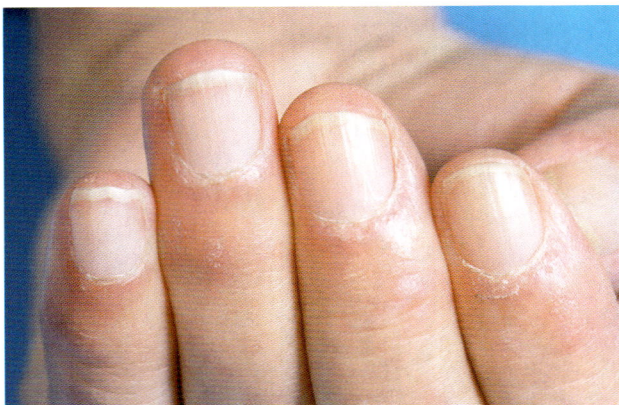

Figure 10–42 □ Dermatomyositis. Ragged cuticles seen with nail fold telangiectasia and mild periungual erythema. Examination of the hands and the periungual area is an essential part of the physical examination for any patient with suspected dermatomyositis as these sites provide many diagnostic clues.

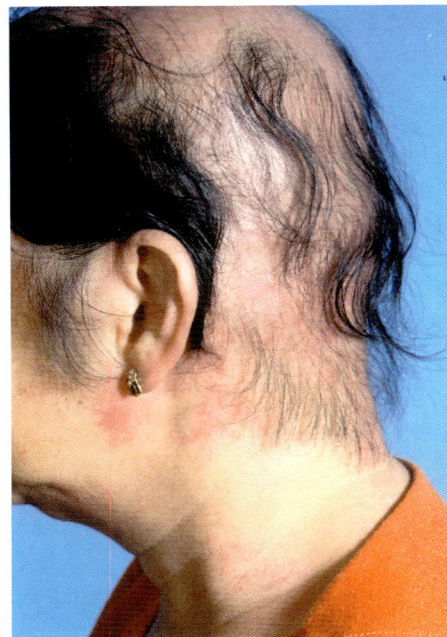

Figure 10–43 □ Dermatomyositis. Diffuse, extensive non-scarring alopecia in a patient with amyopathic dermatomyositis. Some violaceous patches are seen at the hairline and upper neck. Other scalp lesions seen in dermatomyositis include psoriasiform rashes and poikiloderma. Scarring alopecia is rare.

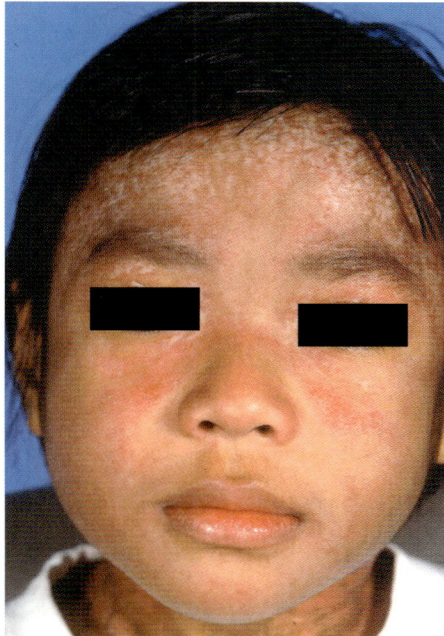

Figure 10–44 □ Juvenile dermatomyositis. This patient has violaceous erythema over the cheeks and nasal bridge and symmetrical, lilac-colored heliotrope erythema over both upper eyelids. Poikiloderma is present on the skin of the forehead. In contrast to adult dermatomyositis, juvenile dermatomyositis is not associated with an increased risk of malignancy.

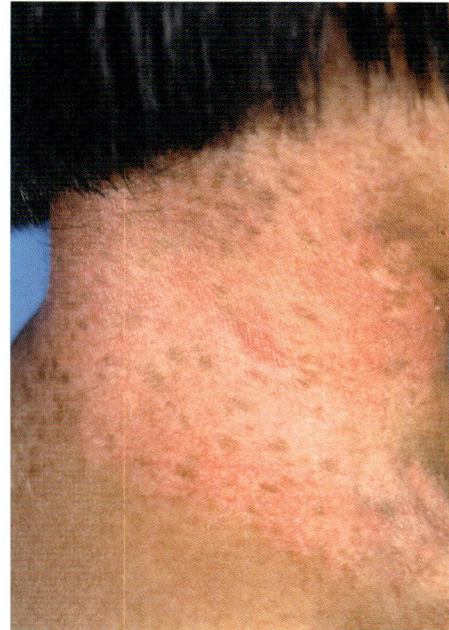

Figure 10–45 □ Juvenile dermatomyositis. Poikilodermatous changes over the posterior and lateral neck of the patient in Figure 10–44. Note the clear demarcation between the sun-exposed and non-exposed areas.

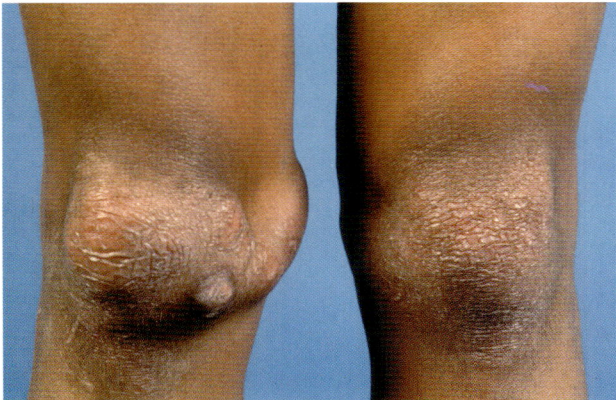

Figure 10–46 □ Juvenile dermatomyositis – calcinosis cutis. Calcinosis cutis presenting as painless hard swellings over the right knee. Note the background rash consisting of symmetrical atrophic erythematous plaques over the knee joints. Calcinosis is more commonly seen in juvenile dermatomyositis compared to the adult variant. Complications include ulceration, secondary infection and, occasionally, loss of joint mobility.

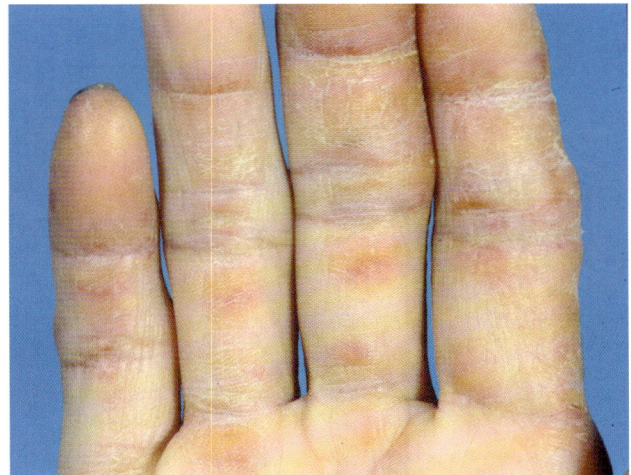

Figure 10–47 □ Dermatomyositis – mechanic's hands. Hyperkeratotic areas over the palmar aspect of the fingers and palm of a patient with dermatomyositis resembling callosities due to repeated friction. This sign has been associated with the presence of anti-Jo1 antibodies.

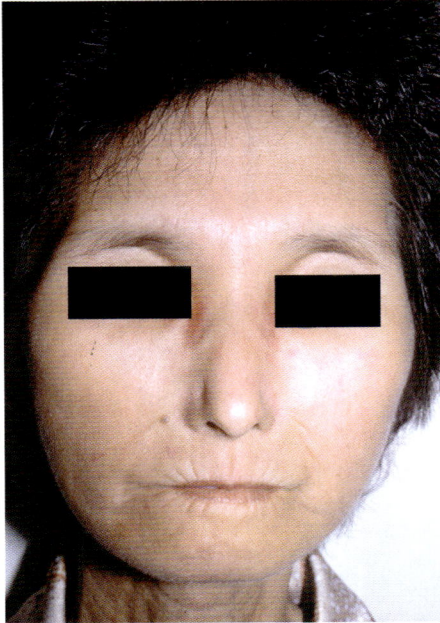

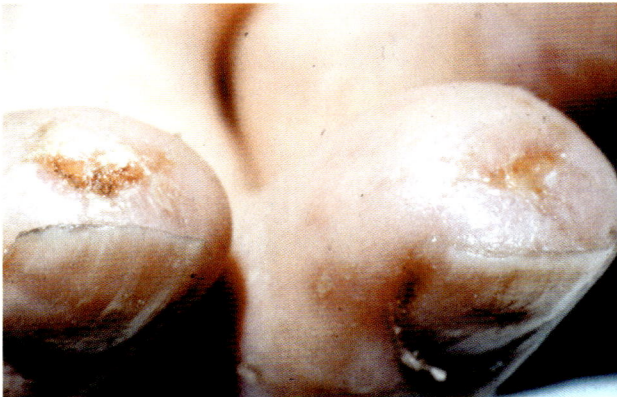

Figure 10–49 □ Systemic sclerosis – pigmentary changes. Characteristic widespread patchy pigmentary changes on the trunk. A rim of perifollicular hyperpigmentation is seen with surrounding depigmentation and hypopigmentation giving a "salt and pepper" appearance. The underlying skin is thickened and sclerotic.

Figure 10–48 □ Systemic sclerosis. Taut smooth waxy appearance of the facial skin seen in systemic sclerosis with typical beaked nose and radial furrowing around the mouth. Other cutaneous manifestations include sclerodactyly, ragged cuticles, nail fold telangiectasia, Raynaud's phenomenon, matted telangiectasia, and digital pits. Systemic involvement includes pulmonary fibrosis, malignant hypertension, intestinal dysmotility, and renal impairment. Anti-topoisomerase (anti-Scl-70) antibodies are usually positive.

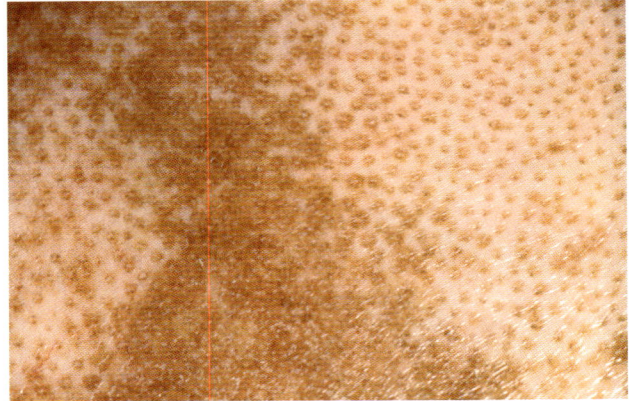

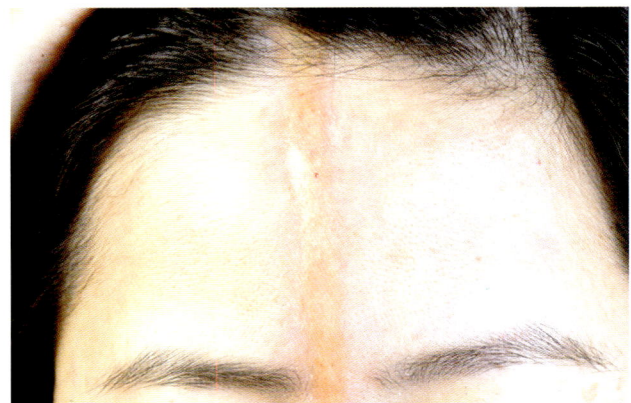

Figure 10–50 □ Systemic sclerosis – digital ulcerations. Painful digital ulceration and pits seen in systemic sclerosis. These can be secondary to underlying obliterative vascular changes or calcinosis with necrosis and ulceration. Note the atrophy of the terminal finger pulps.

Figure 10–51 □ Linear scleroderma – en coup de sabre. A narrow, depressed, linear sclerotic vertical band on the forehead of a patient with the en coup de sabre variant of linear scleroderma. Usually confined to the scalp and forehead, it often results in scarring alopecia. The fibrosis may extend to the subcutaneous tissues and in severe cases, involvement of the underlying bone can occur as well as hemiatrophy of the facial structures.

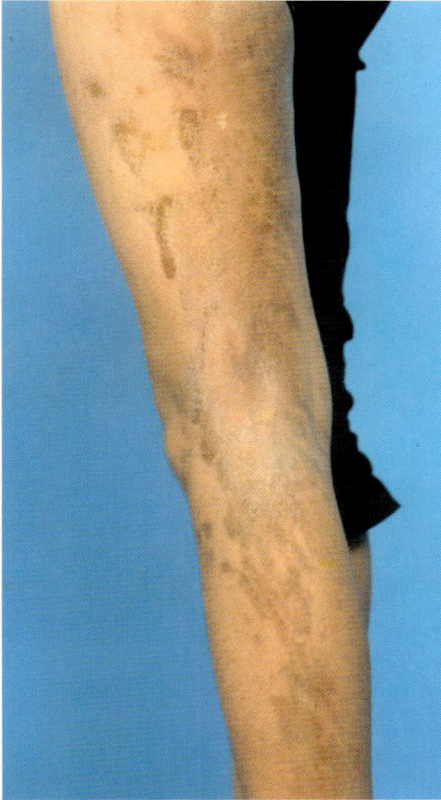

Figure 10–52 □ Linear scleroderma. A broad, linear, band-like sclerotic plaque affecting this patient's left leg, extending from the upper thigh to the lower posterior calf. Extension over the joints can lead to restriction of joint motion. In children, linear scleroderma of the limbs can affect limb development leading to limb-length discrepancy, contractures, and disability.

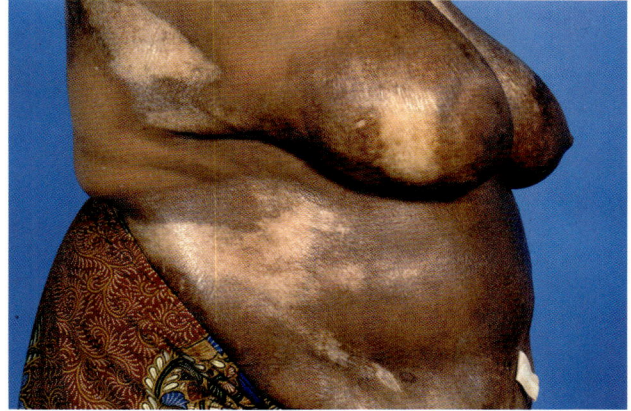

Figure 10–53 □ Generalized morphea. Multiple hypopigmented sclerotic plaques over the trunk. Lesions are ill-defined and indurated in the initial phase, whilst older lesions gradually become softer with residual hyperpigmentation. However, hypopigmentation can also be seen as evident here, especially in racially pigmented patients such as Indians. Destruction of the underlying hair follicles and pilosebaceous glands is permanent and the skin appears smooth and shiny.

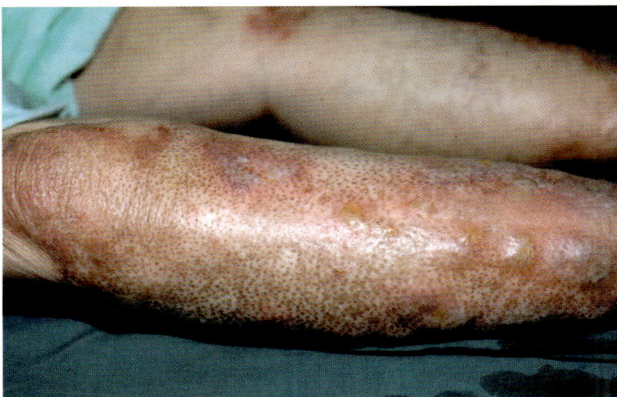

Figure 10–54 □ Bullous morphea. Several tense bullae arising from a sclerotic indurated plaque with prominent pigmentary changes. These tense subepidermal bullae appear to develop as a result of subepidermal edema secondary to lymphatic obstruction from the underlying sclerodermatous process. Other possible causes of bulla formation in a patient with morphea include an inflammatory bullous lichen sclerosus-like process and a superimposed autoimmune skin disease such as epidermolysis bullosa acquisita.

Figure 10–55 □ Lichen sclerosus et atrophicus – extragenital. Well-demarcated, ivory-colored macules and papules over the trunk, one lesion showing prominent wrinkling. Lesions of lichen sclerosus are asymptomatic and may exhibit keratotic follicular plugging. Occasionally, bullae may develop. In the later stages of the disease, atrophy occurs and lesions may have a wrinkled appearance.

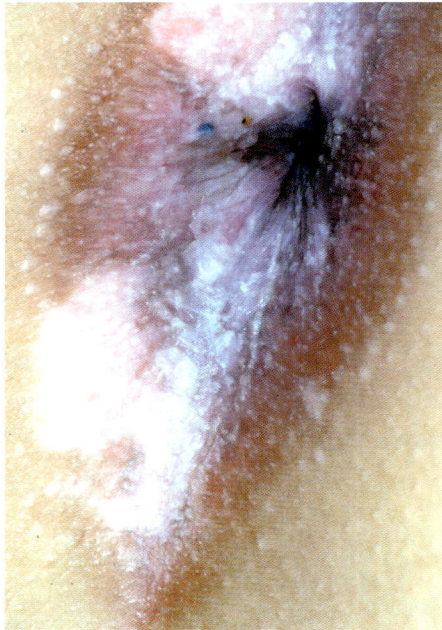

Figure 10–56 ☐ Lichen sclerosus et atrophicus – anogenital. White patches and plaques affecting the perianal skin. Telangiectasia and purpura are commonly seen. At times, vesicles, which may be hemorrhagic, are also present. Patients may experience soreness or itch. In females, extensive lesions can lead to the "figure-of-eight" deformity with sclerotic lesions encircling the vulva and anal orifice, resulting in stenosis of the introitus.

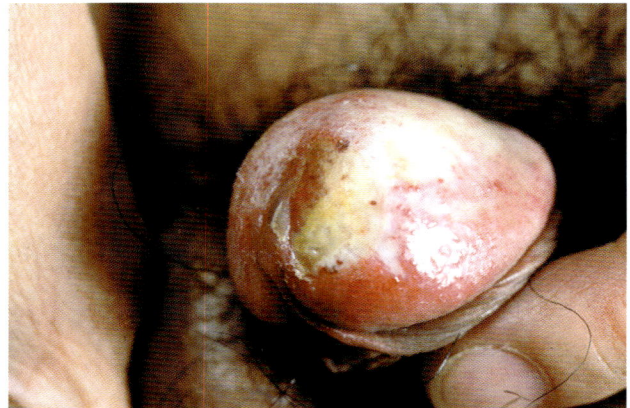

Figure 10–57 ☐ Lichen sclerosus et atrophicus – balanitis xerotica obliterans. Hypopigmented scarred atrophic areas on the glans penis with purpuric macules, telangiectasia, and erythema seen on the surrounding mucosa. Painful, erosive lesions may be seen in severe cases. Complications include meatal stenosis and acquired phimosis which is a common presenting symptom when the prepuce is involved.

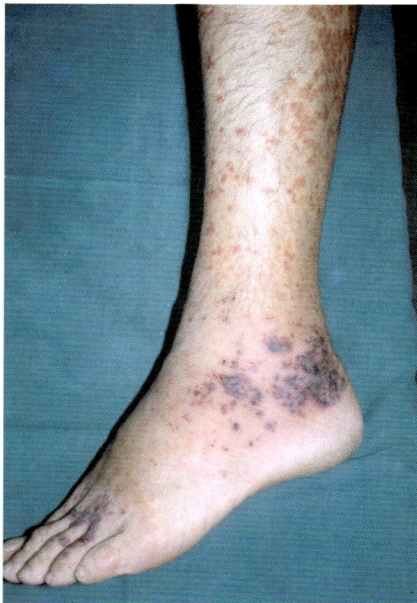

Figure 10–58 ☐ Leukocytoclastic vasculitis (cutaneous small vessel vasculitis). Palpable purpura and purpuric macules on the lower leg with necrotic, dusky areas. Hemorrhagic blisters and ulceration may be seen. Biopsy should be performed on a fresh lesion that is less than 48 hours old. Underlying causes include infection, drugs, connective tissue diseases, and systemic vasculitides and rarely, malignancy.

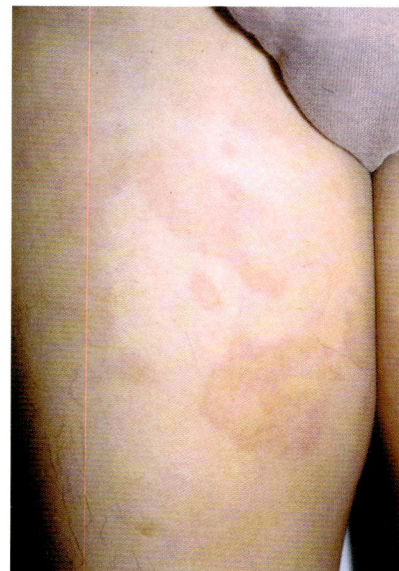

Figure 10–59 ☐ Urticarial vasculitis. Resolving polycyclic annular urticarial plaques with post-inflammatory hyperpigmentation. In contrast to urticaria, lesions of urticarial vasculitis tend to be burning or painful, more persistent, lasting more than 24 hours and they usually resolve with hyperpigmentation. Systemic features like arthralgia and fever may be present. Patients may be subdivided into normocomplementemic and hypocomplementemic urticarial vasculitis. Systemic lupus erythematosus is an important underlying cause that should be excluded.

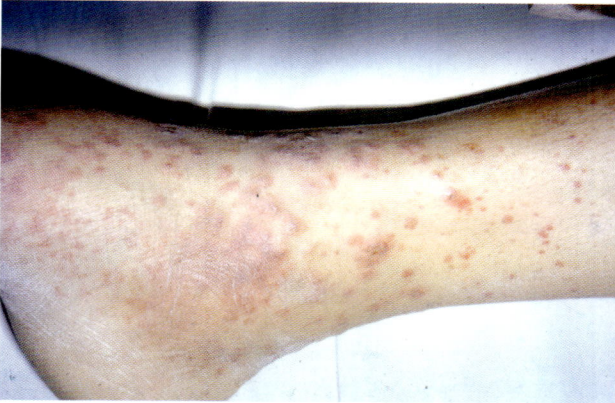

Figure 10–60 □ Henoch-Schönlein purpura. Palpable purpura over the lower leg. Classically extending up to the buttocks, direct immunofluorescence is diagnostic, showing granular IgA deposition in the small blood vessels. Associated signs and symptoms include colicky abdominal pain and polyarthralgia. Patients should be screened for hematuria which indicates underlying glomerulonephritis. Although classically described in children, adults can be affected as well. Recurrences are common.

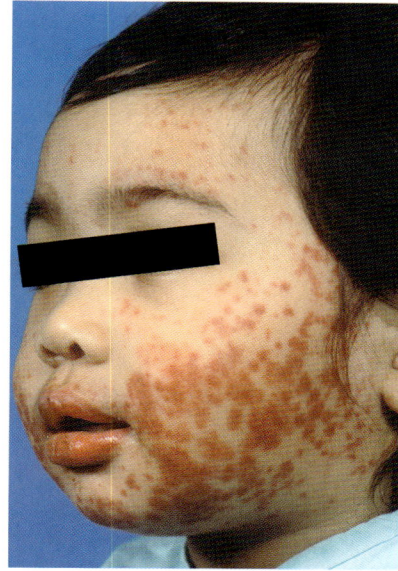

Figure 10–61 □ Acute hemorrhagic edema of infancy (Finkelstein's disease). Multiple purpuric macules, papules, and plaques seen over the cheeks of a young child. The characteristic central purpuric area surrounded by a paler urticarial border is seen in several lesions. There is also confluence of the smaller lesions to form larger polycyclic plaques. Despite the dramatic cutaneous lesions, the child appears clinically well and non-toxic which is typical of this condition. This is a form of leukocytoclastic vasculitis which tends to affect children below the age of three.

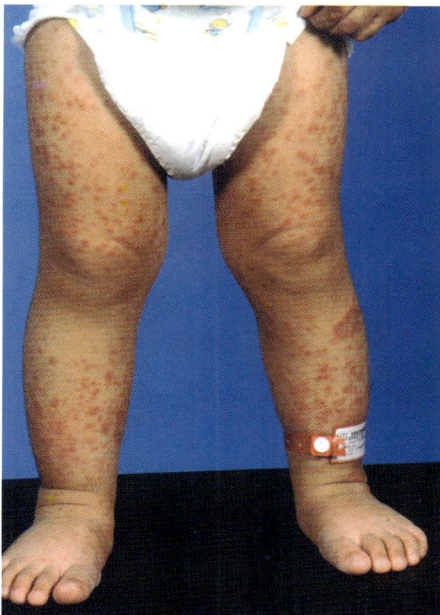

Figure 10–62 □ Acute hemorrhagic edema of infancy (Finkelstein's disease). Symmetrically distributed urticarial purpuric plaques and papules over the lower limbs. There is no ulceration or necrosis and the lesions are non-tender. The trunk and mucous membranes are usually spared. The condition is self-limiting and usually resolves in two to three weeks with post-inflammatory hyperpigmentation.

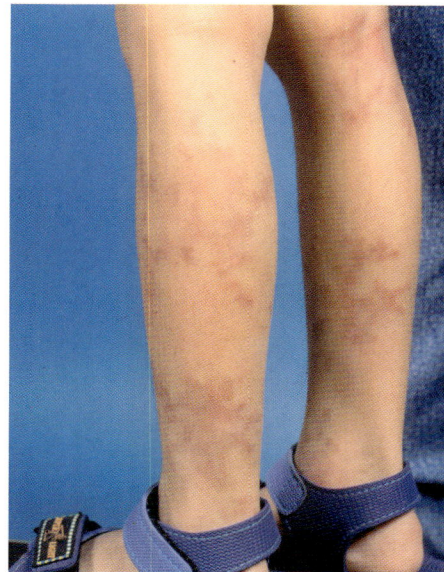

Figure 10–63 □ Polyarteritis nodosa (PAN). Prominent patchy livedo reticularis with a "star-burst" appearance associated with small tender cutaneous nodules which appear to lie along the lines of vessels. These cutaneous findings may be seen in benign cutaneous PAN which has a chronic relapsing benign course with no visceral involvement and also in systemic PAN. Necrotizing vasculitis affecting the medium-sized arteries in the dermis and subcutaneous fat is seen on histological examination of the skin.

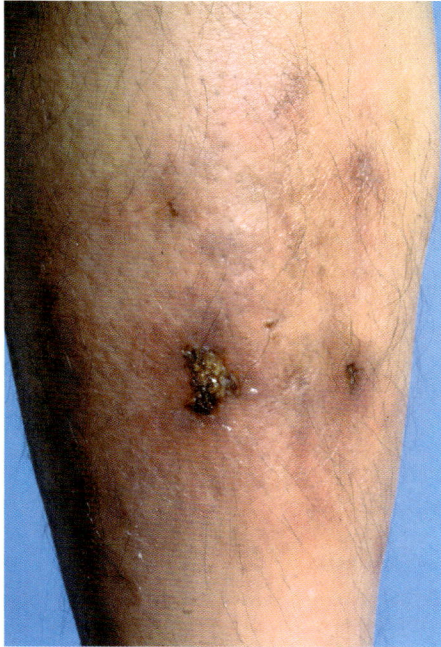

Figure 10–64 □ Polyarteritis nodosa. Painful vasculitic ulcers over the shin of a patient with benign cutaneous PAN. There is necrotic ulceration centrally with an inflamed purpuric border. Lesions heal with depressed scarring and post-inflammatory hyperpigmentation.

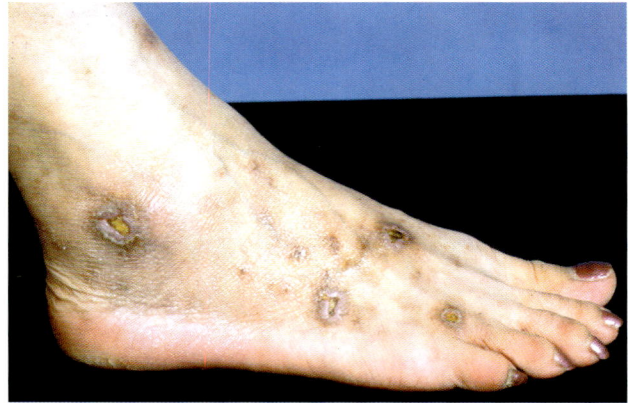

Figure 10–65 □ Cutaneous polyarteritis nodosa – hepatitis B associated. Multiple painful vasculitic ulcers over the dorsum of the foot of a patient with cutaneous PAN that is associated with underlying hepatitis B infection. Interestingly, chronic active hepatitis B infection is more commonly seen with systemic PAN rather than cutaneous PAN.

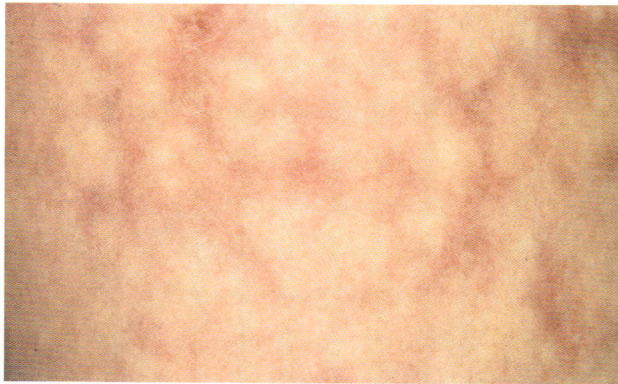

Figure 10–66 □ Livedo reticularis. Reticulate, net-like, erythematous mottling over the thigh. Although commonly idiopathic, secondary causes of livedo reticularis include polyarteritis nodosa, antiphospholipid syndrome, cryoglobulinemia, thrombocythemia, hypercalcemia associated with renal disease and cholesterol crystal emboli. "Secondary livedo reticularis" is often patchy and may be asymmetrical.

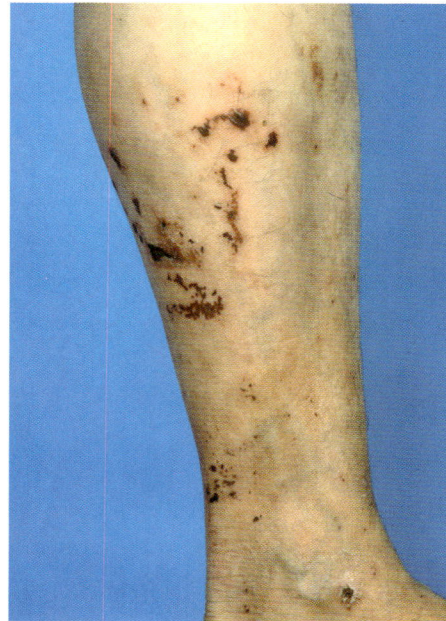

Figure 10–67 □ Churg-Strauss syndrome. Necrotic palpable vasculitic lesions in a patient with worsening adult-onset asthma, severe hypereosinophilia, fever, arthralgia, and renal impairment. Anti-myeloperoxidase autoantibodies (pANCA) were positive. Churg-Strauss syndrome is a multisystemic eosinophilic vasculitis affecting the small- and medium-sized vessels. Skin lesions include palpable purpura, urticarial wheals, necrotic vasculitic lesions, livedo reticularis, erythematous macules and papules, and deep-seated subcutaneous nodules.

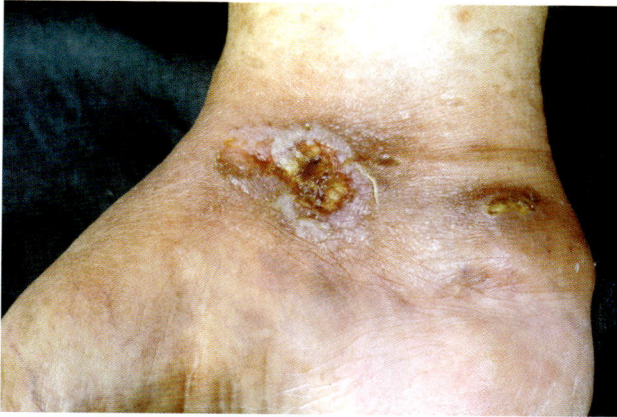

Figure 10–68 □ Rheumatoid vasculitis. Tender, necrotic ulcer with inflamed edges over the medial malleolus in a patient with active rheumatoid arthritis and underlying ankle joint destruction. Other cutaneous manifestations of rheumatoid arthritis include rheumatoid nodules, palpable purpura, digital infarcts, pyoderma gangrenosum, and rheumatoid neutrophilic dermatosis.

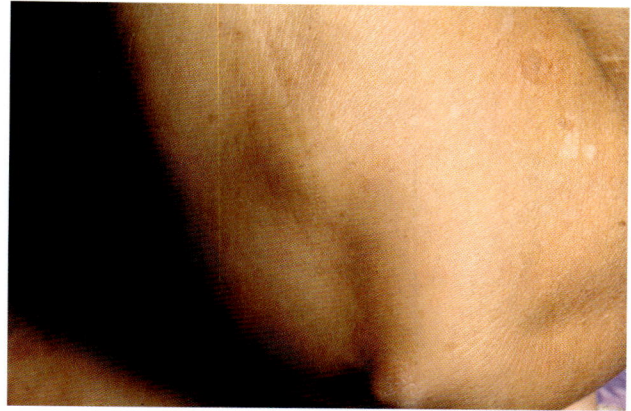

Figure 10–69 □ Rheumatoid nodules. Firm, non-tender, mobile, skin-colored subcutaneous nodules over the elbow which is a classical site of involvement. Rheumatoid nodules may be present at other sites, particularly those subject to repeated trauma and may ulcerate with trauma. Rheumatoid nodules are associated with more severe arthritis and high titres of rheumatoid factor. Palisading granulomas are seen on histological examination.

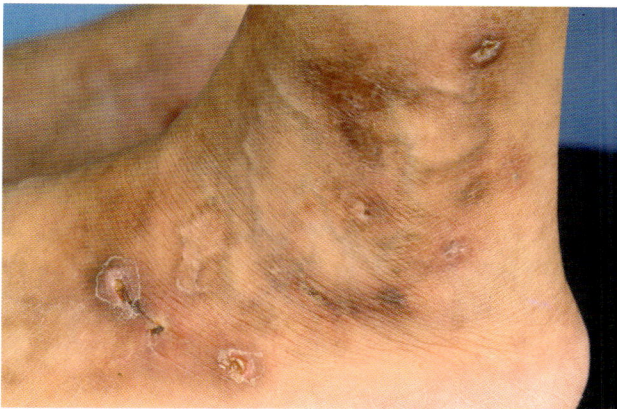

Figure 10–70 □ Livedoid vasculitis. Several healing vasculitic ulcers with typical dusky purpuric edges over the dorsum of the foot. At the region of the lateral malleolus, a porcelain-white atrophic scar (atrophie blanche) is seen as well as a dusky purpuric macule just inferior to it. Classical histological findings are segmental hyalinization of dermal vessel walls, endothelial proliferation, and vascular thrombi. It was previously thought to be an occlusive vasculopathy but is now accepted as a form of lymphocyte-mediated vascular injury causing a procoagulant effect, resulting in skin infarcts.

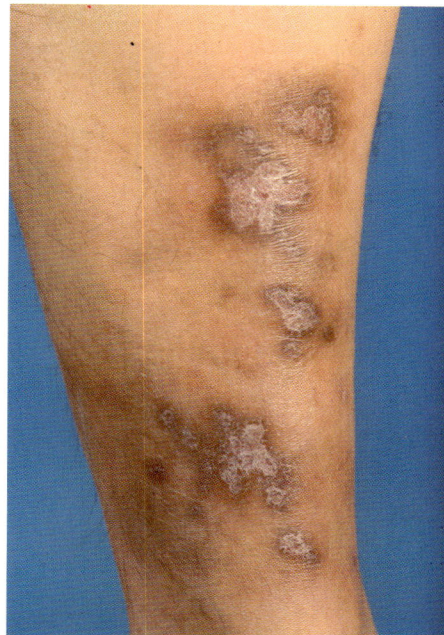

Figure 10–71 □ Nodular vasculitis (Erythema induratum). Resolving nodules over the calves with some atrophic scarring secondary to previous ulceration. Erythema induratum or nodular vasculitis is a chronic relapsing nodular eruption affecting the backs of the lower legs. In contrast to erythema nodosum, the lesions often ulcerate and heal with depressed scars and tend to occur on the calves rather than the shins. There is some evidence to suggest that it is a tuberculide, and hence, a search for an underlying infection with *Mycobacterium tuberculosis* is warranted, especially in endemic areas.

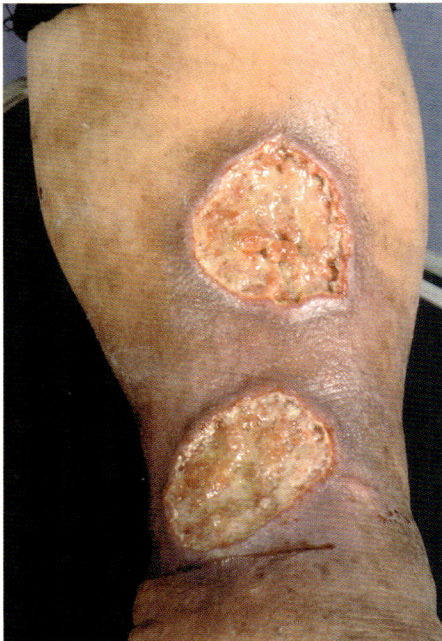

Figure 10–72 □ Pyoderma gangrenosum. Two large necrotic leg ulcers with characteristic bluish undermined edges. Pyoderma gangrenosum usually begins as an inflamed papule that rapidly suppurates, causing a painful inflammatory ulcer that extends peripherally. It is a neutrophilic dermatoses that is associated with systemic conditions such as inflammatory bowel disease, paraproteinemia, rheumatoid arthritis, and myeloproliferative disorders. Pathergy can sometimes be demonstrated.

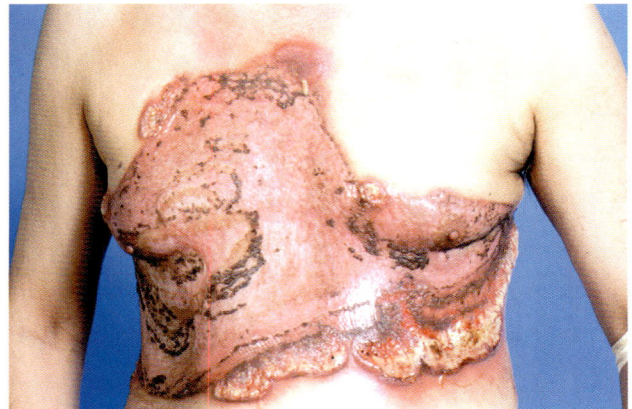

Figure 10–73 □ Pyoderma gangrenosum. Extensive ulceration involving the entire width of the anterior trunk of a patient with idiopathic pyoderma gangrenosum. Note the cribriform scarring over the healed areas as well as the active necrotic inferior edge with typical violaceous overhanging borders. In the assessment of the patient with suspected pyoderma gangrenosum, other causes of cutaneous ulceration must be ruled out and an evaluation for any associated systemic disorders should be performed.

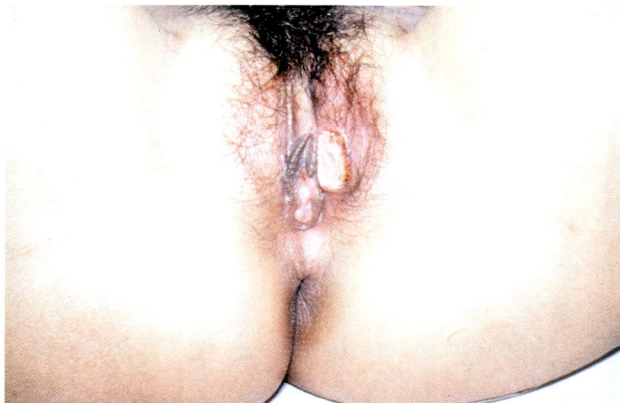

Figure 10–74 □ Behcet's disease – genital aphthous ulcers. Single, large, painful, aphthous ulcer on the labia majora. In males, genital aphthae occur on the scrotum and penis. Behcet's disease is a syndrome consisting of recurrent oral and genital aphthous ulcers and ocular disease. Other cutaneous manifestations include papulopustular lesions, acneiform eruptions, erythema nodosum, necrotizing vasculitis, superficial migratory thrombophlebitis, and pathergy.

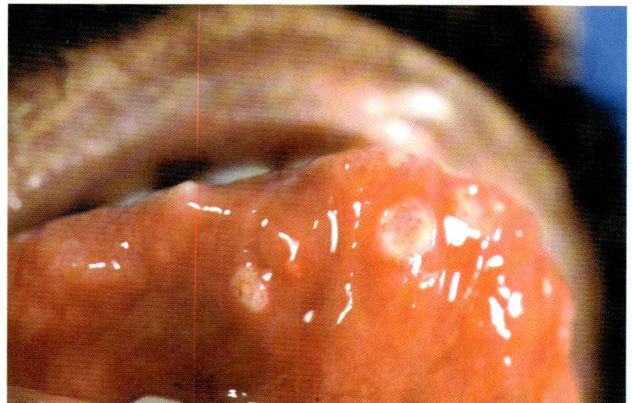

Figure 10–75 □ Behcet's disease – oral aphthous ulcers. Multiple painful, aphthous ulcers seen on the tongue. They are identical to simple oral aphthous ulcers but tend to be multiple and recurrent. The ulcers may occur on the lips, tongue, buccal mucosa and occasionally on the gums, palate, and posterior pharynx.

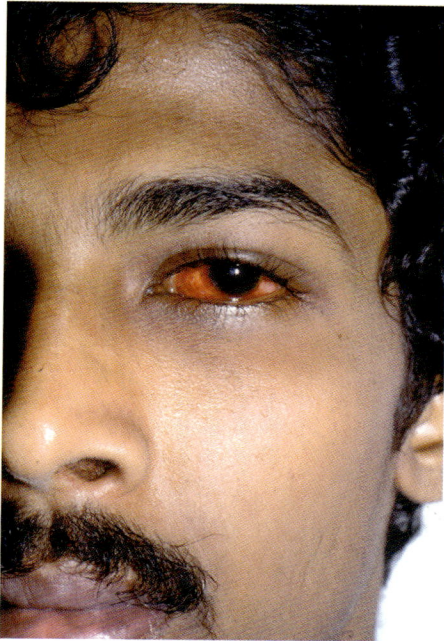

Figure 10–76 □ Behcet's disease – acute anterior uveitis. Acute anterior uveitis presenting as a painful red eye, which is the most common ocular complication seen in Behcet's disease. Other associated eye problems include hypopyon, posterior uveitis, and retinal vasculitis. Blindness is the major cause of morbidity in Behcet's disease. Non-deforming arthritis and, less commonly, neurological involvement may also be seen in this condition.

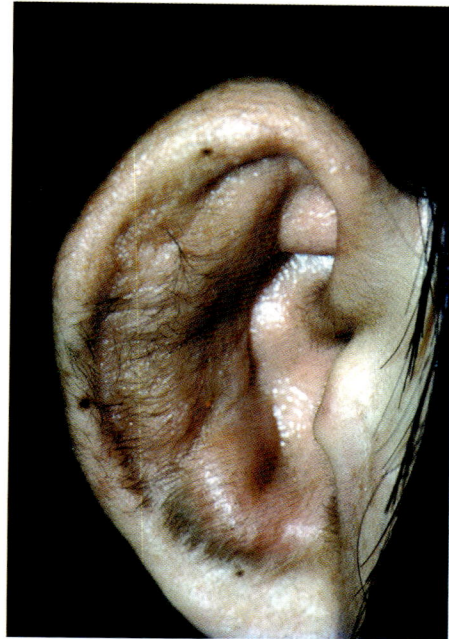

Figure 10–77 □ Relapsing polychondritis. Swelling and mild erythema seen over the cartilaginous areas of the ears, especially over the antihelix. The ear is the most common site of involvement. Advanced disease results in the classical "cauliflower" ear deformity as shown. Note the characteristic sparing of the earlobe. Other clinical manifestations of this condition include arthritis, nasal chondritis resulting in the saddle nose deformity, episcleritis and iritis, tracheitis with secondary tracheal stenosis, deafness due to middle ear ossicle degeneration, and aortitis.

Adverse Drug Eruptions

Leow Y.H.

DEFINITION

Adverse drug eruption (ADR) is part and parcel of clinical practice, as an unexpected adverse event may occur when medication is prescribed. It may arise from intrinsic factors pertaining to pharmacodynamics and pharmacogenetics, but it often arises from immunological or idiosyncratic events. ADR may occur in most normal individuals when given in sufficient doses or duration, viz. overdosage, secondary effects, side effects, and drug interaction. These are usually largely predictable and preventable ADR that should not be catastrophic if the physician exercises great caution. The more feared ADR are hypersensitivity reactions that can present in a small number of individuals as unpredictable idiosyncratic and immunological drug reactions. They represent a small subset of patients but constitute important considerations in clinical practice.

ADR occurs as commonly in Asia as in other parts of the world. However, traditional medication that is unique to the indigenous culture of the region co-exists with medication based on Western models. It is still largely unstudied and may prove to be challenging to interested physicians practising in this part of the world.

INCIDENCE AND PREVALENCE

ADR has been defined by the World Health Organisation as any noxious, unintended, and undesirable effect of a drug that occurs at doses used in humans for prevention, diagnosis, and treatment.

It is difficult to determine the actual incidence and prevalence of ADR in any given population or community as almost all ADR reporting regulatory bodies in different countries rely on voluntary reporting of an ADR event by the specific attending physician. Information collected may not be exhaustive or entirely accurate. However, useful information and statistics can still be collated to reflect trends of ADR seen in a specific community. The other determining factor is the differing prescribing patterns in different communities and countries. Medications that are commonly used in our part of the world may differ significantly from what are commonly prescribed in the West, thus forbidding direct comparison.

PATHOGENESIS AND CLASSIFICATION

Clinicians have actively been trying to simplify the management strategy and protocol, to classify all immunological drug eruptions into neat subcategories that fit the four hypersensitivity types as described by Gell and

Coombs, *viz*. Type I – Immediate hypersensitivity reactions (urticaria, angioedema); Type II – Cytotoxic reactions (pemphigus-like); Type III – Immune complex reactions (urticaria-vasculitis); and Type IV – Delayed type hypersensitivity reactions (allergic contact dermatitis). The first three involve drug-specific antibodies, and the last drug-specific T-lymphocytes. However, this is probably an oversimplified and unrealistically ideal system of classification, as some ADRs may fit well into this classical classification, e.g. IgE mediated urticarial drug eruption. In some instances, they only have features suggestive of fitting into this classification, e.g. maculo-papular drug eruption as akin to an allergic contact dermatitis. However, in others, the eruption does not fit into this neat classification at all, e.g. Stevens-Johnson syndrome, toxic epidermal necrolysis (SJS-TEN).

There has been recent interest in the role of interaction between virus and drug in the host. The most classical example is maculo-papular rash that occurs in susceptible individuals who are given amoxycillin in the presence of infectious mononucleosis. Emerging evidence also points to human herpes virus 6 (HHV6) reactivation associated with drug hypersensitivity syndrome or DRESS (drug rash with easinophilia and systemic symptoms) and its role in the modification of drug metabolism and development of drug reaction.

SPECIFIC ADR

ADR arising from prescribed medication based on the Western model probably does not differ significantly in Asia from what is reported in the West. However, ADR may arise from indigenous medication unique to the rich multicultural setting of Asia. Traditional medication, otherwise known as alternative medication based on the Western model, is often considered as being more natural and thus perceived as less likely to cause ADR. Different ethnic or racial populations have their own potpourri of medication that is akin to homeopathic medication, e.g. the Indian Ayuverdic medication, Malays' Jamu, and traditional Chinese herbal-based medication. ADRs that arise from the use of these medications are often unpredictable and difficult to assess as the cause of the ADRs may be related to an adulterated component of the medication, e.g. addition of Western medication into the supposedly traditional concoction, or it may arise solely from some unstudied and uncontrolled use of herbal remedy. The actual incidence and prevalence of these ADRs are indeed difficult to define.

EVALUATION

De-challenging or stopping the suspect drug that has caused the ADR will be the most logical first step in management. Many medico-legal savvy physicians will adopt the "better safe than sorry" approach to management. However, therein lies the possibility of labeling the patient to be allergic to multiple drugs, sometimes unnecessarily depriving the patient of an entire class of medication.

Evaluation of ADR should thus be holistic and requires the attending physician to address these few basic questions at the outset, namely, is this rash an ADR? If yes, what is the most likely offending drug? Detailed exhaustive history-taking and physical examination are crucial steps in the management. A few factors are critical in making the diagnosis: detailed documentation of clinical circumstances whereby medication was given, temporal sequence between taking of medication and onset of rash, relationship between skin reactions and dosage of medication, previous exposure history, and lesion characteristics.

INVESTIGATIONS

There has been a plethora of literature on different diagnostic tests and strategies for the investigation of ADR. Numerous tests have been propounded to be useful, *viz.* prick testing for immediate hypersensitivity, patch testing for maculo-papular drug eruption and fixed drug eruption (FDE), radioallergosorbent test (RAST) for IgE mediated ADR, lymphocyte blast transformation, provocative drug challenge, etc. However, the actual positive and negative predictive values of most of these tests are not known, as data on actual correlation between the accuracy of the results of these investigations and clinical outcome are lacking.

TREATMENT

Pharmacological therapy is usually quite standard in the treatment of numerous ADRs, *viz.* the use of topical corticosteroid and antihistamines for milder ADRs. Use of systemic corticosteroid is an established therapy in severe FDEs and DRESS. However, there are emerging data on the benefits of using immunomodulators, like cyclosporin A and even intravenous immunoglobulins, in the management of SJS-TEN.

In the face of mild ADRs with no systemic involvement, it is possible to re-challenge to confirm clinical suspicion of ADR. However with severe ADRs like SJS-TEN and DRESS, it is best to avoid onset and consider suitable alternative therapy. In centers whereby desensitization is available, it may be feasible to induce "tolerant" state in affected patients with this treatment strategy of gradual reintroduction of incremental doses of a drug over a period of time. However the beneficial effect of desensitization is not permanent.

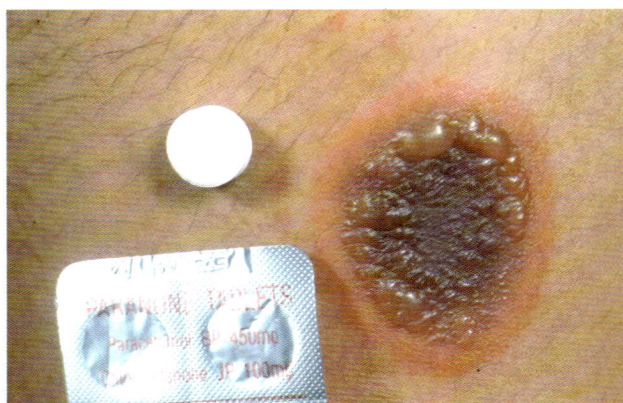

Figure 11–1 □ Fixed drug eruption due to chlormezanone. This is the classical appearance of fixed drug eruption. The lesion shows erythematous swelling, with central bulla formation and hyperpigmentation. In this case, the incriminating drug is chlormezanone that is found in paranone, an analgesic/muscle relaxant that also contains paracetamol.

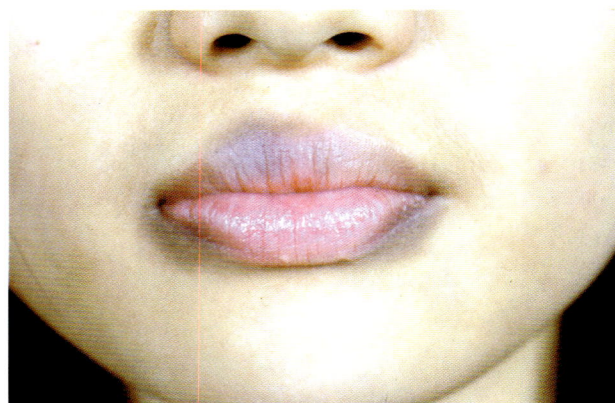

Figure 11–2 □ Fixed drug eruption due to mefenamic acid – lip. The lip is another common presentation of fixed drug eruption. Initial presentation of pruritic erythematous swelling at the lip with the adjacent vermilion border, usually resolves with hyperpigmentation. This clinical presentation can be easily reproduced, upon re-challenge to the same drug. Differential diagnoses to be considered include endogenous cheilitis, contact cheilitis, and angioedema.

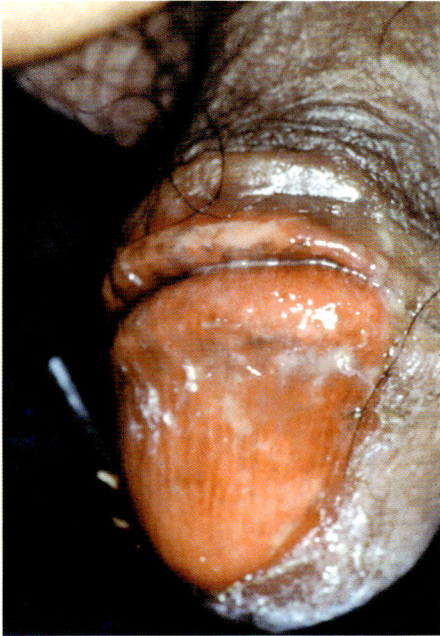

Figure 11–3 □ Fixed drug eruption due to cotrimoxazole – penis. The penis is another common site of involvement of fixed drug eruption. It can present as painful penile blisters that progress onto ulcers. It may be eaasily mistaken as a possible sexually transmitted penile ulcer to the clinician, before the final correct diagnosis is considered.

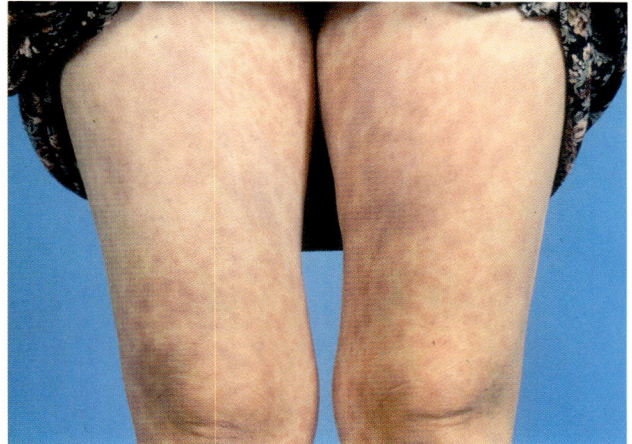

Figure 11–4 □ Maculo-papular drug eruption due to cotrimoxazole. Symmetrical erythematous macules, patches, and papules are seen on the patient's thighs. It is usually rather extensive, with involvement of the trunk, extremities, and possibly the face. Rash usually appears seven to 14 days after ingestion of the incriminating drug.

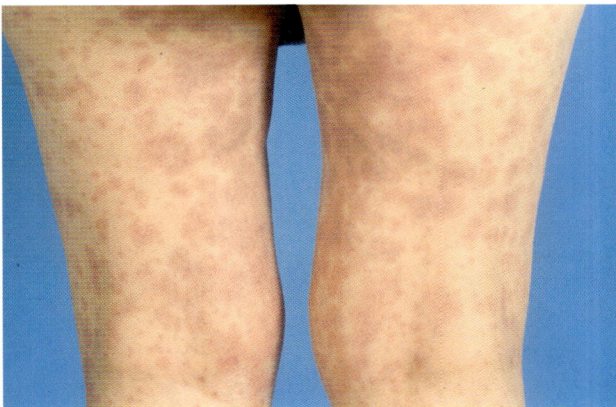

Figure 11–5 □ Maculo-papular drug eruption due to cotrimoxazole. This is the close-up view of the patient's rash. Viral exanthem is often the most commonly considered differential diagnosis, as both conditions also present with sudden onset of pruritic symmetrical extensive patches and plaques.

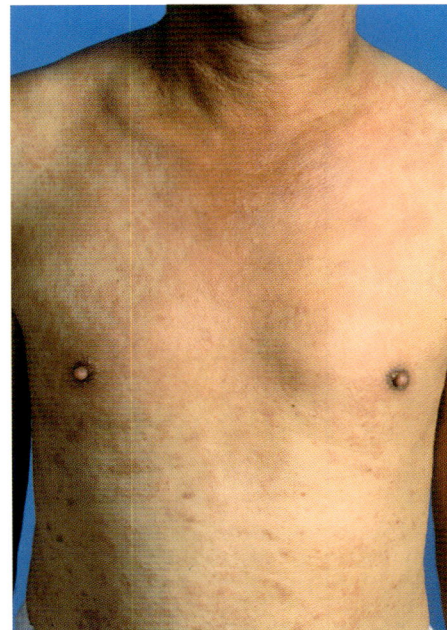

Figure 11–6 □ Maculo-papular drug eruption due to allopurinol. Scattered erythematous patches and plaques are seen on this patient. It is important to investigate for any systemic involvement, *viz.* full blood count, liver function, and renal function, as drug hypersensitivity syndrome can also present with maculo-papular rash.

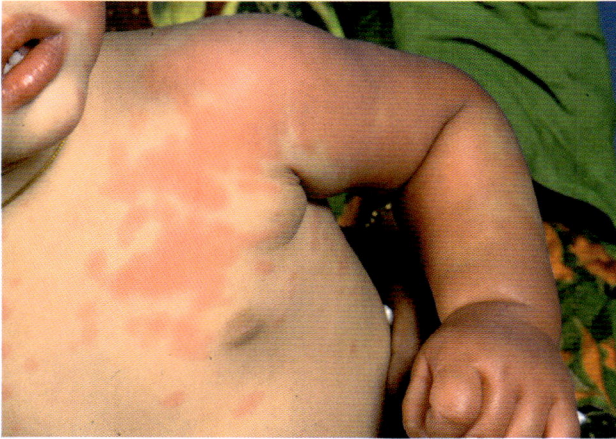

Figure 11–7 □ Urticarial drug eruption due to amoxycillin. Pruritic erythematous swelling and plaques are seen on this child, after being re-challenged with amoxycillin in the clinic. Reaction usually occurs within the first two hours of ingestion of medication. It must be performed under close supervision in a medical institution, as the condition may be associated with other symptoms, like angioedema, wheezing, and anaphylaxis. Delayed reaction, though uncommon, may occur within six hours of ingestion of medication. Re-challenge or drug provocation is performed to exclude other causes of the eruption, rather than to confirm the definitive diagnosis, as the procedure may be risky.

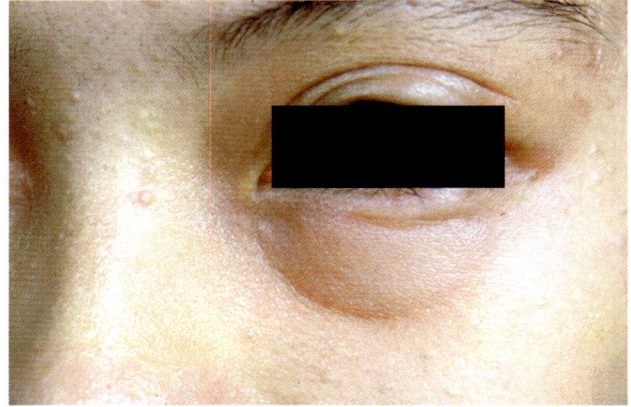

Figure 11–8 □ Angioedema due to amoxycillin. Swelling is noted on the lower and upper eyelids of the patient. Associated swelling of the lip, wheezing, throat or tongue swelling, and angioedema may also occur concomitantly in this immediate type I hypersensitivity reaction. Facilities for resuscitation should be available if the need arises.

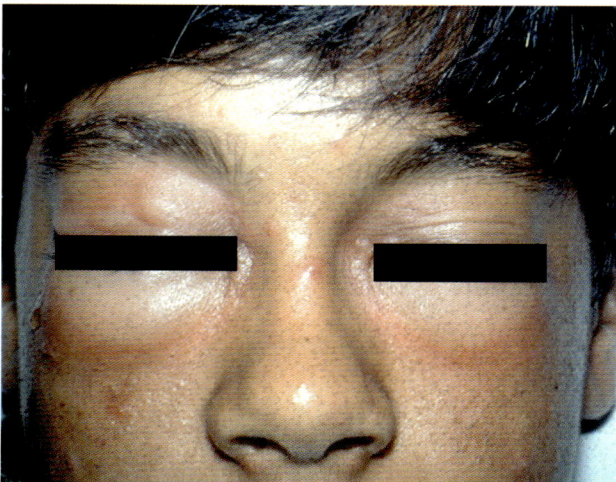

Figure 11–9 □ Angioedema due to aspirin. This patient presents with marked eyelid swelling following ingestion of aspirin. It was previously thought that this is a classical prototype of immediate type I hypersensitivity reaction. However, there are experts who classify this reaction as anaphylactoid, as it is thought that this is not truly an immunological event, but occurs as a result of interference with the prostaglandin metabolism by non-steroidal, anti-inflammatory drug (NSAID).

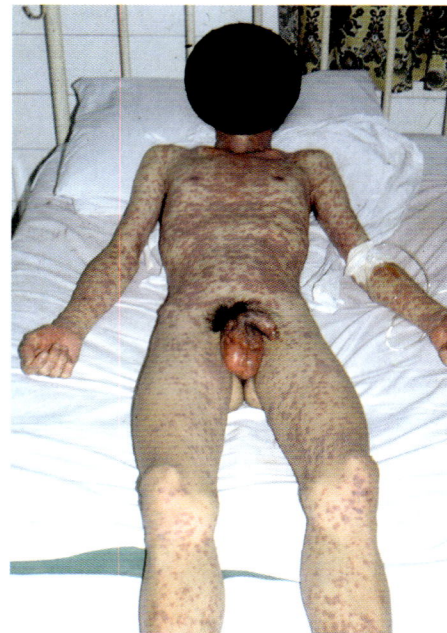

Figure 11–10 □ Stevens-Johnson syndrome. A rather moribund patient with marked mucosal involvement affecting both the oral-genital areas and extensive targetoid lesions on the glabrous skin. Drugs are one of the most common causes of this dermatological emergency.

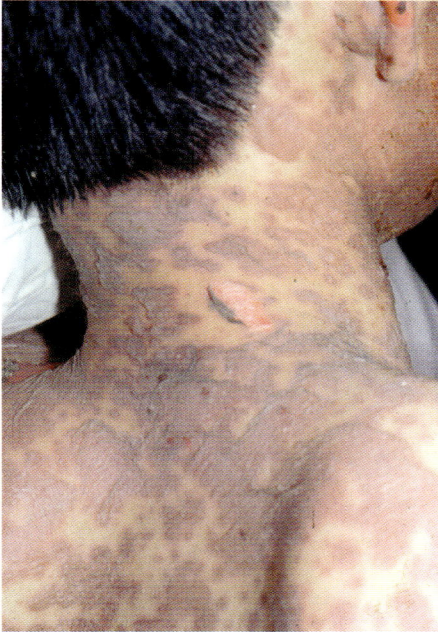

Figure 11–11 □ Stevens-Johnson syndrome. A close-up view of the targetoid lesions on the neck and shoulder. The classical appearance of the skin lesion is an erythematous plaque or patch with bullous center. If only similar lesions are seen on the glabrous skin without any mucosal involvement, erythema multiforme will be the term that best describes this clinical picture.

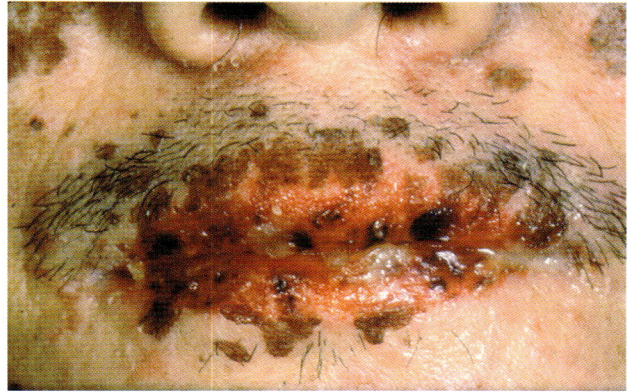

Figure 11–12 □ Stevens-Johnson syndrome due to allopurinol. Marked gingivostomatitis is seen on this patient. An important differential diagnosis to consider will be herpes simplex gingivostomatitis. Cutaneous lesions tend to improve and heal more rapidly than the mucosal lesions. It is important to check thoroughly for other mucosal surface involvement, namely, anogenital, conjunctiva, and nasal surfaces.

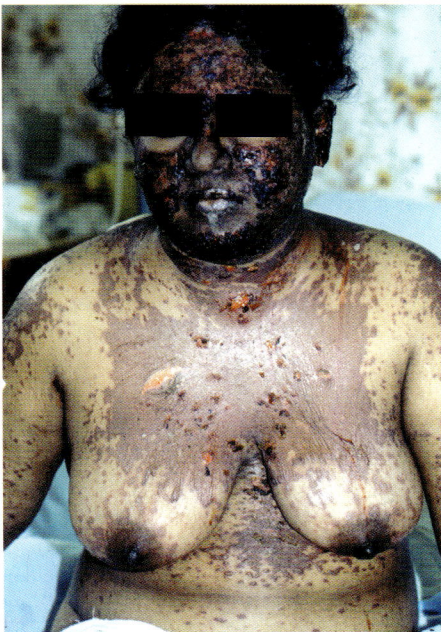

Figure 11–13 □ Toxic epidermal necrolysis due to phenytoin. Extensive erosions are seen on the patient's face, trunk, and limbs. Toxic epidermal necrolysis (TEN) is thought to be in the same spectrum as the Stevens-Johnson syndrome, with more extensive body surface involvement. It is not easy to differentiate the two in the more advanced phase of the disease.

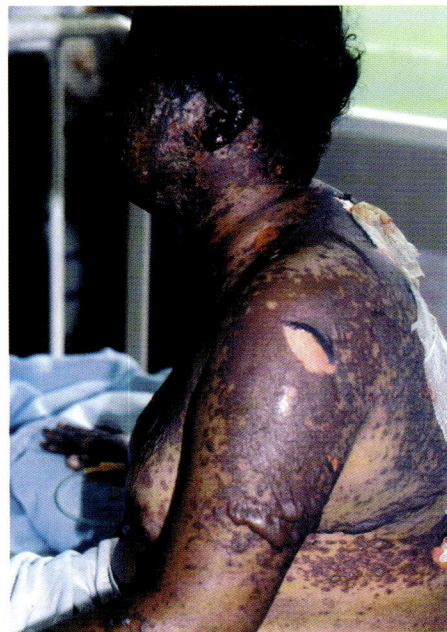

Figure 11–14 □ Toxic epidermal necrolysis due to phenytoin. Large blisters are seen on the patient's left arm. As opposed to the Stevens-Johnson syndrome, target lesions are usually not seen in the early phase of the disease. Instead, tender erythematous patches with subsequent development of flaccid blisters are seen during the early phase of the disease.

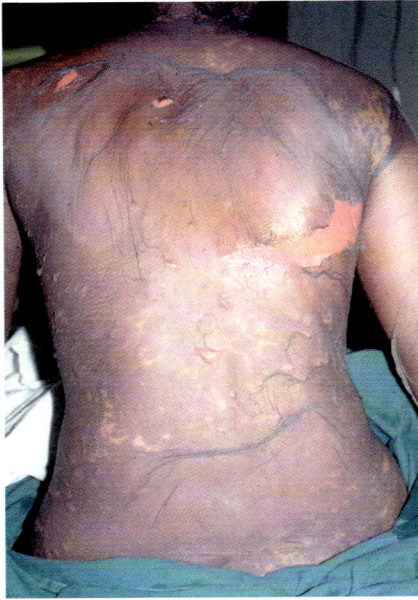

Figure 11–15 □ Toxic epidermal necrolysis – late phase. In the later phase of the disease, blisters coalesce, forming erosions and large sheets of epidermolysis, resembling injuries from burns. Patients may require special burns nursing care as they often succumb to septicemia as a consequence to extensive muco-cutaneous involvement.

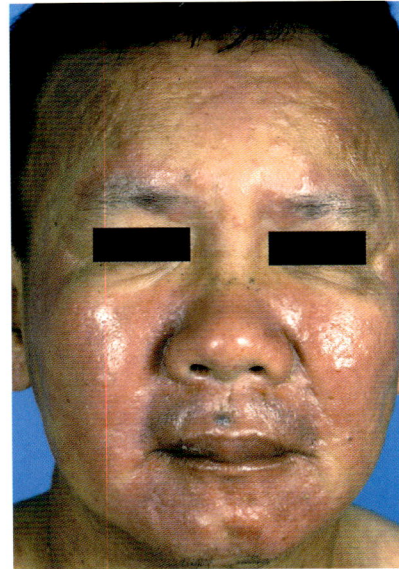

Figure 11–16 □ Drug hypersensitivity syndrome due to allopurinol. Swollen erythematous plaques are seen on this patient's face. The onset of this syndrome may be delayed up to two to four weeks after ingestion of the culprit medication. Clinical differential diagnoses of this syndrome will include viral exanthem, hypersensitivity syndrome of other etiology, and maculo-papular drug eruption. A high index of suspicion is required to make the diagnosis.

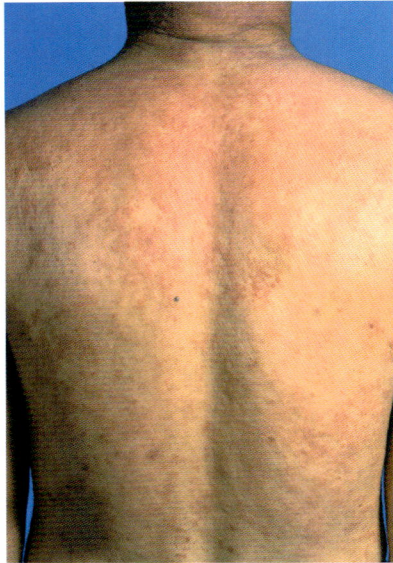

Figure 11–17 □ Drug hypersensitivity syndrome due to allopurinol. Symmetrical erythematous papules and plaques are seen on the trunk. The syndrome may be indistinguishable from the more innocuous maculo-papular drug eruption by examining the skin alone. Systemic investigations, namely, complete or full blood count, liver function, and renal function tests, are imperative to elucidate any associated systemic involvement.

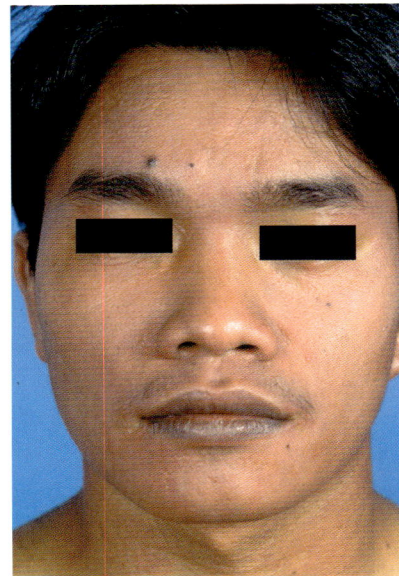

Figure 11–18 □ Drug hypersensitivity syndrome due to dapsone. Another patient with extensive symmetrical erythematous papules and plaques on his face, trunk, and extremities. The patient is also clinically jaundiced from underlying drug-induced hepatitis, as demonstrated by the yellowness of his sclera. Drug-induced hepatitis is one of the most commonly associated systemic organ involvements of this syndrome. The other synonym for this syndrome is **D**rug **R**ash with **E**osinophilia and **S**ystemic **S**ymptoms (DRESS). Other possible systemic features that may occur include blood abnormalities, namely, eosinophilia, atypical lymphocytes, pneumonitis, carditis, and renal involvement.

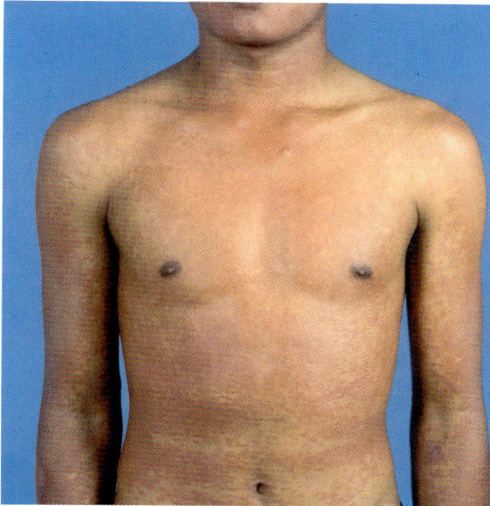

Figure 11–19 □ Drug hypersensitivity syndrome due to dapsone. This is an idiosyncratic drug eruption. Dapsone was given as part of the treatment for Hansen's disease. It is thought that this particular syndrome to dapsone could have been avoided if a lower dosage of the medication was used in the initial phase of treatment, when given in situations other than the treatment of leprosy.

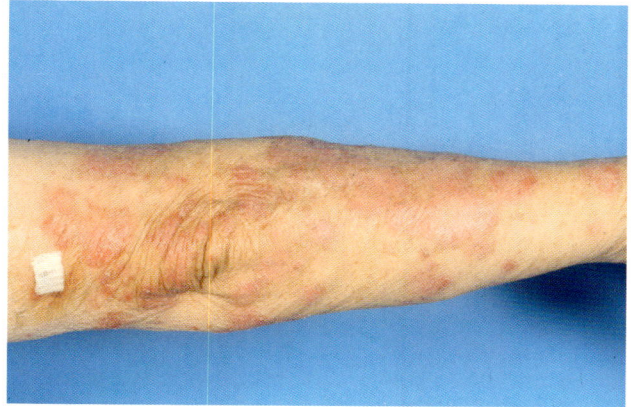

Figure 11–20 □ Psoriasiform drug eruption due to propranolol. Scaly erythematous plaques are seen on the patient's arm and forearm. Differential diagnoses of the lesions include psoriasis vulgaris (plaque-type psoriasis), psoriasiform drug eruption, and other papulosquamous eruption with atypical features, like sebo-psoriasis, pityriasis lichenoides. Skin biopsy can be used as an adjunct to rule out the other differential diagnoses.

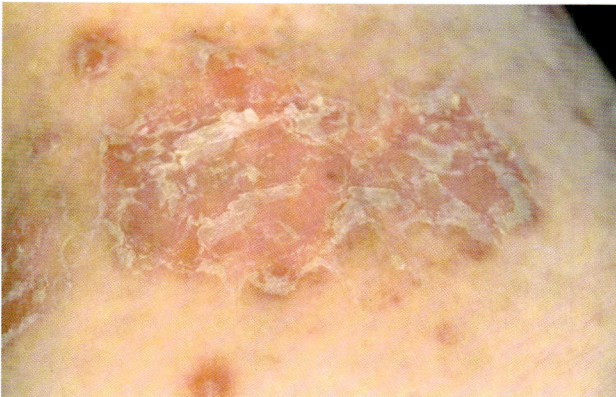

Figure 11–21 □ Psoriasiform drug eruption due to propranolol. A close-up view of the scaly red plaque. Important clues to the diagnosis will be a positive history, suggesting the temporal sequence and relationship between ingestion of medication and onset of rash, resolution of rash upon de-challenge (withdrawal of drug), and recurrence of rash upon re-challenge (provocation).

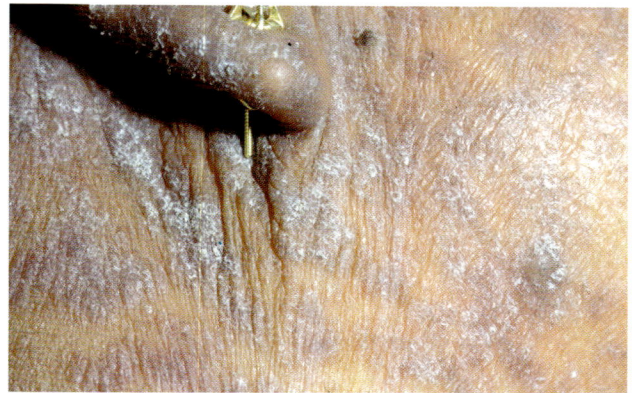

Figure 11–22 □ Lichenoid drug eruption due to allopurinol. Violaceous, scaly lichenoid papules and plaques are seen on the patient's face and neck. Clinically, these lesions may be indistinguishable from idiopathic lichen planus. Skin biopsy may not be pathognomic, but may be useful for eliminating other differential diagnoses of cutaneous lichenoid eruptions.

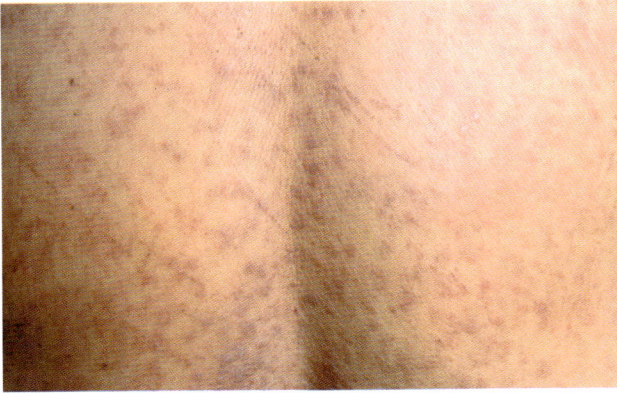

Figure 11–23 □ Lichenoid drug eruption due to allopurinol. Extensive symmetrical, violaceous, scaly lichenoid papules are seen on this patient's trunk. Important keys to diagnosis will be a positive temporal history and relationship between ingestion of medication and onset of rash, resolution of rash upon de-challenge, and recurrence of rash upon re-challenge (drug provocation).

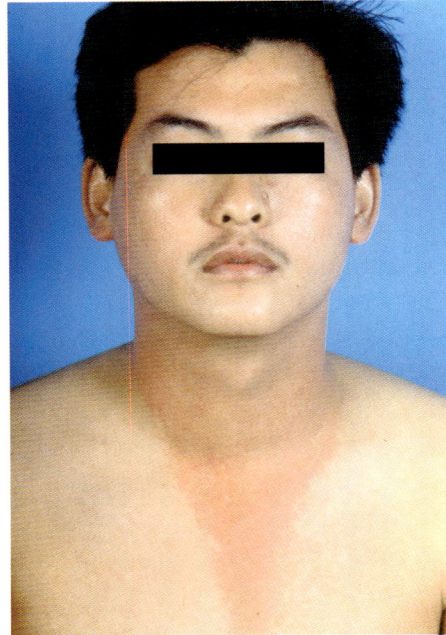

Figure 11–24 □ Photosensitive drug eruption due to griseofulvin. Distinctive photodistributed rash is seen on the patient's face, ears, and V of the anterior neck. Griseofulvin, a commonly prescribed anti-fungal agent, is both a photosensitizer and phototoxic agent. It is important to consider other differential diagnoses before arriving at the diagnosis of drug-related, photodistributed rash.

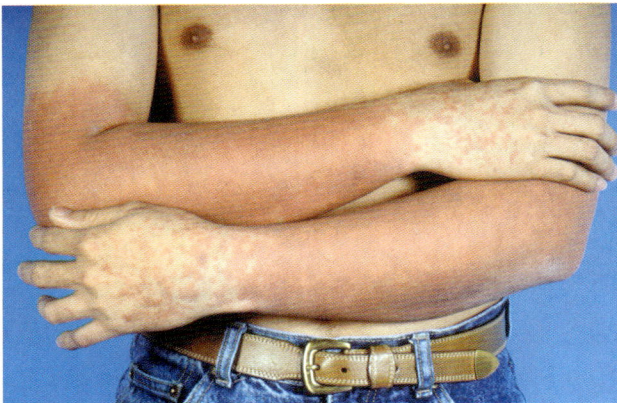

Figure 11–25 □ Photosensitive drug eruption due to griseofulvin. Erythematous plaques are seen on the patient's forearms, hands, and arms with distinctive "lines" between covered and exposed parts of the upper limbs. Important differential diagnoses to consider include photo-allergic contact dermatitis, photo-irritant contact dermatitis, primary photodermatoses like polymorphous light eruption, and connective tissue disease.

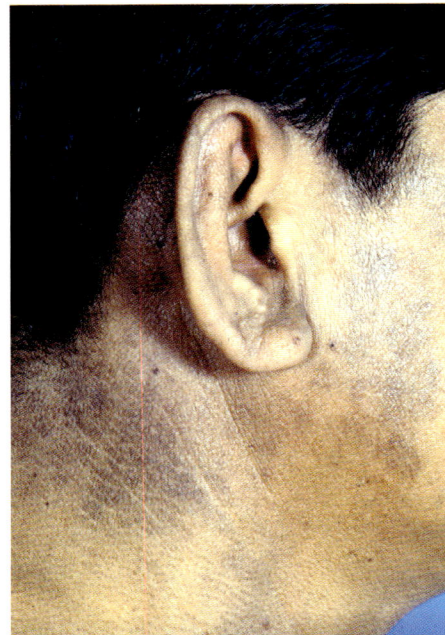

Figure 11–26 □ Photosensitive drug eruption due to quinine. Dusky erythematous to brown plaques are seen on this patient's ears, lateral face, and neck. Lesions are still distinct one month after withdrawal of drugs. It is often not easy to derive a definite diagnosis of photosensitive drug eruption, without considering other differential diagnoses.

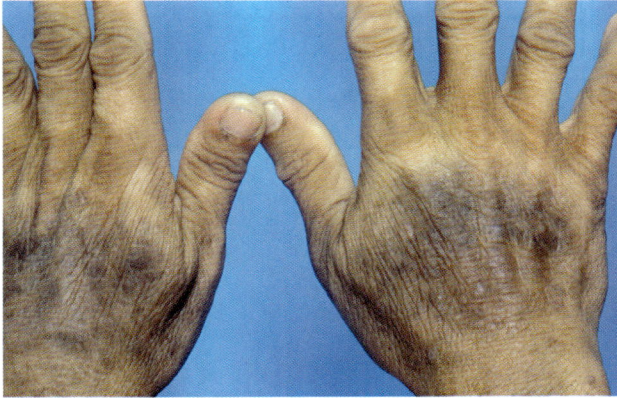

Figure 11–27 □ **Photosensitive drug eruption due to quinine.** Dusky, brown plaques are seen on the dorsal hands. Important investigations to consider include skin biopsy (routine histology and direct immunofluorescence), connective tissues disease screen, photo-patch test, and photo-test. An exhaustive history documenting the temporal sequence between the drug and onset of rash, response to de-challenge, and re-challenge to the suspected drug are imperative for making the final diagnosis.

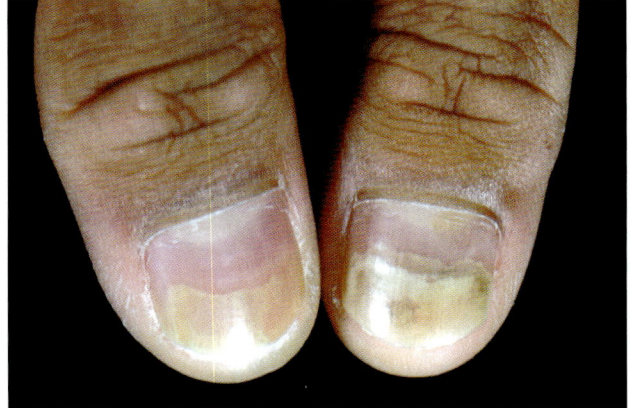

Figure 11–28 □ **Photo-onycholysis from doxycycline.** This is an unusual idiosyncratic reaction to tetracyclines. Other differential diagnoses to consider include psoriasis (nails), onychomycosis, and traumatic onycholysis. It is important to rule out the other differential diagnoses that are amenable to specific treatment. This condition is otherwise benign and will resolve spontaneously upon withdrawal of the causative drug.

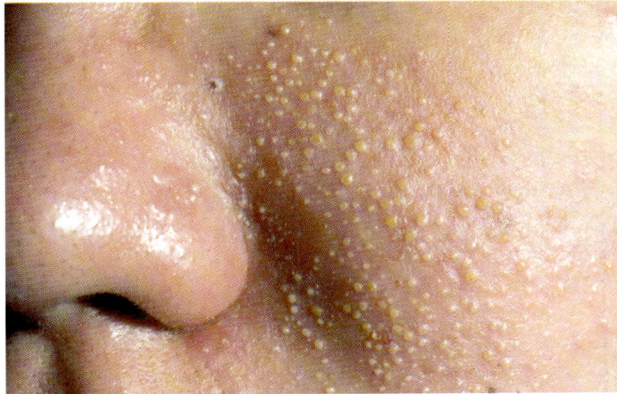

Figure 11–29 □ **Pustular drug eruption due to chlorpromazine.** Monomorphic pustules are seen on this patient's left cheek. Before making this diagnosis, it is important to consider other common differential diagnoses of facial pustular eruption, like acne vulgaris, corticosteroid-induced acne, pustular contact reactions, and Ofuji's eosinophilic folliculitis.

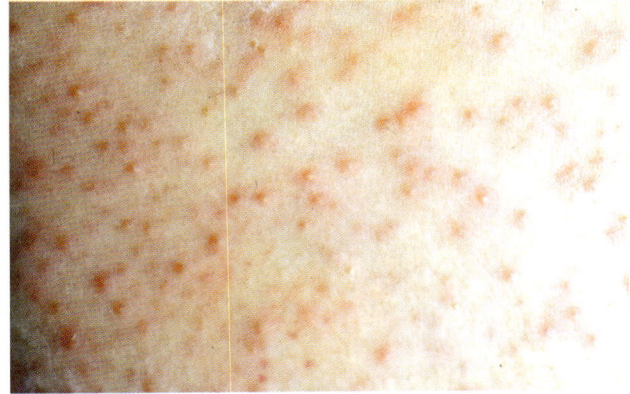

Figure 11–30 □ **Pustular drug eruption due to chlorpromazine.** A close-up view of the monomorphic pustules on this patient's face. Principles of management include detailed exhaustive history, exclusion of other differential diagnoses, trial of standard acne therapy, clearance of lesions upon withdrawal of suspected drug, and recurrence of lesions upon re-challenge with the suspected medication.

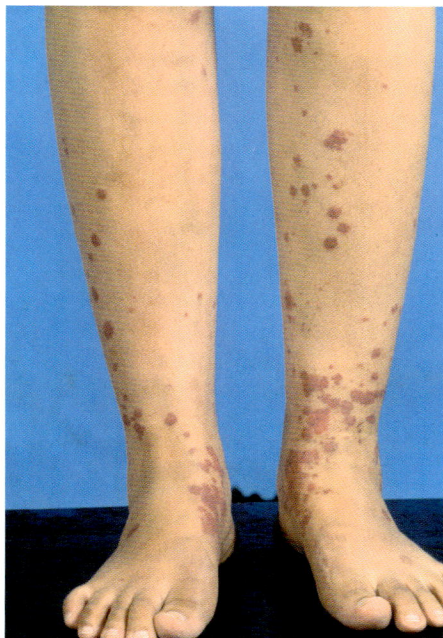

Figure 11–31 □ Vasculitic drug eruption due to propyl-thiouracil. Purpuric plaques are seen on the patient's legs and ankles. It is not possible to make a definite diagnosis at the first consultation. Other more common differential diagnoses of purpuric or ecchymotic lesions on the lower extremities will have to be excluded before arriving at this diagnosis.

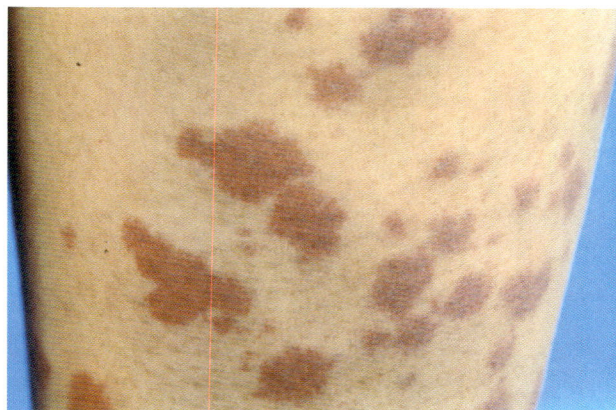

Figure 11–32 □ Vasculitic drug eruption due to propyl-thiouracil. This is a close-up view of the purpuric, ecchymotic plaques on the leg. Important clinical differential diagnoses to consider will include pigmented purpuric dermatoses (primary capillaritis), cutaneous vasculitis, underlying collagen vascular disease, Henoch-Schönlein purpura, and viral infection-related vasculitis.

Pregnancy Dermatoses

Lee J.S.S., Wong S.N., and Chong W.S.

Many physiological changes occur during pregnancy. As the fetus develops in-utero, the mother's body also undergoes immunological, endocrinological, vascular, and metabolic changes. Cutaneous manifestations in pregnancy can be classified as physiological skin changes during pregnancy, pre-existing dermatoses exacerbated by pregnancy, and specific dermatoses of pregnancy.

PHYSIOLOGICAL SKIN CHANGES
(Figures 12–1 to 12–3)

Increased vascularity and hyperaemia occur during pregnancy. Palmar erythema and spider angiomas are commonly seen, as are leg varicosities due to increased intra-abdominal pressure from the gravid uterus. Vascular tumors, such as hemangiomas, may enlarge, and pyogenic granulomas occur more frequently.

Hyperpigmentation may occur due to raised levels of melanocyte stimulating hormone, oestrogen, and progesterone in pregnancy. This is usually seen in the linea nigra, genitals, and areolae. Moles and freckles can also darken, but the color can regress postpartum. Melasma may first present or worsen during pregnancy or the postpartum period.

Striae gravidarum presents during pregnancy as pink, atrophic, cutaneous bands on the abdomen, thighs and, occasionally, the breasts. They fade postpartum to form pale, atrophic lines. Hormonal factors, such as adrenocortical hormones and estrogens, coupled with increased stress on the connective tissue due to distension of various parts of the body, may contribute to its formation.

Other changes seen during pregnancy include pruritus gravidarum, relative increase in anagen hairs with subsequent increase in telogen hairs postpartum, increase in sebaceous and eccrine gland activity, and decrease in apocrine gland activity.

PRE-EXISTING DERMATOSES EXACERBATED BY PREGNANCY

Numerous dermatoses are exacerbated during pregnancy. These include inflammatory conditions such as atopic dermatitis and psoriasis, infective conditions like tuberculosis and candidiasis, and autoimmune conditions such as lupus erythematosus, pemphigus vulgaris, and systemic sclerosis. Certain skin tumors, such as melanomas, keloids, and dermatofibromas, may enlarge during pregnancy. These conditions are covered in their respective chapters of this atlas.

SPECIFIC DERMATOSES OF PREGNANCY (Figures 12–4 to 12–10)

Polymorphic Eruption of Pregnancy

Polymorphic eruption of pregnancy was formerly known as pruritic urticarial papules and plaques of pregnancy (PUPPP). It usually occurs in the first pregnancy and starts in the third trimester with an average duration of six weeks. It rarely recurs in subsequent pregnancies. There is usually intense pruritus. The eruption consists of urticarial red papules and plaques, less commonly vesicles and target lesions. They are usually found on the abdomen and striae with sparing of the umbilicus. They can spread to the limbs. Histology of skin lesions shows perivascular lymphohistiocytic infiltrates with eosinophils, and direct immunofluorescence is negative. Treatment is with potent topical steroids.

Pemphigoid Gestationis

Formerly known as herpes gestationis, it is a rare autoimmune, blistering condition occurring in the second or third trimester of pregnancy. Autoantibodies against BP180 antigen and BP230 antigen of the basement membrane are found. Clinically, there are pruritic vesiculobullous lesions, with a peri-umbilical predilection. There is a subepidermal blister on histology, and direct immunofluorescence of perilesional skin shows linear IgG and C3 along the basement membrane zone. Indirect immunoflourescence of the patient's serum may be positive for antibodies against the basement membrane in a roof pattern. Management is with oral prednisolone. Prognosis is generally good, but small-for-dates infants have been reported with this condition. It may recur in future pregnancies.

Impetigo Herpetiformis

This rare dermatosis has the clinical features of acute pustular psoriasis, precipitated by pregnancy. There may or may not be a prior history of psoriasis. It occurs in the third trimester, and presents as erythematous patches and plaques with pustulation at the margins. Lesions commonly affect the flexures and trunks. The patient is often acutely ill with fever and constitutional symptoms. Blood investigations show a raised total white cell count, raised erythrocyte sedimentation rate, and hypocalcemia. Histology is similar to that of pustular psoriasis, with subcorneal neutrophilic aggregates. Treatment is with systemic corticosteroids. This condition often recurs in subsequent pregnancies at an earlier gestation and with increased severity. Stillbirth and placental insufficiency can sometimes occur.

Prurigo of Pregnancy

This condition is often associated with a personal history of atopy. It often occurs in the second or third trimester of pregnancy, and presents as excoriated, erythematous papules on the abdomen and extensors of the limbs. Direct immunofluorescence is negative in this condition. Treatment is symptomatic with topical glucocorticoids, emolients, and antihistamines. Lesions usually abate post-partum, and the condition does not usually recur in subsequent pregnancies.

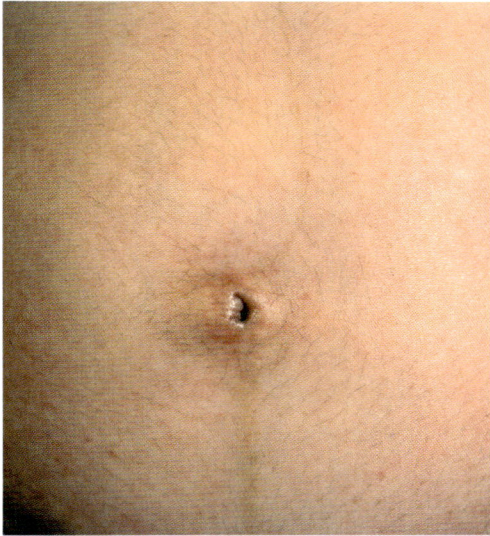

Figure 12–1 □ Linea nigra. The midline of the abdomen of this 34-week pregnant Chinese female is hyperpigmented. Linea nigra is a common feature seen in pregnancy, and occurs when there is hypermelanosis of the linea alba. This hyperpigmentation often fades after parturition.

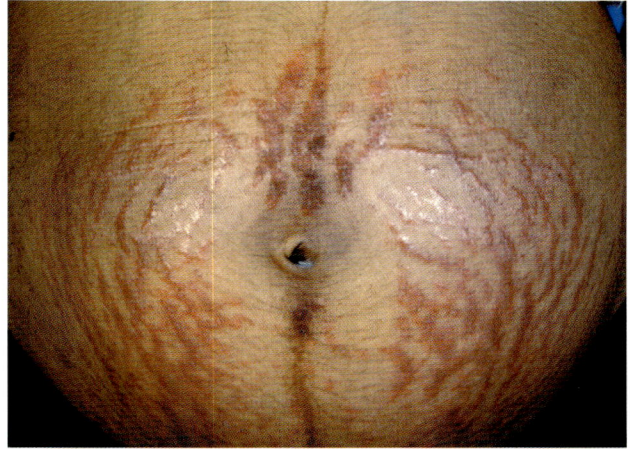

Figure 12–2 □ Striae gravidarum. This 19-year-old Malay female has purplish-red striae over both sides of the anterior abdomen. Striae gravidarum are irregular linear scars, or stretch marks, arising on the abdomen, breasts, and thighs during the later stages of pregnancy.

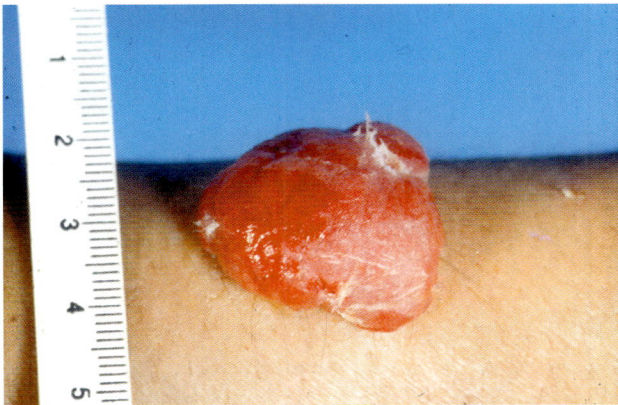

Figure 12–3 □ Pyogenic granuloma in pregnancy. There is a red, vascular nodule with some surface erosion over the lower limb of this female who is in her third trimester of pregnancy. There is increased incidence of pyogenic granulomas in pregnancy as there is hyperaemia and increased tendency toward vascular proliferation during gestation. This rapidly developing vascular lesion often occurs over sites of trauma. It may bleed upon irritation or spontaneously. Treatment is with surgical excision, with electrocautery of the base.

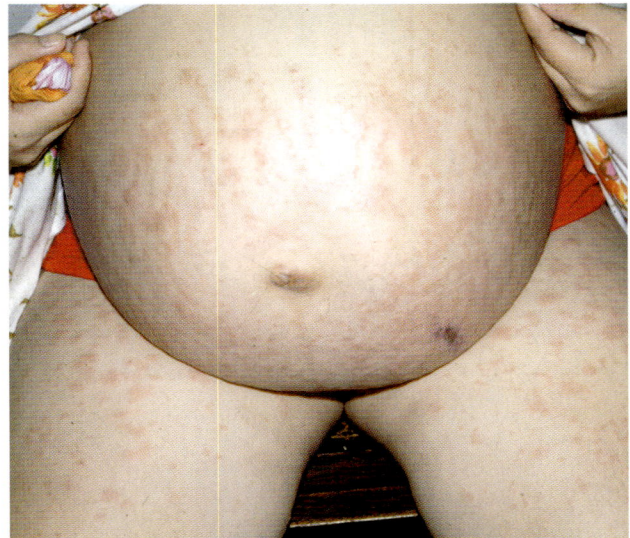

Figure 12–4 □ Polymorphic eruption of pregnancy. This Chinese female has numerous urticarial papules on the abdomen and thighs, particularly along the abdominal striae. Polymorphic eruption of pregnancy presents as itchy papules, plaques, urticarial wheals, and vesicles in the third trimester, or rarely, a few days postpartum. It commonly begins in abdominal striae, and affects primigravidae. The eruption disappears soon after parturition. Treatment with topical glucocorticoids provides symptomatic relief.

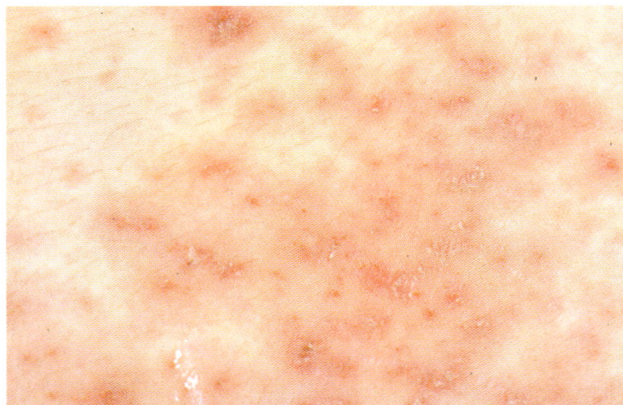

Figure 12–5 □ Polymorphic eruption of pregnancy. A close-up view of lesions seen in another Chinese female shows a polymorphic eruption of papules, vesicles, and erosions. Increased incidence of this disorder has been described in twin and triplet pregnancies, and abdominal distension may play a role in its development. Microchimerism, or the harboring of fetal DNA or cells within the mother, has recently been implicated in the etiology of this disorder.

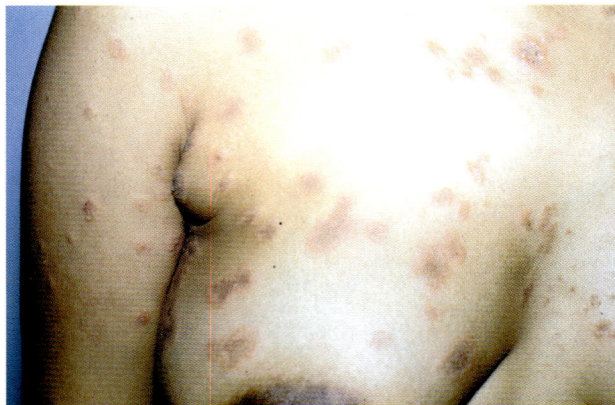

Figure 12–6 □ Pemphigoid gestationis. This pregnant Malay lady has erythematous papular lesions with tense vesicles over the chest and upper limbs. Pemphigoid gestationis is a rare, autoimmune bullous dermatosis, occurring most frequently in the second and third trimesters of pregnancy. Lesions start as itchy, erythematous wheals with subsequent development of vesicles and bullae. These lesions often spread from the umbilical area and can involve the thighs and limbs. It recurs at an earlier gestational age in subsequent pregnancies. Treatment is with systemic corticosteroids.

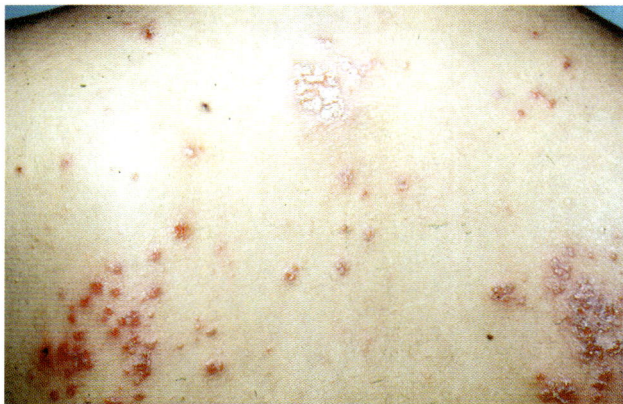

Figure 12–7 □ Pemphigoid gestationis. This pregnant Chinese lady has papules and vesicles over the upper back. Abnormal expression of major histocompatibility class (MHC) II molecules in the placenta may incite the process, followed by cross-reactivity with a cutaneous antigen and subsequent development of vesiculation. There is increased association with HLA-B8, DR3, and DR4.

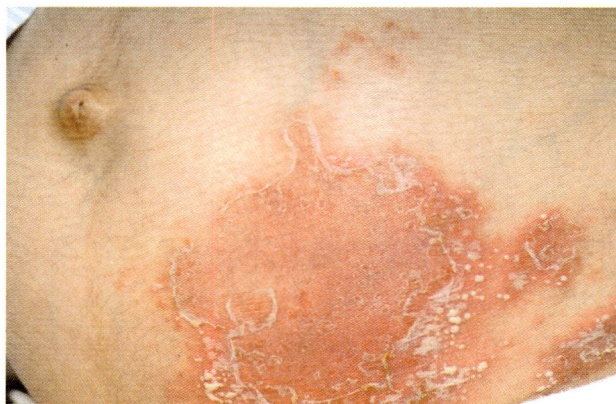

Figure 12–8 □ Impetigo herpetiformis. This pregnant Chinese female has an erythematous plaque over the abdomen, with pustules and exfoliation seen at the active edges. Impetigo herpetiformis resembles generalized pustular psoriasis and presents as erythematous areas with pustulation, often arising symmetrically from flexural regions in the third trimester of pregnancy.

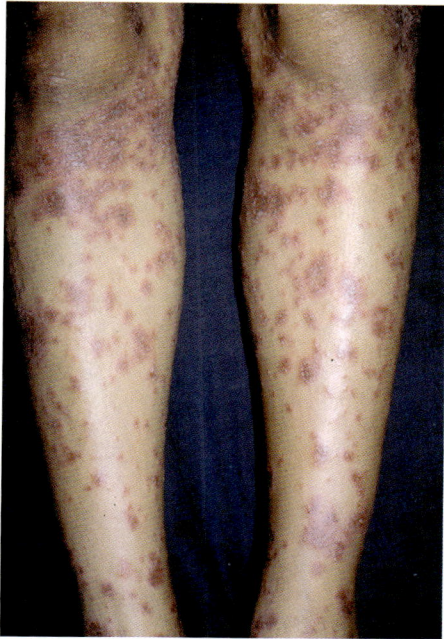

Figure 12–9 □ Impetigo herpetiformis. Multiple erythematous plaques studded with pustules are seen on the lower limbs of this pregnant Malay lady. Impetigo herpetiformis often improves or abates with parturition, but it usually recurs in subsequent pregnancies. As most systemic immunosuppressants are contraindicated in pregnancy, systemic glucocorticoid therapy is the treatment of choice.

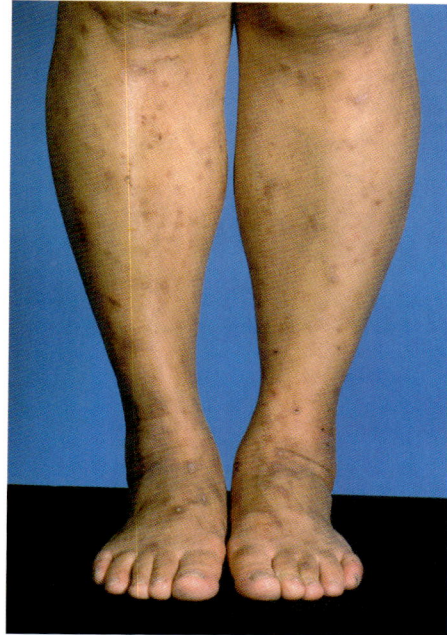

Figure 12–10 □ Prurigo of pregnancy. At 18 weeks gestation, this Chinese lady presents with itchy, excoriated papules and nodules over both lower limbs for one month. She has a history of atopic eczema. Prurigo of pregnancy often presents from the fourth month of pregnancy onward. There are excoriated papules associated with eczematous patches mainly over the extensor aspects of the limbs. They resolve after delivery, and may be associated with a personal history of atopy. Treatment is with topical glucocorticoids.

Cutaneous Manifestations of Endocrine and Metabolic Disorders

Chua S.H.

Whilst endocrine disorders originate from internal glands and organs and the consequences are primarily metabolic and biochemical in nature, skin manifestations associated with endocrine disorders are common and may occasionally be the initial presentation to the clinician. For example, patients with Cushingnoid features, suggesting an underlying hypercortisolic state, may first be referred to the dermatologist for the problem of striae and easy bruising. Cutaneous features may also assist in confirming the diagnosis of a suspected endocrine disorder pending results of the laboratory work-up. For example, pretibial myxoedema in a patient with a goiter, exopthalmos, distal tremors, and tachycardia can confirm the diagnosis of Graves' disease even before the results of the thyroid function and thyroid autoantibodies tests are known. As with other internal or systemic diseases with cutaneous manifestations, the dermatologist should be aware of them so as to evaluate for the possibility of an underlying disease state upon presentation of a characteristic skin lesion. Only then will the patient be given appropriate corrective treatment and not just symptomatic treatment.

ENDOCRINE DISORDERS
(Figures 13–1 to 13–20)

Cutaneous manifestations are present in a host of endocrine disorders. They range from being subtle, often overlooked by the patient, e.g. pallor in hypopituitarism, onycholysis in thyrotoxicosis, to being striking and of major concern to the patient, e.g. hyperpigmentation in Addison's disease, pretibial myxoedema in Graves' disease. Endocrine disorders with distinctive skin manifestations include Cushing's syndrome, Addison's disease, thyrotoxicosis, hyperandrogenism, and diabetes mellitus.

The striking features of Cushing's syndrome (Figures 13–10 to 13–14) are moon facies, buffalo hump, supraclavicular fat pads, centripetal obesity, and abdominal striae. It is not uncommon that such patients are first referred to a dermatologist for evaluation in view of the prominent skin features. In Addison's disease (Figures 13–18 and 13–19), the skin is hyperpigmented, mostly over sun-exposed areas but involvement of the mucosae, tongue, and palmer creases often causes much concern and distress to the patient. Thyrotoxicosis (Figures 13–15 and 13–16) may lead to multiple cutaneous manifestations; some are subtle – mild hair loss and onycholysis – while others are striking such as pretibial myxoedema. Conditions leading to hyperandrogenism in females present as difficult-to-control acne vulgaris, hirsutism, and signs of virilization (male pattern hair loss, clitoromegaly). Diabetes mellitus is a common endocrine disorder with frequent skin manifestations (Figures 13–1 to 13–9); the most common in long-standing diabetes is diabetic dermopathy or shin spots which results from microangiopathy. Less common skin manifestations include diabetic bulla, necrobiosis lipoidica, scleredema, and acanthosis nigricans.

METABOLIC DISORDERS

Hyperlipidemia, a common metabolic disorder, results in deposition of lipids in the skin causing xanthomas of varying morphology (Figures 13–21 to 13–23). Whilst the skin lesions may have minimal clinical consequence, the associated cardiovascular risk may be great and hence further evaluation and specific management of the hyperlipidemia may be required.

STRENGTH OF ASSOCIATION

The strength of association between a skin manifestation and an underlying endocrine or metabolic disorder is variable. Strong associations include xanthomas and hyperlipidemia, pretibial myxoedema and Graves' disease, hyperpigmentation and Addison's disease, hirsutism and hyperandrogenism in females, diabetic dermopathy and microangiopathy in long-standing diabetes mellitus. Weaker associations include necrobiosis lipoidica and diabetes mellitus, granuloma annulare and diabetes mellitus, xanthelasma palpebrarum and hypercholesterolemia. The value of knowing the strength of association will determine how aggressive one evaluates an underlying endocrine disorder – a thorough evaluation and work-up is necessary for a skin presentation with strong association with an underlying endocrine or metabolic disorder.

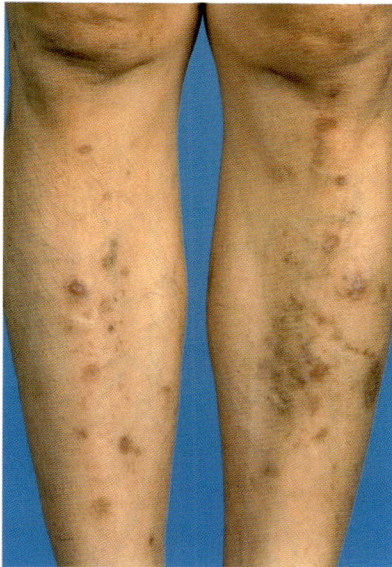

Figure 13–1 □ Diabetic dermopathy. These range from multiple oval-shaped, erythematous to hyperpigmented lesions on the shins. Early lesions are papular in nature with superficial scaling. The lesions progress slowly to slightly depressed atrophic pigmented scars. Lesions tend to be multiple and may be mildly pruritic. Superimposed excoriations may be present.

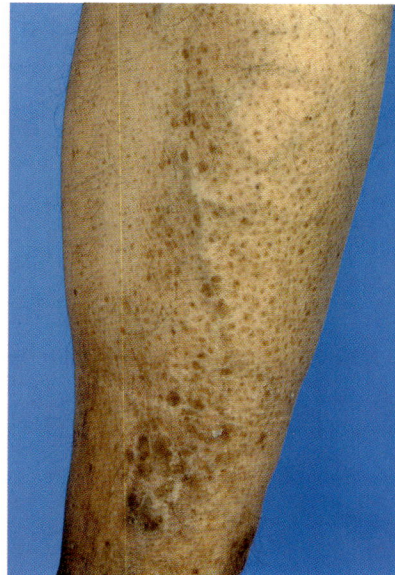

Figure 13–2 □ Diabetic dermopathy. Also known as diabetic shin spots, they result from microangiopathy associated with long-standing diabetes mellitus. Histologically, the vessel walls are thickened (PAS positive) and changes in the dermal collagen are present. Their presence should initiate further evaluation for other diabetic microangiopathic complications such as retinopathy and glomerulopathy.

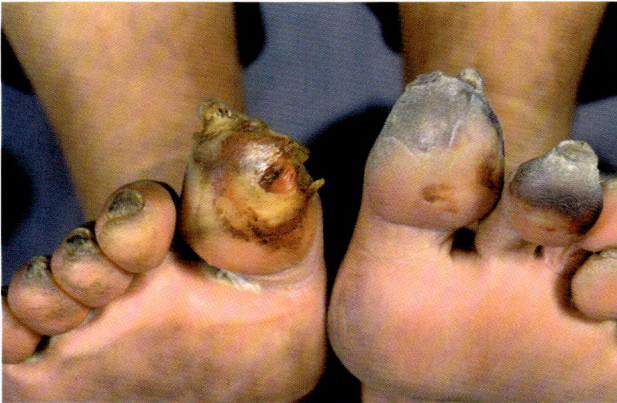

Figure 13–3 □ Diabetic foot ulcers. Foul-smelling, painful, dusky-appearing, "wet" gangrene involving the toes. Diabetic foot ulcers arise as a result of angiopathy and peripheral neuropathy. The ulcer often originates from a minor, unrecognized trauma or a neglected fissured callosity. Complicating bacterial infection results in necrosis and "wet" gangrene. The complicating bacterial infection may extend to the underlying bone causing osteomyelitis as well.

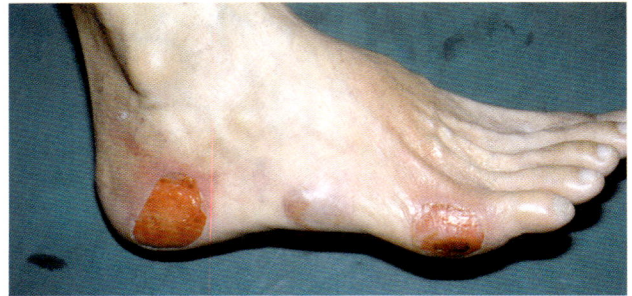

Figure 13–4 □ Diabetic bullae. Recurrent spontaneous blisters occurring on the foot. The size of the blisters ranges from a few millimeters to several centimeters in diameter. The lesions are usually intraepidermal and resolve spontaneously over a period of weeks with no resulting scar formation.

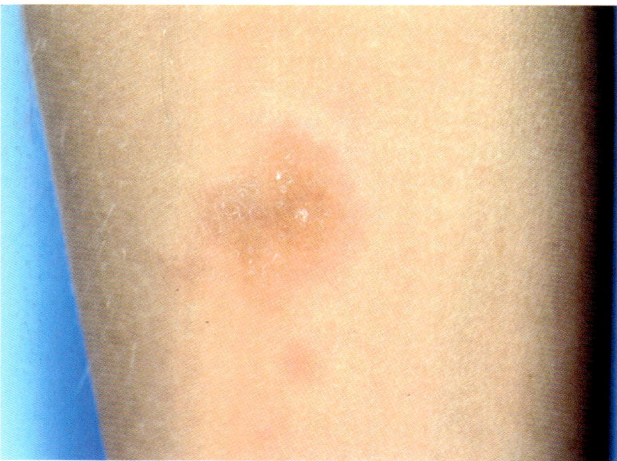

Figure 13–5 □ Necrobiosis lipodica – early lesion. Firm, indurated, erythematous plaque over the anterior shin. Fifty to 75% of patients with necrobiosis lipodica have diabetes mellitus, although less that 0.5% of patients with diabetes have necrobiosis lipodica. Mainly females in their 20s to 40s are affected. Lesions of necrobiosis lipodica may be complicated by ulceration. Treatment with potent topical corticosteroids or intralesional corticosteroids is often tried although results are generally unsatisfactory.

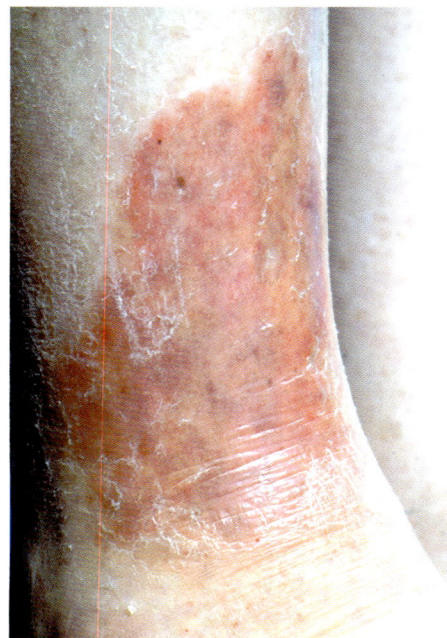

Figure 13–6 □ Necrobiosis lipodica – late lesion. Well-established lesion of necrobiosis lipodica presenting as an irregular, well-defined, brownish-red indurated plaque with central atrophy or sclerosis. The plaque has a glazed appearance and prominent surface telangiectases. Histology is characteristic with degeneration of dermal collagen with a lymphohistiocytic response, microdroplet lipid accumulation, and mucin deposition.

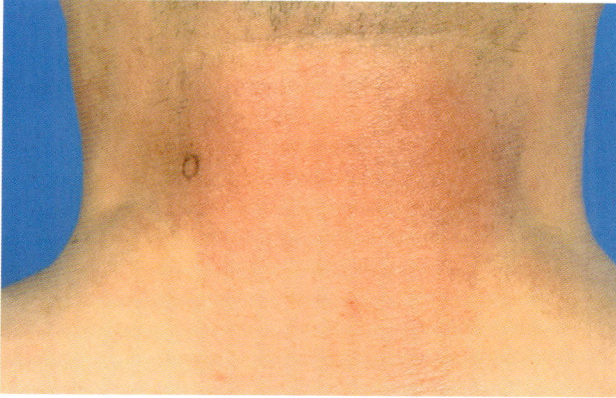

Figure 13–7 □ Scleredema. Non-pitting and firm mildly erythematous induration over the nape of the neck. The induration blends gradually with the surrounding normal skin without clear demarcation. The overlying epidermis is normal. Scleredema is associated with diabetes mellitus as well as after streptococcal infection. Post-infectious scleredema has a better prognosis and may resolve spontaneously after several months.

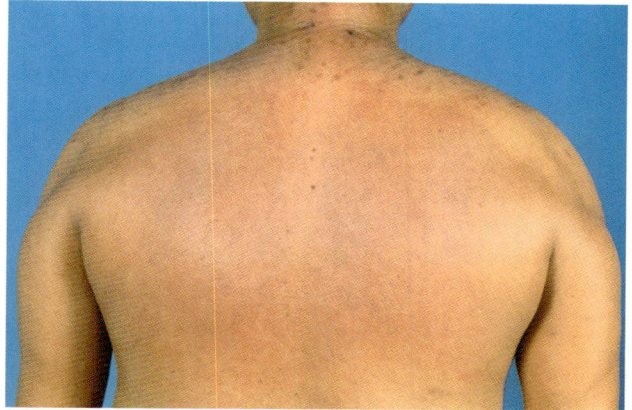

Figure 13–8 □ Scleredema. A more extensive case of scleredema involving the middle and upper back of an adult diabetic patient. Scleredema associated with diabetes tends to be persistent and is not related to the severity or degree of diabetic control. Histology reveals swelling and splitting of the dermal collagen bundles from excessive deposition of acid mucopolysaccharides.

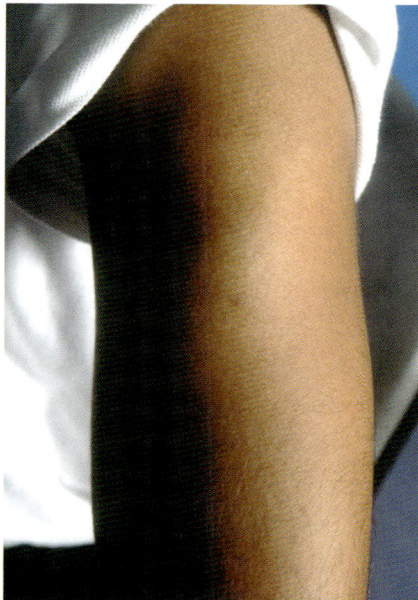

Figure 13–9 □ Fat hypertrophy. Lipohypertrophy at the insulin injection sites on the upper arm of a young man with insulin-dependent type I diabetes. Lipohypertrophy is associated with human insulin injections and may be persistent even after the injections are stopped and the site of injection changed. This complication can be avoided by regularly rotating the sites of injection.

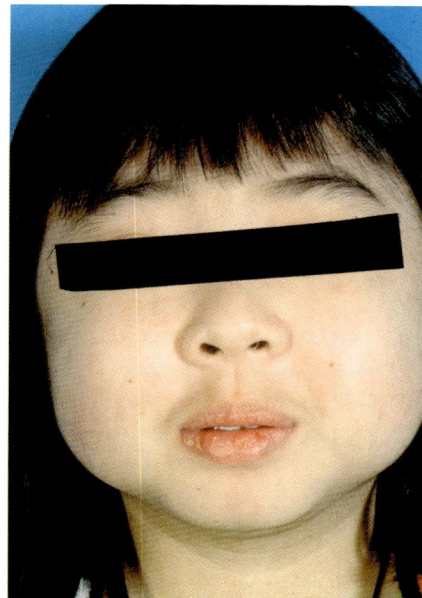

Figure 13–10 □ Cushingnoid facies. The redistribution of fat in Cushing's syndrome results in the typical rounded features of the face (moón facies). This is often accompanied by additional features of skin-thinning, facial telangiectases, and steroid acne. Patients with Cushingnoid facies suggestive of a hypercortisolic state require a full endocrinologic evaluation to determine the cause of the hypercortism as well as other complications, e.g. osteoporosis, diabetes, and hypertension.

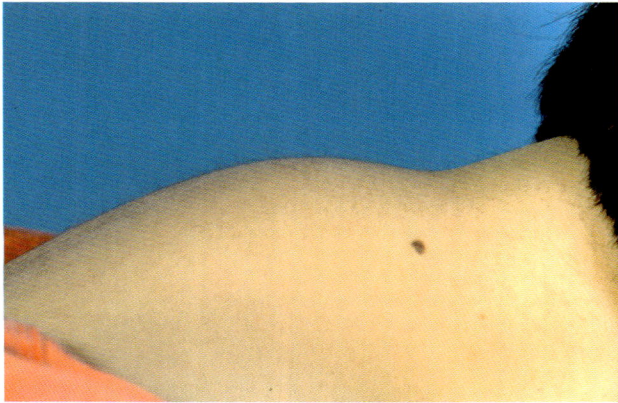

Figure 13–11 □ Cushing's syndrome – buffalo hump. Another typical appearance in Cushing's syndrome resulting from the deposition of fat over the clavicles and nape of the neck. The centripetal fat deposition in Cushing's syndrome causes truncal obesity, which is contrasted by the rather slender limbs resulting from wasting of the proximal muscles.

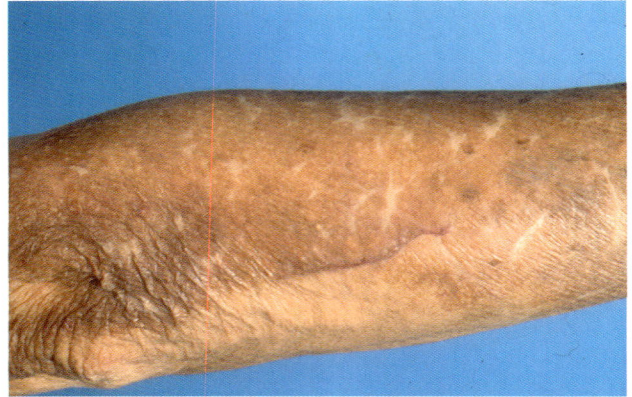

Figure 13–12 □ Cushing's syndrome – skin atrophy and easy bruising. Hypercortism also results in skin-thinning, fragility, and easy bruising. These features are also seen after prolonged application of superpotent topical steroids to the skin. Denudation of the skin occurs after minor trauma which heals slowly leaving significant pigmentation that is slow to resolve. These features are most prominent over exposed skin, e.g. forearms subjected to frequent minor unintentional trauma.

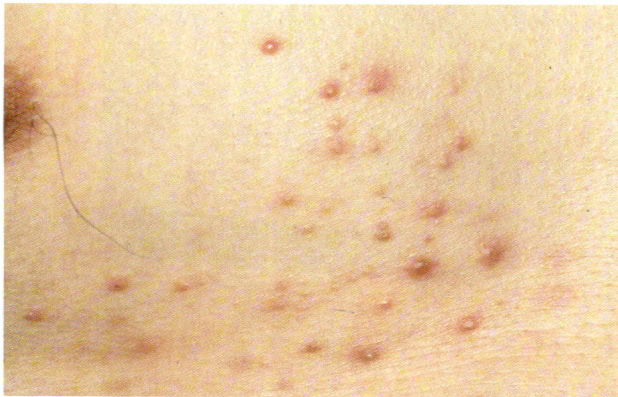

Figure 13–13 □ Steroid acne. Multiple monomorphic papules and pustules on the chest of a patient with iatrogenic Cushing's syndrome. Acne seen in Cushing's syndrome appears monomorphic and is commonly distributed over the upper trunk although the face is frequently affected as well. The onset of acne may be sudden and eruptive, similar to that seen in those with pityrosporum folliculitis. Steroid acne is also seen after prolonged use of topical steroids on the skin.

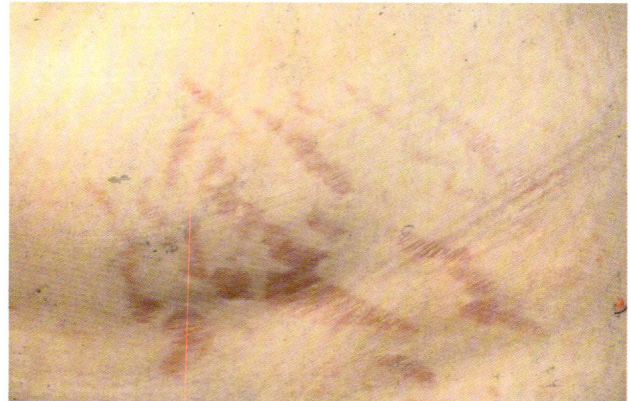

Figure 13–14 □ Purplish striae in Cushing's syndrome. Multiple linear striae with a purplish hue over the lower abdomen. Striae occurring in Cushing's syndrome are distinguished by their characteristic purplish coloration in contrast to the pinkish coloration of physiological striae. Common sites of occurrence include the lower abdomen, inner aspects of the upper arms and thighs, and lower buttocks. This manifestation of Cushing's syndrome results from the impaired synthesis of dermal collagen and mucopolysaccharides.

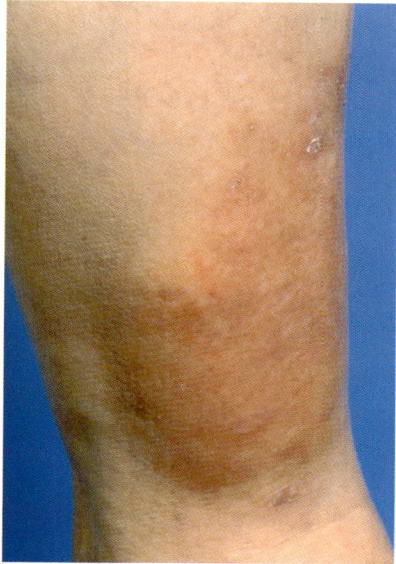

Figure 13–15 □ Pretibial myxoedema – circumscribed variant. Reddish-brown, indurated, circumscribed plaque over the antero-lateral aspect of the lower shin. The lesion is non-pitting with prominent follicular openings. Established lesions take on a peau d'orange appearance. Pretibial myxoedema is essentially a mucinous infiltrative dermopathy seen in less than 5% of patients with Graves' disease. In addition to the circumscribed form seen here, other variants include diffuse and elephantiasic (most severe) forms.

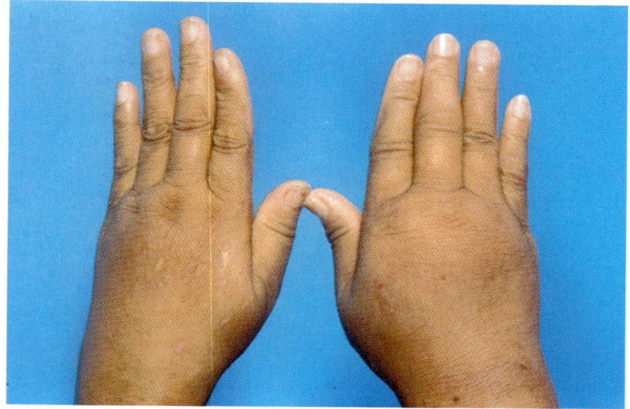

Figure 13–16 □ Pretibial myxoedema – diffuse variant. Diffuse, reddish-brown, firm, non-pitting swelling over the dorsum of both wrists, hands, and fingers. Whilst the pretibial site is the most common site of Graves' dermopathy, other unusual sites have been well-described. TSH receptor antibodies appear to play an important role in the pathogenesis of pretibial myxoedema as well as opthalmopathy. Treatment is difficult; potent corticosteroids applied under occlusion are most commonly tried, with some success in controlling the lesion.

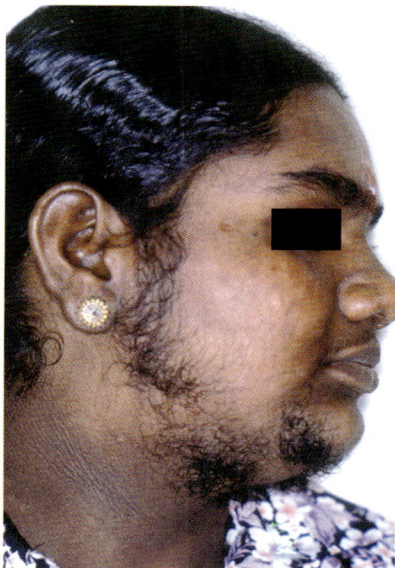

Figure 13–17 □ Polycystic ovary syndrome. Facial hirsutism in a 28-year-old Indian female with polycystic ovary syndrome. The increased density and male-pattern distribution of hairs (e.g. over the face, breasts, and lower abdomen) in hirsutism result from hair follicles response to androgenic stimulation and is often seen in endocrine disorders of hyperandrogenism. Such patients usually require further hormonal studies to elucidate the underlying endocrine abnormality. Permanent hair reduction by lasers is now possible and offers good cosmetic results for female patients bothered about their appearance.

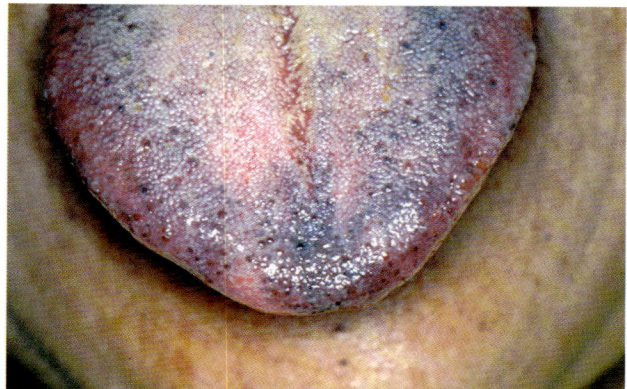

Figure 13–18 □ Addison's disease. Hyperpigmentation of the tongue in Addison's disease (primary adrenal insufficiency). Hyperpigmentation is a prominent feature of Addison's disease and results from the increased secretion of melanotrophic hormones by the pituitary gland. Whilst the hyperpigmentation is most pronounced over the sun-exposed sites, pigmentation of the buccal mucous membranes, tongue, scars, and genitalia is distinctive.

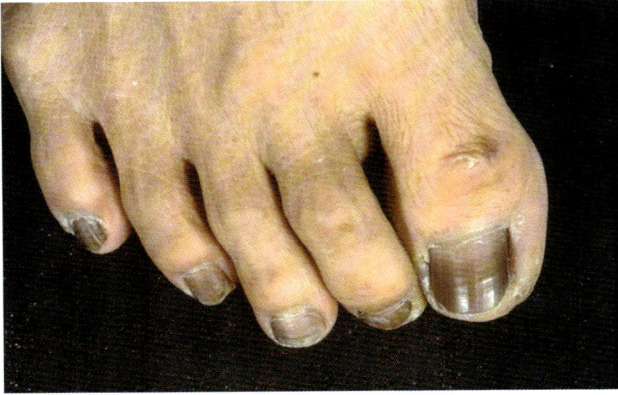

Figure 13–19 □ Addison's disease. Hyperpigmentation under the nails in Addison's disease. Hyperpigmentation occurring in almost all patients with Addison's disease may involve unusual sites such as under the nails, creases of the palms or fingers, and soles, in addition to the mucous membranes and sun-exposed areas of the body.

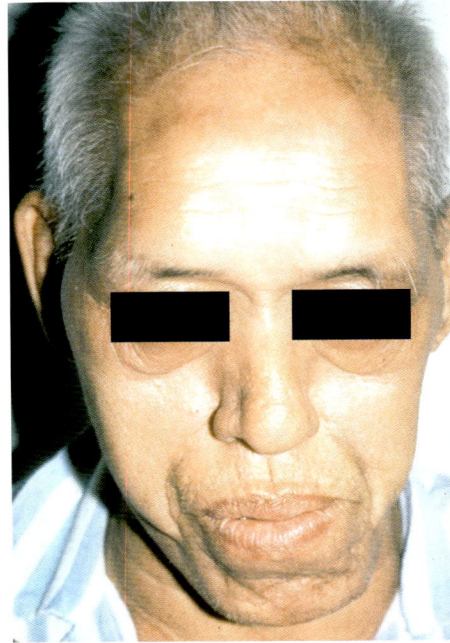

Figure 13–20 □ Acromegaly. Typical facies of acromegaly with frontal bossing, prognatism, thick eyelids, large ears or nose, and thick lips. The facial skin is thickened and seborrheic and the follicular openings are prominent. Macroglossia is typical. The skin features result from the hypertrophy of the skin, subcutaneous tissues, and bone from the stimulating effects of the excess growth hormone.

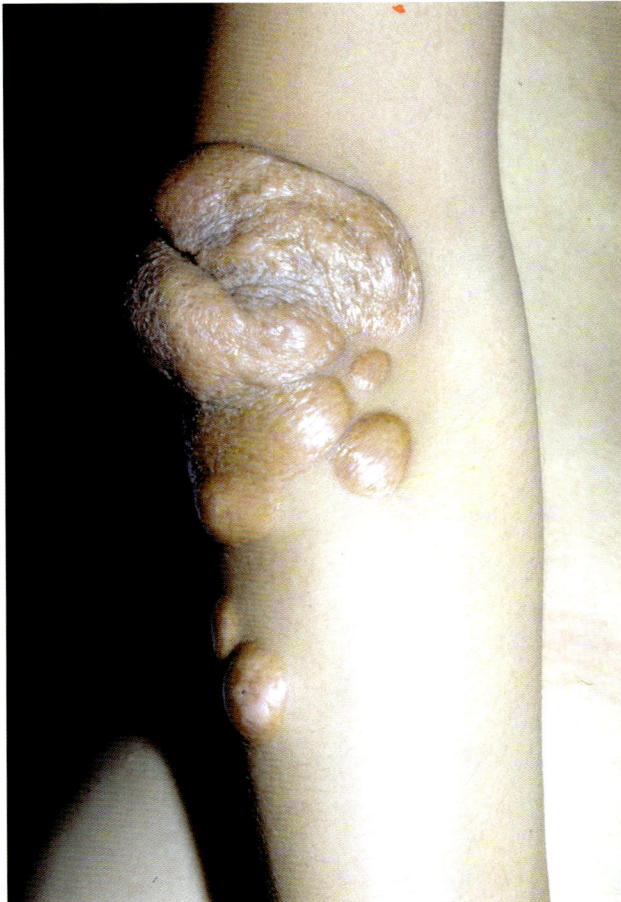

Figure 13–21 □ Tuberous xanthomas. Large plaques and nodules of yellowish-brown, lobulated tumors over the elbow and extensor aspect of the lower arm. The lesions are slowly progressive and painless. Tuberous xanthomas are most commonly seen in hypercholesterolemia and markedly increased levels of LDL. The lesions are associated with significant cardiovascular risk and may persist despite control of the hyperlipidemia.

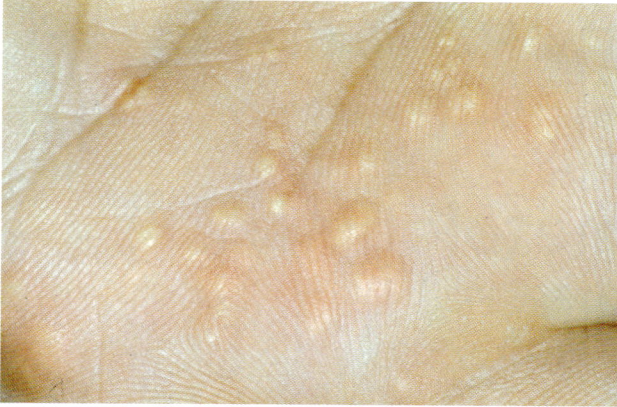

Figure 13–22 ▫ Eruptive xanthomas. Multiple yellowish, dome-shaped, firm papules on the palms. Eruptive xanthomas occur suddenly and can affect any site of the body. These papules may coalesce to form plaques. Eruptive xanthomas are usually associated with hypertriglyceridemia and high concentrations of VLDL and chylomicrons. Patients are at risk of developing acute pancreatitis. Eruptive xanthomas tend to resolve rapidly upon control of the hyperlipidemia.

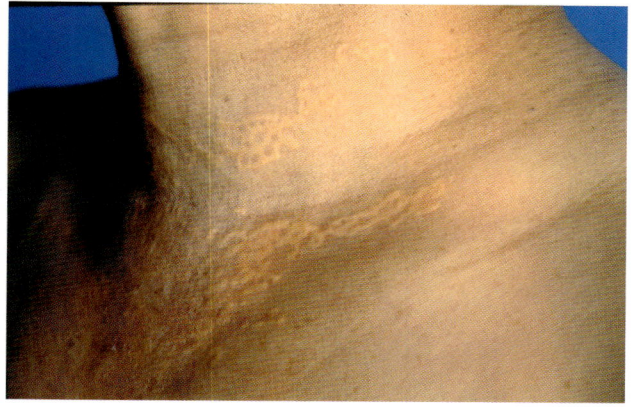

Figure 13–23 ▫ Plane xanthomas. Yellowish, slightly palpable plaques over the antero-lateral neck. Plane xanthomas occur in both primary as well as secondary hyperlipidemias. A full metabolic evaluation by an endocrinologist is needed to classify the lipid disorder. Treatment is directed at lowering the lipid levels to minimize cardiovascular risk.

Psychodermatology

Giam Y.C., Chio M.T.W., and Loh H.T.H.

Psychodermatology involves a spectrum of different types of disorders that straddle the fields of psychiatry and dermatology. At one end of the spectrum, there are patients whose skin disorders have resulted in significant negative psycho-social effects. Conditions like atopic dermatitis, psoriasis, cystic acne, hyperhidrosis, vitiligo, and alopecia have all been documented to be associated with lower self-esteem, physical unattractiveness, depression, emotional stress, anxiety, and social withdrawal. Unfortunately, these impacts are often trivialized or even ignored by their attending doctors.

At the other end of the spectrum, there are patients with primary psychiatric disorders who present with predominantly cutaneous symptoms (e.g. delusion of parasitosis) or signs (e.g. self-inflicted skin lesions) and who refuse referral to the psychiatrist either due to self-denial or fear of the stigma of having a mental illness.

A knowledge of the psychiatric aspect of these disorders and the various psychotropic drugs and psychiatric intervention techniques (e.g. behavioral therapy, stress reduction, and relaxation techniques) that can be used will better equip the dermatologist in managing these disorders or in co-managing these disorders with the psychiatrist.

CLASSIFICATION

These psychodermatological disorders are broadly classified into four groups:

I. Psychophysiological disorders: poor self-image and the resultant psycho-social maladjustments arising from skin disorders such as atopic dermatitis, psoriasis, cystic acne, and hyperhidrosis.

II. Primary psychiatric disorders: patients with an underlying psychiatric disorder, such as obsessive-compulsive disorder, present with secondary self-inflicted skin lesions like neurotic excoriation, factitious dermatitis, trichotilomania, and acne excoriée.

III. Secondary psychiatric disorders: anxiety and depression arising from skin conditions such as alopecia totalis and extensive vitiligo.

IV. Cutaneous sensory disorders: patients with such disorders feel unpleasant sensations of stinging, pricking, and biting but no organic etiology can be established. This group includes conditions such as vulvodynia, glossodynia, and chronic pain syndrome.

TEAM APPROACH

A team approach involving the dermatologist, psychiatrist, social counselor, and nurse practitioner is best suited to manage these difficult disorders in a holistic manner. It is critical for the dermatologists to deliver optimal care with a non-judgmental, accepting, and helpful demeanour. The attending dermatologist must take an empathic stance and convey hope to patients, constantly demonstrating a willingness to help and to encourage patients not to give up.

Management

In the management of such disorders, the physician will need to handle both the physiological aspects and the psychological aspects of the disorder. Knowledge of psychotropic medication, such as fluoxetine, risperidone, and olanzepine, can enhance the physician's therapeutic armamentarium. Psychoeducation and support, psychotherapy ranging from behavioral conditioning techniques to supportive and insight-oriented psychotherapy, are helpful. The effects on the patient can be dramatic, improving not only the skin, but also overall well-being and health.

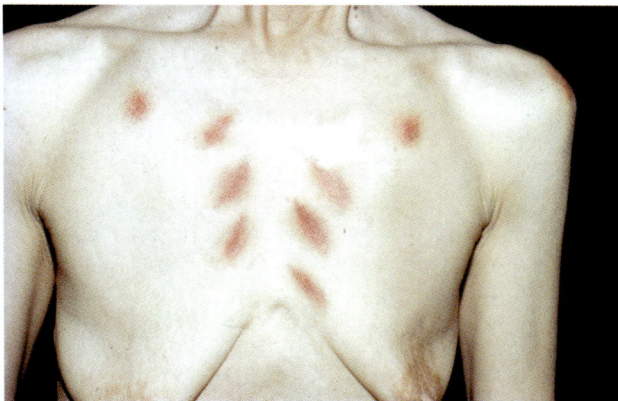

Figure 14–1 □ Factitious dermatitis. Bizarre, multiple linear, geometrical erosions and scars are seen on the chest of this elderly Chinese female. No underlying skin dermatosis is present. She has factitious dermatitis, a manifestation of an underlying primary psychiatric disorder.

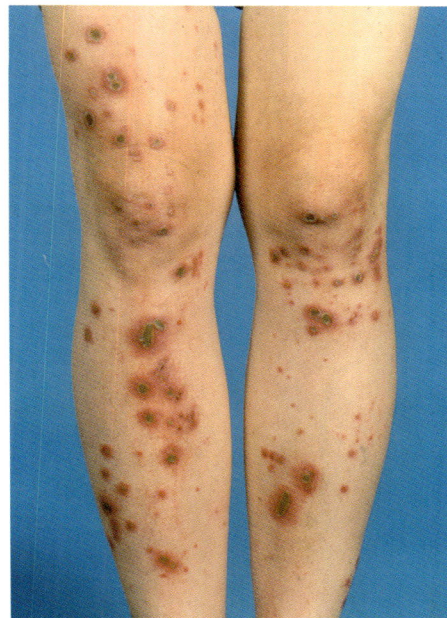

Figure 14–2 □ Neurotic excoriation. This 46-year-old Chinese female has neurotic excoriations. The patient describes an unconscious compulsive urge to use her fingers and finger nails to pick and dig at her skin on her legs, and knowingly removing the scabs of the healing erosions. The patient is aware of her actions but feels powerless to stop. Neurotic excoriation is associated with an underlying primary psychiatric disorder, most commonly obsessive-compulsive disorder. Other associated psychiatric disorders include depression, anxiety, and body dysmorphic disorder.

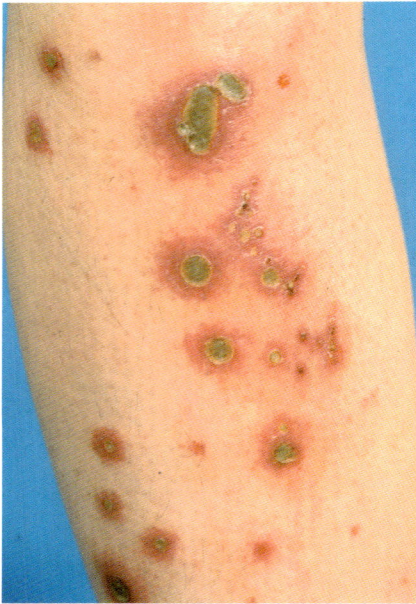

Figure 14–3 □ Neurotic excoriation. This is a close-up view of the lesions shown in Figure 14–2. There are multiple erosions with surrounding reactive inflammation on the edge. The skin surrounding the lesions is normal. The erosions are of multiple sizes and depths, reflecting the different duration of the lesions.

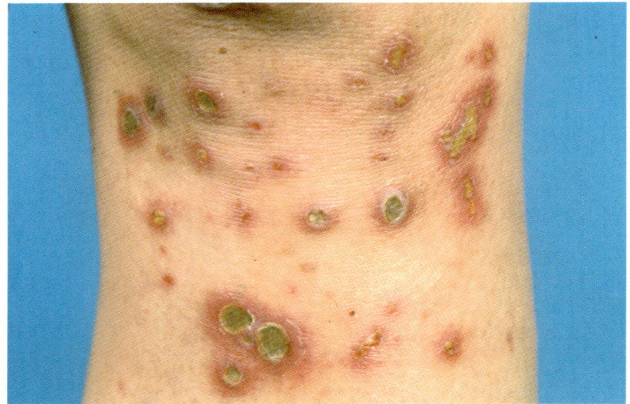

Figure 14–4 □ Neurotic excoriation. The excoriated lesions are often on the easily accessible parts of the body as in this case. As the morphology and distribution of the skin lesions are not specific for neurotic excoriations, careful initial and repeated evaluations to exclude an underlying skin dermatosis, e.g. atopic dermatitis, or systemic disease, e.g. uremia, that may cause pruritus should be carried out.

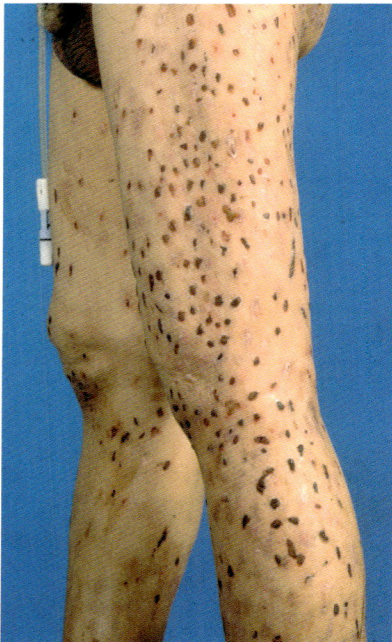

Figure 14–5 □ Neurotic excoriation. This 52-year-old Chinese male with end-stage renal failure, complained of focal sensation especially on his left legs, leading to picking and gouging of his skin. He has multiple erosions with crusted scabs on his lower legs. Despite the underlying uremia, the focal nature of the excoriations and his underlying anxiety disorder suggests the diagnosis of neurotic excoriation.

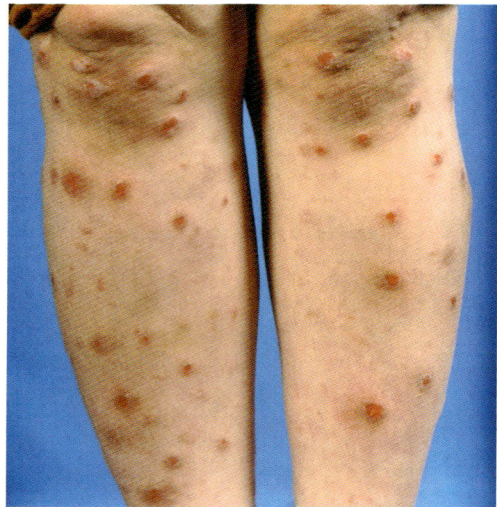

Figure 14–6 □ Neurotic excoriation. This 14-year-old child has multiple excoriations on her lower legs. Despite the lack of symptoms, she picks compulsively at pieces of skin which she describes vaguely as "not feeling right" or "looking right". Neurotic excoriation can occur at any age. In children, an underlying adjustment disorder or a dysfunctional family relationship including physical and emotional abuse needs to be considered.

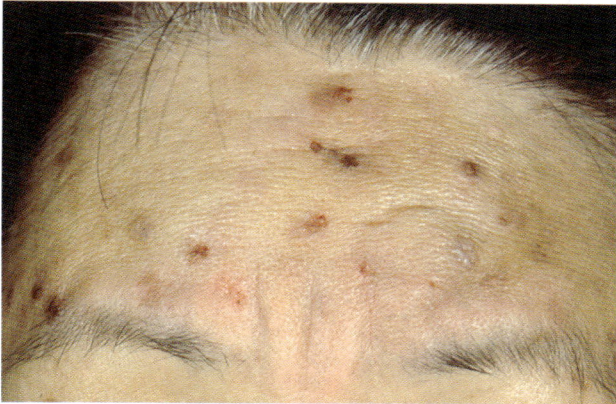

Figure 14–7 □ Neurotic excoriation. This elderly Chinese female had picked at colloid milia on her forehead, resulting in multiple excoriations and scars. She suffered from anxiety disorder, complained of restlessness, worried incessantly, felt "stressed out", and was unable to relax. Treatment of neurotic excoriation is often difficult. It is important to establish a constructive patient-therapist alliance. Her condition has improved with treatment with alprazolam in conjunction with behavioral modification therapy to increase her awareness of her ritualistic behavior.

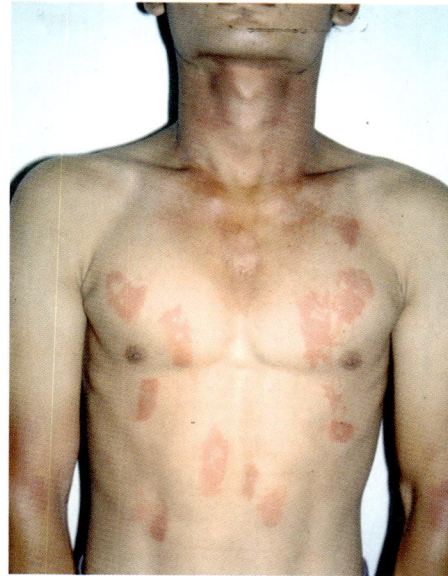

Figure 14–8 □ Dermatitis artefacta. This young Chinese male, a conscript in the military service, used a piece of stone covered with a rough cloth to rub vigorously on skin on his chest and abdomen resulting in frictional swelling, bruising, and erosions. He repeatedly requested to be excused from physical training in the military service. Self-inflicted skin lesions to feign a genuine dermatological illness in the hope of a secondary gain, is a form of Munchausen syndrome. This malingering may achieve a short spell of rest as doctors puzzle over the diagnosis.

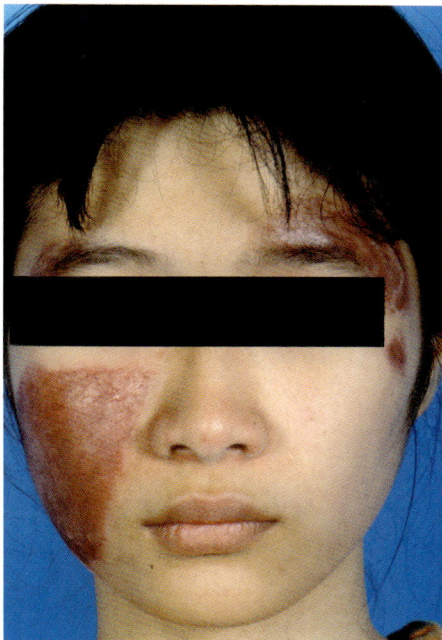

Figure 14–9 □ Dermatitis artefacta. This young Chinese female presents with a well-demarcated, bizarre triangular-shaped, erythematous plaque on her left cheek, and a similar lesion over her left eyebrow. She has denied any contactant exposure despite repeated questioning, although a separate interview with her family members has revealed that she had used garlic to rub her face. Patients with dermatitis artefacta often deny causing the skin lesions in contrast to patients with neurotic excoriation. The spectrum of lesions can range from minor excoriations to large gangrenous lesions. Clues to the diagnosis include the bizarre pattern of the skin lesions and the presence of normal, unaffected skin immediately adjacent to the lesions.

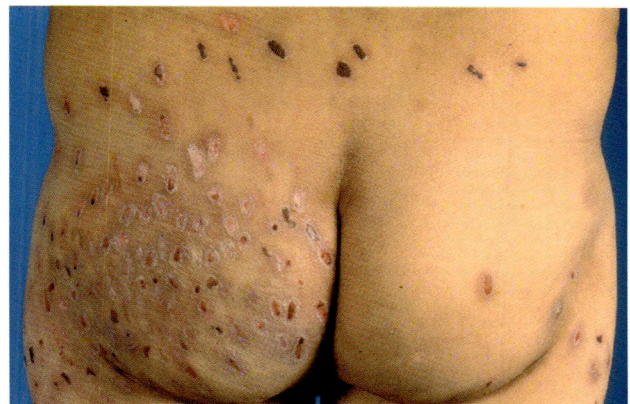

Figure 14–10 □ Dermatitis artefacta. This middle-aged Chinese male presents with multiple blisters, erosions, and scars on his buttocks, which he claims, appeared suddenly without any preceding sign and symptoms. The appearance of the lesions suggests self-inflicted cigarette burns. This vagueness and inability to provide reasonable details on the history of the skin lesions (i.e. a "hollow history") are very characteristic of dermatitis artefacta.

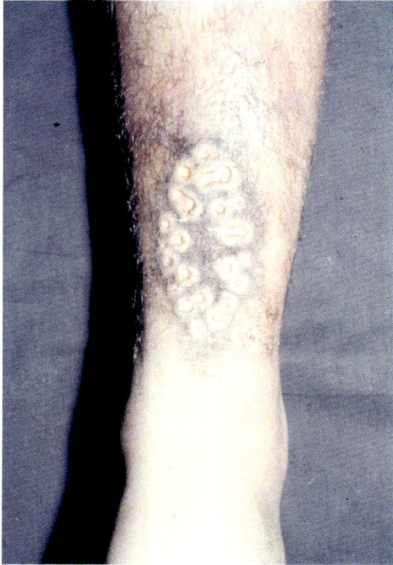

Figure 14–11 □ Dermatitis artefacta. This middle-aged Malay male had similarly used cigarette butts to create multiple burns on his left lower shin. Multiple psychiatric disorders are associated with dermatitis artefacta, including schizo-affective disorders, mono-symptomatic hypochondriacal psychosis (MHP), mental deficiency, anxiety disorders, depression, personality disorders, and body dysmorphic disorders. Monosymptomatic hypochondriacal psychosis is a delusion of being diseased. It overlaps closely with dermatitis artefacta. A full psychiatric evaluation by a psychiatrist is most helpful. Anti-psychotic medication, such as pimozide and risperidone in combination with cognitive-behavioral therapy, is useful.

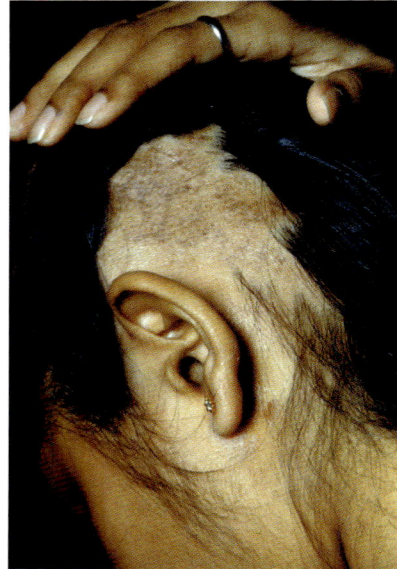

Figure 14–12 □ Trichotilomania. This young Eurasian female admitted to plucking her hair over the left temporal scalp region over a period of several months. There is a well-demarcated, geometrical area of non-scarring alopecia with re-growth of short hairs. This condition is most common amongst females, especially at the onset of puberty though it can occur at any age. Trichotilomania is an impulse control disorder, and pruritus may be a cue to pulling.

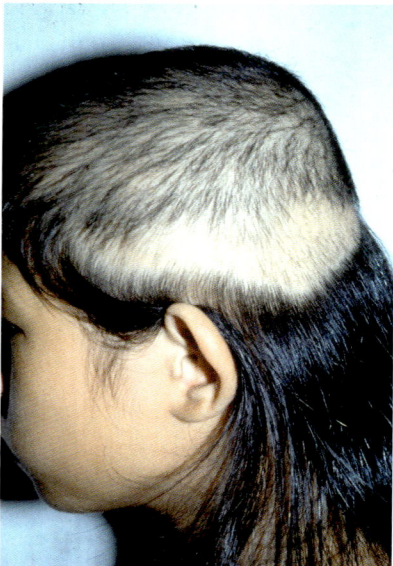

Figure 14–13 □ Trichotilomania. A tonsural pattern of trichotilomania is seen here in this young Chinese female. Patients may use their fingers or devices, such as tweezers, to selectively pluck out hairs on the scalp, eyebrows, or any area of the body. Often, the episode of pulling occurs in response to negative affective cues or during sedentary activity such as reading. A history of childhood trauma is significantly higher amongst persons with trichotilomania.

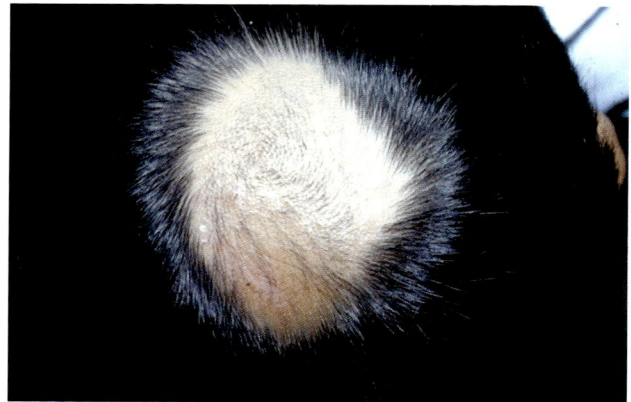

Figure 14–14 □ Trichotilomania. In this case, the tricho-tilomania resembles alopecia areata at the vertex of the scalp of a middle-aged Chinese female. The diagnosis is obvious in this case as the patient acknowledges her hair pulling habit. In cases of trichotilomania, where there is denial of hair pulling, a careful evaluation is needed to exclude alopecia areata. A scalp biopsy is sometimes required in difficult cases. Characteristic findings are traumatized hair bulbs, trichomalacia, and catagen hairs.

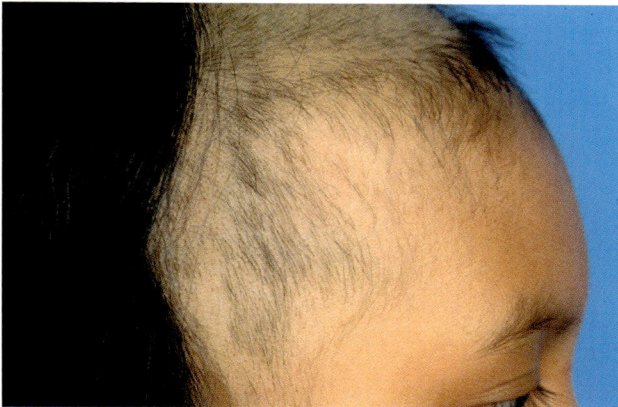

Figure 14–15 □ **Trichotilomania.** This young Malay female presents with hair loss on her frontal scalp secondary to trichotilomania. Patients with trichotilomania commonly have co-morbid mood or anxiety disorders especially obsessive-compulsive disorder. In young children, it may signify a difficult family relationship with physical or emotional abuse. A number of neurological disorders, such as tics or Tourette's syndrome, may result in hair pulling.

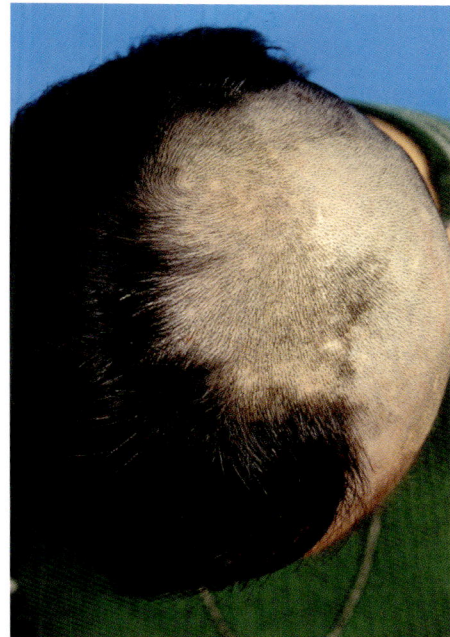

Figure 14–16 □ **Trichotilomania.** This young Chinese female presents with alopecia on the left side of her scalp. The alopecia is non-scarring with evidence of re-growth of hair.

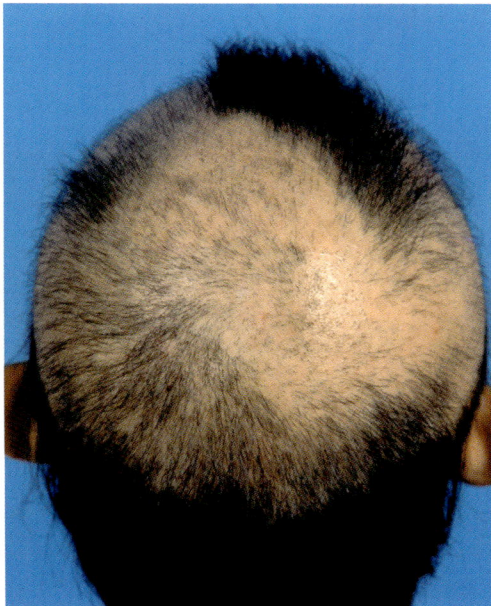

Figure 14–17 □ **Trichotilomania.** Trichotilomania does occur in male patients though far less frequently. This young Chinese male presents with a tonsural pattern of hair loss. Other causes of hair loss, such as alopecia areata, androgenic alopecia, syphilis, traction alopecia, need to be considered. Once the diagnosis is made, treatment of this condition often requires the input of the psychiatrist for full evaluation of underlying psycho-social issues, pharmacotherapy, and psychotherapy.

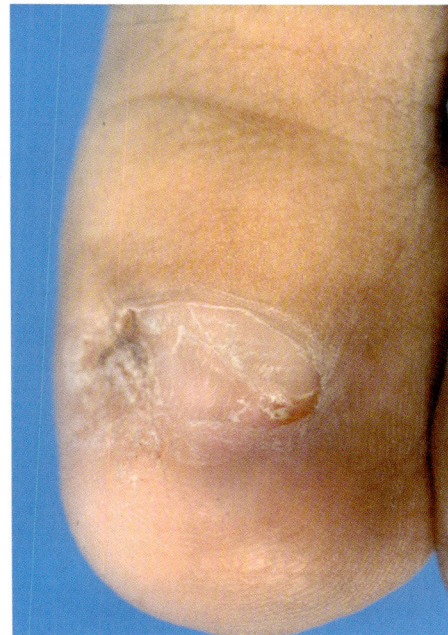

Figure 14–18 □ **Onychotilomania.** This patient's nails are repeatedly being self-avulsed regularly. Psycho-social stress like moving to a new home, severe illness, or death of a close relative can be the triggers.

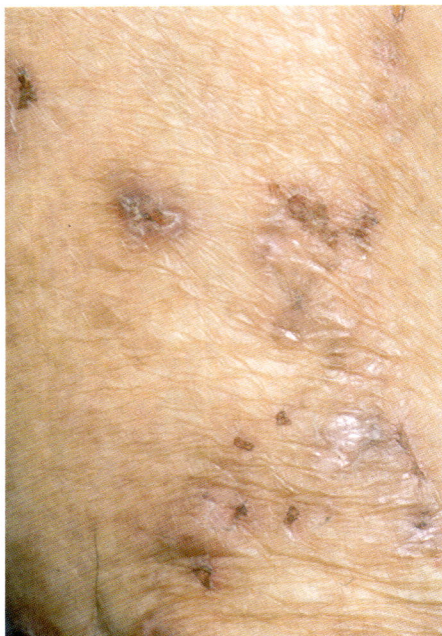

Figure 14–19 □ Delusional parasitosis. This is a form of monosymptomatic hypochondriacal psychosis characterized by an encapsulated delusion of parasitic infestation of the skin. This is in contrast to schizophrenia where there are multiple delusions and deficits in other mental functions. This elderly Chinese male thinks there are worms crawling under his skin and depositing their eggs there. He picks at his skin in an attempt to catch the worms, resulting in multiple erosions and healed scars on accessible parts of his body. He would bring whatever he "caught" in a container to the medical consultation (the so-called "match-box" sign). Other than this particular delusion, the patient is otherwise rational and can function normally.

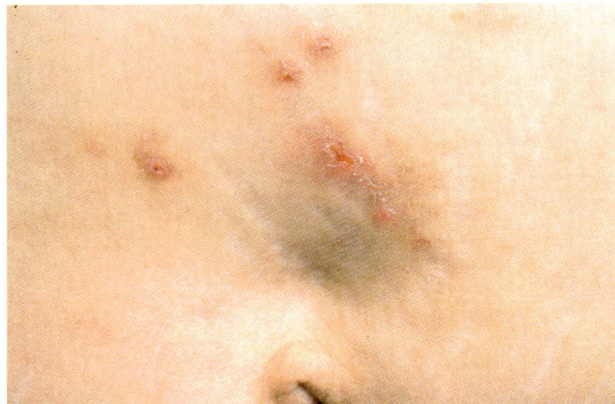

Figure 14–20 □ Delusional parasitosis. This picture illustrates self-induced linear erosions and hyperpigmented scars on the abdomen of an elderly patient who believed that he had parasitic infestations. Careful history-taking and physical examination are always essential to exclude organic causes such as scabies and uremic pruritus. A skin biopsy may sometimes be useful to clarify the issue with the patient though excessive investigations and treatments themselves may reinforce the delusion.

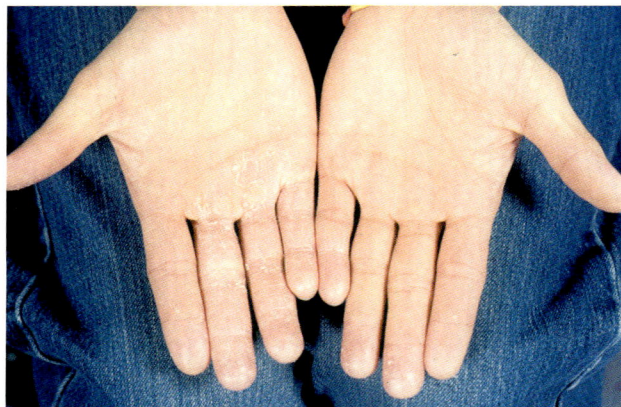

Figure 14–21 □ Obsessive-compulsive disorder. This female patient has developed cumulative irritant contact dermatitis on her hands after excessive, ritualistic hand washing due to her obsessive-compulsive disorder. She washes her hands more than 20 times a day with each session lasting more than 20 minutes. She understands the damage that excessive washing is doing to her hands but the extreme anxiety arising from not washing her "dirty" hands prompts her to do it. Serotonin dysfunction is suggested, and drug therapy with fluoxetine as well as cognitive behavioral therapy is beneficial.

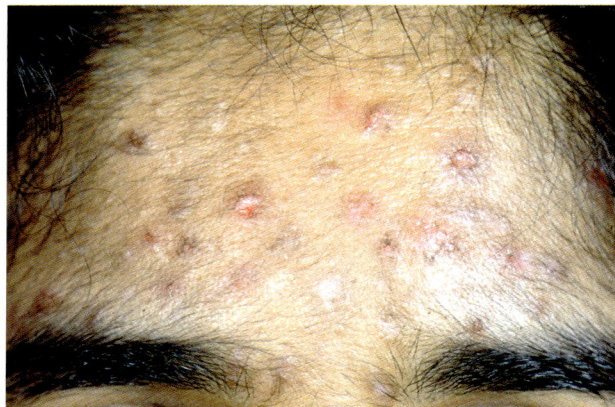

Figure 14–22 □ Acne excoriée. This is a form of neurotic excoriation, where the underlying primary psychiatry disorder is often an obsessive-compulsive disorder (OCD). Scarring from excoriation, pigmentary changes, and disfigurement can result as illustrated on the forehead of this young Indian female patient. Behavioral and psychotherapeutic intervention together with anti-OCD medication, such as fluoxetine and paroxetine, are often needed to reduce the compulsive urge to pick at the acne.

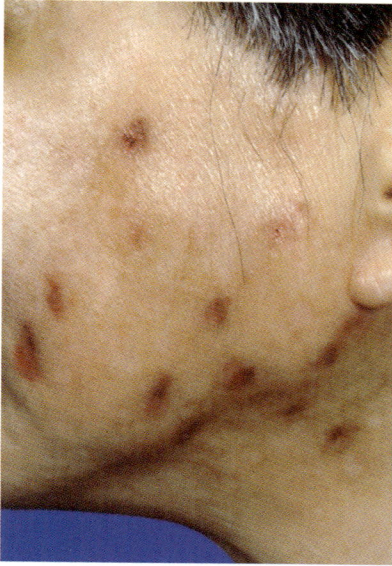

Figure 14–23 ▫ Acne excoriée. Acne excoriée may occur in patients with other psychiatric disorders such as schizophrenia and depression. This female patient suffers from schizophrenia. She has developed a delusional fixation with acne on her face, and picks at the lesions repeatedly resulting in hyperpigmented, excoriated papules and nodules on her cheeks. For such a patient, anti-psychotic medication is the mainstay of treatment.

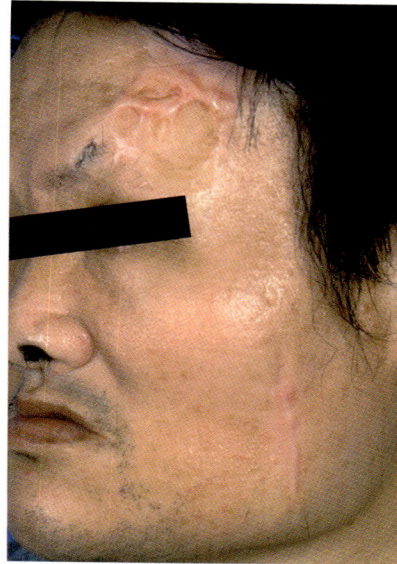

Figure 14–24 ▫ Mental retardation related disease – self-induced lesion. This middle-aged male presents with multiple linear and geometrical erosions on his face and legs which when healed, will leave pink, hypertrophic scars. Whilst initially denying self-inflicting the lesions, careful questioning reveals the use of a sharp bamboo stick to cause the skin lesions. This patient is mildly subnormal and suffers from a combination of depression and personality disorder. Direct confrontation with the patient rarely achieves satisfactory outcome; gaining the trust of the patient is often needed before the full history can be obtained.

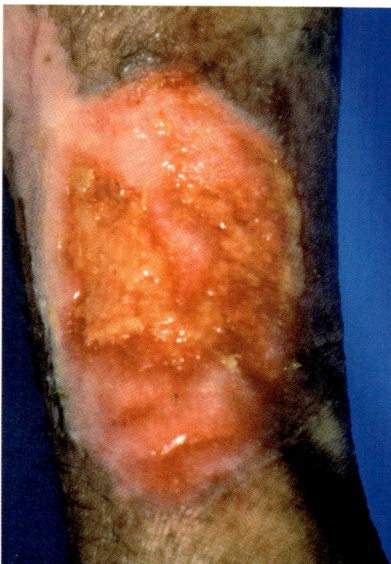

Figure 14–25 ▫ Mental retardation related self-induced lesion. This elderly man, who is intellectually sub-normal, has repeatedly picked at the ulcer on his shin, resulting in a chronic non-healing wound. Whilst any underlying psychiatry disorder needs to be treated, good wound care is still essential for wound-healing. Secondary infections need to be treated, and in chronic cases, careful regular reviews are important to detect the development of a squamous cell carcinoma.

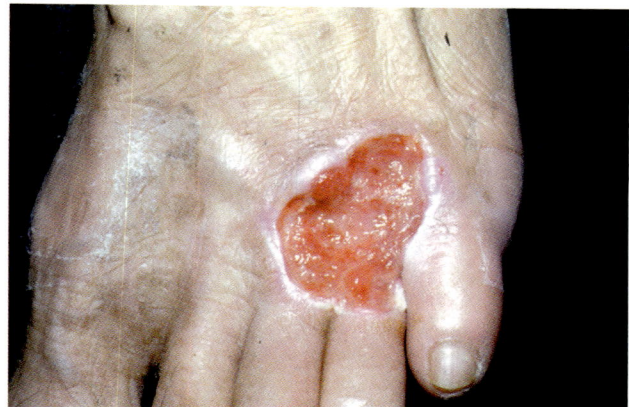

Figure 14–26 ▫ Mental retardation related self-induced lesion. This elderly man has a chronic non-healing wound on the dorsum of his foot due to repeated self-induced trauma. A closer examination revealed the presence of a fleshy, friable nodule arising from the wound. A biopsy revealed squamous cell carcinoma.

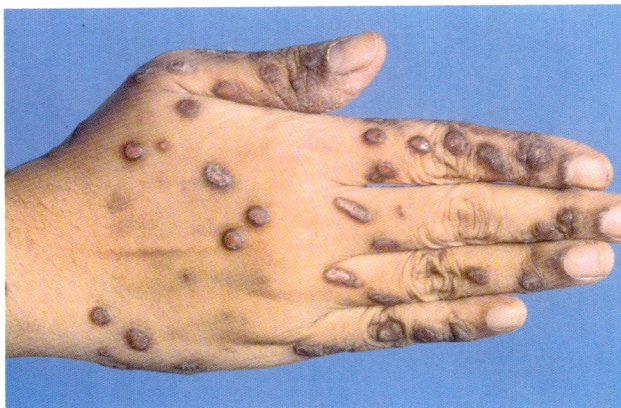

Figure 14–27 □ Prurigo nodularis. This middle-aged Indian female has developed prurigo nodularis. She has multiple discrete hyperpigmented excoriated nodules on the dorsum of her hand. She described intense itch, which led to vigorous scratching with subsequent lichenification and thickening of the excoriated sites. Whilst the primary pathophysiology is not entirely understood, prurigo nodularis is thought to be a neurodermatitis induced or exacerbated by underlying psychiatric disorders.

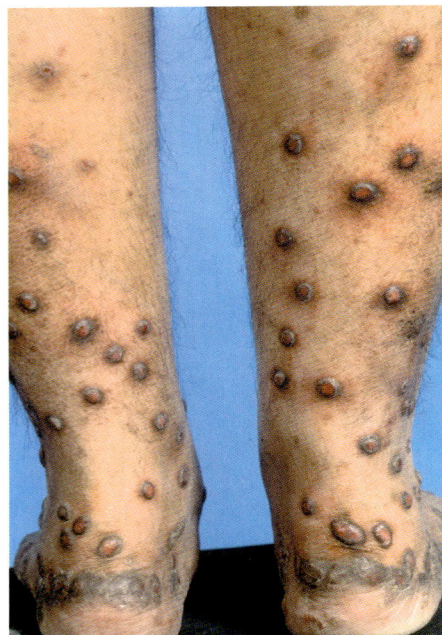

Figure 14–28 □ Prurigo nodularis. Lesions on the legs of the woman in Figure 14–27. The distribution is often on the easily accessible parts of the body. The nodules can be very persistent and rarely resolve spontaneously. Treatment measures include the use of potent topical steroids under occlusion, intralesional steroids, and anxiolytic drugs. Hypnosis may be tried.

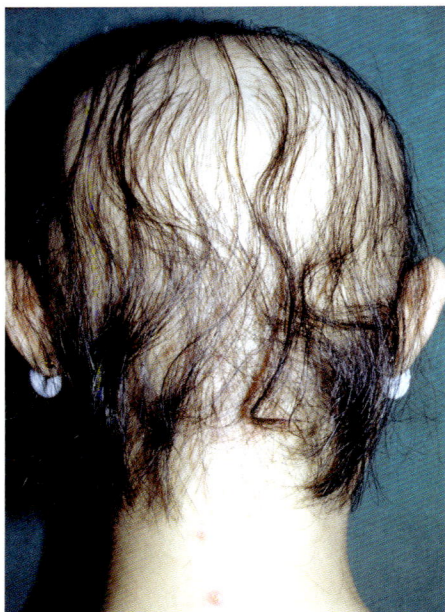

Figure 14–29 □ Psychophysiological disorder – alopecia totalis. This female had developed alopecia totalis. She became depressed and socially withdrawn. To her, it was disfiguring. Her activity level dropped and she was unable to cope with work. However, treatment with topical immunotherapy using diphencyprone restored her hair growth in six months and renewed her self-esteem.

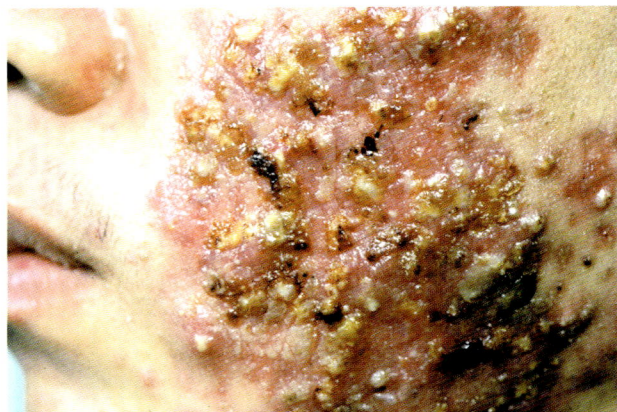

Figure 14–30 □ Psychophysiological disorder – cystic acne. This 22-year-old Chinese male had cystic acne and the disfigurement caused him to be depressed, with low self-esteem. He refused to socialize and had suicidal thoughts. Systemic isotretinoin improved his severe acne within six months. Cognitive behavior therapy helped in his case as well.

Cosmetic Dermatology

Ang P. and Goh B.K.

Cosmetic dermatology is the aspect of dermatology that deals with skin conditions that do not cause any significant morbidity or functional disability. These conditions may be left alone if desired or are treated mainly for the enhancement of the patient's appearance. Correct identification and characterization of these conditions are the pre-requisites for subsequent effective treatment. Cosmetic dermatology is a growing and challenging aspect of dermatology. Better recognition, improved practitioner's skills, more effective and safer medical technological advances and equipment all contribute to the dermatologist's ability to enhance the appearance with minimal side effects, complications, and downtime.

Cosmetic dermatological conditions in the Asian skin may be broadly classified into four main categories:

I.   Hyperpigmentation
II. Benign small growths
III. Scars
IV. Wrinkles

HYPERPIGMENTATION
(Figures 15–1 to 15–12)

Hyperpigmentation is a common problem in Asia. The Asian skin is more prone to develop pigment both constitutionally and reactively.

The common acquired cosmetic pigmentary problems encountered are freckles, lentigines, melasma, Hori's nevus, and post-inflammatory hyperpigmentation. Nevus of Ota and Ito are pigmented birthmarks that occur almost exclusively in Asian-Oriental skin for which effective laser treatment now exists.

Hyperpigmentation may be treated with topical lightening agents and/or lasers. The outcome of treatment depends on the depth of pigment and the pathophysiology. Epidermal pigmentation such as freckles, lentigines, and melasma respond to topical lightening agents whilst dermal pigmentation such as Hori's nevus and nevus of Ota do not. The advancements in lasers over the last two decades, especially with the use of selective photothermolysis to produce Q-switched pigment lasers, have resulted in safe and effective treatment for many conditions such as solar lentigines, ephelides, Hori's nevus, and nevus of Ota. The treatment of other pigmentary conditions, like melasma, however, remains a challenge.

BENIGN SMALL GROWTHS
(Figures 15–13 to 15–24)

These are growths which may be epidermal, such as seborrheic keratoses; dermal, such as dermatofibroma, or in the fat, such as lipoma.

The choice of treatment depends on the location of the lesion. Epidermal lesions may be removed with methods like electrosurgery and cryotherapy with minimal risk of scarring. Lesions in the upper dermis, such as syringomas, can be ablated with the carbon dioxide laser. Lesions in the deeper dermis and fat, such as dermatofibroma and lipoma, will need excision. Lesions like syringomas, sebaceous hyperplasias, and seborrheic keratoses tend to recur.

SCARS (Figures 15–25 to 15–32)

Scars may result from trauma, surgery, or disease, e.g. chicken pox and acne. They may be flat, atrophic, hypertrophic, or keloidal. The initiating damage is at the level of the reticular dermis or deeper. Scars cannot be removed, only improved upon.

Flat scars are best left alone or may be revised surgically with Z plasty to release tension on surrounding skin structures, or with the W plasty to break up the linearity.

Acne scars are usually atrophic and these may be subdivided into rolling, box-car, or pitted. Options for atrophic acne scars depend on the depth of scarring. Rolling and box-car acne scars can be treated with a combination of chemical peeling, microdermabrasion, dermabrasion, or filler injection. They are also the most common indication for laser resurfacing and non-ablative laser rejuvenation in Asia, in contrast to the West, where perioral and periorbital wrinkles are the main indications. Deep pitted acne scars are best treated with scar excision and/or subcision.

Hypertrophic and keloidal scars are more common over the chest, back, shoulders, jawline, and earlobes. There is also a familial tendency and they are most commonly treated with intralesional steroid injections. Very large keloids may be debulked with surgical excision or ablative laser, followed by intralesional steroid injections to minimize recurrences.

Erythematous or pigmented scars will improve slowly with time; the erythema may be lightened with the use of the pulsed dye laser.

WRINKLES (Figures 15–33 to 15–36)

Wrinkles are a sign of aging, especially photo-aging. In Asia, fair skin is considered desirable; most Asians avoid the sun if possible and do not actively seek a tan. Thus, photo-damage, actinic keratoses, and wrinkles are much less severe than in the West. Wrinkles can be classified into dynamic or resting.

Dynamic wrinkles appear in patients in their late 20s and are obvious when certain muscles are used. For example, "crow's feet" at the corners of the eyes when smiling is due to the contraction of the orbicularis oculi. Dynamic wrinkles are effectively treated with botulinum toxin injection. This toxin weakens the muscle for three to four months and decreases the appearance of wrinkles during muscle contraction.

Resting wrinkles are those that are present even when there is no muscle contraction. These are more pronounced with age and are secondary to progressive degeneration and atrophy of supporting structures like collagen, fat, and bone. Resting lines may be subdivided into fine or deep. Fine resting wrinkles can be treated with topical retinoids, chemical peeling, microdermabrasion, laser resurfacing, or non-ablative laser rejuvenation. Deeper resting lines may be augmented with fillers, such as collagen, autologous fat, and synthetic substances like hyaluronic acid.

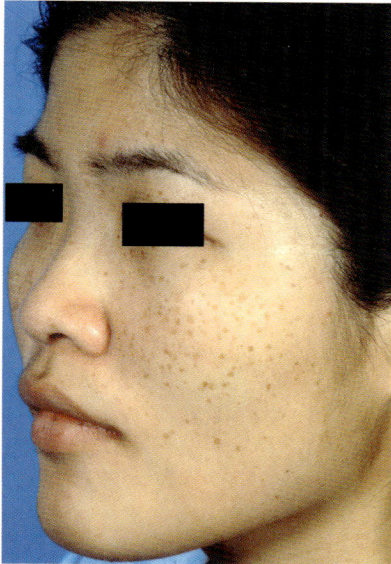

Figure 15–1 □ Ephelides (freckles). Ephelides are small, tan-brown macules occurring on sun-exposed areas only. Ephelides fluctuate in intensity, size, and number in accordance with the amount of sun exposure. Histologically, there is hypermelanization in the basal layer of the epidermis. The number of melanocytes is normal but the melanosomes are elongated and rod-shaped. Ephelides are benign but many Asians desire their removal or lightening for cosmetic reasons. Treatment options include topical lightening agents, intense pulsed light therapy, and pigment-specific laser treatment.

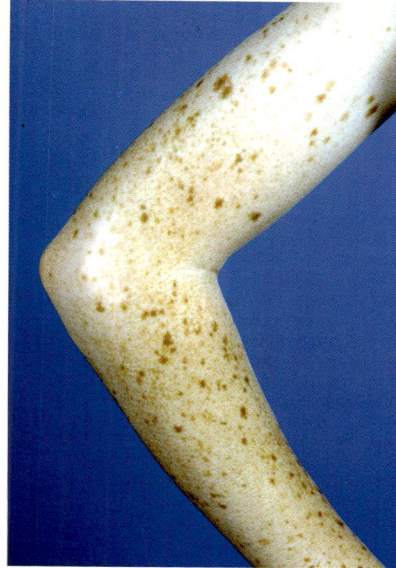

Figure 15–2 □ Lentigo simplex. This arises in childhood and presents as small well-defined pigmented macules on any skin surface as well as mucous membranes. The pigmentation is uniform throughout the lesion, varying from light brown to black. They are not limited to sun-exposed areas as in ephelides and solar lentigines. They may be unilateral and dermatomal (segmental lentiginosis, partial unilateral lentiginosis).

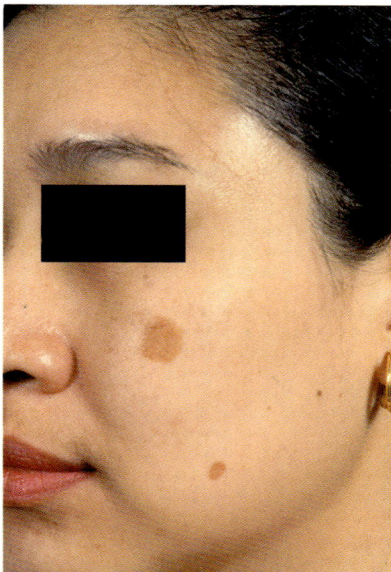

Figure 15–3 □ Solar lentigines. These are acquired lentigines as a result of age and cumulative sun exposure. They are brown macules of varying sizes and pigmentation. The sites of distribution are sun-exposed areas like the face and forearms. Histologically, they are similar to lentigo simplex. Solar lentigines may be treated with lightening creams, cryotherapy, intense pulsed light therapy, or pigment-specific lasers. The treatment response to laser and intense pulsed light is similar as that for ephelides.

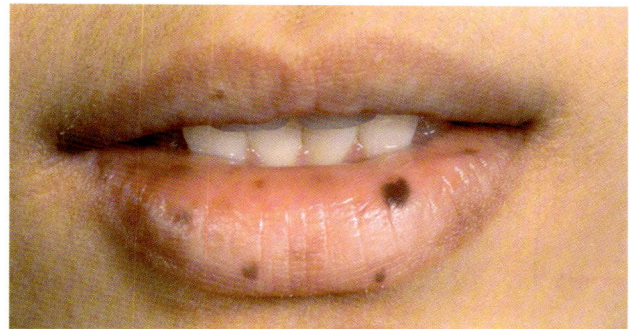

Figure 15–4 □ Labial melanotic macules. These occur in 3% of the population, predominantly women and on the lower lip. They are often isolated or may be part of the Laugier-Hunziker syndrome, which is associated with oral mucosal lesions and melanonychia striata. The response to pigment-specific laser is good, requiring one or two treatments.

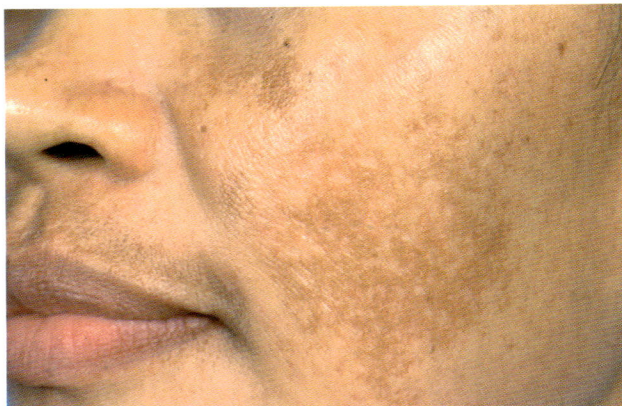

Figure 15–5 □ Melasma. Melasma is an acquired hyperpigmentary disorder, more common in middle-aged women. It is very common in Orientals, Hispanics, and Blacks. The estimated prevalence is 40% in females and 20% in males. Clinically, there are bilateral, symmetrical, ill-defined light brown to gray brown patches over the sun-exposed areas, especially the malar, mandibular, and centrofacial regions. It is due to a combination of sun exposure, hereditary, and hormonal influences. Histologically, melasma may be predominantly epidermal, dermal, or mixed. In the epidermal type, there is increased melanin in the melanocytes in the basal and suprabasal layer. In the dermal type, there are dermal melanophages. In the mixed pattern, there are features of both.

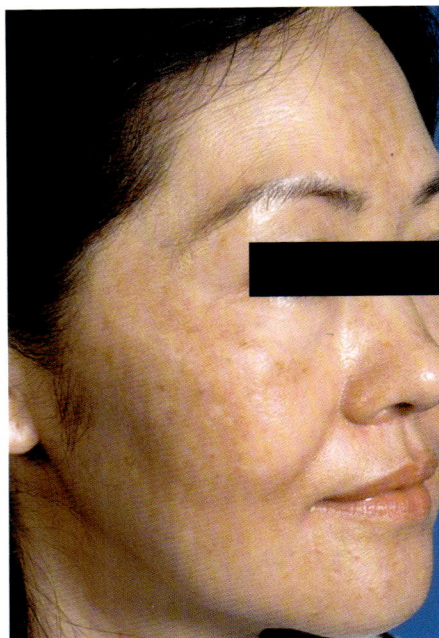

Figure 15–6 □ Melasma. First line treatment involves sunscreens and topical lightening agents. If these fail, second line treatment with deep chemical peels, Q-switched pigment lasers or intense pulsed light may be attempted. However, the response to these are unpredictable or poor, or may even worsen the pigmentation.

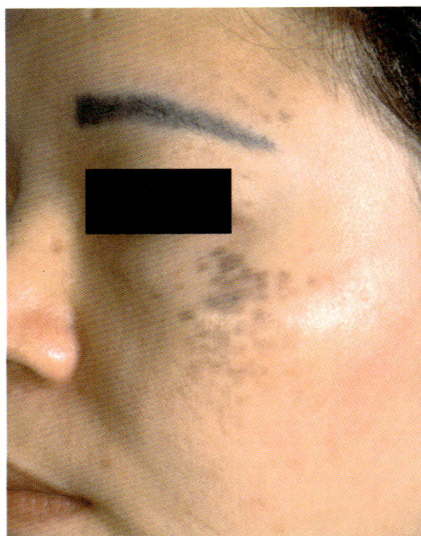

Figure 15–7 □ Hori's nevus (acquired bilateral nevus of Ota-like macules). This is a common acquired symmetrical pigmentary disorder occurring in Asian women. The age of onset is in the 20s or 30s and there may be a family history. The prevalence is 0.8 to 2% of Asian women and is usually bilateral. Clinically, there are light brown to bluish macules over the forehead, temples, eyelids, malar regions, nasal alae, and nasal root. Early Hori's nevus has a light brown color similar to ephelides. As it progresses, Hori's nevus becomes less discrete and confluent and assumes a slate-gray to dark brown color.

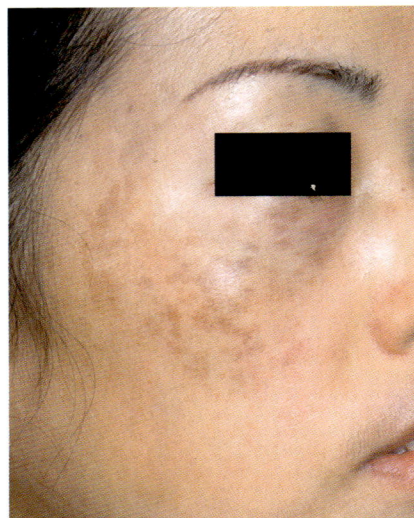

Figure 15–8 □ Hori's nevus. Histologically, there are increased bipolar and irregular melanocytes in the upper and middle dermis. Topical treatment is unsatisfactory. For effective treatment, multiple sessions of Q-switched pigment-specific lasers at two to three monthly intervals are required. Both short and longer wavelength lasers in isolation or combination have been used with success. Short wavelengths, e.g. 532 nm, may help by causing transepidermal elimination of the dermal pigment or by removing superficial overlying normal melanin that may interfere with longer wavelength treatment, e.g. 1,064 nm of the deeper component.

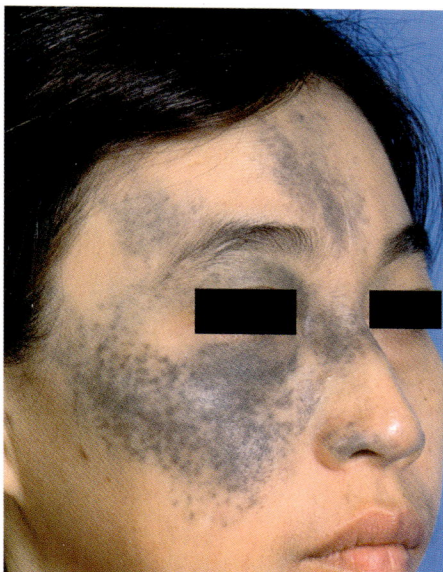

Figure 15–9 □ Nevus of Ota. This lesion affects predominantly females and presents as slate-gray or blue-black macules on the facial area innervated by the first and second divisions of the trigeminal nerve. It may be present at birth or during teenage years. Significant lightening can be achieved with pigment-specific lasers such as the Q-switched Nd YAG laser. Multiple treatments are required.

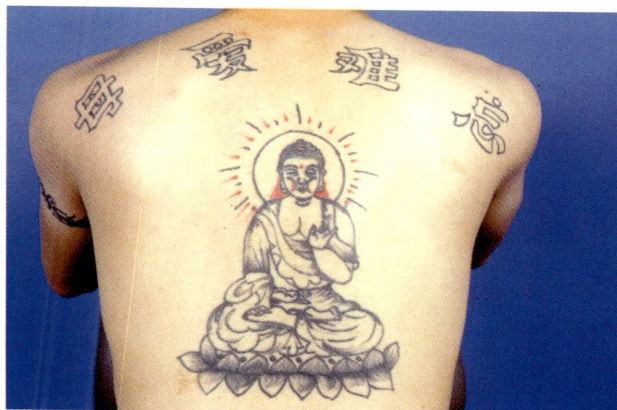

Figure 15–10 □ Tattoos. By innoculating insoluble pigments into the skin, permanent figures or inscriptions of various colors are produced. Tattoos may be for decorative, religious, cosmetic, or symbolic reasons.

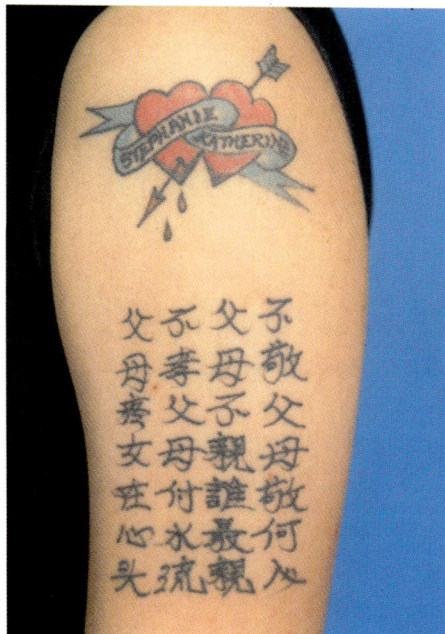

Figure 15–11 □ Tattoos. Tattoos can be safely and effectively removed with the use of Q-switched pigment-specific lasers. The response to laser treatment depends on the color, depth, and density of pigment. Blue-black tattoos are the easiest to remove compared to red, yellow, and green tattoos. Professional tattoos, which are denser, deeper, and more uniform are more difficult to remove compared to amateur tattoos.

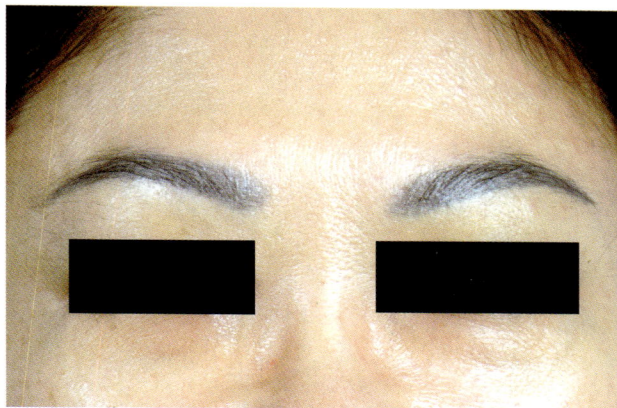

Figure 15–12 □ Eyebrow tattoos. In many parts of Asia, many women acquire eyebrow tattoos for cosmetic enhancement. Some seek laser removal later because of dissatisfaction with the results or when the tattoos acquire a greenish hue over the years.

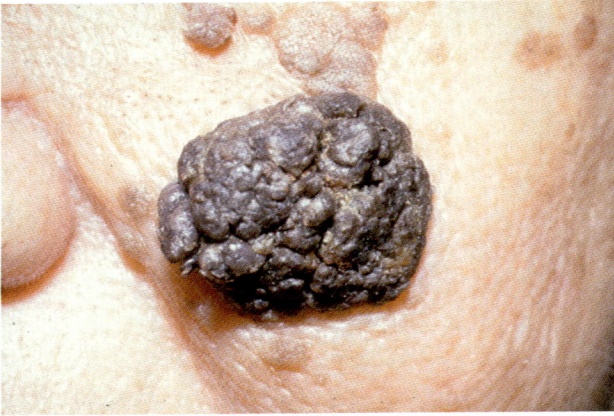

Figure 15–13 □ Seborrheic keratosis. These are benign, brown to black, sessile, warty papules or plaques, commonly involving the scalp, face, and extremities. The onset is generally when a person is in his or her 30s. Removal can be easily performed with curettage, cryotherapy, shave excision, or electrosurgery.

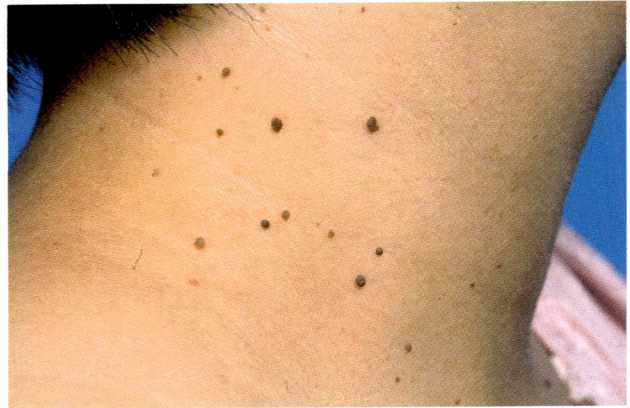

Figure 15–14 □ Skin tags. These are small, flesh-colored to brown, pedunculated papillomas, seen frequently on the neck, axillae, and eyelids. They may increase in numbers during pregnancy or weight gain. Histologically, the lesions show hyperplastic epidermis enclosing a dermal stalk of loose collagen fibres. They can be left alone or removed by snip excision and electrodessication.

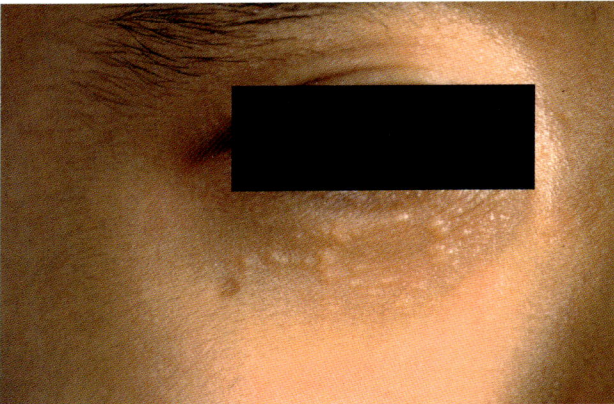

Figure 15–15 □ Syringomas. These are benign adnexal tumors of well-differentiated eccrine sweat ducts. Lesions are usually multiple and appear as small, skin-colored, smooth papules. They often occur symmetrically on the face, particularly around the eyes, of genetically predisposed individuals. Predominantly women are affected, and the lesions begin at puberty. Syringomas may be removed with electrosurgery or ablative laser, e.g. carbon dioxide laser. However, the recurrence rate is high.

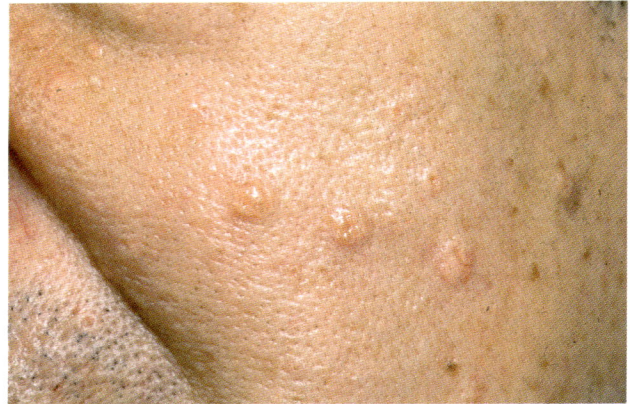

Figure 15–16 □ Sebaceous hyperplasias. Lesions are small, dome-shaped, yellow papules. A central umbilication is characteristic. They are composed of hyperplastic mature sebaceous glands communicating with the surface by a dilated follicular infundibulum. The lesions occur on the forehead and cheeks during adult life, and may be confused with basal cell carcinomas. Sebaceous hyperplasia may be removed with electrosurgery or ablative laser. However, the recurrence rate is high.

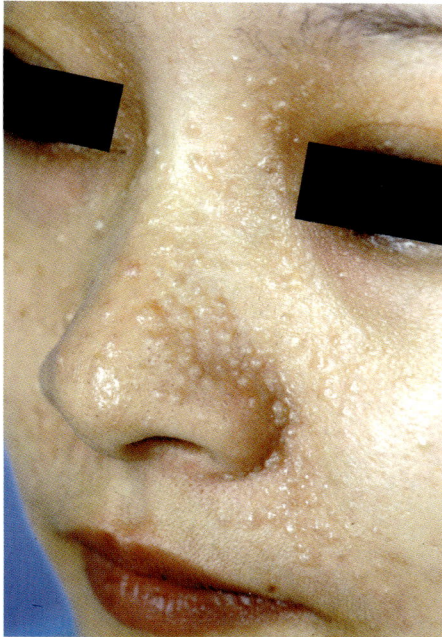

Figure 15–17 □ Trichoepithelioma. Multiple trichoepitheliomas is a disfiguring, autosomal dominant condition. Multiple skin-colored, often telangiectatic, pearly papules or nodules appear after puberty. The lesions frequently occur on the nasolabial folds, upper lip, and eyelids. Solitary lesions can be confused with basal cell carcinomas. Laser resurfacing may help to improve the appearance of the lesions. The recurrence rate is high.

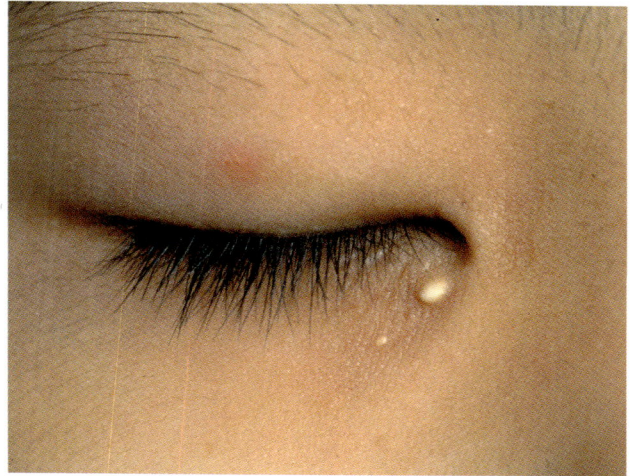

Figure 15–18 □ Milia. These are small 1 to 4 mm keratinous cysts occurring mostly on the face, especially around the eyes, and appear as white or cream-colored papules. They may develop without a predisposing condition or as a result of a blistering process like bullous pemphigoid or epidermolysis bullosa. Milia may be incised gently and expressed, or removed with light electrodessication.

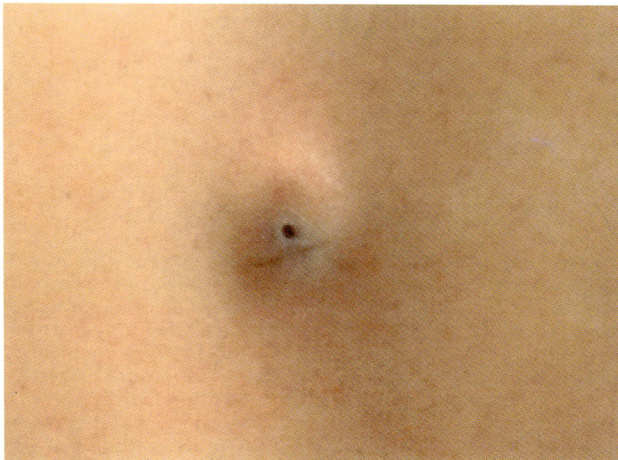

Figure 15–19 □ Epidermal cyst. This is a dome-shaped, smooth cystic swelling, often with a central punctum that may extrude cheesy keratinous contents. It is attached to the overlying normal skin. It may occur spontaneously or as a result of innoculation injuries. The cyst may rupture and induce a foreign body inflammatory reaction resulting in fibrosis and adhesion to the surrounding tissues. Multiple epidermal cysts are a feature of Gardner's syndrome. Histologically, the cyst is lined by stratified squamous epithelium containing a granular layer. Epidermal cysts may be excised.

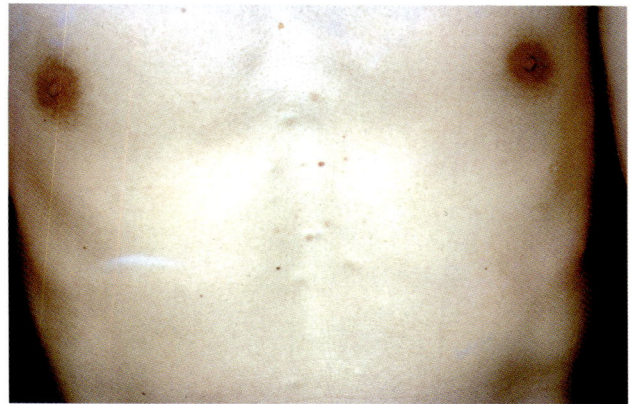

Figure 15–20 □ Steatocystoma multiplex. This is an autosomal dominant condition presenting at or after puberty. The lesions consist of multiple small, smooth-surface, yellowish papules, located principally on the chest, proximal parts of the limbs, and axillae. The cysts are lined with squamous epithelium with flattened sebaceous lobules. The contents are yellow and in liquid form. Treatment is by excision but may be precluded by the sheer number of lesions.

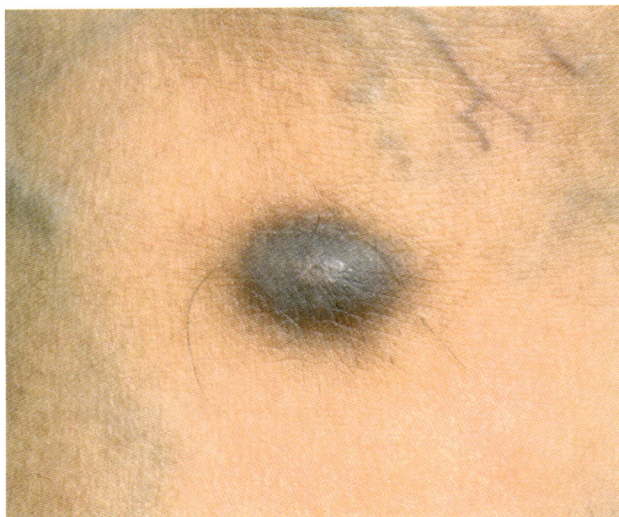

Figure 15–21 □ Dermatofibroma. This is a smooth, firm, dome-shaped, red-brown nodule, occurring mostly on the limbs. It represents a fibrohistiocytic reaction to a previous skin injury, like an insect bite or blunt trauma. Typically, a depression is created over the lesion when it is grasped gently ("dimple sign"). The lesion is benign and may involute within a few years. However, it is usually excised for diagnostic or cosmetic reasons.

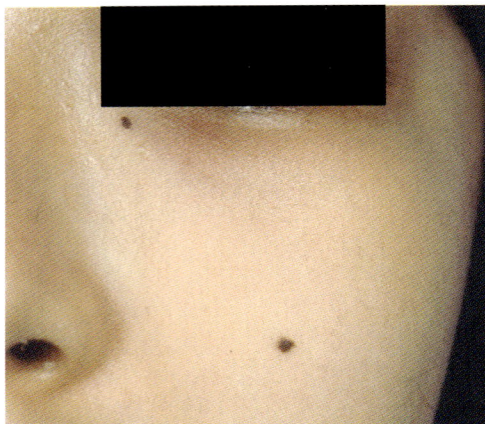

Figure 15–22 □ Junctional melanocytic nevus. This is an acquired melanocytic nevus occurring in the first few decades of life. Clinically, it presents as a smooth, hairless, dark-brown or two-toned macule and can be slightly raised. Histologically, nests of nevocytes are found in the lower epidermis, usually within the epidermal ridges. Many Asians, especially the Chinese, request removal of moles at certain sites which are considered unlucky, e.g. those below the eye and those on the shoulders. Junctional melanocytic nevi may be removed by ablative laser or excision.

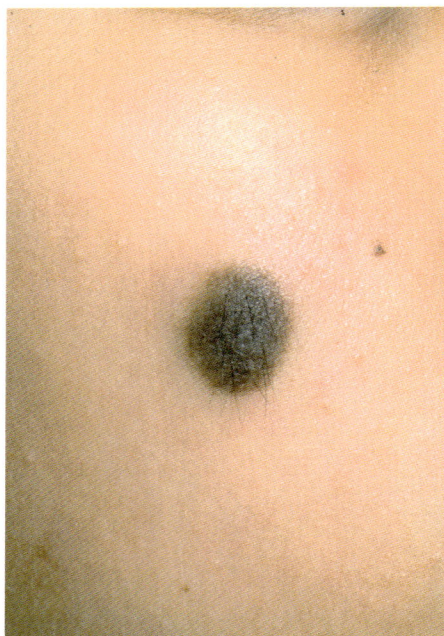

Figure 15–23 □ Congenital melanocytic nevus. These are any moles presenting below the age of one year. The risk of malignancy depends on the size. Small- (less than 1.5 cm) and medium-sized (1.5 to 20 cm) lesions can be left alone or excised. Giant lesions (more than 20 cm) have a lifetime risk of malignant change of 4 to 6%. These should be excised with skin grafting. The use of pigment-specific laser is controversial because the lesion is not completely removed with the possibility of masking future malignant changes. There is also a theoretical possibility of laser-induced carcinogenesis, which has not been clinically demonstrated.

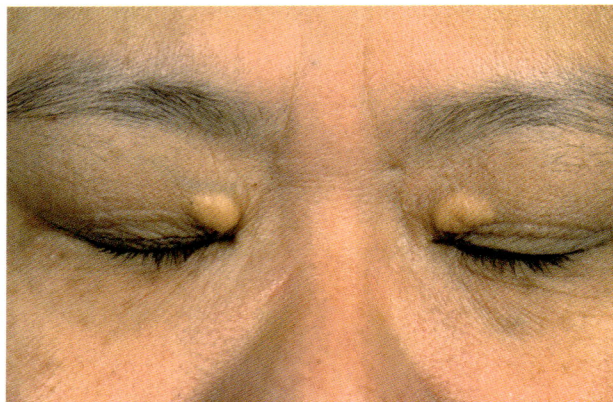

Figure 15–24 □ Xanthelasma palpebrarum. This is the most common form of xanthoma, usually presenting at middle age. The lesions consist of chamois or orange-colored plaques on the eyelids, especially near the inner canthi. Although they can be a feature of familial hyperlipoproteinemia, half or more of the patients are normo-lipemic. Excellent cosmetic results can be obtained with surgical excision for smaller lesions. Electrosurgery, ablative laser vaporization, and trichloroacetic acid cauterization can also be performed.

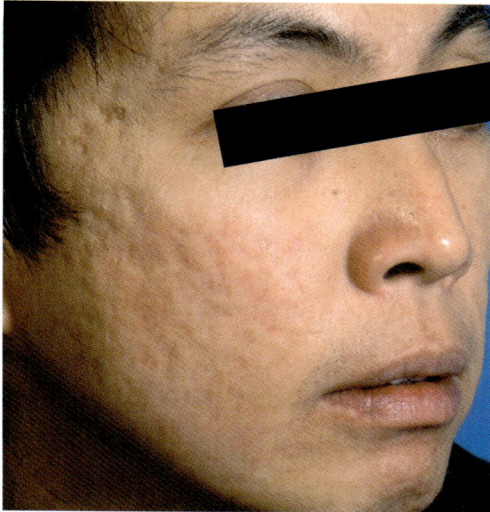

Figure 15–25 □ **Acne scars – box-car and rolling.** Severe inflammation in acne vulgaris can result in disfiguring scars. Atrophic acne scars may be classified into box-car, rolling, and pitted scars. Rolling scars are due to fibrous tethering of dermis to the subcutis. Box-car-type scars are round to oval depressions with clearly defined, vertical borders. These may be improved with laser resurfacing, non-ablative laser rejuvenation, chemical peeling, microdermabrasion, or filler injection.

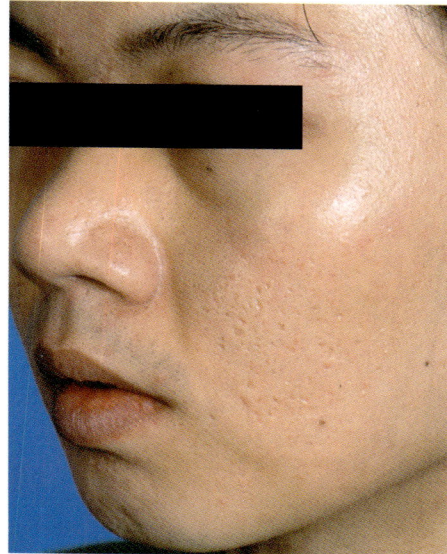

Figure 15–26 □ **Acne scars – pitted.** This patient has predominantly ice-pick scars on her cheeks. Ice-pick scars are narrow, sharply marginated epithelial tracts that extend vertically or conically to the deep dermis or subcutis. Because of their depth, excision, and/or subcision is the mainstay of treatment.

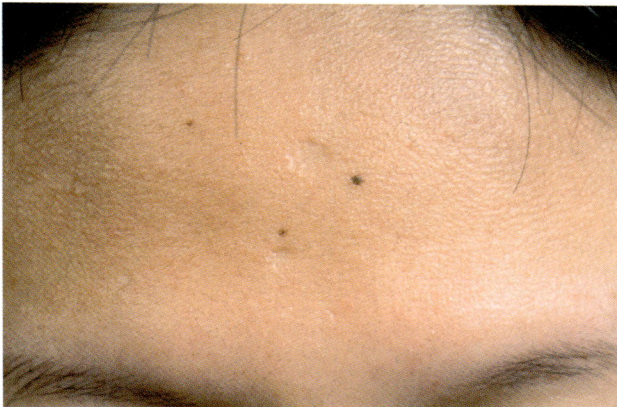

Figure 15–27 □ **Chicken pox scars.** These are usually of the box-car type. They are usually larger than acne scars and found on the face. They may be improved as with box-car and rolling acne scars.

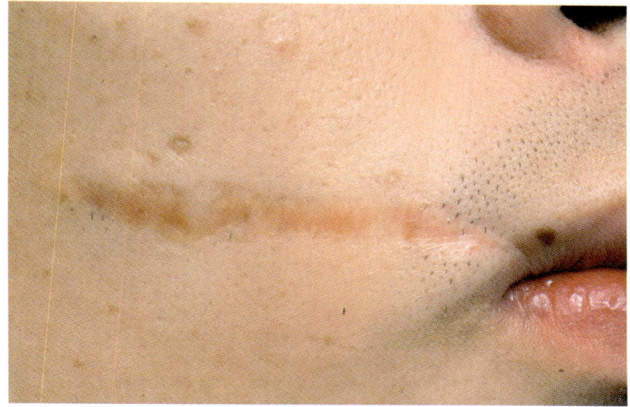

Figure 15–28 □ **Traumatic scar.** This patient had a laceration on her face as a result of a road traffic accident. The injury has resulted in a linear, slightly depressed, atrophic scar. Scar revision using dermabrasion, CO_2 laser, or non-ablative laser resurfacing has shown variable success.

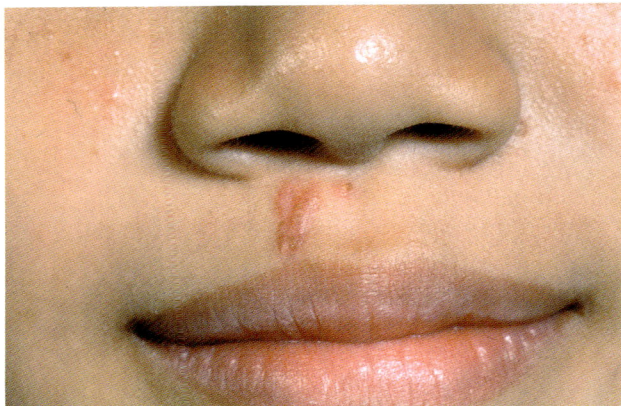

Figure 15–29 □ Hypertropic scar. This represents an overgrowth of connective tissue during wound healing. It appears as a raised, firm, smooth-surface lesion. Unlike a keloid, which spreads beyond its confines, a hypertrophic scar remains within the limits of the traumatized area. It may regress over time when broad bundles of hyalinized collagen shrink and line parallel to the epidermal surface. Hypertrophic scars can be flattened with potent topical steroids or intralesional steroid injections.

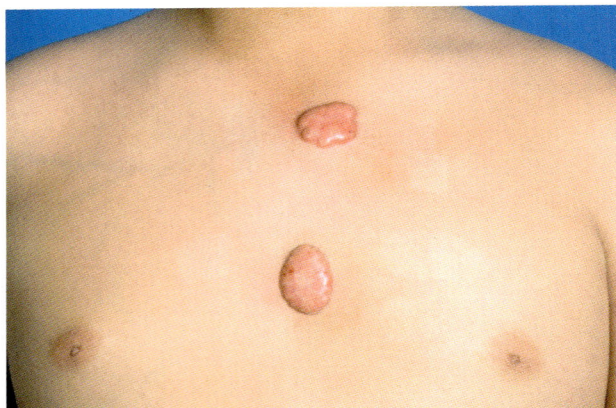

Figure 15–30 □ Keloids. These are exaggerated growths of scar tissue in areas of previous skin injury. They are due to a preponderance of collagen production during the phases of wound healing. On the chest, the lesions usually arise from acne or chicken pox. They appear as raised, firm, rubbery plaques with a flat surface.

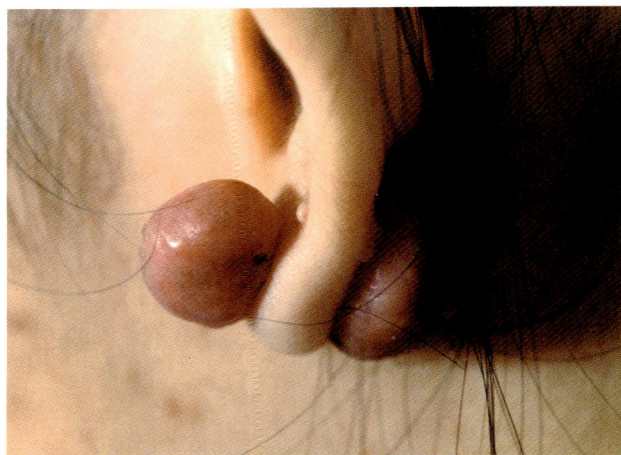

Figure 15–31 □ Ear lobe keloids secondary to ear piercing. Keloids on the ear lobe tend to be pedunculated. They may be debulked first with surgery or laser followed by intralesional steroid injections to minimize recurrences.

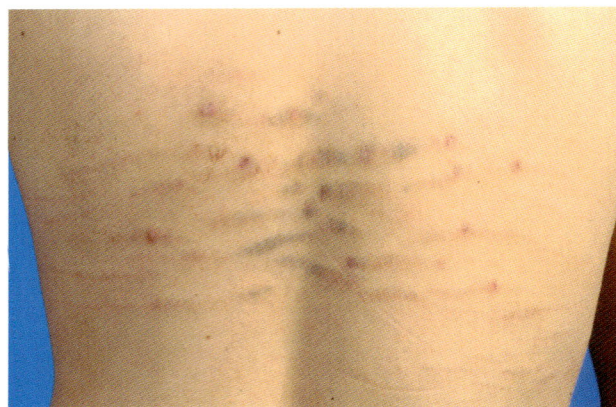

Figure 15–32 □ Striae distensae. Striaes are stretch marks. Clinically, they consist of erythematous and slightly depressed, linear atrophic streaks. These striaes have occurred over areas of distension during pubertal growth spurts. Erythematous striae may be lightened with pulsed dye laser. The new excimer laser may be promising for the tanning of white striae.

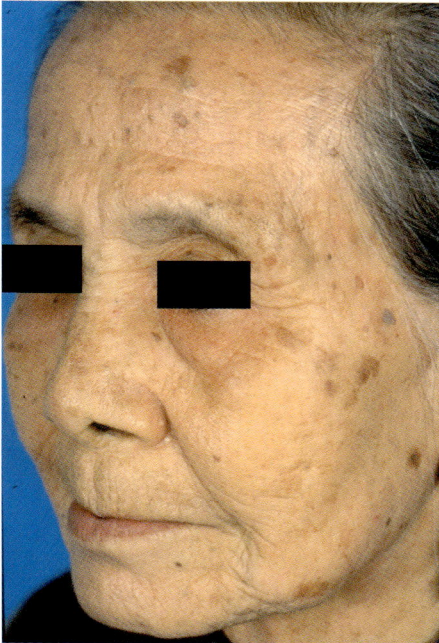

Figure 15–33 □ Photo-aging. Photo-aging in Asian skin presents as dyspigmentation, keratoses, dryness, wrinkling, and a thickened, pebbly skin texture (elastosis). In severe elastosis, deep furrows are seen. Premalignant neoplasia and malignancies may develop as a result of the chronic photo-damage.

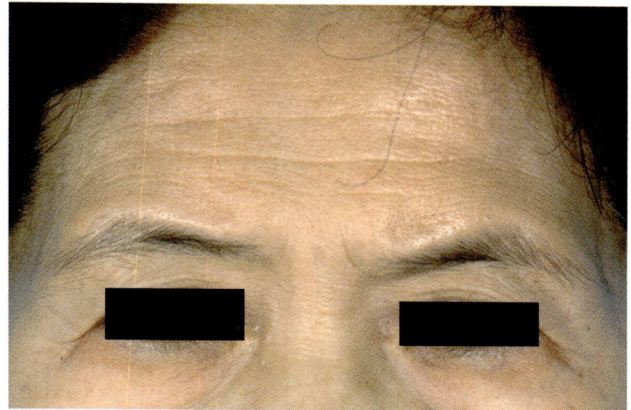

Figure 15–34 □ Forehead lines. These are common dynamic wrinkles secondary to the contraction of the frontalis muscles. They are often more severe in males because of their larger muscle mass.

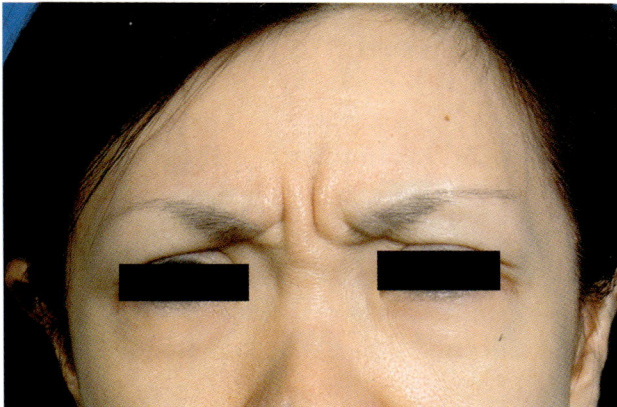

Figure 15–35 □ Glabellar frown lines. These are due to the contraction of brow depressors (corrugators, procereus) during subconsious frowning. They may be treated with injection of botulinum toxin as well as fillers.

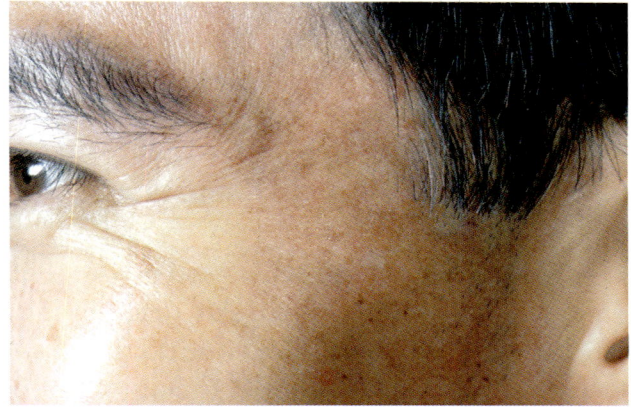

Figure 15–36 □ "Crow's feet". These are due to the contraction of the lateral portion of the orbicularis oculi. Botulinum toxin injections are quite effective in treating them. However, the effects of botulinum toxin injections are temporary and only last for three to four months, although with subsequent injections, the effects may last up to six months.

Miscellaneous Dermatoses in Asians

Seow C.S. and Kwah R.Y.C.

Asians are a diverse group of people. They consist of people from South Asia, which includes the subcontinent region of Pakistan, India, and Sri Lanka; Southeast Asia, (Singapore, Malaysia, Indonesia, the Philippines, and Thailand); and East Asia (encompassing amongst others Japan, Korea, and China). In these regions, the Fitzpatrick skin types III, IV, and V predominate.

Skin conditions that are distinct to Asians may stem from either unique cultural practices or inherent genetic differences. This chapter will highlight several interesting dermatoses in Asians that may not be covered adequately in the preceding chapters.

DERMATOSES DUE TO CULTURAL PRACTICES (Figures 16–1 to 16–11)

There is diversity in the beliefs and practices of Asians. As a result of these differences, some unique dermatological conditions can sometimes be encountered. It is important to know the signs and symptoms associated with these practices in order for a proper diagnosis to be made and appropriate treatment instituted. Some of these conditions include bruising of skin secondary to traditional medicinal therapy with cupping, scar sarcoidosis from kavadi procession, traction alopecia in Sikhism, chronic arsenic poisoning from the use of

traditional medications or drinking of well water contaminated with arsenic, and foreign bodies implanted into the genitals.

Cupping

This is a traditional Oriental therapy whereby a jar is attached to the skin to cause local congestion through partial vacuum created by burning a material within the jar. The therapy has the function of warming and promoting the free flow of *qi* (internal energy) and blood through the meridians, dispelling dampness, alleviating swellings and pains. Indications for treatment with cupping include rheumatic pain caused by "dampness", gastrointestinal disorders, and pulmonary disorders such as cough and asthma. Cupping is performed via two main methods: "fire throwing" and "fire twinkling". The former involves throwing a piece of ignited paper or an alcohol-soaked cotton ball into a cup, then rapidly placing the mouth of the cup firmly on the skin at the desired location. The latter method involves heating the interior of the cup with an ignited cotton ball, which has been soaked with 95% alcohol. The cup is then placed at the selected position. This therapy will result in bruising of the skin. Sometimes, cupping may be combined with bloodletting, whereby a needle pricks the skin at the selected site. This treatment can sometimes result in infection at the site.

Post-kavadi Scar Sarcoidosis

Devotees of Lord Muruga take a vow to offer Him a kavadi for the purpose of tiding over or averting a great calamity. The kavadi varies in shape and size, from a simple wooden stick with two baskets at each end slung across the shoulders, to the costly palanquin structure, elaborately decorated with flowers and peacock feathers. Some of these kavadis are attached to the bodies of the kavadi-carriers by hooks or spears. As sarcoidosis occurs more frequently in the Indian ethnic group, wound sites from a kavadi carriage can become complicated by scar sarcoidosis which takes on a striking and distinct pattern.

Traction Alopecia in Sikhs

Sikhism is a monotheistic faith that emphasizes the teachings of honesty, compassion, humility, piety, social commitment, and religious tolerance. The word "Sikh" is derived from the Sanskrit word *shishya* which means disciple, learner, and seeker of truth. One of the practices of Sikhism is *kes* or unshorn hair that is regarded as a symbol of saintliness. The keeping of hair in its natural state is regarded as living in harmony with the will of God, and is a symbol of the Khalsa brotherhood and the Sikh faith. Hair is an integral part of the human body created by God and Sikhism calls for its preservation. The shaving or cutting of hair is considered a taboo in Sikhism.

Another practice involves the *kangha* or comb. A Sikh must comb his hair twice a day and tie his turban neatly. The Gurus wear turbans and command the Sikhs to do likewise for the protection of their hair and the promotion of social identity and cohesion.

Due to the practice of keeping facial and scalp hair, traction alopecia (marginal and non-marginal) may sometimes occur.

Chronic Arsenic Poisoning

Inorganic arsenic has been used in medicine for over 2,500 years. The most widely used form is the Fowler solution which contains 1% potassium arsenite and is used for treatment of psoriasis. Arsphenamine was for many years the standard treatment for syphilis. Melarsoprol is an organoarsenic compound used to treat infections caused by *Trypanosoma cruzei*. In Asia, arsenic was also a component of many traditional treatments such as traditional Chinese herbal balls, Korean herbal preparations used to treat hemorrhoids, and kelp supplements. It was a component of a traditional Chinese medication for asthma (called "Sin-Luk" pill) in Singapore. Stricter regulations over the past decades have fortunately abolished the presence of most of these arsenic-containing traditional medicines. Well water contaminated with arsenic still poses health problems in some Asian countries such as Bangladesh and Thailand.

The skin changes develop years to decades later. They consist of pigmentation, keratosis, Bowen's disease, basal cell and squamous cell carcinomas. The disease process remains active and progresses as the patient ages.

DERMATOSES DUE TO GENETIC DIFFERENCES (Figures 16–12 to 16–22)

Asians, due to their genetic make-up, may also present with different dermatological conditions such as pigmentary disorders, Ofuji's disease, papuloerythroderma of Ofuji, Kimura's disease, and primary cutaneous lichen amyloidosis.

Ofuji's Disease (Eosinophilic Pustular Folliculitis)

Three variants of this disorder have been described: classic (as originally described by Ofuji), HIV-associated, and infantile variants.

The classical form described by Ofuji occurs mainly in the Japanese and Orientals. This condition usually presents as papulopustules, with or without plaques, with a predilection for the face and the trunk. Peripheral extension with central clearing is often noted. The lesions may heal with post-inflammatory hyperpigmentation. Peripheral leukocytosis and eosinophilia may be seen. At present, the etiology remains unknown. Treatment with oral indomethacin appears to be effective for most patients, although a chronic relapsing course is to be expected.

Kimura's Disease

This is a benign disorder, a consequence of abnormal proliferation of lymphoid follicles and vascular endothelium. Its pathogenesis is unknown. It has no known potential for malignant transformation. Findings include solitary or multiple, firm, subcutaneous masses, which are usually located on the head or neck. The parotid region is the most common site. These lesions can be large and disfiguring. Marked lymphadenopathy can also be found. Kimura's disease has to be differentiated from angiolymphoid hyperplasia with eosinophilia

(AHLE), which is a benign condition but presents as papules on the head and neck.

Conservative management is appropriate in Kimura's disease if it is asymptomatic and non-disfiguring. Otherwise, systemic corticosteroids, cyclosporin, and radiotherapy have been reported to be beneficial, although recurrences occur in 20 to 25% of patients.

Papuloerythroderma of Ofuji

A rare condition that presents with pruritic lesions but spares the skin folds, resulting in alternating bands of involved and uninvolved skin. This is known as the "deck chair" sign. It has been reported to be associated with neoplasms, such as lymphomas and visceral carcinomas, which must be screened for if this condition is diagnosed.

Primary Cutaneous Amyloidosis

This entity comprises macular, papular, and nodular varieties. It is postulated to arise from focal epidermal damage with consequent keratinocyte degeneration. The arms, legs, neck, and interscapular region are common sites of involvement.

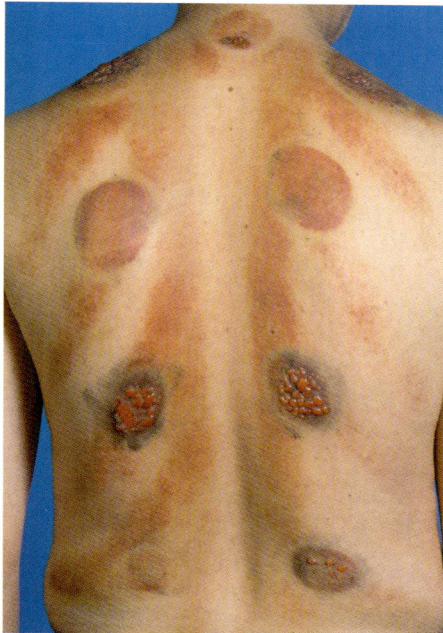

Figure 16–1 □ Cupping. Cupping is a form of traditional Chinese treatment used to regulate the flow of *qi* or "internal energy". This therapy can result in bruising of the skin. Sometimes, thermal injury may occur when the ignited material placed in the cup comes in contact with the skin. Blisters may result as evident in these pictures.

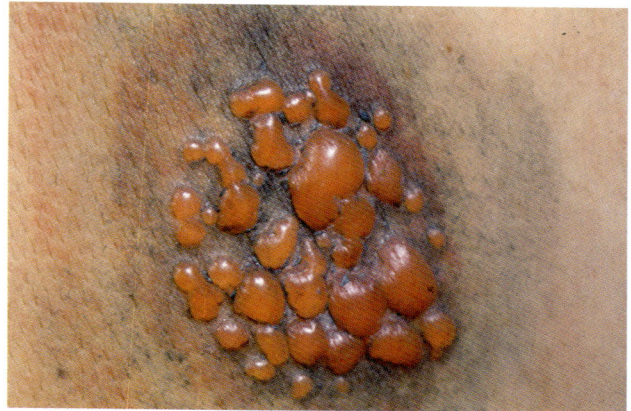

Figure 16–2 □ Cupping. A closer view of the lesions, revealing multiple tense blisters.

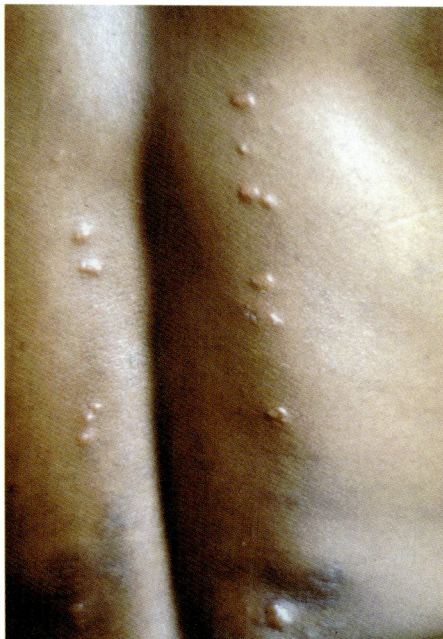

Figure 16–3 □ Post-kavadi scar sarcoidosis. Neat, parallel rows of dermal nodules developing over puncture wounds due to hooks of the kavadi being pierced into the skin during the Thaipusam festival. Initially thought to be keloids, a skin biopsy demonstrated epitheloid granulomas forming naked tubercles, confirming the diagnosis of scar sarcoidosis. The lesions resolved with intralesional corticosteroid injections.

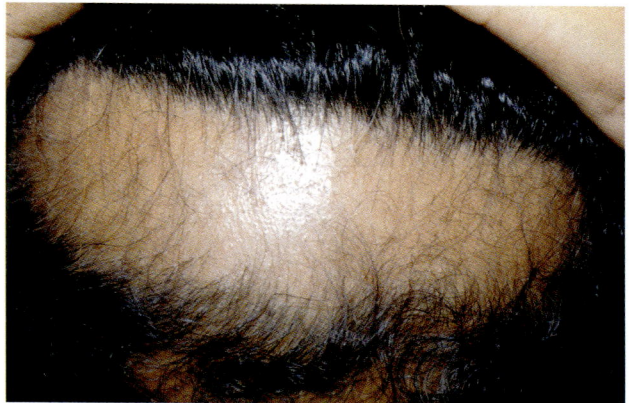

Figure 16–4 □ Traction alopecia in a Sikh. Hair loss in the occipital and frontal region of the scalp of a 35-year-old Sikh who ties his long hair beneath the turban. In Sikhism, hair is not to be removed throughout life. The scalp hair is kept from falling in front of the face by pulling it tightly over the head. The beard is also pulled tightly into a bun in the submandibular region. There are two patterns of traction alopecia: marginal alopecia (alopecia linearis frontalis) and non-marginal alopecia (chignon alopecia).

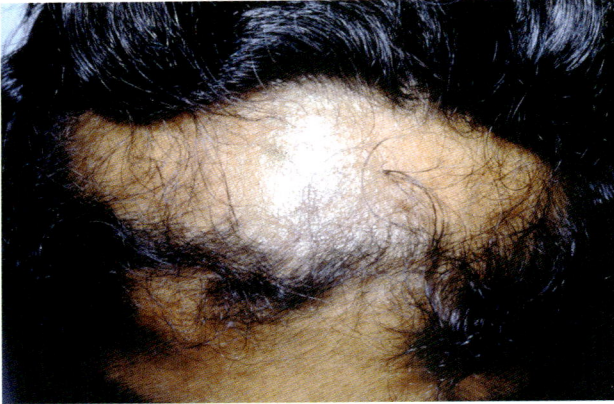

Figure 16–5 □ Traction alopecia in a Sikh. Traction alopecia tends to follow a series of events. Initial presentation includes pruritus and perifollicular erythema. These may be accompanied by hyperkeratosis, simulating a seborrheic picture. Pustules and scales can also develop. Eventually, an abundance of broken hairs can be found. With persistent traction, follicular atrophy results, producing thinner, fine, and short hair as evident in this picture

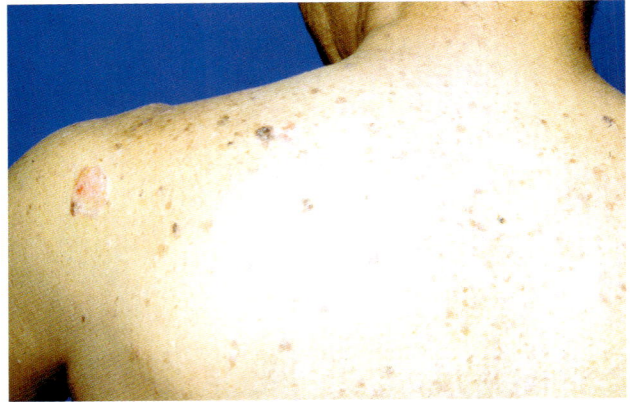

Figure 16–6 □ Chronic arsenic poisoning – arsenical keratosis. Arsenical compounds may be ingested through consumption of traditional medication or from drinking contaminated water. This picture demonstrates multiple pigmented keratotic plaques distributed diffusely on the back of this 55-year-old Chinese male. He has a history of drinking well water that is contaminated with arsenic. Chronic arsenic poisoning causes skin pigmentary changes and hyperkeratotic lesions on the skin called arsenical keratoses. Arsenical keratoses are usually multiple and typically occur at sites of friction and trauma, especially on the palms and soles.

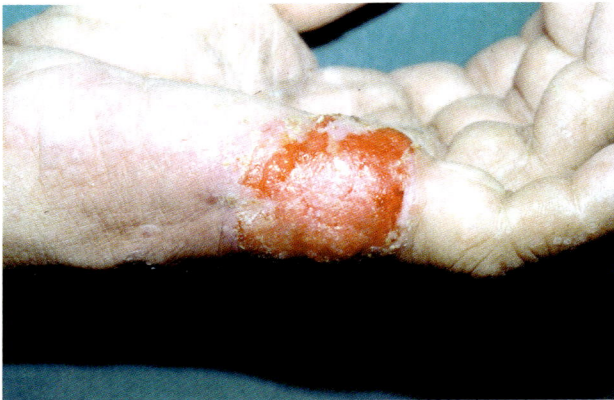

Figure 16–7 □ Chronic arsenic poisoning – Bowen's disease. This picture shows the development of Bowen's disease in a previous arsenical keratotic lesion on the palm of a 55-year-old Chinese male. The lesion appears as an erythematous, scaly, slightly indurated plaque. Chronic arsenic poisoning can cause Bowen's disease, squamous cell carcinoma, and basal cell carcinoma of the skin. The average latency period for the development of skin cancers in chronic arsenic poisoning is about 14 to 20 years.

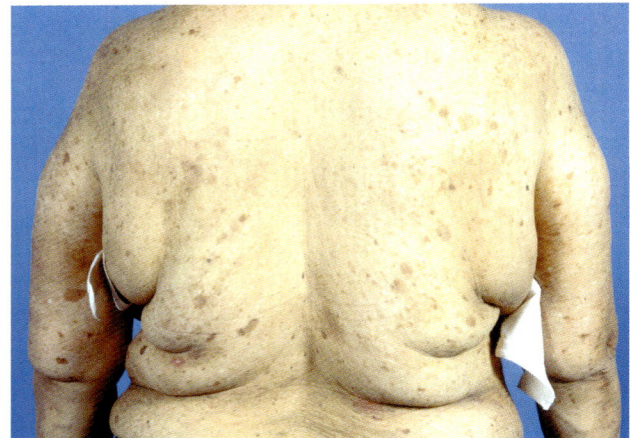

Figure 16–8 □ Chronic arsenic poisoning – arsenical keratoses and Bowen's disease. This 64-year-old Malay female has multiple arsenical keratoses and Bowen's disease on her back. She has a history of drinking well water contaminated by arsenic. Oral retinoids may be helpful in treating arsenic-induced cutaneous lesions and reducing the risk of cutaneous and internal malignancy formation. Surgical removal or local destruction, e.g. by cryotherapy, is usually the treatment of choice.

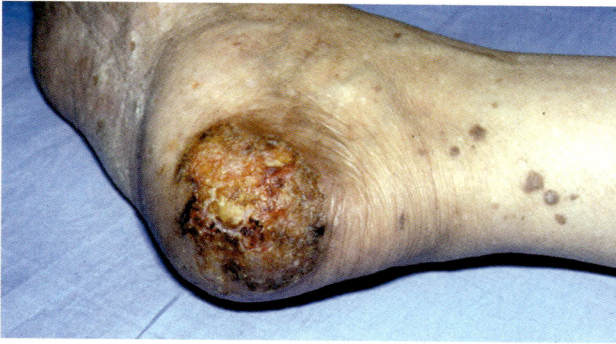

Figure 16–9 □ Chronic arsenic poisoning – squamous cell carcinoma. Squamous cell carcinoma can be a complication of arsenical keratosis. In this picture, the arsenical keratotic lesion on the heel of the foot has undergone malignant transformation into a squamous cell carcinoma. There is a non-healing ulcer with everted margins and a necrotic base.

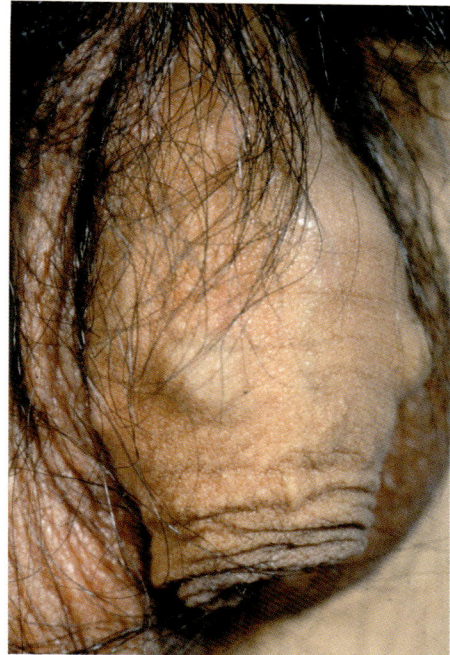

Figure 16–10 □ Foreign bodies in penis. In an attempt to augment their sexual prowess, some men resort to implanting foreign objects in their penis. This 35-year-old Thai male has three pearls implanted around the corona. They are regularly spaced out and they are stony hard and mobile.

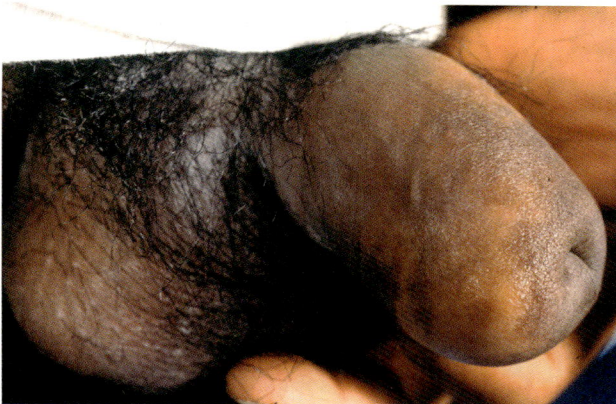

Figure 16–11 □ Foreign bodies in penis. Some men try injecting concoctions into the penis to augment its size as shown in this picture. A concoction of olive oil and paraffin has been injected under the skin of this 28-year-old man's penis in an attempt to enhance the girth of the penis. With time, foreign body granulomas may form.

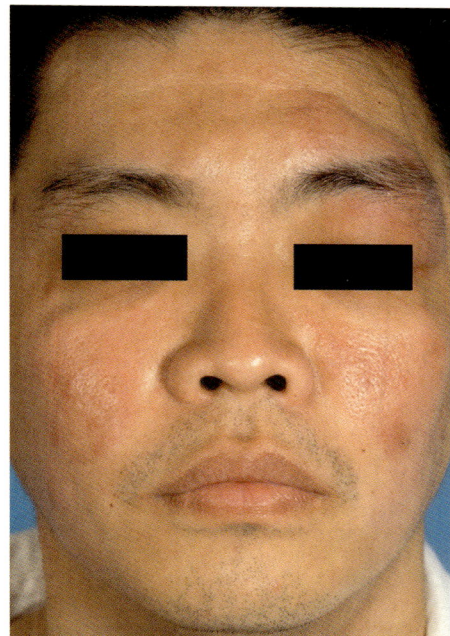

Figure 16–12 □ Ofuji's disease (eosinophilic pustular folliculitis). This benign inflammatory dermatosis, most commonly reported in the Japanese and Orientals, present with sterile follicular papulopustules that show peripheral extension and central clearing as visible in this picture. The face and upper trunk are most commonly affected. The disease runs a chronic relapsing course.

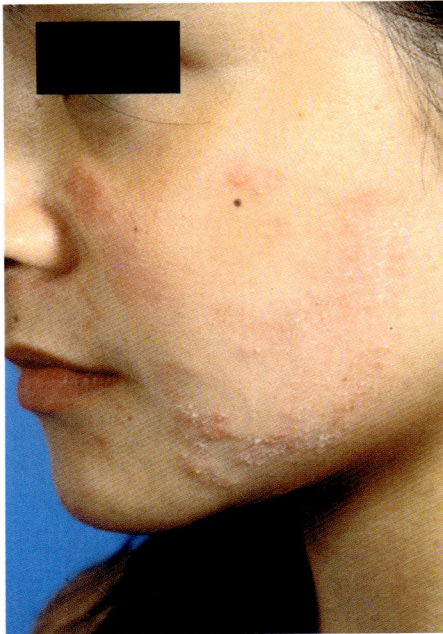

Figure 16–13 □ Ofuji's disease. This is a close-up view of the follicular papulopustules with peripheral extension and central clearing. The condition responds well to oral indomethacin although relapses are common.

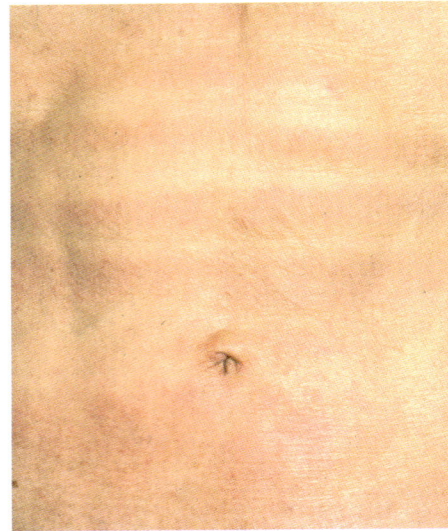

Figure 16–14 □ Papuloerythroderma of Ofuji. This is a rare condition which presents as widespread erythematous, flat-topped papules, with a striking sparing of body folds ("deck-chair" sign), as shown in this picture. Papuloerythroderma of Ofuji is a distinct clinical entity with a polymorphous etiology which frequently includes an association with cutaneous T-cell lymphoma or visceral malignancy. PUVA, oral corticosteroids, and UVB in combination with topical corticosteroids have been reported to be beneficial therapeutic modalities.

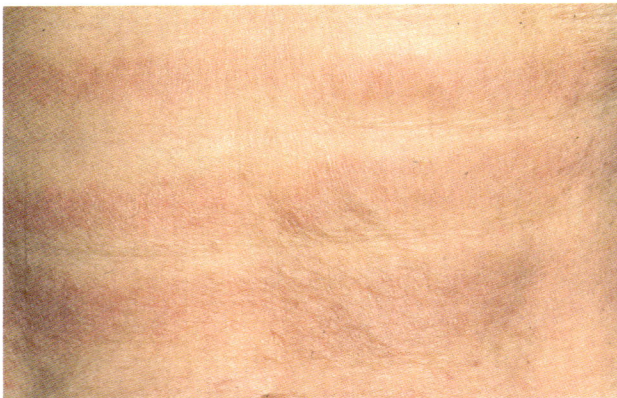

Figure 16–15 □ Papuloerythroderma of Ofuji. This is a close-up view of the affected area demonstrating the striking sparing of the body folds. This 72-year-old Chinese patient also has an underlying non-Hodgkin's lymphoma which was detected upon subsequent malignancy screening.

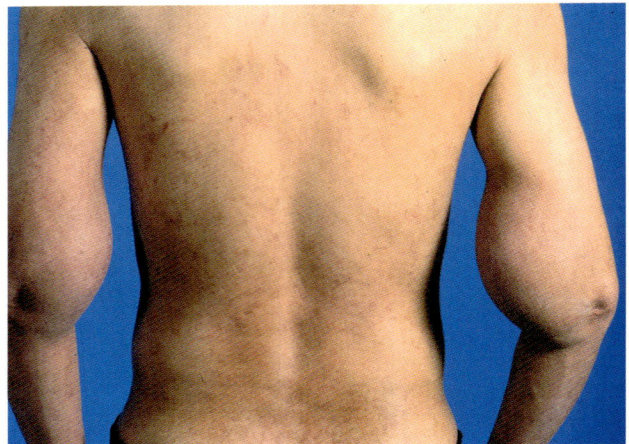

Figure 16–16 □ Kimura's disease. This picture shows multiple soft tissue masses involving both upper limbs of a 52-year-old Chinese male. Kimura's disease (KD) is a chronic inflammatory soft tissue disorder often presenting as swollen soft tissue or enlarged lymph nodes. KD is rare, and most reported cases involve Asians. Histologically, these lesions are characterized by a constellation of features: deep inflammation with vascular proliferation, lymphoid follicles, and marked infiltration of eosinophils.

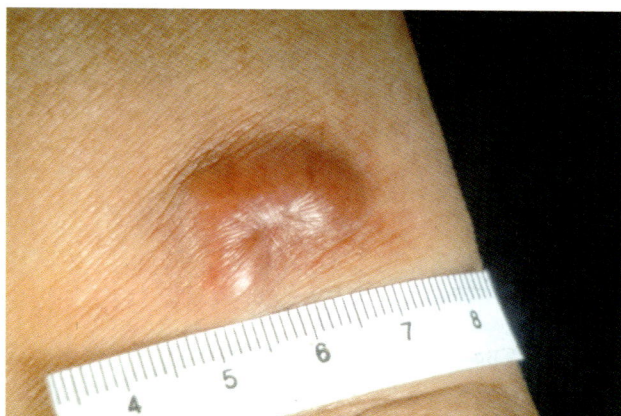

Figure 16–17 □ Kimura's disease. This patient with KD presents with a solitary, firm, subcutaneous mass which is painless and asymptomatic. The disease is characterized by a triad of painless subcutaneous masses in the head or neck region, blood and tissue eosinophilia, and elevated serum Immunoglobulin E levels. The pathogenesis is poorly understood and treatments are unsatisfactory. KD is associated with allergic conditions such as asthma, rhinitis, and eczema.

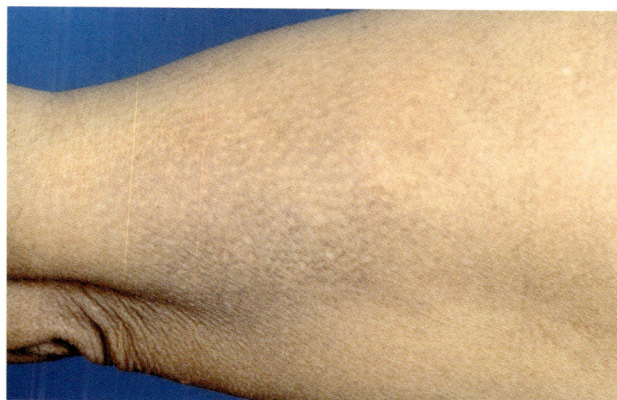

Figure 16–18 □ Primary cutaneous amyloidosis – macular variant. Primary cutaneous amyloidosis refers to deposition of amyloid in apparently previously normal skin with no evidence of deposits in internal organs. It occurs as a primary event and is not associated with an underlying chronic disease. The macular variety shows a lace-like pigmentation with rippled appearance as present on the arms of this middle-aged Indian lady. Macular amyloidosis is the most common variant of primary cutaneous amyloidosis seen in Asian-Indians. This condition affects females three times more frequently than males.

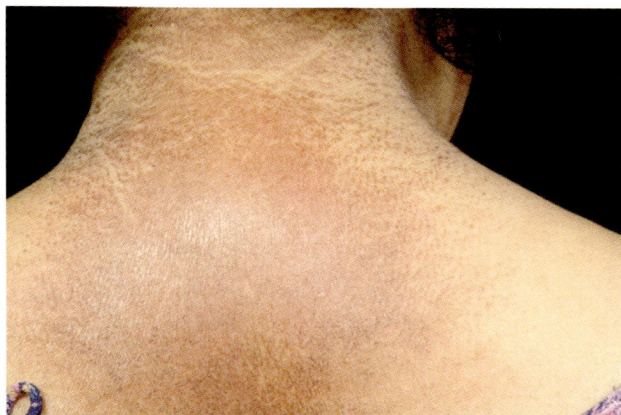

Figure 16–19 □ Macular amyloidosis – upper back. This is a common area of involvement. It may easily be confused with other eczematous conditions such as seborrheic dermatitis. However, close examination will usually reveal discrete brownish macules.

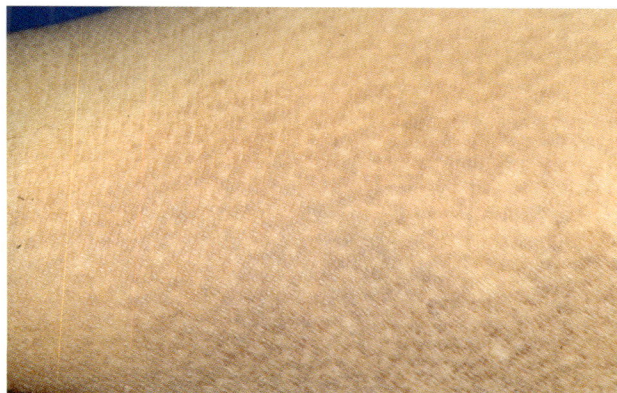

Figure 16–20 □ Primary cutaneous amyloidosis – macular variant. This close-up view of an arm clearly reveals the "rippled" pattern of the pigmented macules.

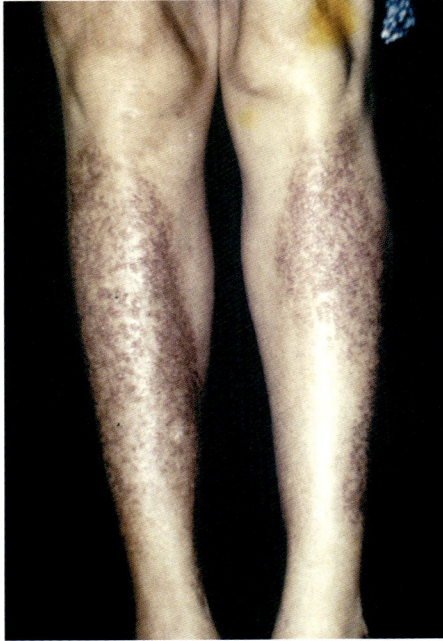

Figure 16–21 □ Primary cutaneous amyloidosis – papular variant. Papular lichen amyloidosis is the most common variant of primary cutaneous amyloidosis seen in Asian-Chinese. It resembles the skin of a lychee fruit. It presents as reddish-brown hyperkeratotic papules on the pretibial surfaces. Other sites that can be involved include the forearms and thighs. Pruritus is a prominent symptom. Most cases are sporadic although familial cases have been reported.

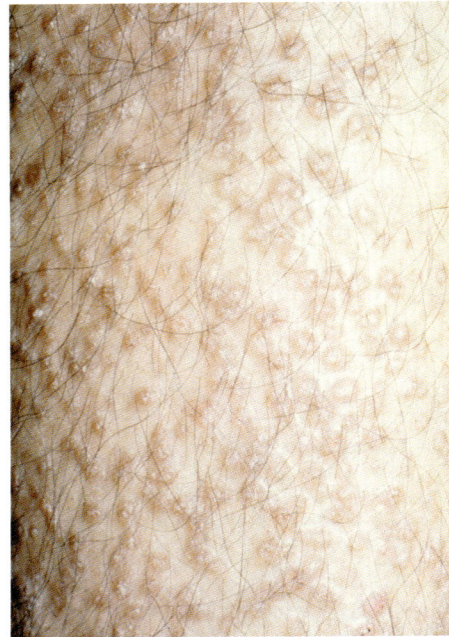

Figure 16–22 □ Primary cutaneous amyloidosis – papular variant. A close-up view of the lesions, clearly demonstrating the hyperkeratotic pigmented papules. The amyloid deposited in the skin binds to anti-keratin antibodies. These deposits also contain sulfhydryl groups, suggesting altered keratin as a source of these deposits. The actual pathogenesis is yet unknown although some have postulated that the deposition of amyloid is the result of itching and scratching.

Sexually Transmitted Infections and Non-STI Genital Dermatoses

Sen P. and Chan R.K.W.

Dermato-venereology as a specialty is practised in most parts of the world, *viz.* Europe (excluding the UK and Ireland), Asia, the Middle East, Africa, and most of Latin America. The dermatologist is well-positioned to diagnose and manage sexually transmitted infections (STIs) as these infections present with mucocutaneous lesions which the dermatologist is most familiar with.

Approximately one-third of the world's population lives in Asia with China, Indonesia, and India comprising some of the most populous nations. There exists a tremendous cultural diversity and this transcends through to the level of sexual practices. For example, in Asian cultures, there is a common factor as regards male dominance in sexual beliefs and practices, and this has been cited to be a reason for the high rate of STIs in the region. Complicating this are the influences of tradition, religion, migration, and politics which have strong effects on the prevalence and expression of STIs. For example, open and frank discussion about sex is still taboo in many Asian cultures and STIs are often attributed to immoral and perverted sexual practices. This results in poorly developed sex education in schools and poor health-seeking behavior, both of which hinder STI prevention and control.

The first part of this chapter covers the STIs (Figures 17–1 to 17–54), whilst the latter part covers the common non-STI genital dermatoses (Figures 17–55 to 17–79) which may be misdiagnosed or suspected to be STIs by doctors unfamiliar with their presentation.

STI-RELATED GENITAL DERMATOSES

Genital Ulcers (Figures 17–1 to 17–28)

Bacterial STIs, both ulcerative (syphilis, chancroid) and non-ulcerative (gonorrhoea, *Chlamydia trachomatis*), are still prevalent in many Asian countries. In the more developed parts of the region, however, traditional bacterial infections are becoming much less common, and replaced by those infections caused by viral pathogens.

Syphilis (Figures 17–1 to 17–18) is a systemic infection caused by *Treponema pallidum*. With the exception of mother-to-child transmission, syphilis is predominantly spread by direct contact with infectious lesions. Primary syphilis usually occurs two to six weeks following infection. It is characterized by a single or, less often, multiple, painless, indurated ulcer (chancre) at the site of inoculation. Secondary syphilis occurs two to six months following primary syphilis. This stage is characterized by variable mucocutaneous and systemic signs such as symmetrical non-pruritic rashes, mucous membrane lesions, patchy alopecia and generalized lymphadenopathy.

Latent syphilis is an asymptomatic phase with no clinical signs of organ involvement. Tertiary syphilis occurs five to ten years after secondary syphilis and includes benign tertiary syphilis characterized by gumma formation, cardio-vascular syphilis, and neurosyphilis.

Genital herpes (Figures 17–19 to 17–23) is caused by *Herpes simplex virus*, usually HSV type 2 but also by type 1. Transmission of the virus can occur through genital to genital, mouth to genital, genital to anal, or mouth to anal contact. The first episode of genital herpes is often severe, presenting with multiple grouped vesicles which rupture easily leaving painful erosions and ulcers. In the male, the lesions occur mainly on the prepuce and subpreputial areas of the penis; and in the female, on the vulva, vagina, and cervix.

Healing of uncomplicated lesions takes two to four weeks. Recurrent attacks are less severe than first-episode genital herpes. Groups of vesicles or erosions develop on a single anatomical site and these usually heal within ten days. Recurrences average five to eight attacks annually and are more frequent during the first two years of infection. Genital herpes caused by HSV1 generally recurs infrequently. It is now recognized that the majority of persons with HSV infection have mild, unrecognized, or subclinical disease and are unaware of the infection. They may shed the virus intermittently in the genital tract, thus unknowingly transmit the infection to their partners.

Patients presenting with lesions on the anogenital region should be questioned on sexual exposure and travel history. The possibility of chancroid, lymphogranuloma venereum, and granuloma inguinale (Figures 17–24 to 17–28) should be suspected if there has been sexual exposure in areas where these infections are still prevalent. Chancroid is a STI caused by the bacterium *Hemophilus*

ducreyi. This infection is very uncommon in Singapore, but still common in parts of India and Southeast Asia. The infection presents with one or more painful genital ulcers with a purulent base. The ulcers are usually foul-smelling and appear after an incubation period of 3 to 14 days. Associated inguinal lymphadenopathy (bubo) is common. Lymphogranuloma venereum is a sexually transmitted disease caused by the L1, L2, and L3 serovars of *Chlamydia trachomatis*. It presents with a transient genital ulcer and inguinal lymphadenitis (bubo) which is usually unilateral and becomes fluctuant. The genito-anorectal syndrome presents with lower abdominal pain and dyspareunia in females and homosexual males. Proctocolitis, perineal, and perianal inflammation can occur, resulting in fissures and strictures. Granuloma inguinale is a STI caused by the gram-negative bacillus *Calymmatobacterium granulomatis (Donovania granulomatis)*. This infection is still endemic in India, parts of South America, and Africa. It presents with "beefy", red, granulomatous genital ulcers.

Genital Discharges (Figures 17–29 to 17–47)

Gonorrhoea (Figures 17–29 to 17–37) is caused by *Neisseria gonorrhoeae*. The common sites of infection include the urethra, the endocervix, the rectum, the pharynx, and the conjunctiva. Hematogenous spread results in disseminated gonococcal infection (DGI). Gonorrhoea is clinically characterized by a profuse purulent discharge from the affected mucosal site, often accompanied by local pain or discomfort. However, asymptomatic infection occurs in 10% of urethral infection, in 50% of cervical infection, and in 80% of pharyngeal and rectal infection. Penicillin was thought to be the solution to gonorrhoea but instead bacteria have also evolved, resulting in Asia housing a large amount of antibiotic-resistant gonorrhoea.

Chlamydia trachomatis (Figures 17–38 to 17–43) is a bacterium which can cause a variety of genito-urinary infections, depending on the serotypes. Chlamydial genital infections occur frequently amongst sexually active adolescents and young adults. Lymphogranuloma venereum is caused by serotypes L1 to L3. Serotypes D to K cause non-gonococcal urethritis (NGU), muco-purulent cervicitis, proctitis, epididymitis, pneumonia, and inclusion conjunctivitis in the newborn. Many of the adult infections caused by chlamydia are asymptomatic.

Trichomoniasis (Figure 17–44) is an infection of the genital tract by the protozoan *Trichomonas vaginalis*. Women are the main carriers of the disease. Infected men are usually asymptomatic or may present with NGU.

Genital candidiasis (Figures 17–45 and 17–46) is the infection of the vulva, vagina, prepuce, and glans penis by *Candida albicans* or occasionally by other *Candida* species, *Torulopsis* species, or other yeasts. Female patients complain of vulval pruritus and discharge. Non-specific symptoms include soreness, burning, dyspareunia, and external dysuria. Male patients may complain of penile rash. Examination reveals vulval erythema, fissuring, satellite lesions, and thick curdy discharge in females, or white or red patches on the glans penis in males. Predisposing factors include diabetes mellitus, long-term oral antibiotics, systemic corticosteroids, and oral contraceptives.

Bacterial vaginosis (BV) is a condition resulting from replacement of the normal H_2O_2-producing *Lactobacillus* species in the vagina with high concentrations of anerobic bacteria (e.g. *Prevotella* species and *Mobiluncus* species), *Gardnerella vaginalis*, and *Mycoplasma hominis*. The exact role of sexual transmission in the pathogenesis of BV is unclear. BV may be asymptomatic or present with a foul-smelling, thin homogenous vaginal discharge.

Genital Growths (Figures 17–48 to 17–52)

Over 30 types of *human papilloma virus* (HPV) can infect the anogenital tract. HPV infection occurs as clinical lesions (condylomata acuminata, papular, and flat warts), subclinical lesions and latent HPV infection. Subclinical lesions are often only visible after application of acetic acid and magnification. Latent HPV occurs when HPV DNA can be demonstrated in the absence of clinical or histological evidence of infection.

Molluscum contagiosum is a viral infection caused by a pox virus. Genital molluscum infections in adults are usually sexually transmitted. Individual lesions of molluscum contagiosum are discrete, smooth, pearly, or flesh-colored, dome-shaped papules and are often confined to the genital area. Each papule may have a mildly erythematous base and a central punctum beneath, in which lies a white curd-like core.

Parasitic Skin Infestations (Figures 17–53 to 17–54)

Scabies is an infestation by the mite, *sarcoptes scabiei var. hominis*. The clinical features of scabies are pruritic papules on the genitals, finger webs, wrists, axillae, and buttocks. There is a nocturnal exacerbation of the itch. Family members may have similar symptoms. The mite can be demonstrated by microscopic examination of scrapings from burrows on the skin.

Pubic lice is an infestation of the anogenital region by the crab louse, *phthirus pubis*. In adults, it is usually sexually transmitted and infestation is indicated by the presence of brown adult lice on the pubic skin and by their ova (nits) on pubic hair shafts. Small hemorrhagic spots are also seen on the pubic or genital skin and underwear. The presence of lice or nits recovered from pubic hair confirms the diagnosis.

NON-STI GENITAL DERMATOSES
(Figures 17–55 to 17–79)

These can be categorized into inflammatory conditions and growths (benign and malignant). Non-sexually transmitted genital skin conditions affecting Asian patients may be modified by increased pigmentation as well as the hot and humid conditions in many areas of the body leading to greater itch and excoriations. For example, lesions of psoriasis and lichen planus affecting the anogenital epithelium may appear darker and exhibit more lichenification. Traditional practices to enhance the sexual experience in this region include the introduction of inert substances and objects into the penis, and this should be remembered when one is faced with an unusual clinical situation.

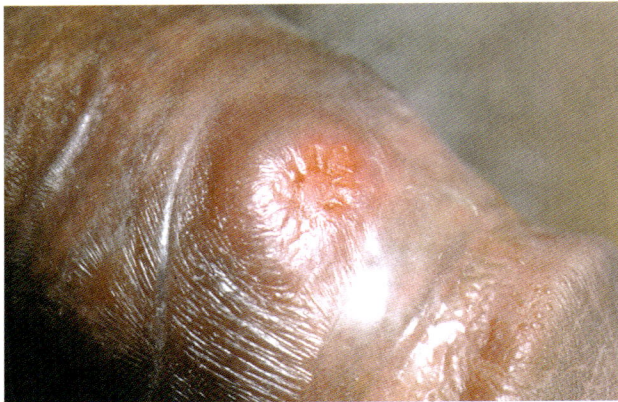

Figure 17–1 □ Primary syphilis – penile chancre. A painless indurated ulcer which characterizes the primary stage of syphilis. It presents following an incubation period usually of between 14 to 21 days and occurs at the site of inoculation. It commonly appears on the penis and starts off as a papule which breaks down and ulcerates.

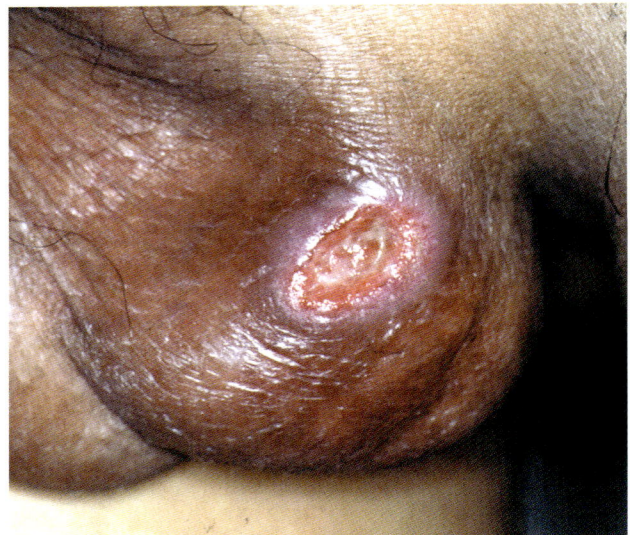

Figure 17–2 □ Primary syphilis – scrotal chancre. The chancre has an indurated edge, with a clean yellow base and feels indurated or "button-like" on palpation. The ulcer may produce a serous exudate, and a swab taken from the base will demonstrate the characteristic "cork-screw" *Treponema pallidum* which exhibits characteristic movements using dark-field microscopy.

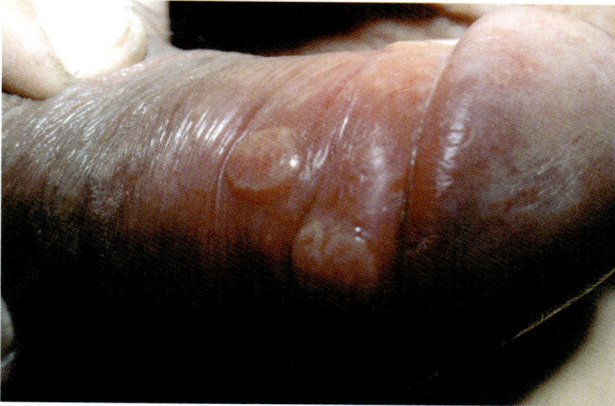

Figure 17–3 □ **Primary syphilis – multiple atypical penile chancres.** Chancres may appear on the genitalia as multiple ulcers. Some of these may have a sloughy appearance when secondarily infected and, in these cases, may present with tenderness and a pus-filled discharge. The differential diagnoses are chancroid and herpes infection which should be excluded with appropriate microbiological investigations.

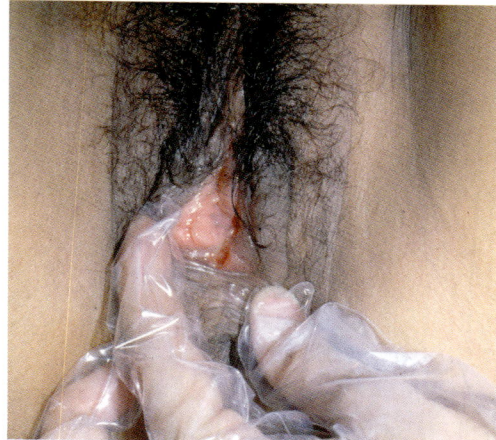

Figure 17–4 □ **Primary syphilis – vulval chancre.** Painless indurated ulcers are seen on the vulva of this female patient. These primary syphilitic ulcers will exhibit spontaneous resolution, and because they are often hidden and painless, tend to be unnoticed by affected females. Treatment of choice for primary syphilis is a single intramuscular injection of benzathine penicillin G 2.4 megaunits.

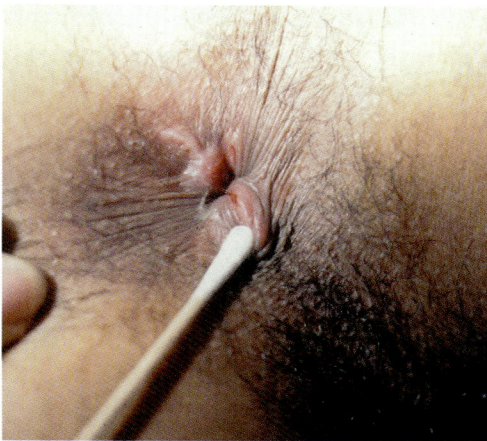

Figure 17–5 □ **Primary syphilis – anal chancre.** This chancre resulted following anal intercourse. Although more commonly presenting on the genitalia, syphilitic chancres can occur on other parts of the body such as the lips, on the buccal mucosa, or even on the hands.

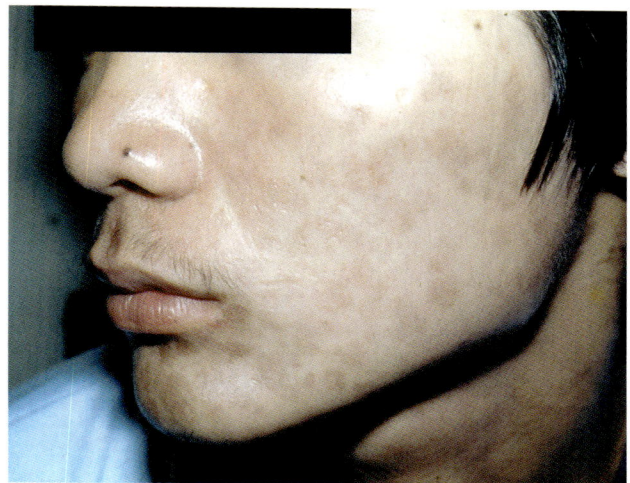

Figure 17–6 □ **Secondary syphilis – early macular rash.** A pink, macular, non-pruritic rash that is not associated with the presence locally of the causative organism. The secondary stage of syphilis occurs approximately six to eight weeks following infection and after the healing of the primary chancre. The treponemes disseminate hematogenously throughout the body in this highly infectious stage, and the VDRL/RPR titres are typically high. As this rash appears rather non-specific, a high index of suspicion is necessary to clinch the diagnosis.

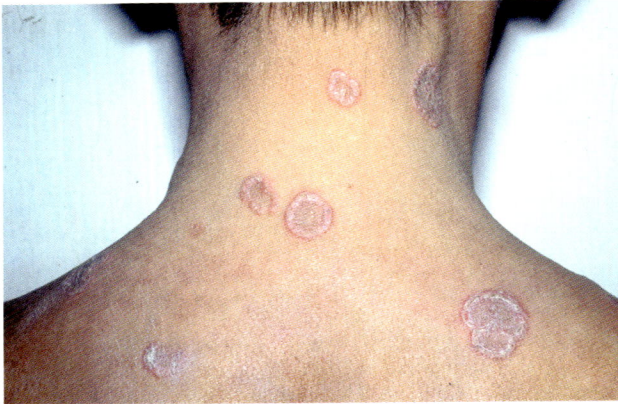

Figure 17–7 □ Annular papulosquamous lesions of secondary syphilis. Following the early macular stage, the lesions become more papular and scaly forming an annular configuration. They are characteristically non-pruritic, coppery-red in color, and symmetrical in distribution. These may be associated with a non-specific, flu-like illness consisting of a low-grade fever, headache, nasal discharge, sore throat, and arthralgia. The lesions are non-scarring and resolve quickly after effective treatment with penicillin.

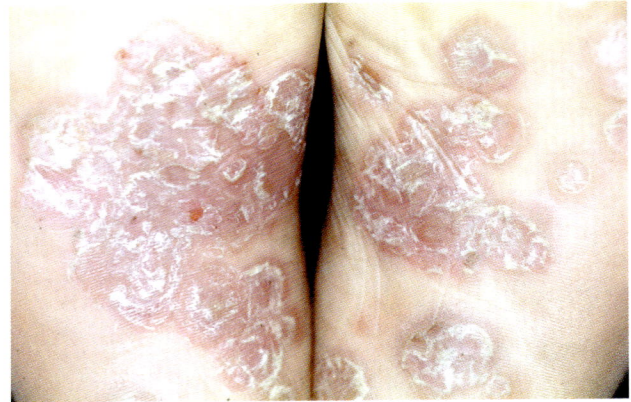

Figure 17–8 □ Secondary syphilis – papulosquamous plantar lesions. These annular, coppery-red, well-demarcated papules and plaques with thick scales may resemble the lesions of psoriasis. They are bilateral and symmetrically distributed and may appear in the absence of truncal involvement. Secondary syphilis has a special predilection for the palms and soles of the feet. These hyperkeratotic lesions on the soles may fissure and involvement of the toe webs may be mistaken for tinea pedis. The lesions on the palms can appear as a combination of macular as well as papulosquamous lesions.

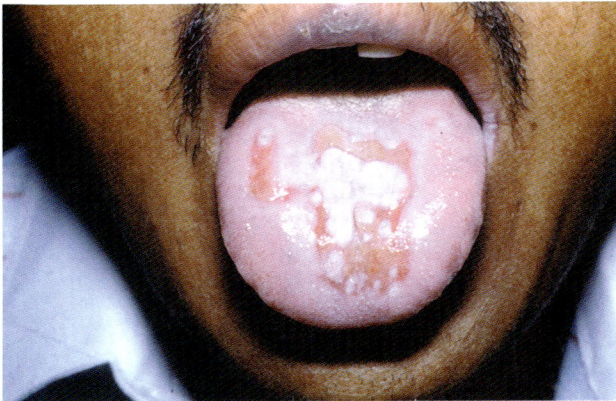

Figure 17–9 □ Secondary syphilis involving the tongue. This appears as sharply demarcated, off-white oval patches on the tongue. The lesions are associated with flattened papillae and may appear ulcerated. These mucosal lesions occur simultaneously with the cutaneous lesions of secondary syphilis and are teeming with spirochaetes.

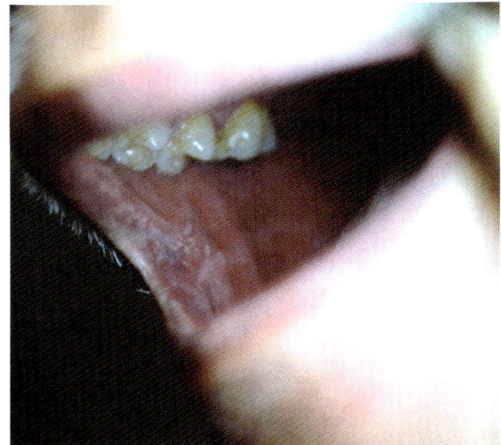

Figure 17–10 □ Secondary syphilis – oral ulcers. Small, white, adherent mucous patches in the form of papules are seen along the right buccal mucosa in this patient who presented with simultaneous papulosquamous rashes on his palms and soles. Contiguous lesions are seen forming serpiginous or "snail-track" ulcers.

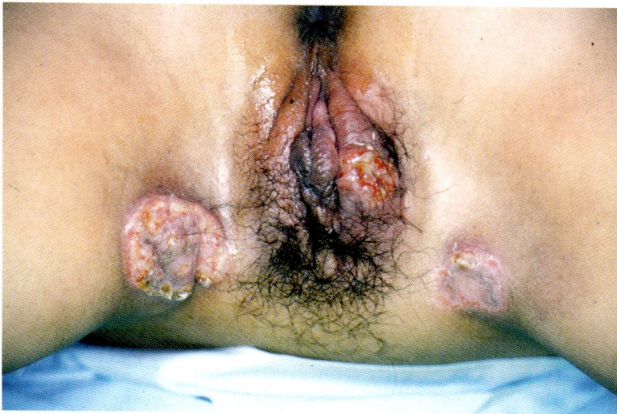

Figure 17–11 □ Condyloma lata affecting vulva and intertriginous sites. The papular lesions of secondary syphilis which occur on the moist areas of the body are called condyloma lata. These consist of eroded weeping papules with a tendency to coalesce and hypertrophy forming large gray lesions. Although commonly occurring on the vulva, they may also be found in other intertriginous sites such as the groin, axillae, inframammary area, the umbilicus, or the toe webs.

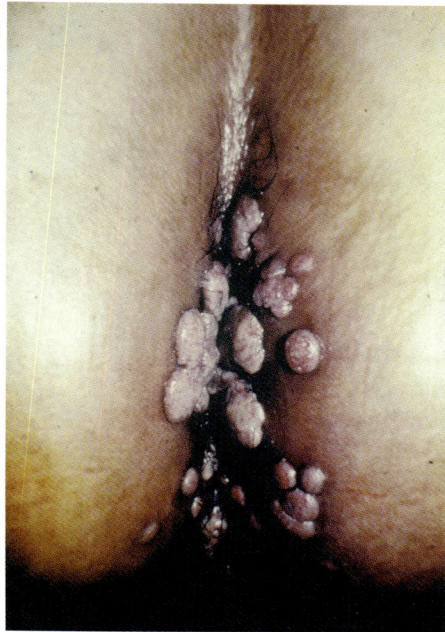

Figure 17–12 □ Perianal condyloma lata. These large eruptions of hypertrophic eroding papules commonly affect the anus and are moist and highly infectious. Dark-ground microscopy will yield *Treponema pallidum*.

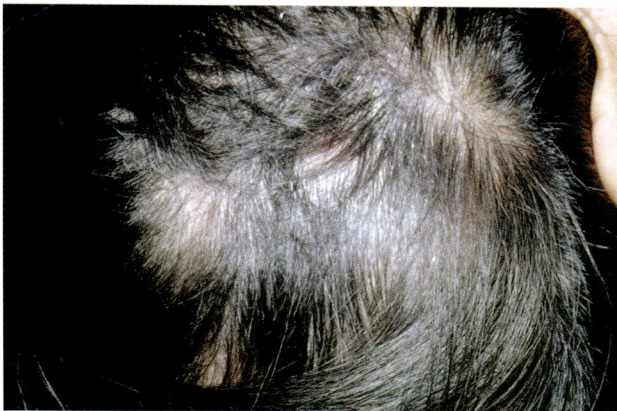

Figure 17–13 □ Secondary syphilis – alopecia. This appears as a patchy, non-scarring alopecia with a characteristic "moth-eaten" appearance. Other manifestations include lymphadenopathy, iritis, headache, and meningismus.

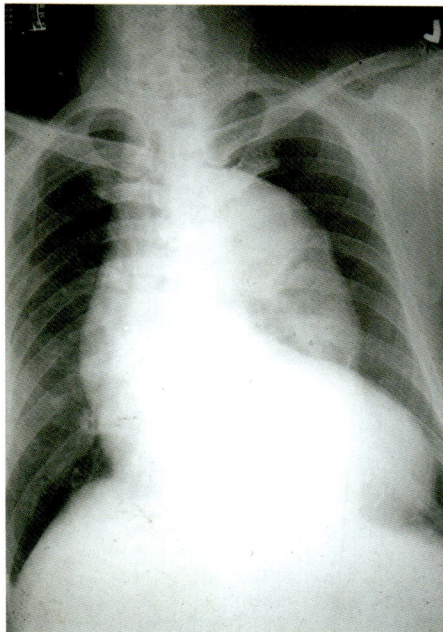

Figure 17–14 □ Aortic aneurysm of cardiovascular syphilis. A large aneurysm of the ascending aorta. Cardiovascular syphilis can lead to uncomplicated aortitis, aneurysms of the thoracic aorta, aortic valvulitis with regurgitation, and stenosis of the coronary ostia. These complications arise when syphilis goes untreated for more than ten years or so.

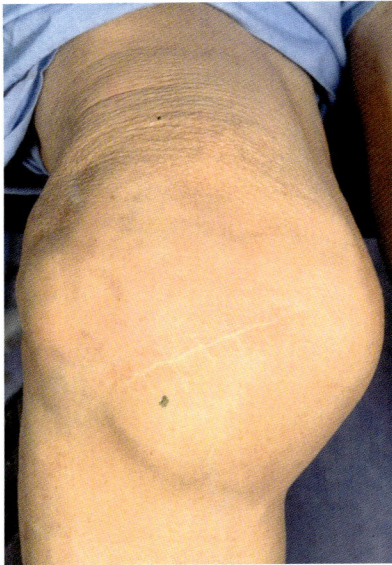

Figure 17–15 □ Charcot's joint of neurosyphilis. A large dystrophic painless knee joint resulting from repeated trauma following untreated syphilis. Neurosyphilis can occur at any stage of syphilis after the primary stage and is not limited to tertiary syphilis. It is classified into asymptomatic, meningeal, parenchymatous, and gummatous. Tabes dorsalis is a form of parenchymatous neurosyphilis affecting the spinal cord and results in, amongst other things, loss of sensation and destruction of the joints (Charcot's joints) by repeated trauma.

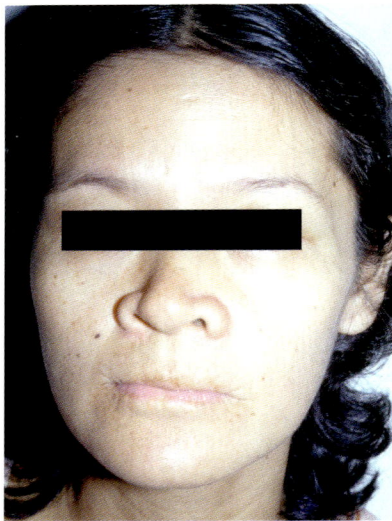

Figure 17–16 □ Early congenital syphilis. Erythematous papulosquamous rash on the palms of this infant. It occurs within the first two years of life. This is seen rarely now with routine antenatal serological screening of expectant mothers. Infections that occur early in pregnancy can result in abortion or stillbirth. The neonate presents with syphilitic rhinitis or "snuffles" and the characteristic bullae or coppery-red papular rash on the palms and soles. In two-thirds of cases, the signs appear in the third to eight week of life.

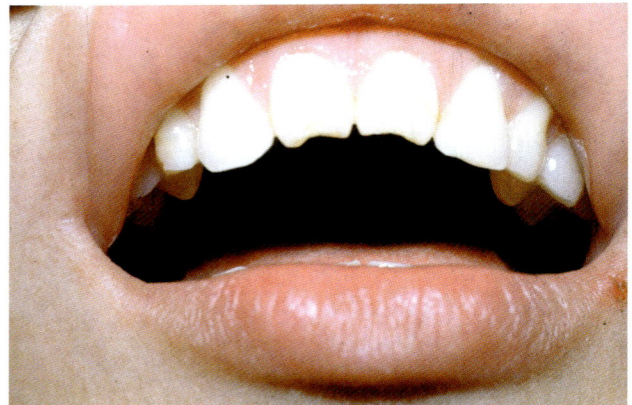

Figure 17–17 □ Late congenital syphilis. A saddle nose, frontal bossing of the forehead, and perioral rhagades are seen in this adult female. The characteristic clinical features and malformations (stigmata) generally appear in children from 5 to 16 years of age. They include perforation of the palate and the collapse of the nose resulting from gummata, frontal bossing of the forehead, and bowing of the tibia secondary to periostitis. Rhagades are seen here as linear scars in the form of "spokes of a wheel", radiating from the angles of the mouth. They can also be found around the eyes, chin, and anus. Interstitial keratitis, short maxillae, protuberant mandibles, a high palatal arch, eighth nerve deafness, and Clutton's joints are other characteristic features.

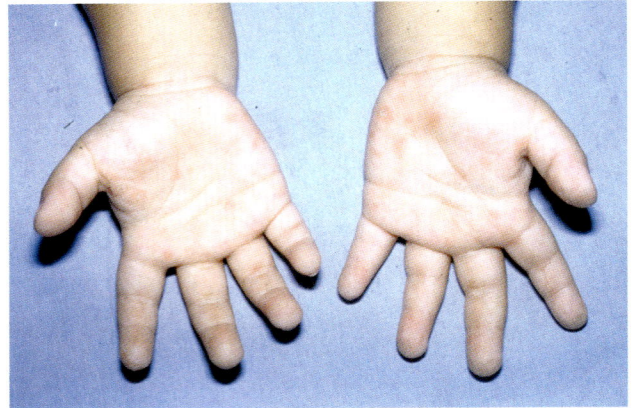

Figure 17–18 □ Late congenital syphilis – Hutchinson's teeth. The incisors and canines of the permanent dentition are small, tapered toward the apex, widely spaced, with a notched biting edge. This is an abnormality of the upper central incisors that occurs after six years of age. They are due to defective development of the permanent teeth buds. The molars can also be affected and are characterized by multiple small cusps in a circle known as "mulberry molars". Hutchinson's triad includes the combination of nerve deafness, abnormal teeth, and interstitial keratitis.

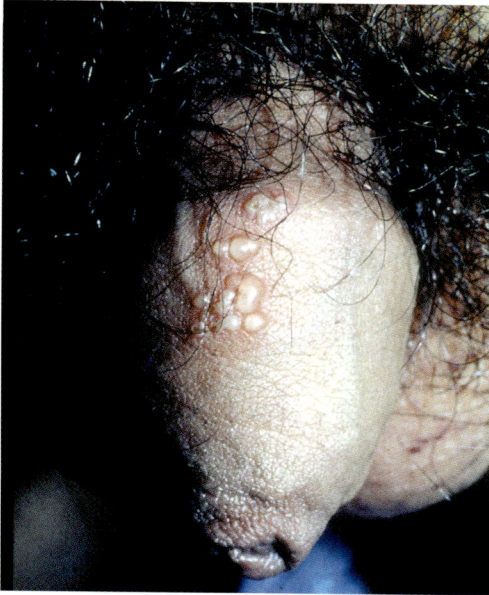

Figure 17–19 □ **Primary genital herpes in a male.** A crop of painful vesicles on the penile shaft. They have progressed to erosions over several days. The first attack is characteristically very painful and occurs within three days to two weeks of exposure to infection. This is associated with tender inguinal lymphadenopathy in about 20% of patients.

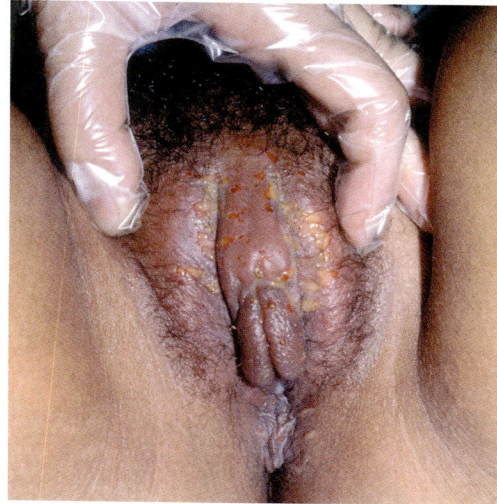

Figure 17–20 □ **Primary genital herpes in a female.** Extensive vesicles and erosions are seen on the vulva of this patient. Herpetic lesions may also be found on the cervix. The first attack may be associated with a mild constitutional disturbance consisting of fever, headache, and myalgia. Dysuria and frank urinary retention can also occur. Symptoms and the formation of new lesions continue with active viral shedding for seven to ten days; complete resolution of lesions occurs after about three weeks.

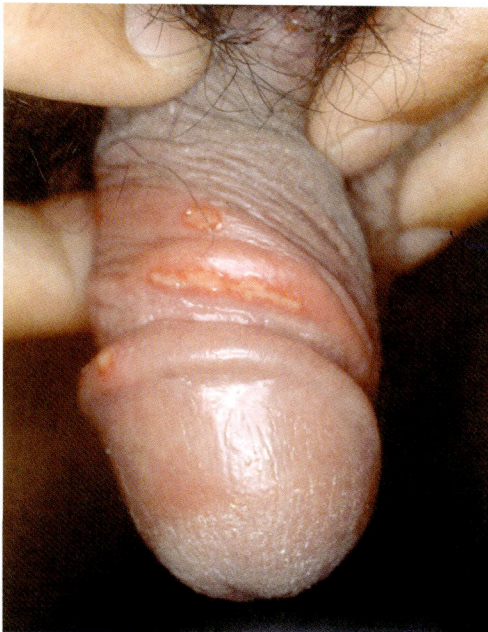

Figure 17–21 □ **Recurrent genital herpes in a male.** These painful grouped erosions are similar in clinical presentation but tend to be less severe than the primary episode. Recurrent attacks occur when the latent herpes virus is reactivated. HSV2 is the aetiological agent in the majority of genital HSV infections. HSV1 infection results in the same acute clinical syndrome but is associated with fewer recurrences.

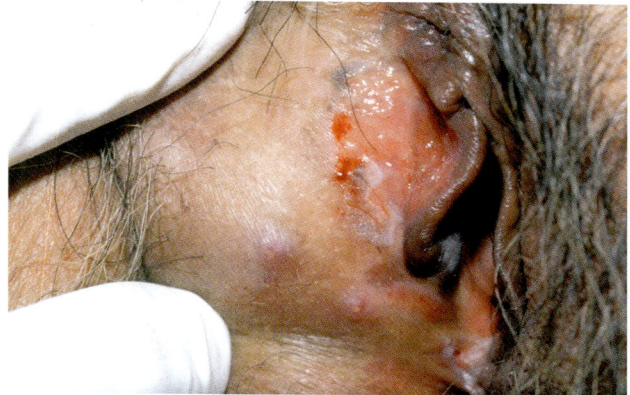

Figure 17–22 □ **Recurrent genital herpes in a female.** Painful erosions on the labia majora. Clinical recurrences of genital herpes infection typically occur within a year of primary infection. This may be associated with factors that promote viral protein synthesis such as stress, trauma, fatigue, and sunlight exposure. Patients typically experience prodromal symptoms of itch, burning, or tingling at the site of the eruption. This is followed by a crop of painful vesicles which progress through stages of ulceration and crusting. The lesions are typically smaller and fewer in number than are seen in the primary disease, and are associated with mild or no constitutional symptoms.

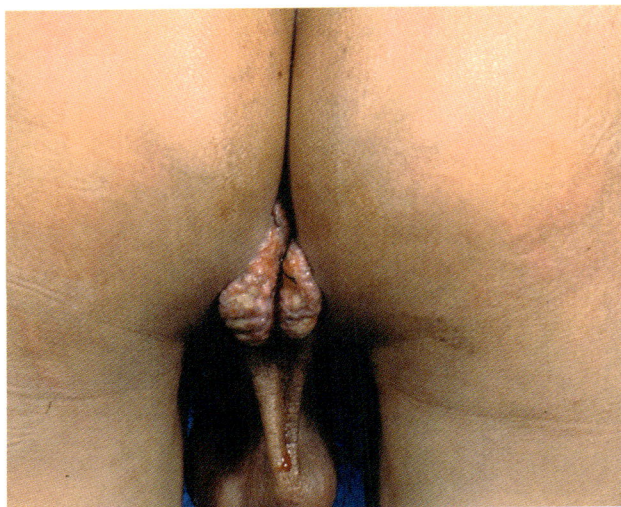

Figure 17–23 □ Recurrent genital herpes – anal. Painful anal erosions in a male who practices anal sexual intercourse. Patients with recurrent anogenital herpes typically experience three to four recurring episodes a year which can be treated with short courses of oral antiviral medications. More frequent recurrences resulting in psycho-sexual problems may require antiviral suppressive therapy.

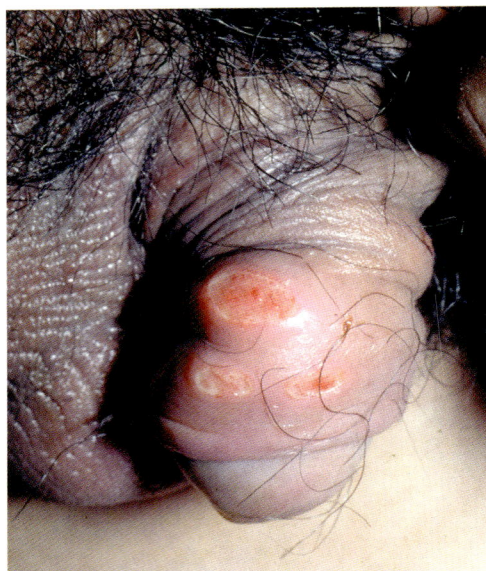

Figure 17–24 □ Chancroid – penile ulcers. Multiple painful, purulent penile ulcers with a foul-smelling discharge. Chancroid is an acute ulcerative STI that is endemic in the tropics and subtropics. It is caused by the bacteria, *Hemophilus ducreyi* and the incubation period ranges from one to seven days. The ulcers have a predilection for the preputial margin, frenulum, and coronal sulcus in males as these are sites of trauma during sexual intercourse through which the organism enters through minor abrasions. Autoinoculation of adjacent skin results in confluent ulcers or "kissing lesions".

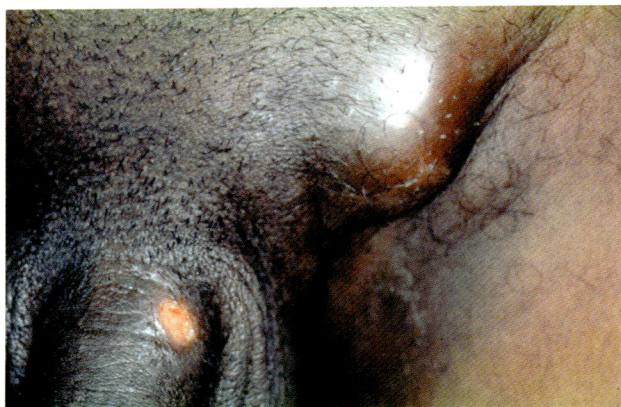

Figure 17–25 □ Chancroid – inguinal bubo. Erythematous, tender, pointing, left inguinal bubo with a solitary penile ulcer. Chancroid is associated with painful inguinal lymphadenitis in about 50% of patients and this tends to occur seven to 14 days after infection. It is usually unilateral but can also be bilateral; it can occasionally be the presenting feature if the ulcer goes unnoticed. The bubo consists of a group of suppurative inguinal lymph nodes matted together. Complications from delayed treatment may result in abscess formation, rupture, and discharging sinuses with scarring.

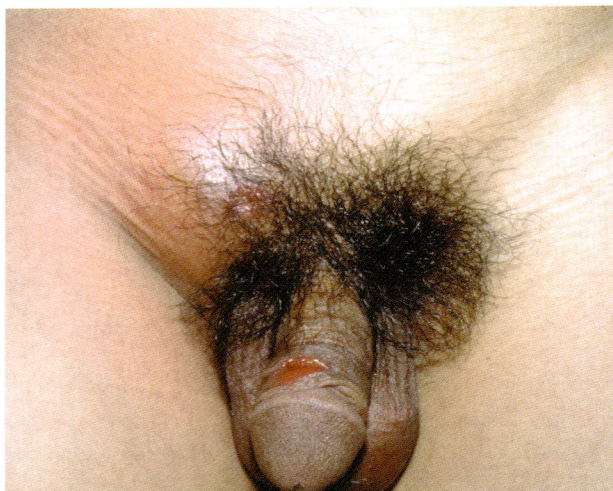

Figure 17–26 □ Lymphogranulomo venereum – primary lesion. Non-tender penile ulcer with right inguinal bubo. This is a systemic STI caused by *Chlamydia trachomatis* serovars L1, L2, and L3. It occurs in the tropics and subtropics. The primary lesion is often transient and goes unnoticed. It consists of a non-tender papule or ulcer commonly on the coronal sulcus or penile shaft that occurs after an incubation period of 3 to 30 days. It may also present as a urethritis if the ulcer is located internally. The primary lesion usually heals without scarring after a few days.

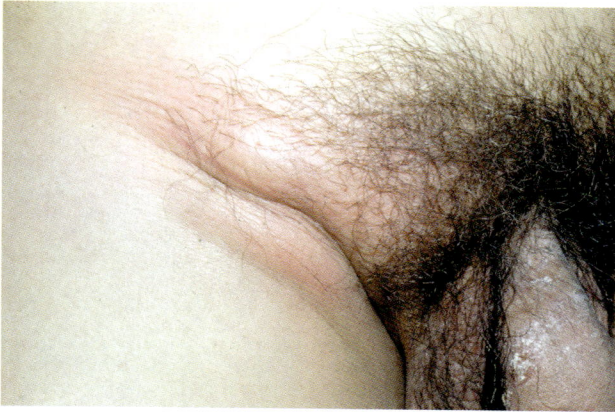

Figure 17–27 □ Lymphogranuloma venereum – inguinal syndrome with "groove sign". Right inguinal and femoral buboes resulting in the "groove sign". The "inguinal syndrome" occurs two to six weeks after the primary stage. Patients present with tender inguinal and/or femoral lymphadenopathy or bubo formation. Involvement of both the femoral and inguinal lymph nodes and separation by the inguinal ligament result in the "groove sign". This stage can be associated with constitutional symptoms and in less than 10% of cases with erythema nodosum. The late manifestations are termed the "genito-anorectal syndrome".

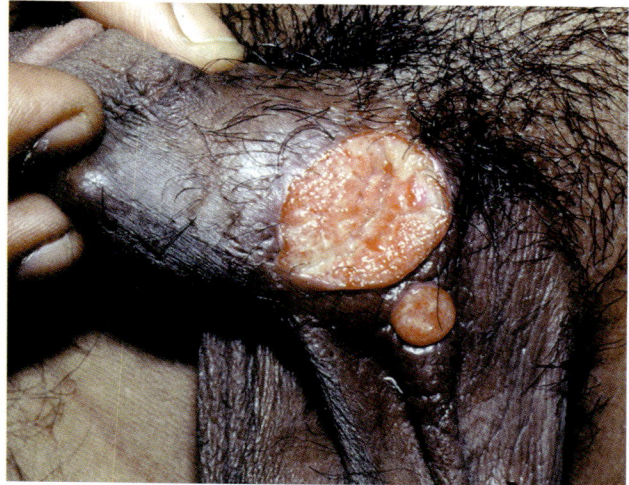

Figure 17–28 □ Granuloma inguinale (Donovanosis) – ulcerovegetative penile ulcer. Two large, painless, clean, "beefy red" ulcers that have a friable base and distinct raised rolled margins. This is a chronic ulcerative and granulomatous STI caused by the gram-negative bacillus, *Calymmatobacterium granulomatis*. The incubation period ranges from one week to three months, and patients may present with four morphological skin lesions: ulcerovegetative, nodular, cicatricial, and hypertrophic types. The ulcerovegetative type is the most common and commences as painless small nodules or papules which break down to form one or more large ulcers. They occur most commonly on the prepuce or coronal sulcus. Subcutaneous spread to the inguinal lymph nodes may result in "pseudobubo" formation.

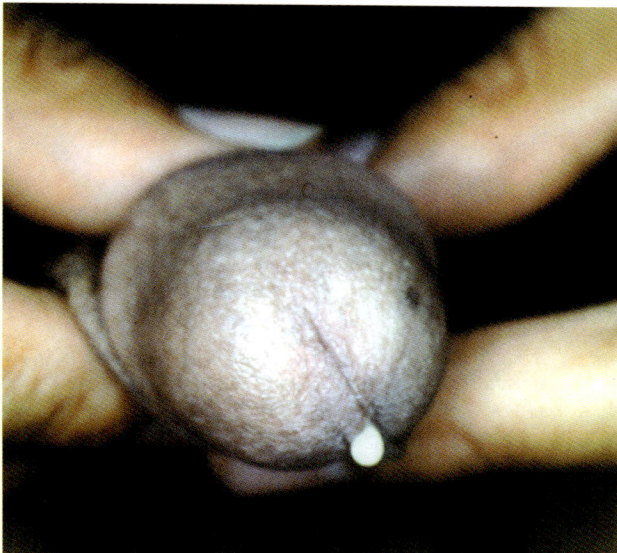

Figure 17–29 □ Gonorrhoea – penile discharge. A thick, yellow mucopurulent or purulent urethral discharge which may be profuse. Gonorrhoea is a STI caused by infection by the gram-negative diplococcus, *Neisseria gonorrhoeae*. It is transmitted by direct inoculation of secretions between mucous membranes. In males, it commonly presents after an incubation period of four to seven days.

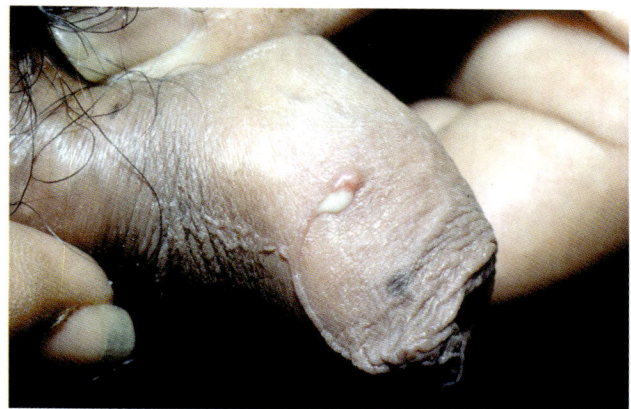

Figure 17–30 □ Gonorrhoea – median raphe sinus infection. An indurated, red, tender swelling on the surface of the penis with a purulent discharge. Purulent gonococcal discharge may present with infections of anatomical anomalies such as a median raphe sinus. Treatment in these unusual sites often requires more intensive regimens than uncomplicated infections.

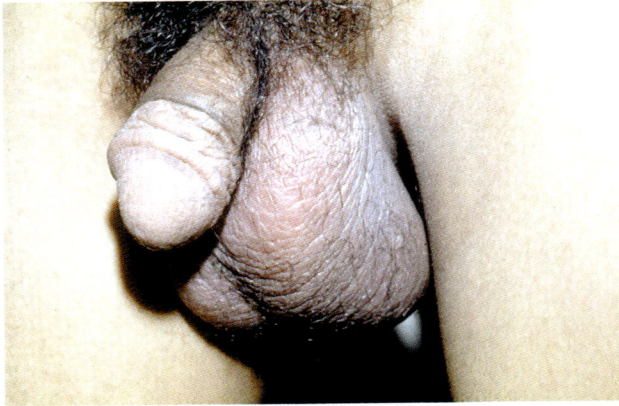

Figure 17–31 □ Gonorrhoea – epididymo-orchitis. This presents as acute pain and swelling of the epididymis and testis; it is characteristically very tender. It results from the spread of gonococcal infection from the urethra and can occur early on in the infection, occasionally being the presenting feature of a gonococcal infection.

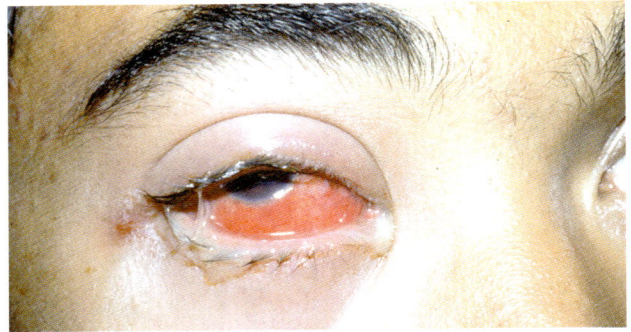

Figure 17–32 □ Gonococcal opthalmia. A thick, sticky, mucopurulent discharge occurring at the margins of the eyelid. It is associated with swelling of the eyelids and erythema of the eye due to subconjunctival hemorrhages. It is caused by autoinoculation of secretions from associated genital infection. If left untreated, corneal ulceration or perforation and panopthalmitis may result.

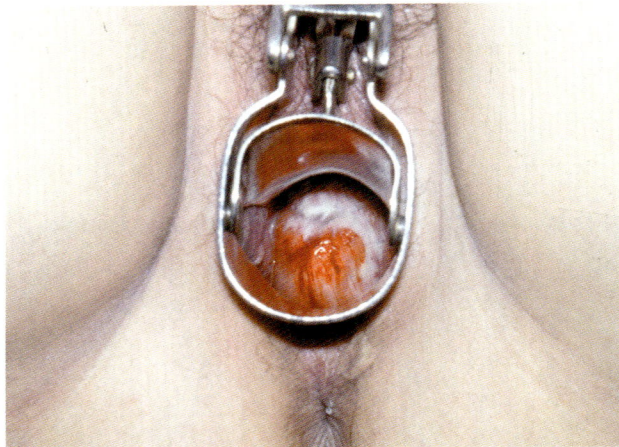

Figure 17–33 □ Gonorrhoea – vaginal and cervical discharge. A mucopurulent or purulent vaginal discharge that may be profuse and even blood-stained. The cervix is seen here to be edematous and inflamed. Contiguous, upward spread of infection may result in endometritis and salpingitis. These complications may result in long-term sequelae of infertility and an increased risk of ectopic pregnancy.

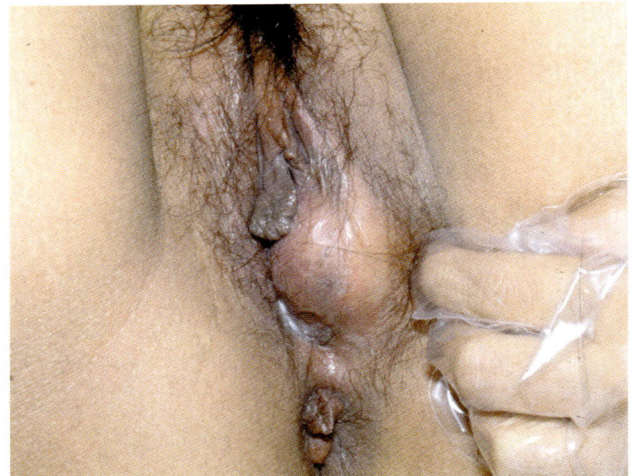

Figure 17–34 □ Gonorrhoea complications – Bartholin's gland abscess. An acutely tender swelling of the Bartholin's gland within the left vulva that has resulted in the formation of an abscess. This is a local complication of gonococcal infection and may require surgical intervention for management.

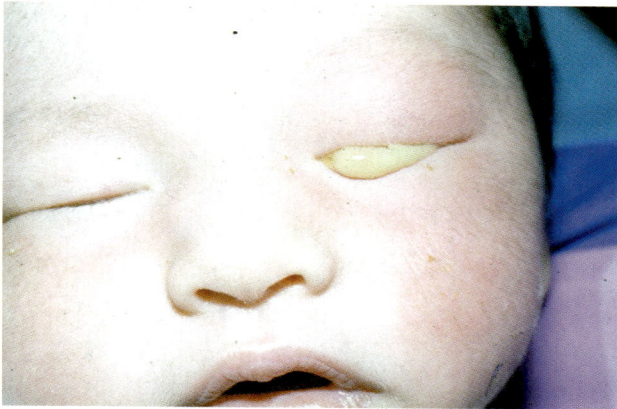

Figure 17–35 □ Neonatal gonococcal opthalmia. A profuse, thick, purulent, yellow discharge from the margins of the eyelid. There is associated edema and erythema of the eyelid and the infant is unable to open his eye as a result. It occurs through inoculation during passage through the birth canal during vaginal delivery in infected mothers and often presents one to seven days after birth.

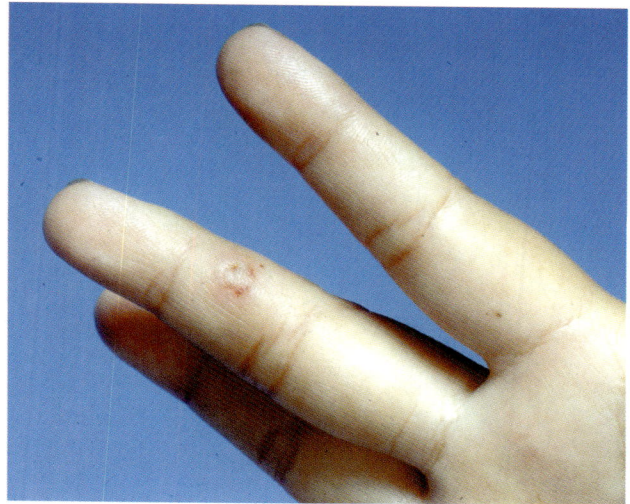

Figure 17–36 □ Disseminated gonococcal infection – septic gonococcal dermatitis. This is seen here as a hemorrhagic pustule with a red halo on the right middle finger. Lesions may also present as macules, papules, vesicles, or bullae, and commonly occur on the limbs as single lesions or in crops. The lesions result from hematological spread of *Neisseria gonorrhoeae* and generally heal within a few days without scarring.

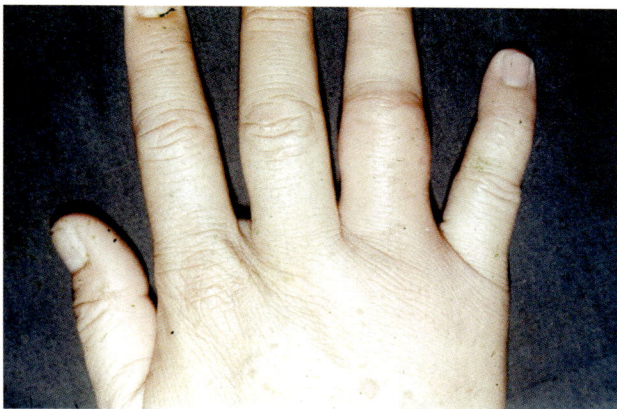

Figure 17–37 □ Disseminated gonococcal infection – septic arthritis. Erythema and swelling are seen around the proximal interphalangeal joint of the right ring finger. It is very tender and the patient may present with associated constitutional symptoms of fever. Culture of the synovial fluid will reveal the presence of the infecting organism. However, blood cultures are often negative.

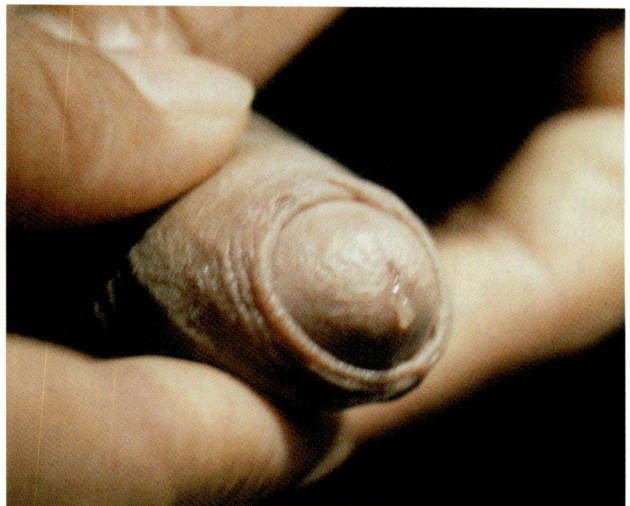

Figure 17–38 □ Non-gonococcal urethritis. A clear, slightly mucoid discharge is seen at the urethral meatus. The discharge is less profuse than that resulting from gonococcal infection and is often associated with dysuria or itch along the urethra. The incubation period may vary from two days to three weeks. *Chlamydia trachomatis* (serovars D-K) is the causative organism in over 50% of cases.

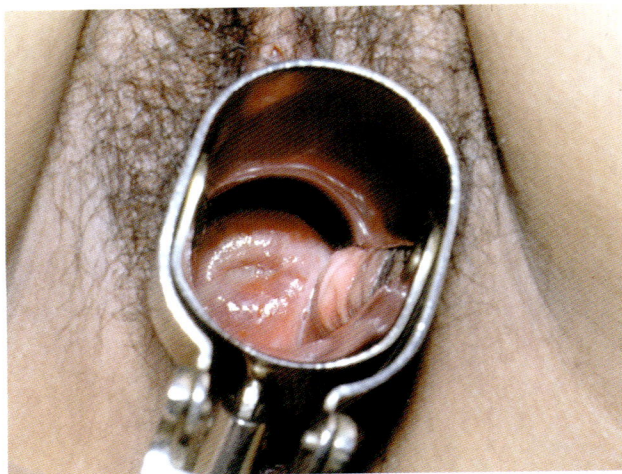

Figure 17–39 ☐ Chlamydial cervicitis. A mucopurulent discharge that appears yellow on a cotton-tipped swab. It is caused by infection by *Chlamydia trachomatis* serovars D-K. There may also be edema, erythema, and contact bleeding on examination of the cervix. However, patients are often asymptomatic and the diagnosis is made after examination and laboratory tests.

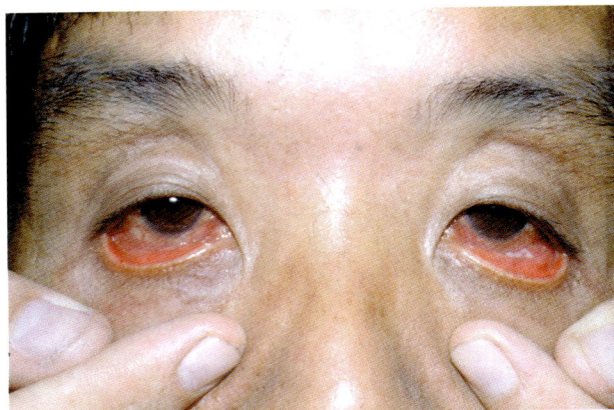

Figure 17–40 ☐ Reiter's disease – iritis. Bilateral conjunctivitis with subconjunctival hemorrhage is seen in this patient. There is also subtarsal hemorrhage. Iritis occurs more commonly in late recurrent attacks of Reiter's disease and occurs in approximately 5% of first episodes. Other ophthalmic complications are anterior uveitis, glaucoma, and keratitis. Reiter's disease consists of a triad of urethritis, arthritis, and conjunctivitis.

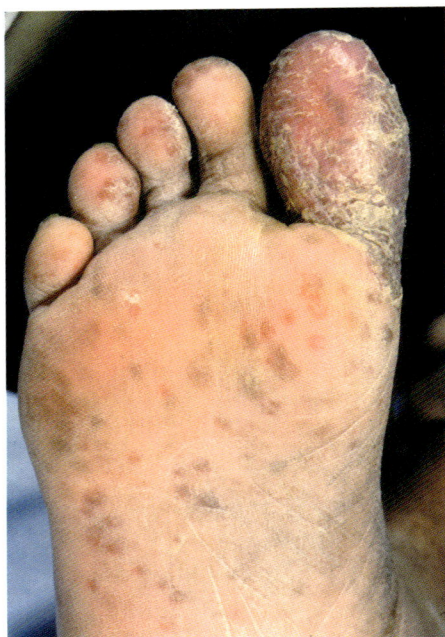

Figure 17–41 ☐ Reiter's disease – keratoderma blenorrhagicum. Hyperkeratotic orange-red papules and plaques are seen on the sole of the foot. Some of the plaques are seen to have a collarette of scales. It most commonly appears on the palms and soles but it can also occur on the scalp and trunk. Keratoderma blenorrhagicum generally appears one to two months after the onset of iritis and arthritis. Differential diagnoses include secondary syphilis and psoriasis.

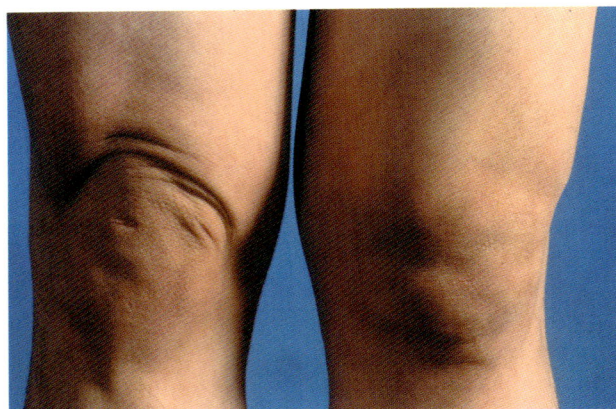

Figure 17–42 ☐ Reiter's disease – peripheral arthritis. There is an asymmetric swelling of the left knee due to a large effusion and an associated erythema and warmth over the joint. This asymmetric pauciarticular arthritis predominantly affecting the lower extremities is characteristically seen in this condition. Other joint involvements are axial arthritis and enthesitis involving the Achilles tendons.

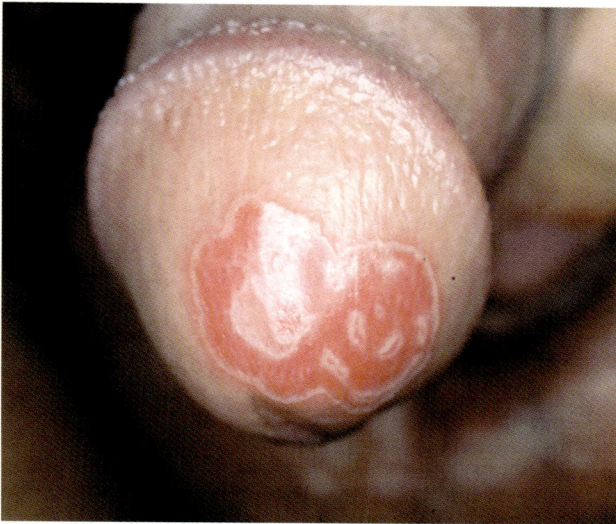

Figure 17–43 □ Reiter's disease – circinate balanitis. Well-demarcated, erythematous, and serpiginous annular lesions with raised margins are seen on the glans penis. The lesions can occur independently of the urethritis. They consist of moist, red erosions which coalesce to form serpiginous borders and are usually non-tender.

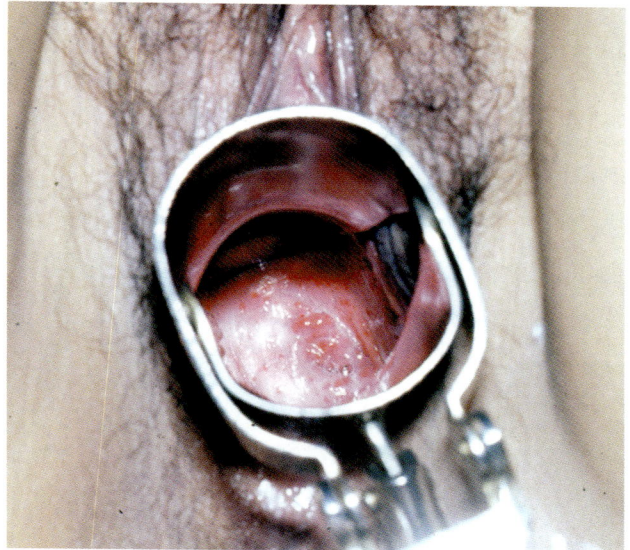

Figure 17–44 □ Trichomoniasis. A frothy, grayish-green discharge that is typically malodorous. It is caused by infection by *Trichomonas vaginalis*. The cervix is studded with punctate bleeding erosions giving it a "strawberry" appearance. Direct microscopy of a wet (normal saline) mount of vaginal secretions will demonstrate the trichomonads.

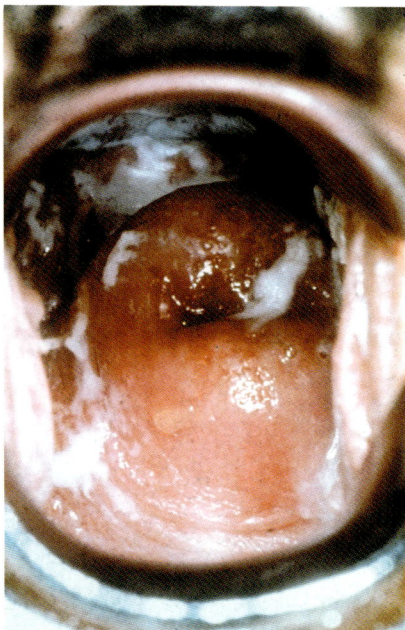

Figure 17–45 □ Vaginal candidiasis. A thick, curdy, white, or yellow vaginal discharge caused by infection by the yeast *Candida albicans*. The patient may complain of associated vulval pruritus or soreness. The infection is predisposed to in pregnancy, diabetes mellitus, or the recent use of oral antibiotics.

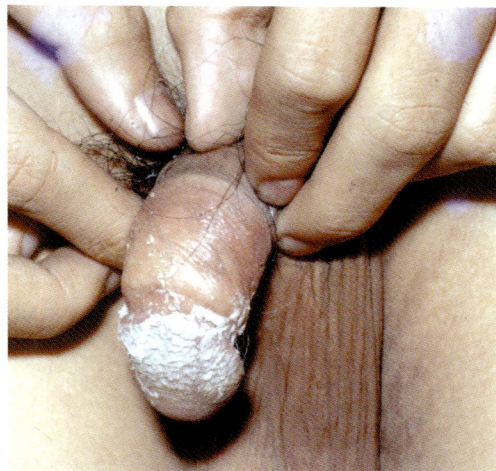

Figure 17–46 □ Candidal balanitis. A thick, white, cheesy coating on the glans penis with adjacent erythema of the penile shaft. This may present with an erythematous papular eruption. This condition is commonly seen in men with diabetes mellitus who have poor blood sugar control. It may occasionally be the presenting feature in a newly diagnosed diabetic.

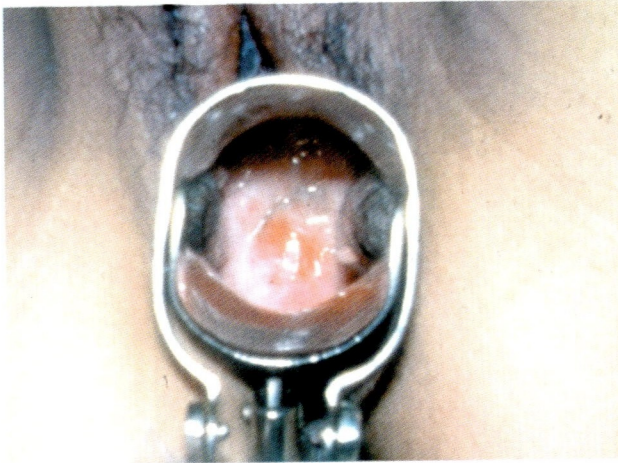

Figure 17–47 □ **Bacterial vaginosis.** A thin, homogenous, gray-white discharge is seen; it is often malodorous and may be associated with itch. The diagnosis is confirmed by the presence of clue cells on microscopy, a positive whiff test, and a pH of more than 4.5. This condition is due to a change in vaginal bacterial flora with a loss of normal lactobacilli and an increase in anerobic bacteria.

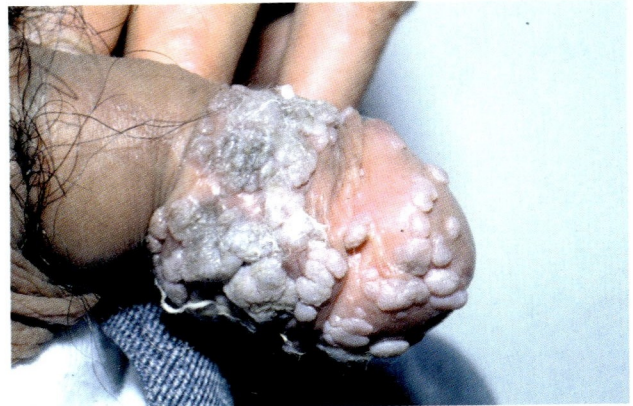

Figure 17–48 □ **Genital warts (condyloma acuminata) – penile.** Extensive grayish-white, verrucous papules are seen on the glans penis, coronal sulcus, and penile shaft. They are clustered together forming a cauliflower-like growth. This is a STI caused by infection with human papilloma virus (HPV).

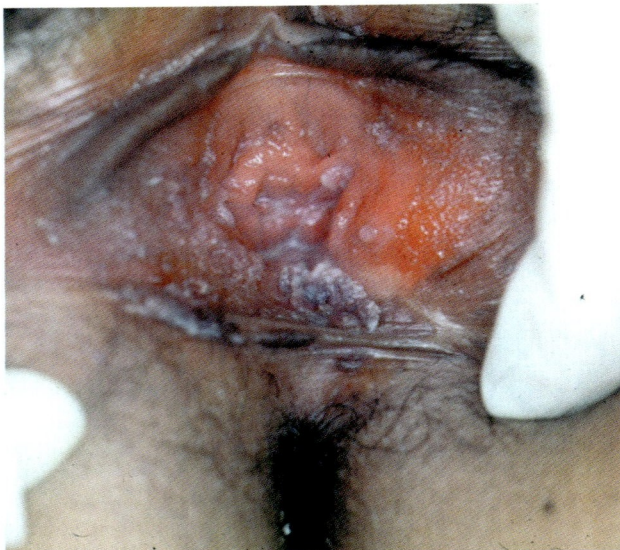

Figure 17–49 □ **Genital warts (condyloma acuminata) – vulvo-vaginal.** Extensive grayish, verrucous papules are seen on the labia majora and minora in this patient. It is caused by sexual transmission of human papilloma virus. HPV types 16, 18, 31, 33, and 35 are associated with an increased risk of cervical cancer and regular (annual) Pap smear examination is recommended to detect dysplastic changes.

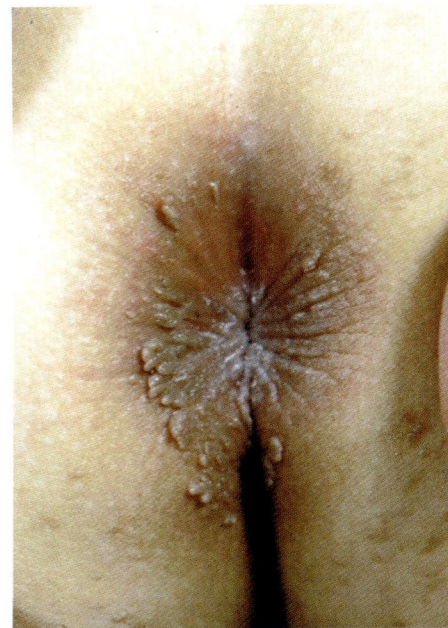

Figure 17–50 □ **Perianal warts.** Small, verrucous papules are seen around the anus. These are transmitted by anal intercourse. A proctoscopic examination should be done to exclude anal and rectal warts. HPV types 16, 18, 31, 33, and 35 are associated with an increased risk of anal cancer. Regular assessment should be performed to rule out malignant change.

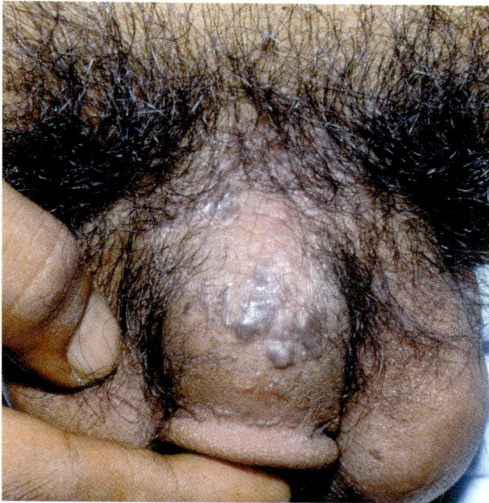

Figure 17–51 □ Bowenoid papulosis. A group of asymptomatic hyperpigmented papules with a flat and sometimes verrucous surface are seen on the dorsal surface of the penile shaft. This is a STI caused by HPV infection, particularly type 16. It is a generally benign condition that spontaneously regresses over several months, but has a distinct histology of Bowenoid dysplasia. A few case reports have associated this condition with malignant invasive transformation.

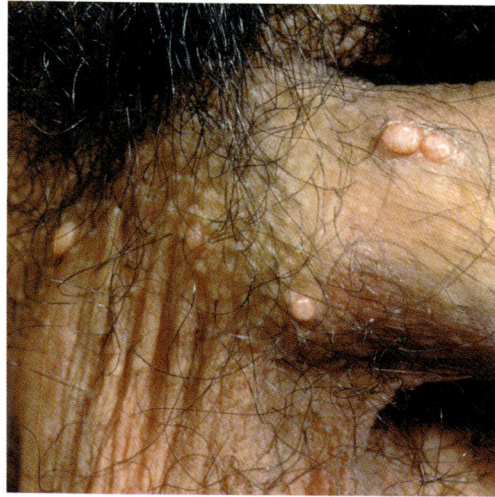

Figure 17–52 □ Molluscum contagiosum – penis and scrotum. Flesh-colored or pinkish, umbilicated papules (1 to 5 mm in diameter) are seen at the base of the penis and on the scrotum. They are spread by direct contact during sexual intercourse and appear after an incubation period of two to eight weeks. It is caused by a pox virus and may resolve spontaneously without treatment after several months.

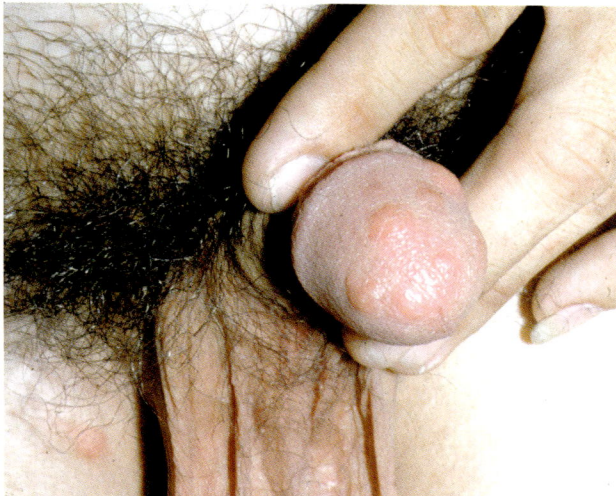

Figure 17–53 □ Scabies. Erythematous papules and nodules are present on the glans penis, scrotum, and groin in this patient. This condition is extremely pruritic and the sex partner of the patient may often complain of similar symptoms. Scabies is spread by close contact as during sexual contact. It is caused by the mite *Sarcoptes scabiei*, which burrows into the skin; the accompanying itch is due to an allergic reaction to the mite.

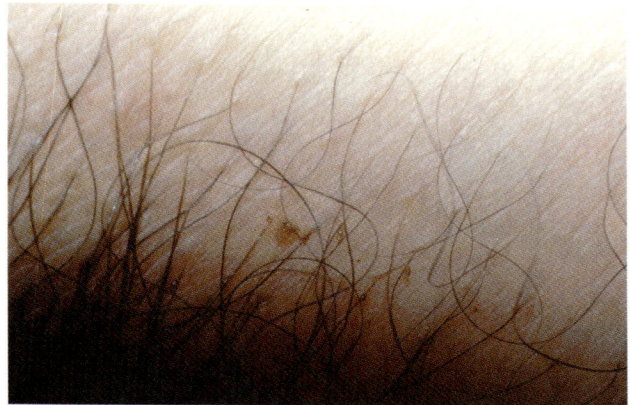

Figure 17–54 □ Pubic lice. Small, gray-white, oval eggs (nits) are seen here attached to the hair shaft. It is caused by the louse *Pthirus pubis*, which is a six-legged creature seen here attached firmly to the genital hair. The crab louse requires human blood to survive and buries its head into a pubic hair follicle. The term "crabs" refers to the crab-like appearance of the louse as seen under a microscope. Small egg sacs or "nits" are seen attached to a pubic hair under magnification. It is a STI and is associated with moderate to severe itch. The louse does not cause a rash but bleeding spots are noticed on undergarments and scratching can result in raw excoriations.

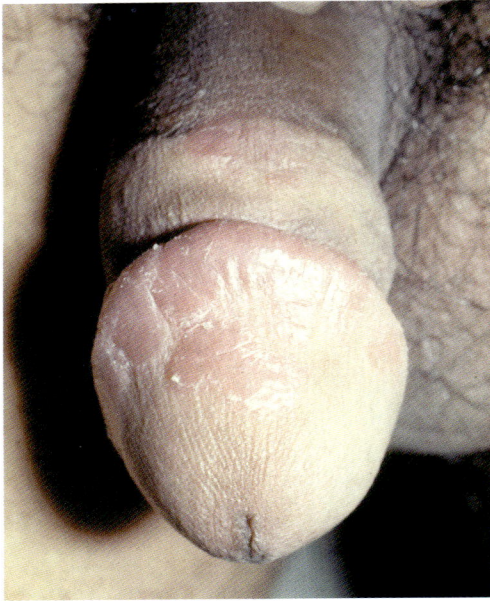

Figure 17–55 □ Psoriasis – glans penis. Well-demarcated, annular, erythematous plaques of psoriasis are seen on the glans penis and penile shaft. This may be associated with psoriatic plaques on other parts of the body which would make the diagnosis easy. However, genital lesions are occasionally the only presenting lesion.

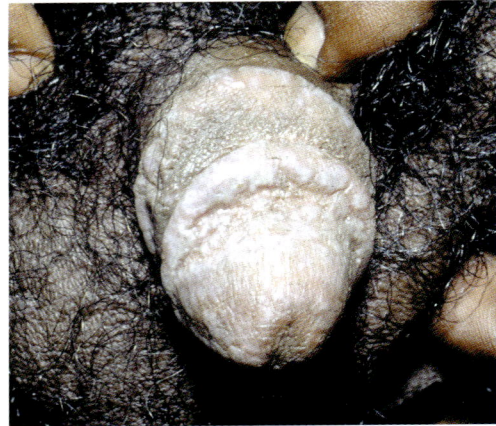

Figure 17–56 □ Lichen planus – glans penis and penile shaft. Violaceous lichenoid papules are seen on the glans penis, coronal sulcus, and penile shaft of this circumcised male patient. Some of the papules are seen to coalesce and there appears to be a fine network of white streaks on the surface (Wickham's striae). These lesions are typically pruritic.

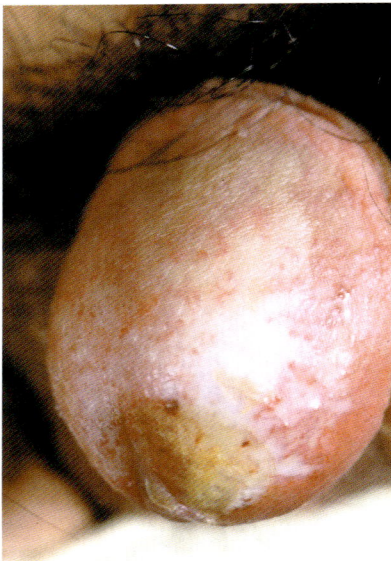

Figure 17–57 □ Lichen sclerosus et atrophicus – penis. The glans penis is seen here to be largely whitish and atrophic with telangiectasia seen at the margin of the lesion. The peri-meatal area is stenosed due to fibrosis. This condition is also known as balanitis xerotica obliterans and patients may present with itch, soreness, or painful erections. There have been reports of squamous cell carcinoma developing.

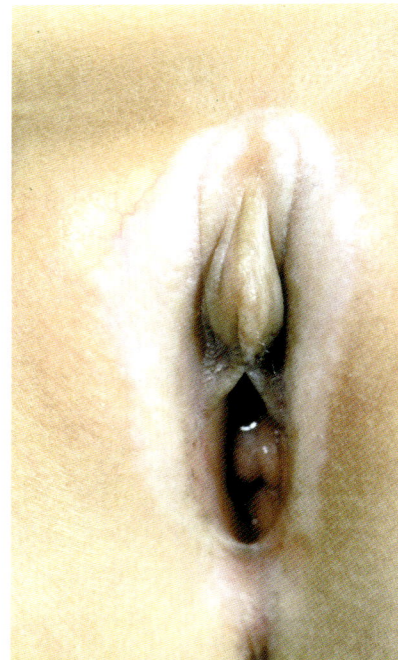

Figure 17–58 □ Lichen sclerosus et atrophicus – vulva. Ivory-white atrophic plaques are seen on the vulva of this young girl. There are telangiectasias seen at the margins on the right side. Symptoms include pruritus and soreness. Progressive disease may cause shrinkage of the labia and stenosis of the introitus. Pre-malignant changes and squamous cell carcinoma may develop in long-standing cases.

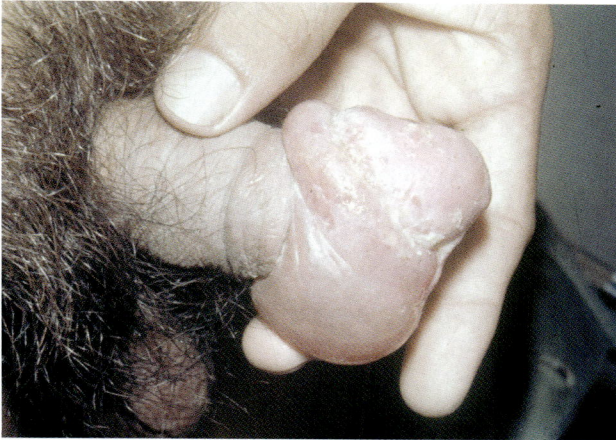

Figure 17–59 □ Balanitis – irritant contact dermatitis to podophyllin. There are erythema and edema of the coronal sulcus with the development of a large blister on the ventral aspect of the penis. This was the result of an irritant contact dermatitis due to excessive application of podophyllin paint used to treat genital warts which are seen here on the glans penis and coronal sulcus.

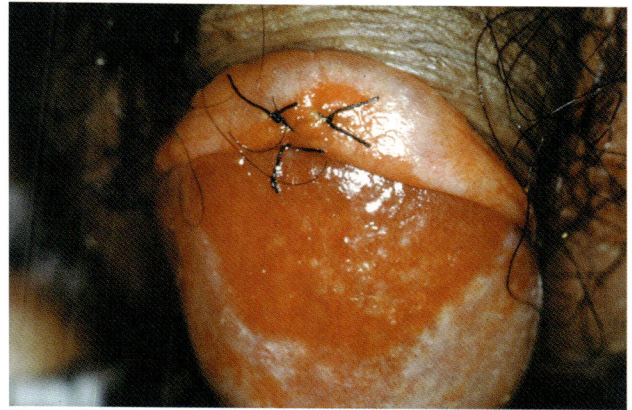

Figure 17–60 □ Zoon's balanitis. A moist, shiny, well-circumscribed, erythematous plaque with white stippling resembling "cayenne pepper" is seen on the glans penis. The lesion is asymptomatic; a biopsy performed revealed dense plasma cell infiltrates, characteristic of this benign condition. Circumcision gives beneficial results in recalcitrant cases.

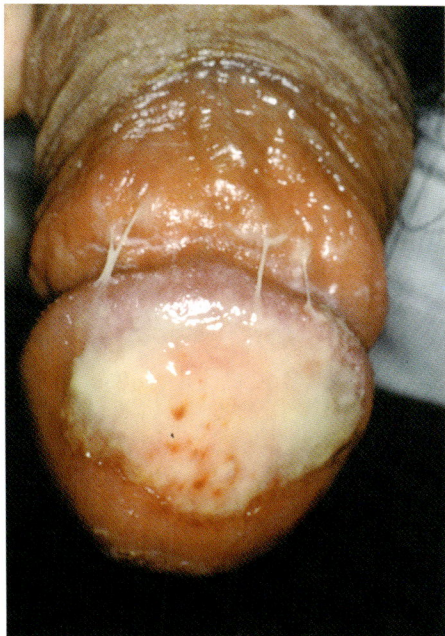

Figure 17–61 □ Erosive balanitis – fixed drug eruption to cotrimoxazole. There is a sloughy, tender erosion on the glans penis with erythema of the adjacent skin. This lesion started off as a blister, occurring three days after the patient had consumed cotrimoxazole. This condition is often misdiagnosed initially as a STI or allergic contact dermatitis due to the use of latex condoms.

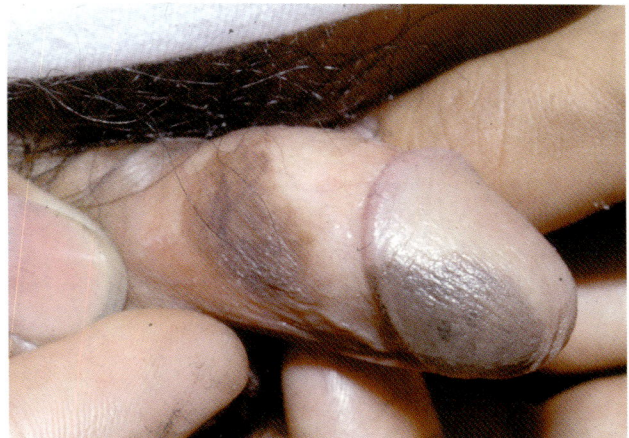

Figure 17–62 □ Fixed drug eruption to aspirin. Brown, pigmented, painful patches appeared five days after the patient had consumed aspirin. The hyperpigmentation persisted for several months and reappeared in the same form and on the same site when the patient consumed aspirin again, thus confirming the diagnosis.

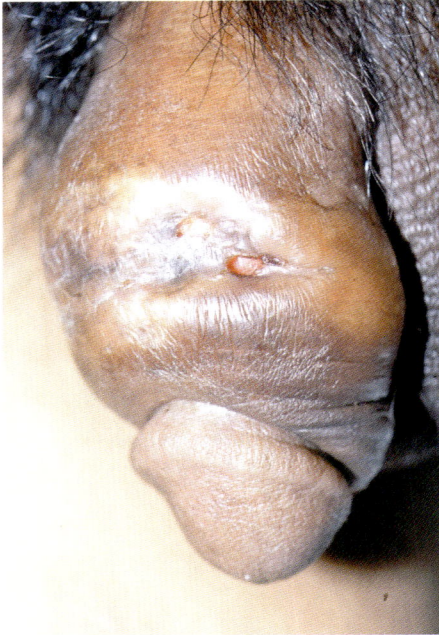

Figure 17–63 □ Foreign body reaction – oleogranuloma. This patient presented with an infected, indurated, hard mass encircling the penile shaft. A biopsy revealed a foreign body granuloma due to the presence of olive oil. On further questioning, this patient revealed that he had self-injected olive oil into his penis two years earlier. This is practiced in some Southeast Asian countries to enlarge the penis.

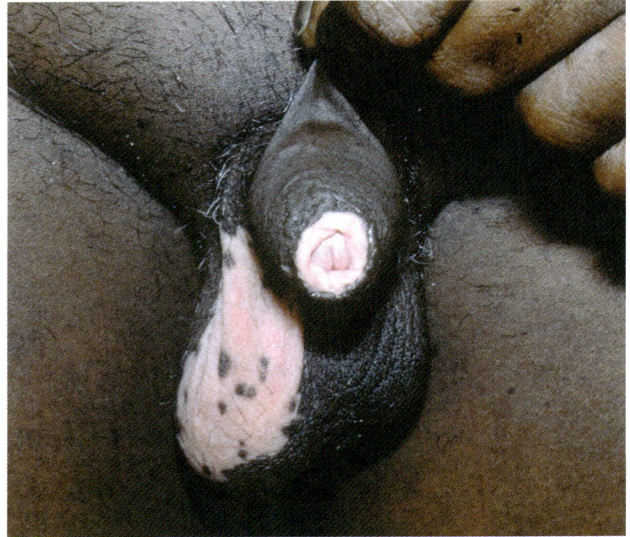

Figure 17–64 □ Vitiligo – scrotum and penis. Ivory-white, depigmented patches are seen over the scrotum, glans penis, and prepuce in this Indian patient. The patches are asymptomatic. The diagnosis is supported by similar lesions elsewhere on the body and the repigmentation may return with the application of topical steroids.

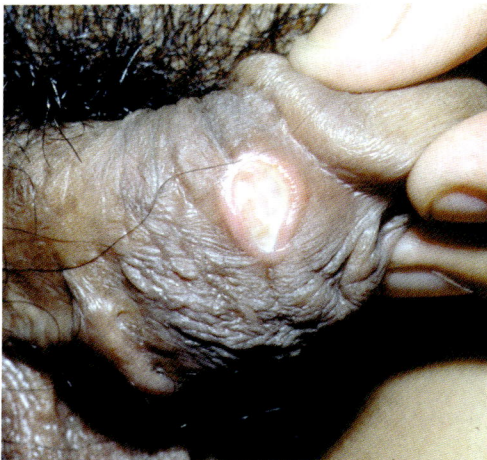

Figure 17–65 □ Behcet's disease – penile ulcer. A single, moderately sized ulcer with a sloughy base and a distinct erythematous raised margin are seen on the penile shaft. The ulcer is very painful, recurrent in nature, and is associated with painful recurrent ulcers on the oral mucosa. Other cutaneous manifestations in Behcet's disease include papulopustular lesions, erythema nodosum, and a positive pathergy test.

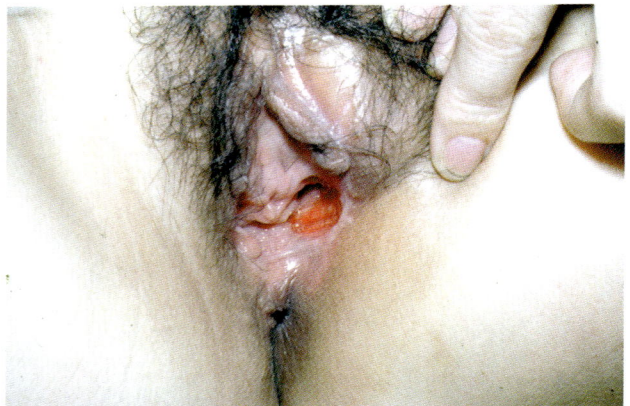

Figure 17–66 □ Behcet's disease – vulval ulcer. There is a large single vulval ulcer with an erythematous margin seen over the left labia majora. This ulcer is exquisitely tender and recurrent and is associated with recurrent oral ulcers. Behcet's syndrome is the association of recurrent orogenital ulceration with eye disease (iridocyclitis and retinal vasculitis).

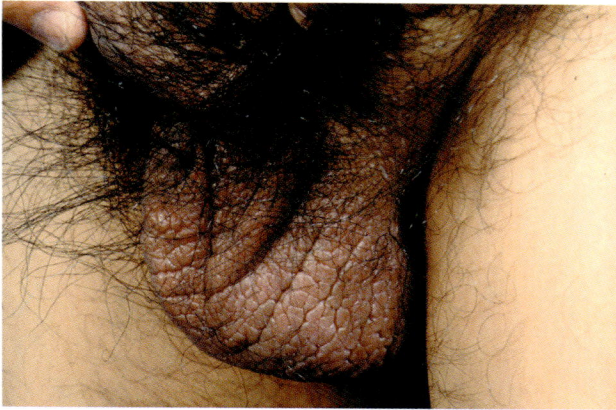

Figure 17–67 □ Lichen simplex chronicus – scrotum.
Thickening, lichenification, erythema with hyperpigmentation is seen over the scrotal skin in this patient. This is a very pruritic condition and results from repeated excoriations and rubbing of chronic eczema of the scrotum. It is treated with topical steroids and oral antihistamines.

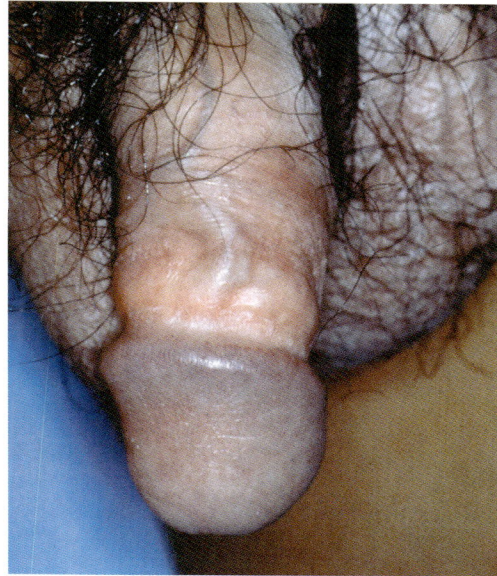

Figure 17–68 □ Sclerosing lymphangitis (lymphocoele) of the penis. A translucent, flesh-colored, cord-like lesion is seen on the shaft of the penis. This is usually asymptomatic and occurs after vigorous sexual activity. Histology will reveal thrombosed lymphatic vessels (likely secondary to trauma). The lesion usually resolves spontaneously within a few weeks.

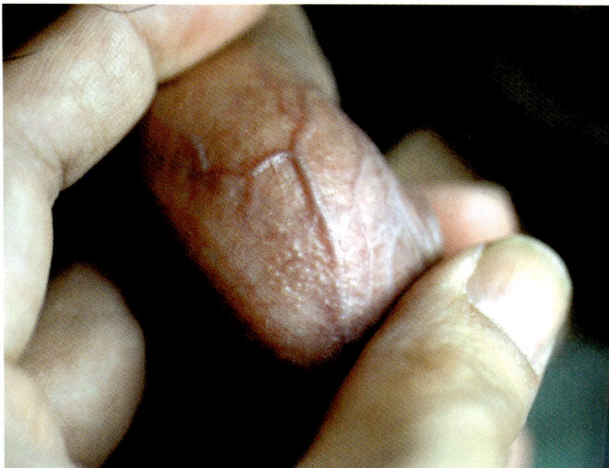

Figure 17–69 □ Fordyce spots. A cluster of tiny white papules is seen in the submucosa of the penile shaft. They are asymptomatic and arise from the presence of ectopic sebaceous glands. They are also seen on the buccal mucosa, lips, and vulva in females. Patients should be reassured that this is a normal finding.

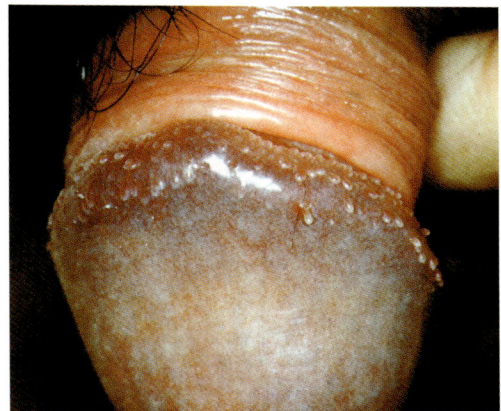

Figure 17–70 □ Pearly penile papules (coronal papilla).
Rows of tiny white papules are seen along the coronal sulcus. These are congenital anomalies consisting of hypertrophic papillae. It is important to reassure patients that these are not viral warts.

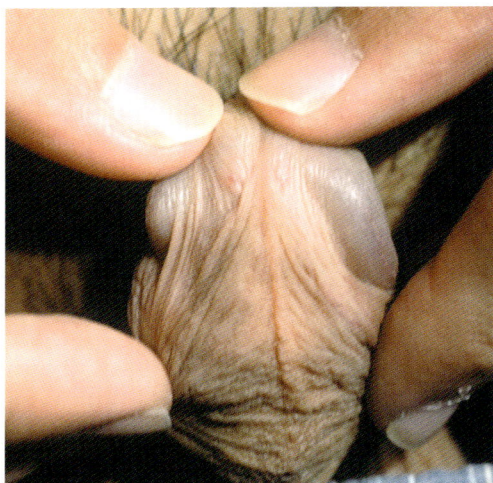

Figure 17–71 □ Tyson's glands. Two tiny flesh-colored glandular structures are seen on either side of the frenulum on the ventral surface of the penis. They are symmetrical and their appearance as para-frenal papules can sometimes be mistaken by patients for warts.

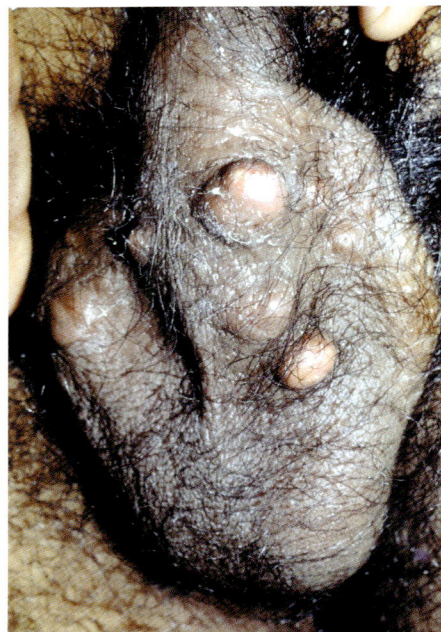

Figure 17–72 □ Scrotal calcinosis. Multiple white or pinkish, subcutaneous, hard nodules are seen underlying the scrotal skin of this patient. They are generally asymptomatic. These are due to abnormal deposits of calcium within the skin with normal serum calcium and phosphate levels. Treatment is by surgical excision.

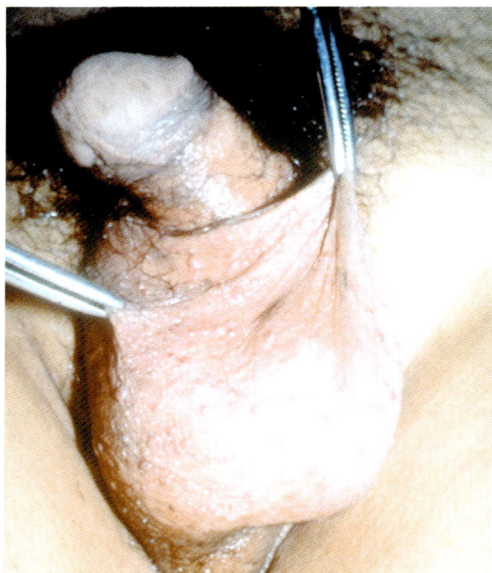

Figure 17–73 □ Scrotal angiokeratomas. Multiple red, angiomatous papules are seen on the scrotum of this patient. They range from 2 to 6 mm in diameter, are hyperkeratotic, and may bleed if traumatized. This is an idiopathic condition.

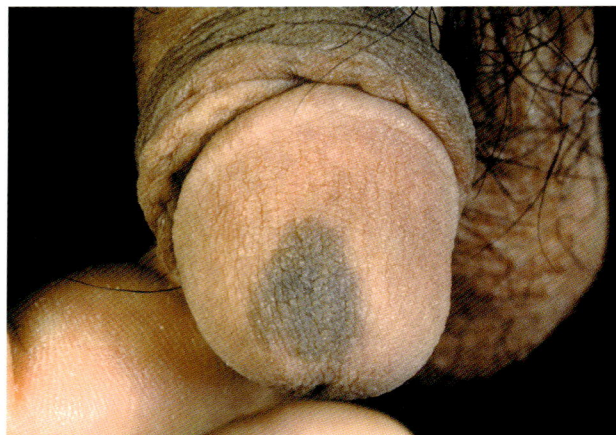

Figure 17–74 □ Benign genital lentiginosis. There is a black macular pigmented area with irregular borders on the glans penis. This uncommon, idiopathic, pigmentary abnormality is usually found over the glans and penile shaft.

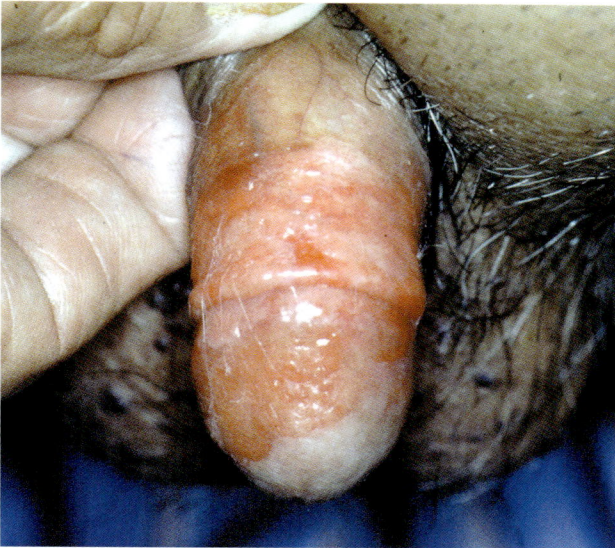

Figure 17–75 □ Erythroplasia of Queyrat. A moist, ulcerative, erythematous plaque with crusting in some areas is seen on the glans penis and penile shaft of this patient. It arises from the squamous epithelial cells of the glans penis or the inner lining of the prepuce and is mostly seen in uncircumcised males. Histology will confirm it to be a squamous cell carcinoma-in-situ.

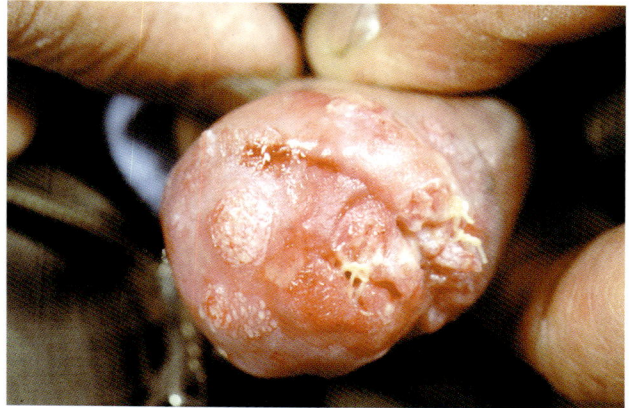

Figure 17–76 □ Squamous cell carcinoma of the penis. Several ulcerative erythematous and sloughy plaques are seen distorting the glans penis of this uncircumcised patient. It is the most common malignant tumor of the penis and is rare in the circumcised male. It spreads to regional lymph nodes. Treatment is with surgery and adjuvant chemotherapy and depends on the stage of the tumor at the time of treatment.

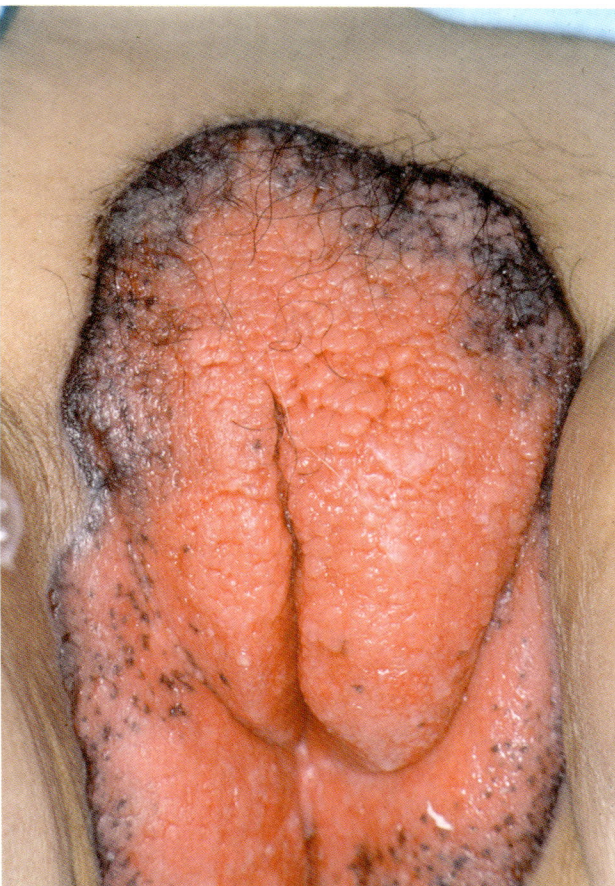

Figure 17–77 □ Squamous cell carcinoma of the vulva and mons pubis. This elderly Chinese patient presents with extensive erythematous, well-demarcated, verrucous plaque affecting her entire vulva and mons pubis. There are scattered ulcerations present throughout the plaque. Histology confirmed the diagnosis of squamous cell carcinoma.

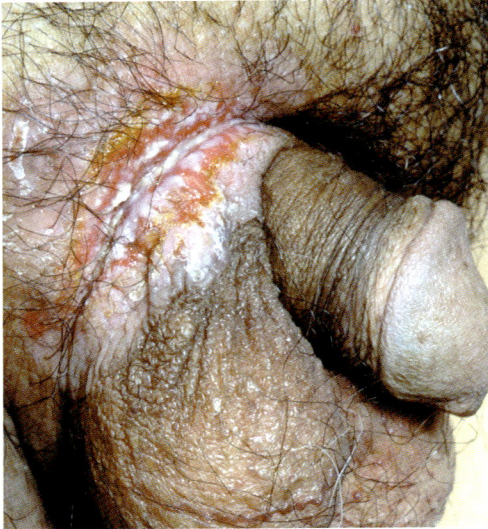

Figure 17–78 □ **Extramammary Paget's disease.** An erythematous and ulcerative plaque with raised margins is seen over the scrotum and pubic area of a 55-year-old male. Biopsy confirmed this to be extramammary Paget's disease. This is characterized clinically by a marginated plaque resembling Paget's disease of the nipple and histologically by the presence of large Paget's cells in the epidermis.

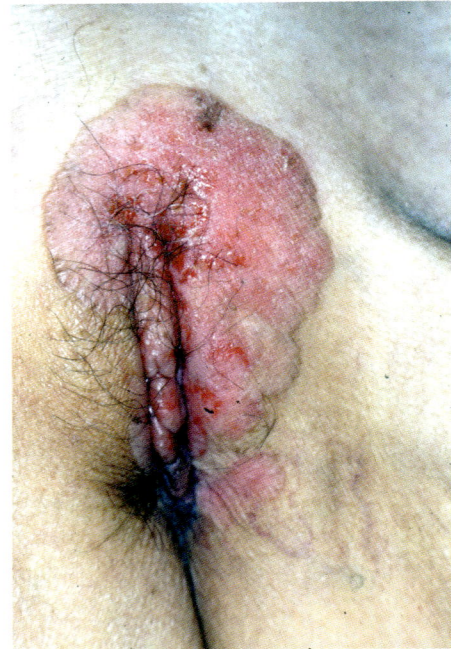

Figure 17–79 □ **Extramammary Paget's disease.** A persistent, well-demarcated, pinkish plaque over the vulva of a 62-year-old female. Patients often complain of itching and a burning sensation over the affected area. Because of the associated itch, patients are often misdiagnosed initially as having lichenified eczema. It is important to examine the cervix and the rectum to exclude a primary carcinoma as this condition may be associated with an underlying malignancy.

Skin Conditions in HIV-Infected Persons

Chan R.K.W. and Sen P.

HIV infection is spreading rapidly in many Asian countries. Treatment of HIV in most Asian nations is costly and inaccessible. Cutaneous complications are a major cause of morbidity amongst infected individuals. These result from (1) infectious agents such as viruses, bacteria, protozoa, or arthropods, (2) inflammatory dermatoses, (3) adverse drug reactions, and (4) neoplasms.

Several opportunistic infections that can have cutaneous manifestations may be geographically determined, e.g. patients originating from Southeast Asia may be infected with *Penicillium marneffei*; this diagnosis should be in the differential diagnosis of any skin eruption in these patients. Pruritic inflammatory conditions have been noted more frequently in some Asian studies. For example, pruritic papular eruption of HIV infection is one of the most common skin manifestations in Asian patients. The use of anti-retroviral drugs in Asia has lagged behind that of developed countries although this is gradually changing. With an increasing number of patients being treated with anti-retroviral drugs, we should expect to see more adverse drug reactions due to these medications.

This chapter covers the wide spectrum of skin conditions that may be seen in HIV-infected persons.

BACTERIAL SKIN INFECTIONS
(Figures 18–1 to 18–6)

Staphylococcal aureus is the most common bacterial pathogen in cutaneous infections; the nasal carriage rate is twice that of HIV negative controls. Clinical features include impetigo, bullous impetigo, ecthyma, papular and plaque-like folliculitis, furuncles and carbuncles, cellulitis, botryomycosis, pyomyositis, and secondary infection of scabies, dermatitis, and central lines. M. *tuberculosis*, M. *avium-intracellulare*, M. *marinum*, M. *chelonaea*, M. *fortuitum*, and M. *kansasii* may cause acneiform papules, indurated crusted plaques, abscesses, matted lymphadenopathy, and sporotrichoid pattern of lesions.

VIRAL SKIN INFECTIONS
(Figures 18–7 to 18–15)

Recurrent anogenital and orofacial HSV infections are very common with increasing immunodeficiency, and herpetic ulcers may be confluent, large, chronic, granulating, and slow to heal. Treatment is with acyclovir, valaciclovir, or famciclovir. However, viral resistance to acyclovir is common, usually due to TK(-) variants, which may also be TK(-) altered, or DNA polymerase-altered variants. In these cases, i/v foscarnet, trifluridine 1% ophthalmic solution, or cidofovir in gel may be used.

Ten to 20% of HIV patients have molluscum contagiosum, especially in advanced disease (CD4 < 200). Clinical lesions are usually multiple and may be large. They commonly occur on the face, eyelids, intertriginous areas, and genitals. Treatment is with liquid nitrogen cryotherapy, electrocautery, and curettage. Recurrences are common.

The prevalence of viral warts is increased. This infection is caused by the human papilloma virus. Anogenital warts are difficult to treat in immunocompromised individuals; treatment is as for non-HIV infected individuals. There is increased incidence of cervical and anal intraepithelial neoplasia and carcinomas in HIV+ individuals. Routine cytologic screening is needed to detect the development of intraepithelial neoplasia and carcinoma.

Oral hairy leukoplakia is specific to HIV infection with rare exceptions. It correlates with moderate-to-advanced immuno-deficiency; the probability of developing AIDS is 48% after 16 months and 83% after 31 months. The lesions are hyperplastic, verrucous, white to gray epithelial plaques, corrugated in appearance comprising parallel rows arranged vertically at the lateral margins of the tongue. The lesions do not scrape off easily. Differential diagnoses include candidiasis, condyloma acuminata, geographic tongue, and leukoplakia. Histology shows acanthosis, marked parakeratosis with formation of ridges and keratin projections, and areas of ballooning cells. The etiology is EBV-induced, benign, epithelial thickening. The lesions may respond to acyclovir.

Varicella zoster virus infection occurs seven times more frequently in HIV-infected persons, and correlates with moderate immuno-deficiency. The lesions are usually uni-dermatomal with uneventful recovery, but may be multi-dermatomal, recurrent, disseminated, or chronic. Treatment is as for non-HIV-infected individuals. Acyclovir resistant strains have been reported.

FUNGAL SKIN INFECTIONS (Figures 18–16 to 18–22)

Candidiasis is the most common opportunistic infection (OI) in HIV infection; almost all patients will have this at some point in the course of the illness. The infection affects oropharyngeal, oesophageal, vaginal, and other mucocutaneous surfaces. This occurs at moderate levels of immunosuppression (CD4 < 400), and often becomes intractable when the CD4 count falls below 100. The clinical features of oropharyngeal disease are asymptomatic infection, soreness, burning, and reduced or altered taste sensation. Four patterns of oropharyngeal candidiasis are described: pseudo-membranous, atrophic, hyperplastic, and angular cheilitis. Oesophageal infection causes odyno-phagia and retrosternal pain. Investigations include KOH preparation and culture. Treatment for symptomatic disease includes topical nystatin mouthwash, amphotericin B lozenges, clotrimazole troches, oral ketoconazole, itraconazole, and fluconazole. Parenteral amphotericin B may be required for resistant cases.

Dermatophytosis occurs in up to 20% of HIV-infected individuals. Clinical features are typically tinea cruris, corporis, faciei, pedis, manuum, or unguium. Infection may be severe and widespread, mimicking seborrheic dermatitis and palmo-plantar keratoderma. Treatment with oral agents is usually necessary.

Cutaneous histoplasmosis may occur in association with pulmonary or disseminated histoplasmosis in patients with advanced immunosuppression. Ten percent of patients with disseminated histoplasmosis have hematogenous spread to the skin. The clinical features are varied, including shallow crusted ulcers, pustules, folliculitis, psoriasiform papules, papulonecrotic plaques, perianal ulceration, mild diffuse dermatitis, disseminated maculo-papular eruption, and pink to red papules of 2 to 6 mm. Diagnosis is made by skin biopsy (fungal stains), crushed tissue specimens, fungal culture for specimens from skin and bone marrow. Treatment is with i/v amphotericin B (drug of choice for disseminated disease). Oral itraconazole may be used for non-meningeal and non-septicemic diseases.

Penicilliosis is the third most common HIV-related OI in Thailand and is caused by the dimorphic fungus, *Penicillium marneffei*, whose natural habitat is in Southeast Asia and China. Clinical features include fever, anemia, weight loss, lymphadenopathy, hepatomegaly, pulmonary, and GIT symptoms. Skin lesions (71%) include generalized papules with umbilication especially on the face, upper trunk, extremities, and palate. Diagnosis is by skin biopsy which reveals septate and elongated yeast forms in macrophages (differential diagnosis is that of histoplasmosis, where there are no septa, and narrow-based unequal budding), and cultures of the blood, bone marrow, skin, stool, and sputum. Treatment is with i/v amphotericin B and itraconazole.

PARASITIC SKIN INFESTATIONS
(Figures 18–23 to 18–25)

The typical clinical features of scabies are seen, but this may affect the face and scalp, areas that are usually spared in HIV-uninfected hosts. Scabies should be a differential diagnosis in all unexplained pruritic eruptions or dermatitis. Norwegian (crusted) scabies is seen in advanced immunosuppression, featuring generalized scaling and marked hyperkeratosis. Treatment is with the usual anti-scabetic agents; post-scabetic dermatitis may persist for several months.

Demodex folliculitis is caused by the saprophytic skin mite, *Demodex folliculorum*. It presents as pruritic follicular papules commonly on the face but it can also occur on the trunk and extremities.

INFLAMMATORY SKIN CONDITIONS
(Figures 18–26 to 18–30)

Seborrheic dermatitis is one of the most common non-infectious manifestations; up to 85% in comparison to 5 to 12% in HIV-uninfected individuals. This is correlated with *Malassezia furfur* colonization; though the exact role of this organism is unclear. Clinical features are typical pinkish-to-red scaly, occasionally greasy patches and plaques on the malar region, eyebrows, scalp, chest, axillae, and groin. The lesions may progress to generalized erythrodermic dermatitis. Plaques may resemble psoriasis, and severity correlates with the degree of immunosuppression. Seborrheic dermatitis may predate other manifestations of HIV infection. Treatment includes use of low to medium potency topical corticosteroids, topical anti-fungals, oral anti-fungals, selenium sulfide, and salicylic acid shampoos.

The incidence of psoriasis is from 1.3 to 6.4% of HIV-infected (compared with 1 to 2% of HIV negative), and the severity is greater in the HIV-infected. Arthropathy is more common and is considered a poor prognostic indicator. Sudden worsening of psoriasis or recent onset of psoriasis may indicate HIV infection in patients with appropriate risk factors. Clinical features include guttate lesions, small to large plaques, inverse pattern, palmoplantar keratoderma, erythrodermic psoriasis, and involvement worsens with immunosuppression. Treatment is with topical corticosteroids, anthralin, coal tar, UVB, and PUVA. Systemic therapy includes oral acitretin, methotrexate (immunosuppressive and marrow suppressive), and cyclosporin (immunosuppressive). Anti-retroviral therapy may reduce severity.

Photosensitive conditions are not uncommon in HIV infection. Chronic actinic dermatitis may be the presenting condition of HIV infection; porphyria cutanea tarda is more common in HIV-infected persons.

ADVERSE DRUG REACTIONS
(Figures 18–31 to 18–35)

Adverse drug reactions (ADRs) are much more frequent in HIV-infected than uninfected patients. This is the result of the increased use of medications as well as an increase in absolute risk. CMV and EBV may predispose to skin reactions analogous to that associated with the ampicillin rash seen in mononucleosis. The most common drugs causing ADRs are cotrimoxazole (TMP-SMX), sulphadiazine, TMP-dapsone, aminopenicillins and anti-TB medications.

PRURITIC SKIN CONDITIONS
(Figures 18–38 to 18–43)

Pruritic papular eruption of HIV is a common finding amongst African (35 to 72%), Haitian (46%), and Asian AIDS patients, but less so amongst the Americans and Europeans. The lesions are small, firm, well-demarcated, skin-colored papules (2 to 4 mm) distributed on the trunk, face, and extremities. They may be acneiform or follicular, and pink to red in color. They do not form plaques and are very pruritic. They are often excoriated and give rise to prurigo-like lesions with post-inflammatory hyperpigmentation. The activity waxes and wanes.

Eosinophilic folliculitis is a non-infective chronic pruritic folliculitis which has been previously confused with eosinophilic pustular folliculitis of Ofuji. It may be within the spectrum of PPE of HIV infection. Clinical features are multiple discrete pruritic urticarial papules, distributed mainly on the trunk, head and neck, and proximal extremities. The lesions are frequently excoriated and crusted.

NEOPLASTIC SKIN CONDITIONS
(Figures 18–44 to 18–47)

HIV-associated or epidemic Kaposi's sarcoma (KS) is the most common neoplasia in HIV infection. It is 20,000 times more common in patients with AIDS than in the general population, 300 times more common than in other immunosuppressed groups. It generally occurs in homosexuals, rarely in heterosexuals, IVDUs, blood transfusion recipients, and hemophiliacs. The putative cause is the human herpes virus type 8 or the KS-associated herpes virus (KSHV). KSHV is thought to be a sexually transmitted pathogen.

Clinical features comprise asymptomatic erythematous macules, bruise-like discoloration, violaceous elevated lesions that are brownish, sometimes scaly, oval, or round, often sited along lines of skin cleavage. The common sites are the lower extremities, upper trunk, head and neck, hard palate, oropharyngeal mucosa, occipital, and periauricular regions. Visceral involvement includes the GIT, kidneys, lymph nodes, liver, and spleen. The nodules coalesce to form firm tumors. KS may precede, develop concurrently with other HIV-related symptoms, or develop late in the course of the disease. The lesions rarely resolve spontaneously. AIDS-KS, though more aggressive than classical KS, is not commonly fatal.

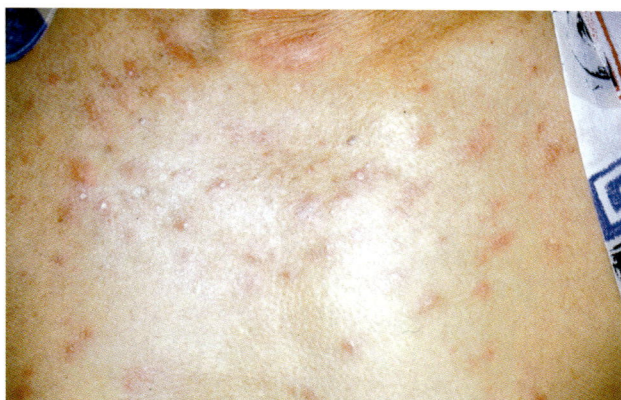

Figure 18–1 □ Folliculitis. Recurrent crops of erythematous follicular papules are seen on the chest of this patient. It responded to courses of anti-staphylococcal treatment. *Staphylococcus aureus* is the most common cause of bacterial infections of the skin, manifesting as folliculitis, furunculosis, carbuncles, or secondary infections of other skin pathologies.

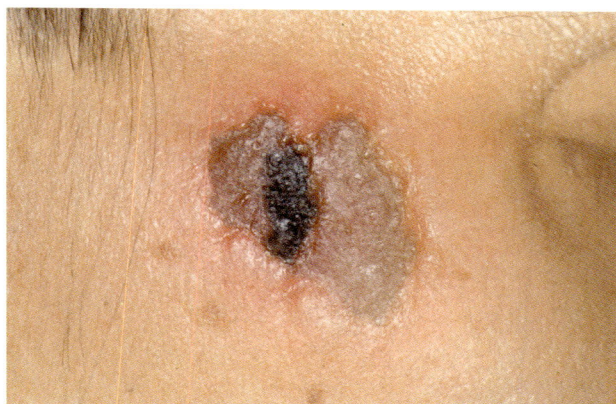

Figure 18–2 □ Ecthyma gangrenosum. A shallow ulceration with a grayish-yellow and black adherent crust and an indurated erythematous margin is seen on the cheek of this patient. This is due to a deeper dermal infection of the skin on the face and will leave an atrophic permanent scar. In this patient, it was caused by *Pseudomonas aeruginosa*.

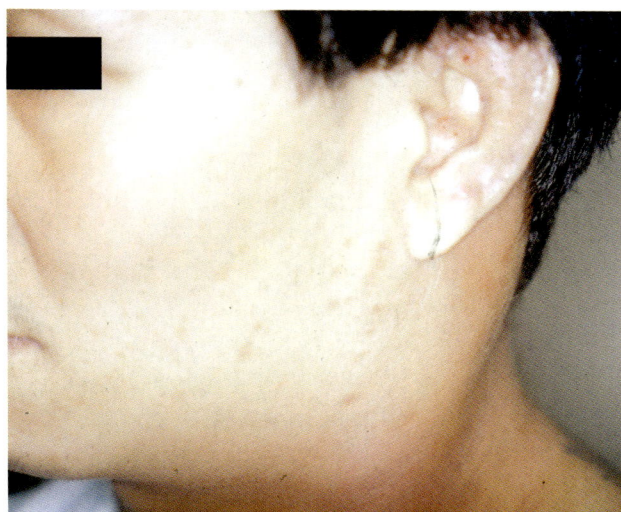

Figure 18–3 □ Pyomyositis. A subacute indolent swelling with minimal inflammation is seen on the neck. This is a deep purulent infection of the muscles by *Staphylococcus aureus*. There may be little leukocytosis or fever. Diagnosis is aided by ultrasound or CT scans. Treatment with antibiotics and surgical drainage is usually required.

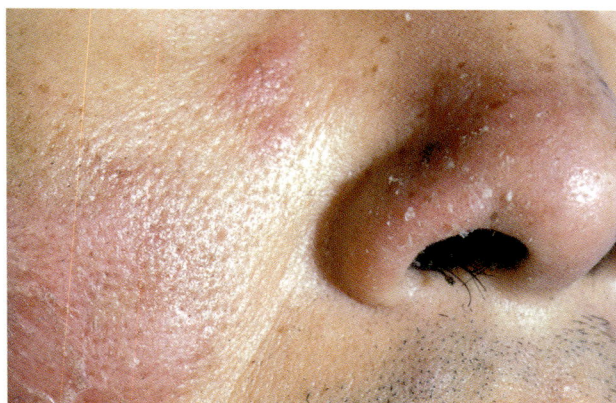

Figure 18–4 □ Cutaneous tuberculosis. Tumid erythematous plaques with some scaling on the nose and cheek. This is a case of lupus vulgaris-like lesions. Mycobacterial infections involving the skin can produce a variety of lesions, ranging from acneiform papules, folliculitis, indurated crusted plaques, abscesses, ulcers, sporotrichoid nodules, to enlarged lymph nodes. Tuberculosis (TB) is the most common systemic, opportunistic infection seen in AIDS patients. Mantoux testing may be falsely negative in anergic HIV-positive individuals.

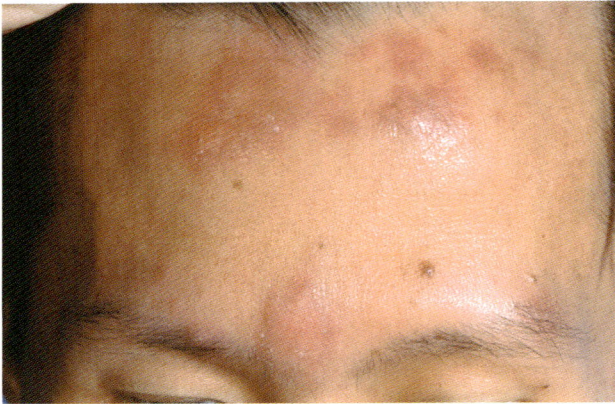

Figure 18–5 ▢ Cutaneous tuberculosis. Erythematous nodules and plaques on the forehead of this patient. This represents another case of cutaneous TB in AIDS. Patients usually respond to the usual anti-TB drugs.

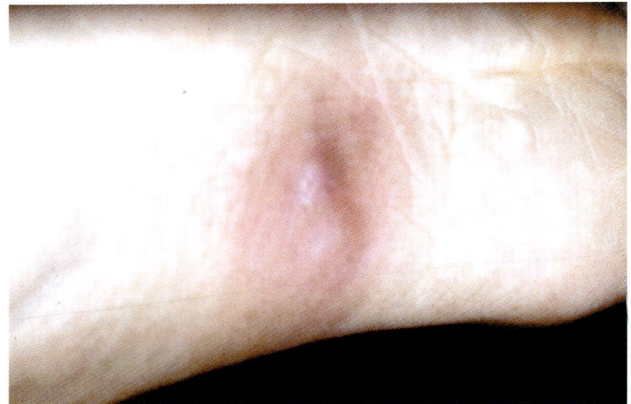

Figure 18–6 ▢ Atypical mycobacterial infection. Erythematous mildly tender nodules and plaques on the sole of the right foot. Infections by non-tuberculous mycobacteria (NTM) species are also seen in AIDS, e.g. *M. avium-intercellulare* (this picture), *M. hemophilum*, and *M. kansasii*. Systemic infection, e.g. lungs, bone marrow, liver, GIT, lymph nodes, is common. Diagnosis is based on isolation of the bacteria from skin or other tissue samples. PCR techniques for rapid diagnosis are being developed and evaluated. Atypical mycobacterial infections usually require a combination of various antibiotic therapies, e.g. clarithromycin and ciprofloxacin, to be given over several months.

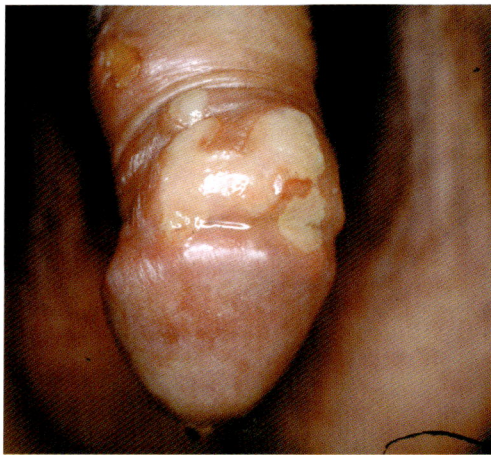

Figure 18–7 ▢ Herpes genitalis. Multiple tender erosions with a slightly sloughy base on the coronal sulcus and penile shaft. Herpes simplex virus infections produce typical herpetic lesions at the usual sites in early HIV infection. However, with increasing immunosuppression, lesions tend to become atypical, some develop chronic deep enlarging ulcers with raised borders. In early HIV infection, herpes will generally respond to regular courses of anti-virals.

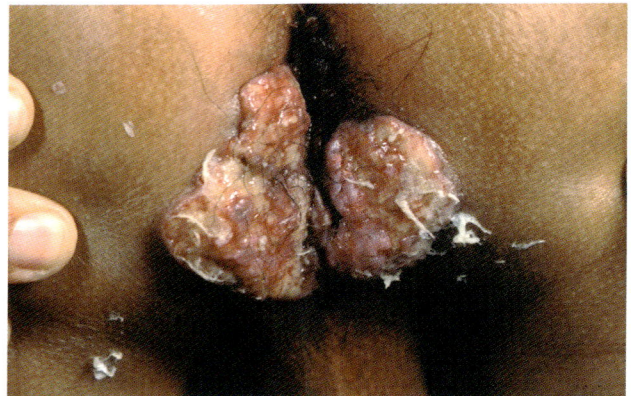

Figure 18–8 ▢ Perianal herpes simplex virus infection. Large chronic perianal ulcers with extensive granulation tissue. Chronic herpetic lesions may be mistaken for other diagnoses as in this case of fungating lesions that resemble human papilloma virus or syphilitic lesions. Resistance to acyclovir and related medications should be suspected in patients with late-stage HIV infection who do not respond to treatment and who have been treated with multiple courses of these medications previously.

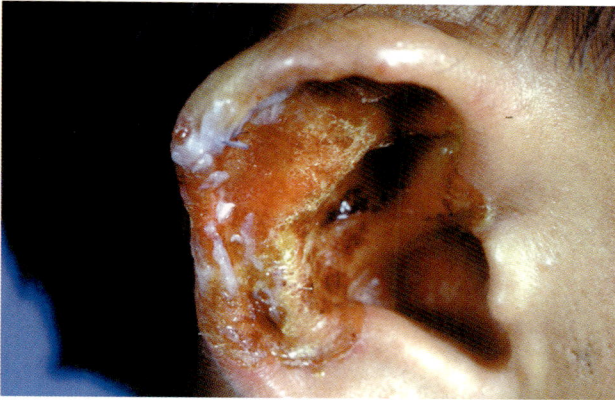

Figure 18–9 □ Herpes simplex virus infection of the pinna. Extensive painful ulceration with a clean base and granulation tissue involving the pinna. Herpes simplex virus infection should be in the differential diagnosis of any ulcerated or crusted lesions in patients with HIV infection. Once the diagnosis is suspected, it can be easily confirmed by viral culture or antigen detection.

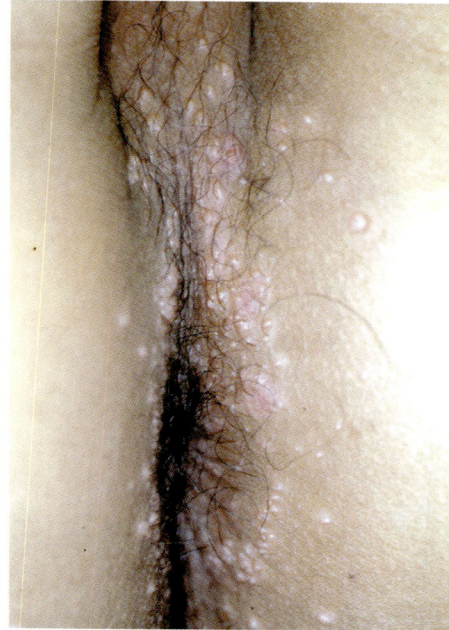

Figure 18–10 □ Molluscum contagiosum. Multiple skin-colored, pearly papules, some with central umbilication, measuring 2 to 5 mm in diameter in the perineum and perianal region. This is caused by a DNA pox virus spread by direct contact. The genital and perianal areas are commonly affected. Diagnosis is made on clinical grounds or by identification of molluscum bodies on a gram-stained smear from the material taken from the center of the papules.

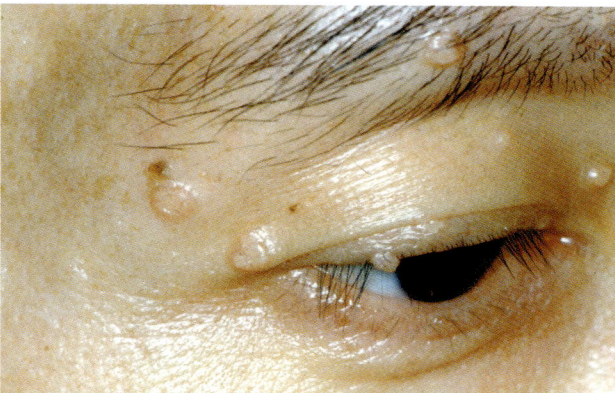

Figure 18–11 □ Molluscum contagiosum. Lesions on the face and around the eyes are typical of molluscum contagiosum in HIV-infected individuals. Treatment is with destruction by liquid nitrogen, tri-chloroacetic acid, cantharidin lotion, curettage, electro-surgery, or imiquimod cream.

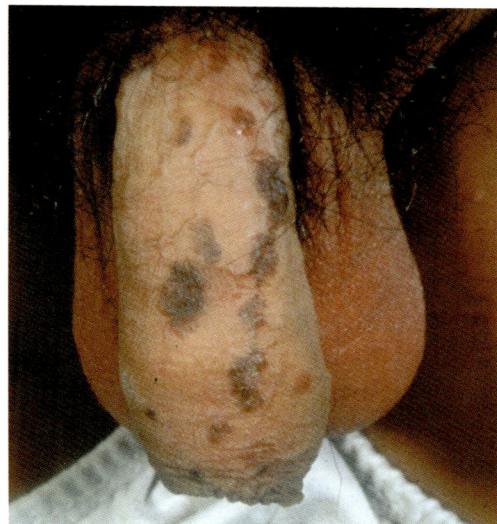

Figure 18–12 □ Bowenoid papulosis. Several hyperpigmented papules and plaques, some with a verrucous surface, on the foreskin of this patient. Genital infection by human papilloma virus (HPV) is a common STI among HIV-infected populations. With increasing immunosuppression, warts may become refractory to treatment. Oncogenic types of HPV are responsible for the increased incidence of cervical and anal cancers in HIV infection. Bowenoid papulosis is a pigmented clinical variant of HPV infection, usually by oncogenic types of HPV.

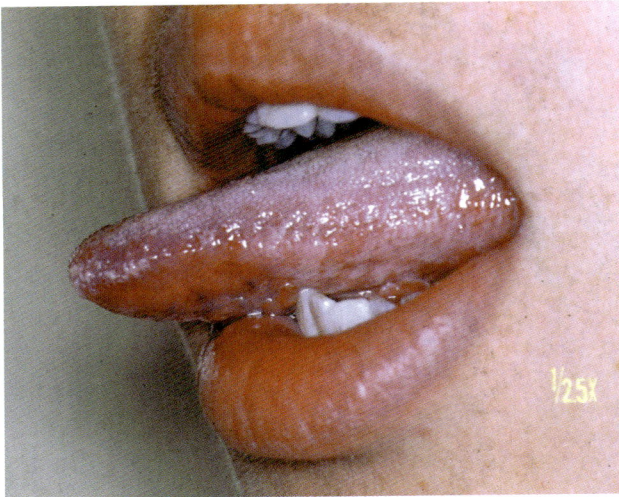

Figure 18–13 □ Oral hairy leukoplakia. Benign, white, corrugated, vertically orientated lesions on the sides of the tongue. These are almost pathognomonic of HIV infection. It is caused by Ebstein-Barr virus (EBV) and is found in patients who are moderately immunosuppressed. The lesions are asymptomatic and do not respond well to any form of therapy.

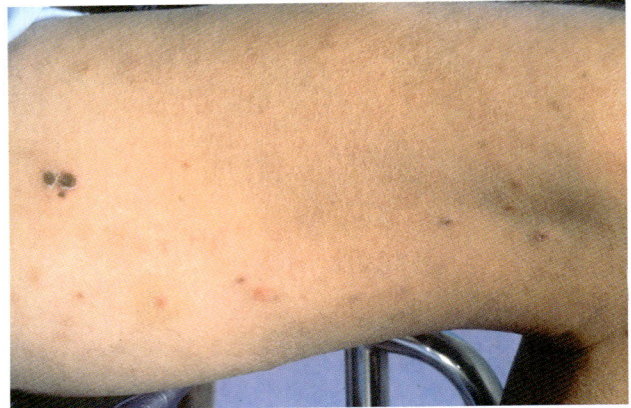

Figure 18–14 □ Disseminated varicella zoster virus infection. Crusted erosions in a dermatomal distribution on the thigh. Reactivation of varicella zoster virus (VZV) as herpes zoster or shingles is common in HIV-infected individuals. Most cases will present with typical dermatomally distributed lesions. With increasing immunodeficiency, it may be multi-dermatomal, and complicated by neuralgia and scarring. Disseminated VZV infection should be suspected when there are chronic or recurrent crops of vesicles.

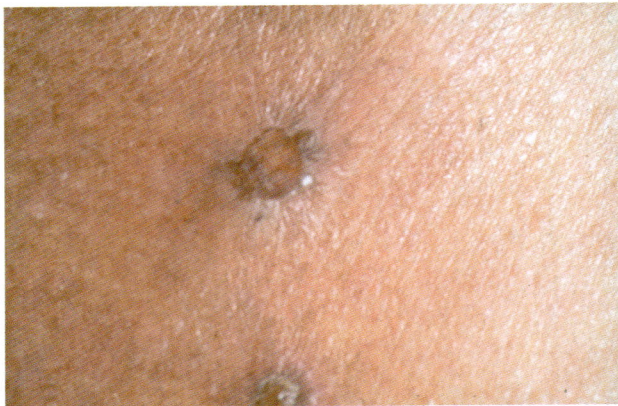

Figure 18–15 □ Varicella zoster virus infection – close up. Two lesions are seen here, one vesicular and the other crusted. A high index of suspicion in cases presenting with sparsely distributed vesicles or papules is necessary to make the correct diagnosis. Biopsy of the lesion and viral culture will clinch the diagnosis. Most persons will respond to regular doses of oral acyclovir. Ophthalmic zoster will usually warrant high intravenous doses of acyclovir.

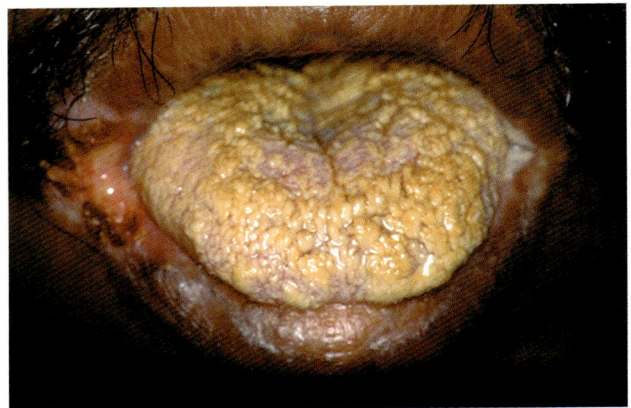

Figure 18–16 □ Oral candidiasis. Extensive yellow adherent material is seen on the tongue with bilateral angular cheilitis. This is the most common HIV-associated opportunistic infection. Infection may extend to the oropharynx and esophagus. Its presence in an adult in the absence of other predisposing factors warrants a HIV test. There are four clinical patterns: pseudomembranous, atrophic, hyperplastic (pictured above), and angular cheilitis. Treatment is with oral anti-fungal agents, supplemented with topical agents.

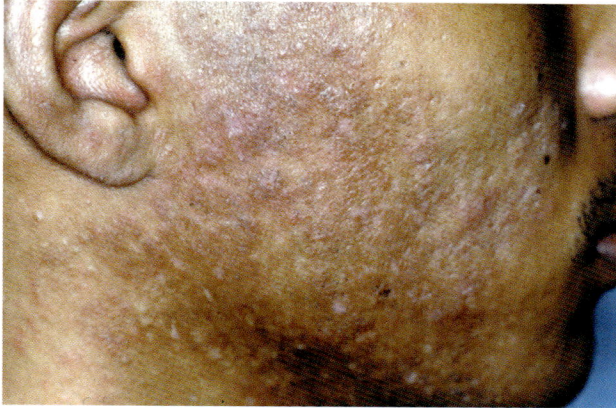

Figure 18–17 □ Tinea faciei. Erythematous, scaly plaques on the cheek and neck. Dermatophyte infection in HIV infection may be extensive, recurrent, and have an atypical appearance. In this patient, it resembles seborrheic dermatitis, a condition commonly found in HIV-infected patients. Detection is easily made by microscopic examination of KOH preparation of a skin scraping.

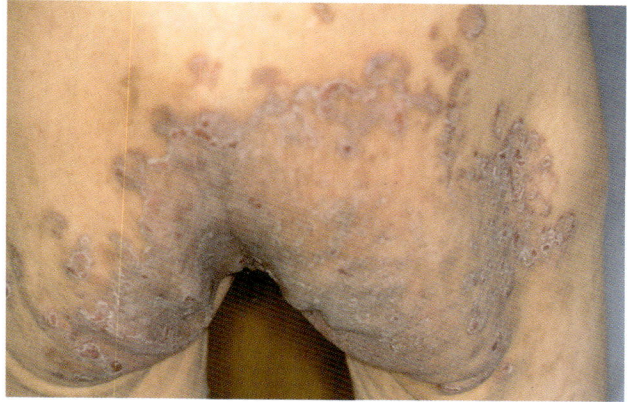

Figure 18–18 □ Tinea corporis. Well-demarcated, pigmented, scaly plaques on the buttocks resulting from extensive tinea corporis in a severely immunosuppressed patient. Such infections are more resistant to treatment than in non-immunocompromised hosts, and will usually require long-term oral anti-fungal agents. Nail infections are typified by proximal white subungual onychomycosis.

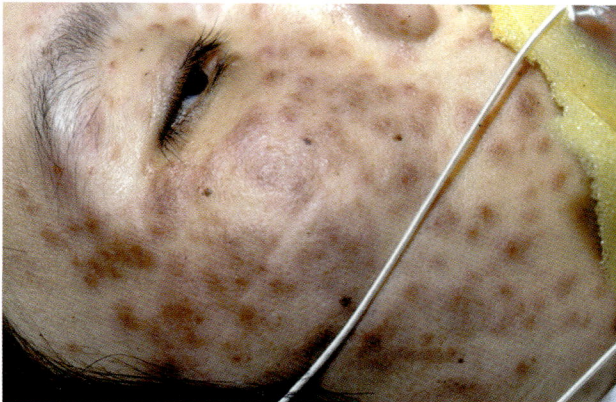

Figure 18–19 □ Histoplasmosis. Erythematous papules, some with purpuric centers, caused by *Histoplasma capsulatum,* a dimorphic fungus, are seen on the face of this moribund patient. Cutaneous lesions occur in 10 to 20% of cases of disseminated histoplasmosis which usually presents with systemic symptoms like fever, weight loss, hepato-splenomegaly, and pulmonary symptoms.

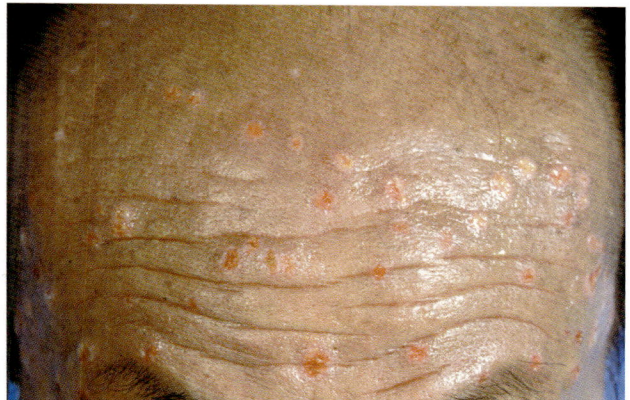

Figure 18–20 □ Histoplasmosis. Skin lesions may also be maculo-papules, ulcerated papules (as in this picture), nodules, pustules, and psoriasiform lesions. Diagnosis is confirmed by finding the small intracellular yeast cells (2 to 5 μ) in tissue smear or biopsy. Treatment is with systemic anti-fungal agents, e.g. amphotericin B, itraconazole, and fluconazole.

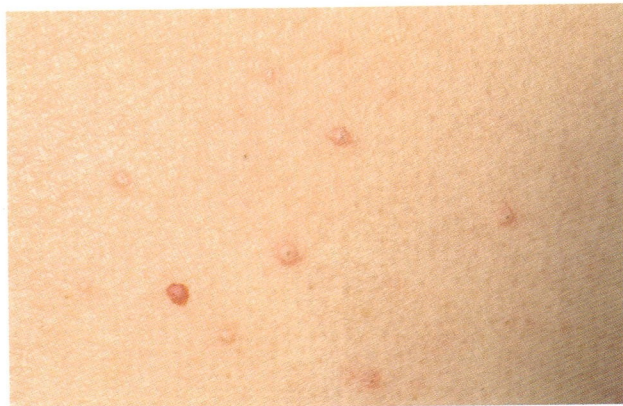

Figure 18–21 □ Penicilliosis. Erythematous papules, some with necrotic central umbilication on the trunk. The single bright-red lesion is a cherry angioma. *Penicillium marneffei*, the causative microorganism, is a dimorphic fungus endemic to Southeast Asia. Disseminated infection causes fever, cough, and a generalized rash, most commonly affecting the face, upper trunk, and arms. Genital and oral lesions have also been reported.

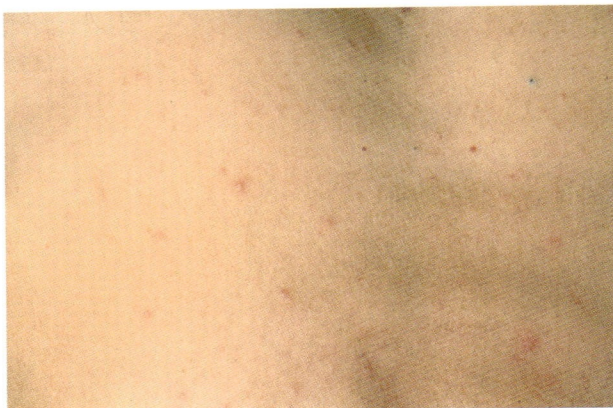

Figure 18–22 □ Penicilliosis. Similar erythematous papules on the chest. The differential diagnoses of a papular eruption in a febrile HIV-infected patient includes cutaneous cryptococcosis, histoplasmosis, mycobacterial infection, penicilliosis, and an adverse drug eruption. Tissue smear or biopsy of the skin lesions will yield small (2 to 4 μm) yeast-like cells that are divided by a septum. The infection responds to amphotericin B and itraconazole.

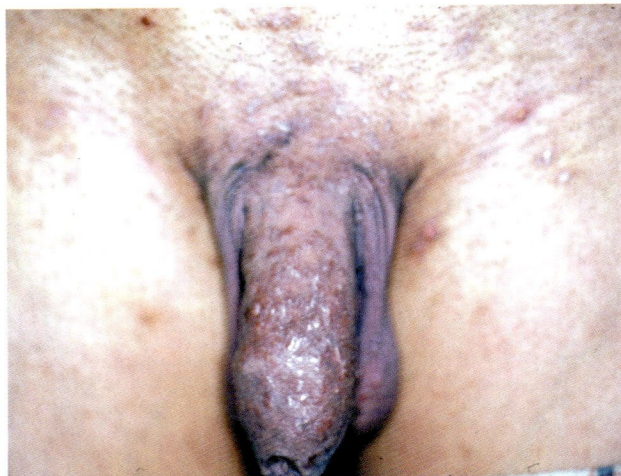

Figure 18–23 □ Scabies. Pruritic erythematous papules with excoriations involving the pubic region and genitalia. This is a common infestation, and immunosuppressed individuals have a high mite burden and are very infectious. Clinical presentation may be typical, affecting sites of predilection, e.g. hands, genitalia, or severe with crusted lesions. Diagnosis for mites is easily made from skin scrapings.

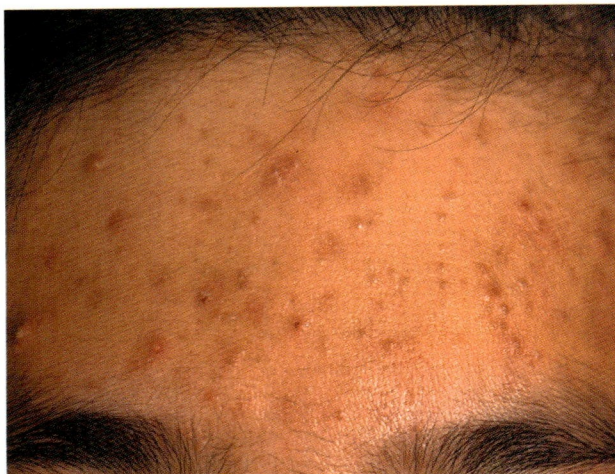

Figure 18–24 □ Scabies. Erythematous papules and nodules on the forehead. Facial involvement in adults is rare in HIV-negative individuals, but is commonly seen in those who are HIV-infected. A high index of suspicion is needed, and diagnosis is occasionally made only after a skin biopsy demonstrates the presence of mites. Treatment is with topical scabietic agents, whilst oral ivermectin is useful for severe cases. Post-scabietic dermatitis and itch may persist for several months.

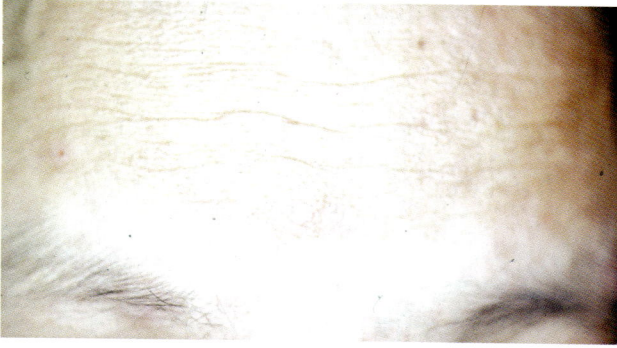

Figure 18–25 □ **Demodicidosis.** Follicular pruritic papular lesions on the forehead. Proliferation of *Demodex* mites within the hair follicles results in a pruritic papular eruption in the seborrheic areas. Diagnosis is usually made incidentally after a skin biopsy. The differential diagnoses are eczema and scabies. Treatment is with permethrin cream.

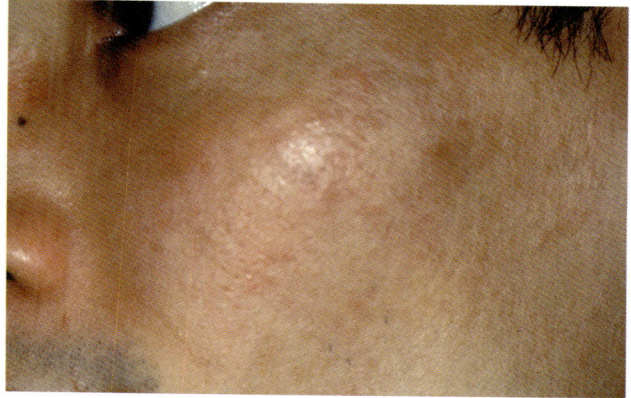

Figure 18–26 □ **Seborrheic dermatitis.** Erythematous, scaly papules and plaques on the cheek. This is commonly found in HIV-infected individuals and may be the result of increased *Malassezia furfur* colonization. The dermatitis affects the cheeks, eyebrows, sides of the nose, scalp, chest, and back. It is treated with anti-fungal and topical steroid preparations, selenium sulphide, and salicylic acid shampoos.

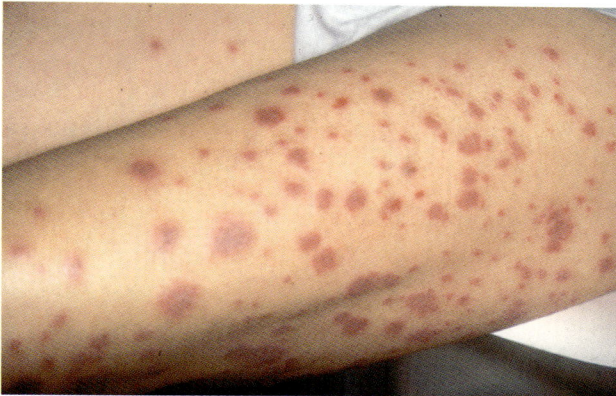

Figure 18–27 □ **Psoriasis.** Well-demarcated, annular, scaly, erythematous plaques on the thighs. Psoriasis is more common in HIV-infected individuals than in the general population (up to 6% versus 2%). In a third of cases, it is present before HIV seroconversion (group 1). In these cases, the disease behaves as in HIV-negative individuals. In two-thirds of cases, psoriasis appears after HIV seroconversion (group 2).

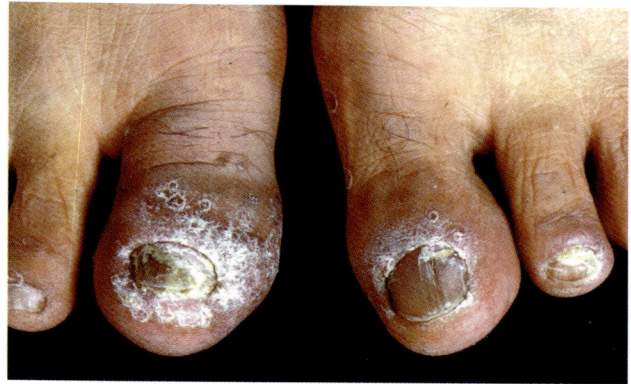

Figure 18–28 □ **Severe psoriatic onychodystrophy.** Thickened dystrophic toe nails with surrounding periungual psoriasis. Psoriasis in HIV-infected persons follows a more severe course, particularly in group 2 cases. Severe nail changes are commonly found.

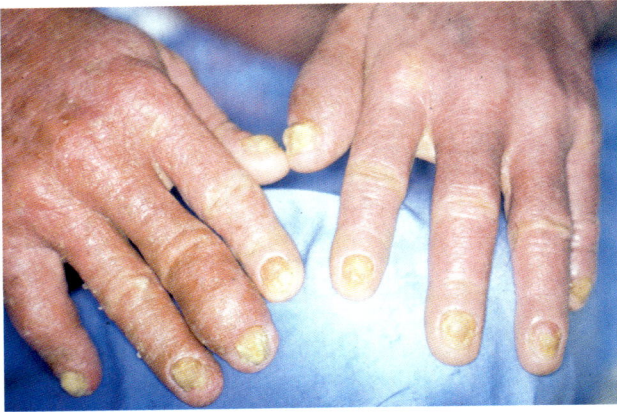

Figure 18–29 □ Psoriatic arthritis. Distal interphalangeal involvement with dystrophic finger nails. Rheumatic changes are commonly seen and usually signal a more aggressive course. Reiter's syndrome – arthritis, conjunctivitis, urethritis – is also more commonly seen and is associated with keratoderma blenorrhagicum on the palms and soles.

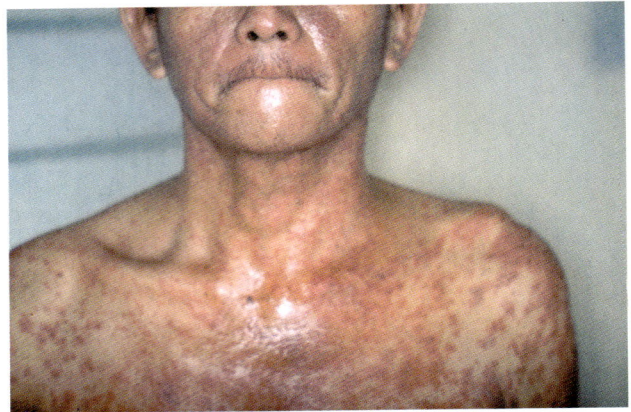

Figure 18–30 □ Unstable psoriasis. The onset of acute eruptive psoriasis or sudden exacerbations in a patient with previous chronic stable plaque psoriasis suggests the possibility of underlying HIV infection if the patient has risk factors.

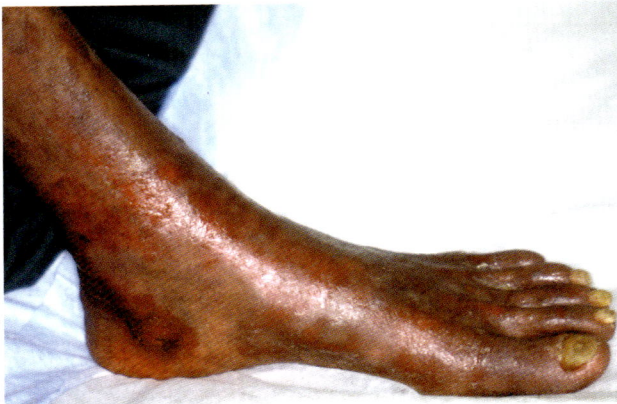

Figure 18–31 □ Psoriasis – methotrexate – induced skin erosions. This patient developed skin erosions soon after starting methotrexate (MTX). Treatment for psoriasis in HIV-infected patients is similar to that for HIV-negative patients except that extra care should be taken when administering immunosuppressive drugs like cyclosporin and MTX. Anti-retroviral therapy has been associated with better control of psoriasis.

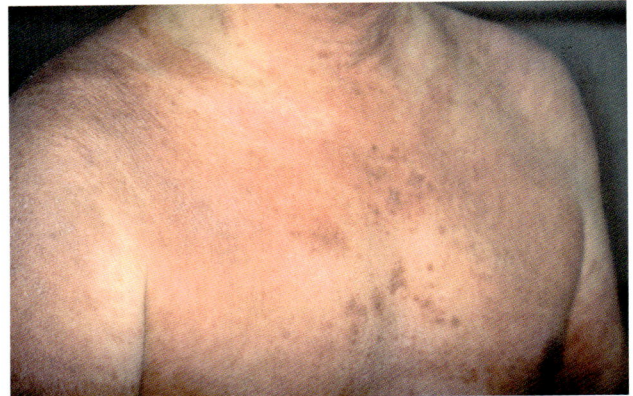

Figure 18–32 □ Adverse drug eruption to cotrimoxazole. This patient has an extensive eczematous eruption on the neck and trunk after taking cotrimoxazole. HIV-infected individuals are especially prone to side effects from anti-microbial and anti-retroviral medications. Cotrimoxazole used in the management of Pneumocystis carinii pneumonia (PCP) is the most common cause; allergy is seen in over 50% of patients taking the medication. Mild reactions can be tolerated and desensitization has been tried. More severe reactions (as in this patient) will require a change of medication and total avoidance in the future.

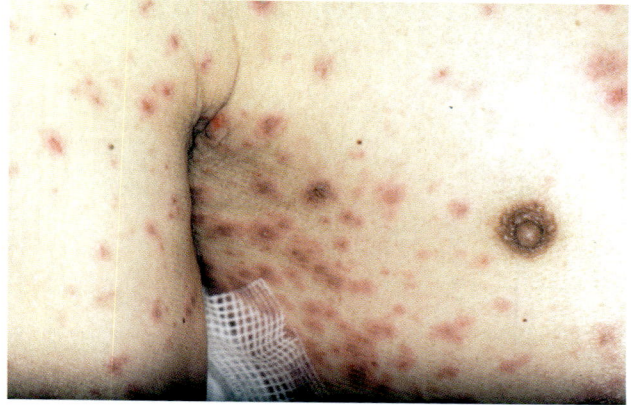

Figure 18–34 ▫ Erythema multiforme due to cotrimoxazole. Erythematous target lesions are seen on the trunk of this patient after taking cotrimoxazole. Progression to Steven-Johnson's syndrome and toxic epidermal necrolysis has been reported to sulphur drugs, anti-tuberculous medications, and to some anti-retroviral medications, particularly nevirapine and amprenavir.

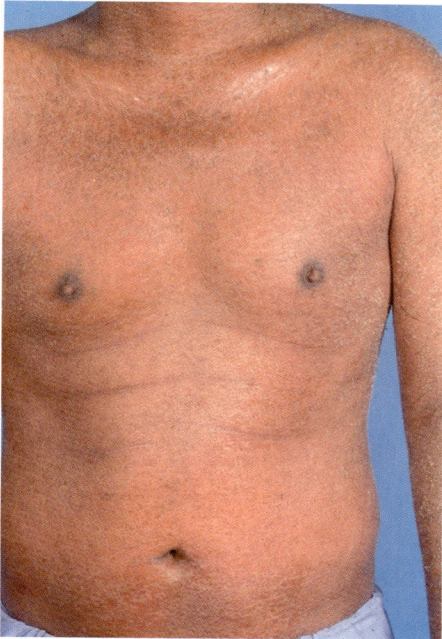

Figure 18–33 ▫ Erythroderma secondary to adverse drug eruption. Erythroderma due to dapsone allergy. Antituberculous medications are another common cause of ADR and often require careful re-challenge to elucidate the offending drug(s).

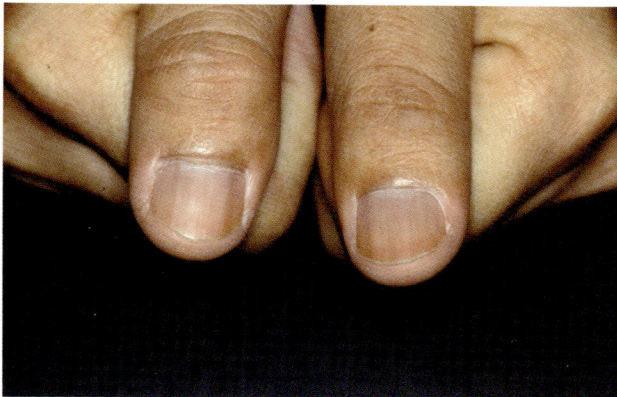

Figure 18–35 ▫ Nail pigmentation. Brown-black longitudinal and transverse linear pigmentation of the nail plates of this patient taking zidovudine (AZT). AZT-induced isolated or generalized hyperpigmentation of the skin and punctate mucous membrane hyperpigmentation have also been described. This pigmentation is due to melanin deposition and may be reversible.

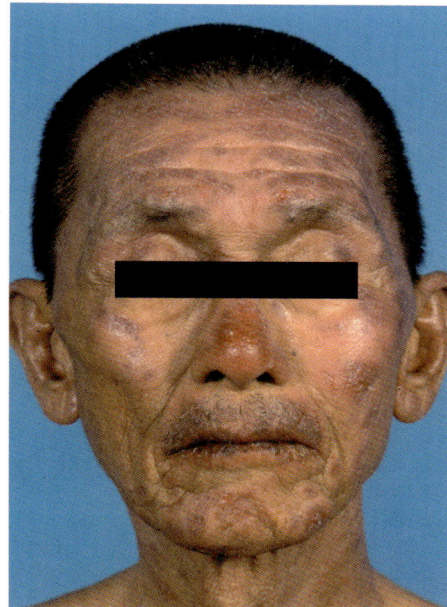

Figure 18–36 ▫ Photosensitivity. Erythematous plaques on the sun-exposed areas (face and neck). Photosensitivity in HIV-infected individuals may be the result of idiopathic chronic actinic dermatitis or may be drug-induced, as in this patient who is sensitive to cotrimoxazole.

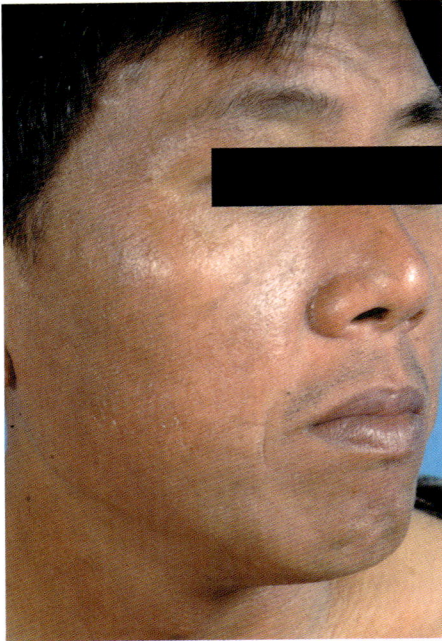

Figure 18–37 □ Porphyria cutanea tarda. Extensive erythema of the face. Porphyria cutanea tarda is another cause of photosensitivity. It is more commonly seen in HIV-infected patients than in the general population. This is the result of abnormal haem metabolism related to hepatitis.

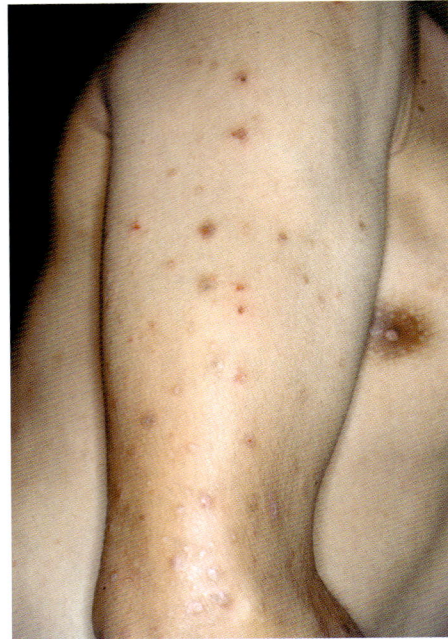

Figure 18–38 □ Pruritic papular eruption of HIV. Erythematous pruritic papules, mostly excoriated, on the arm. Pruritic papular eruption (PPE) is a very common skin condition in HIV-infected patients. The lesions are small, firm, well-demarcated, skin-colored papules. They may also be acneiform or follicular, and they do not form plaques. The lesions occur on the extremities and trunk, less on the face and are very pruritic. Their activity waxes and wanes.

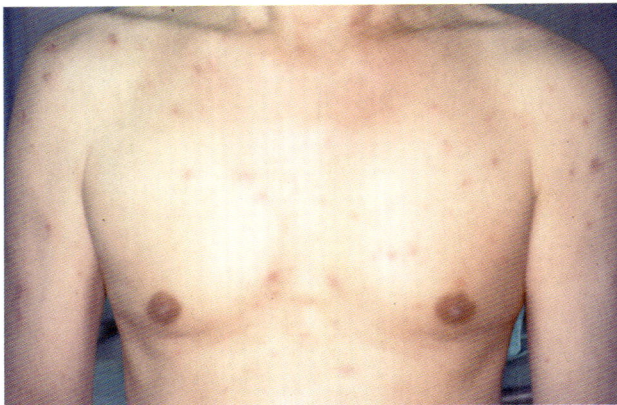

Figure 18–39 □ Pruritic papular eruption of HIV. Skin biopsy of the lesions shows a superficial and mid-dermal perivascular and perifollicular mononuclear cell infiltrate with numerous eosinophils. *Demodex* mites, *Malassezia furfur*, fungi, and bacteria are not associated findings. Treatment is unsatisfactory; strong topical steroids, systemic antihistamines, dapsone, UVB phototherapy, and PUVA photochemotherapy have been tried with limited success.

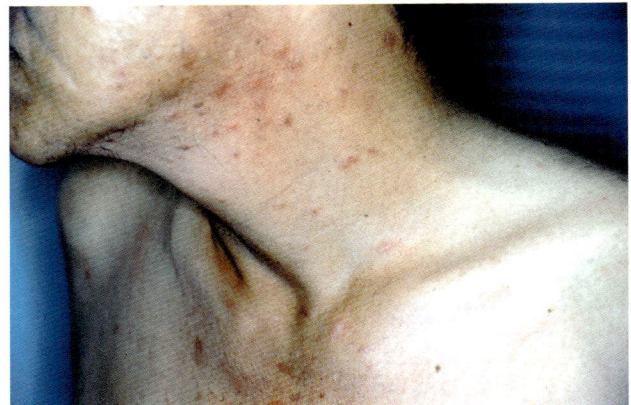

Figure 18–40 □ Eosinophilic folliculitis. Multiple urticarial pruritic follicular papules distributed over the trunk, head and neck, and proximal extremities. This is a non-infective chronic pruritic folliculitis, not to be confused with eosinophilic pustular folliculitis of Ofuji. It may lie within the spectrum of pruritic papular eruption. It is distinguished histologically by perivascular and perifollicular infiltrates with variable numbers of eosinophils.

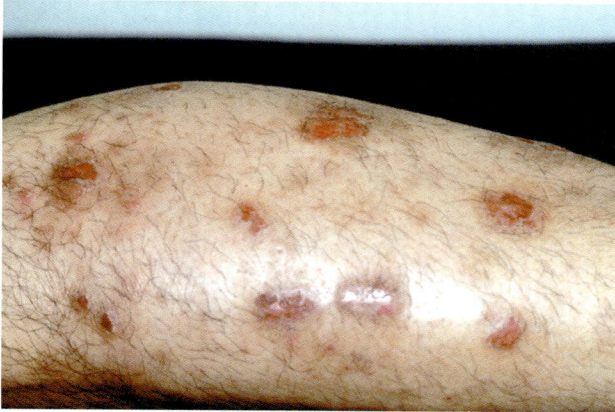

Figure 18–41 □ **Prurigo papules and nodules.** Erythematous pruritic lichenified nodules with excoriations on the forearm. Patients with pre-existing atopic dermatitis may experience worsening of the condition with progressive immunosuppression. Dermatitis is also exacerbated by xerosis and acquired ichthyosis often found in HIV-infected individuals. Chronic excoriations may lead to prurigo papules and nodules.

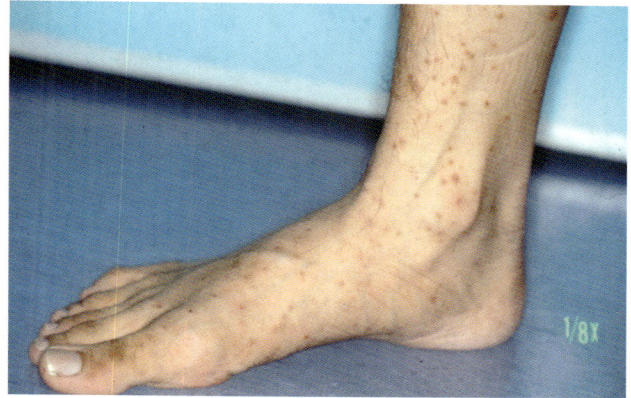

Figure 18–42 □ **Insect bite reaction.** Erythematous pruritic papules on the leg and dorsum of the foot. The differential diagnosis of a pruritic papular rash in an HIV-infected individual is long and includes an insect bite reaction (as was the final diagnosis in this patient), pruritic papular eruption, eosinophilic folliculitis, prurigo simplex, allergic drug eruptions, acneiform eruptions, scabies, and demodicidosis.

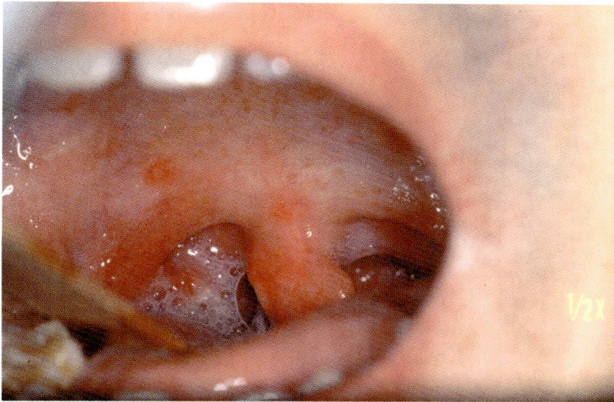

Figure 18–43 □ **Aphthous ulcers.** Multiple tender aphthous ulcers on the soft palate. Chronic severe painful ulcers may occur on the oral mucosa, pharynx, and esophagus. Differential diagnoses include herpes simplex virus infection and cytomegalovirus infection. Treatment ranges from topical corticosteroids, oral colchicine to thalidomide for intractable cases.

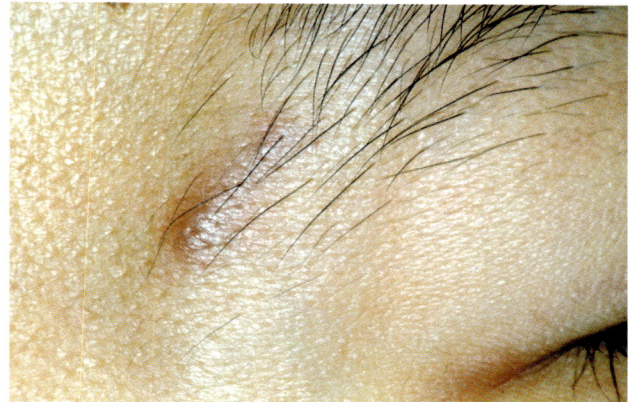

Figure 18–44 □ **Kaposi's sarcoma – early lesion.** Two asymptomatic violaceous papules on the eyebrow. In the pre-HAART era, Kaposi's sarcoma was one of the most common skin manifestations of AIDS. Early lesions start as erythematous macules with a bruise-like discoloration, progressing to violaceous, elevated lesions that may be scaly, oval, or round.

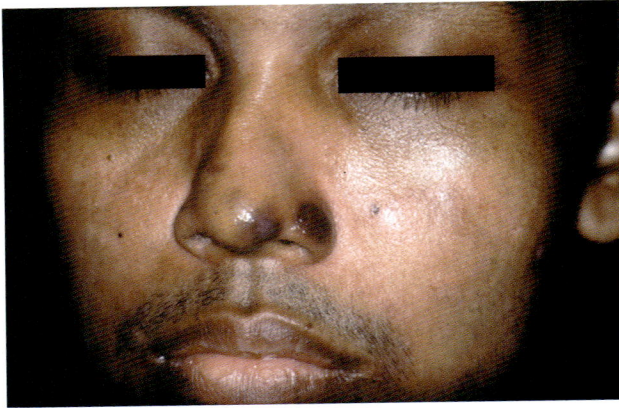

Figure 18–45 □ Kaposi's sarcoma. Violaceous, indurated nodules on the nose. Common sites affected are the lower extremities, upper trunk, head, neck, hand, oropharyngeal mucosa, occipital, and periauricular regions. Facial lesions are particularly disfiguring. Visceral involvement can involve the GIT, lymph nodes, liver, spleen, and kidneys.

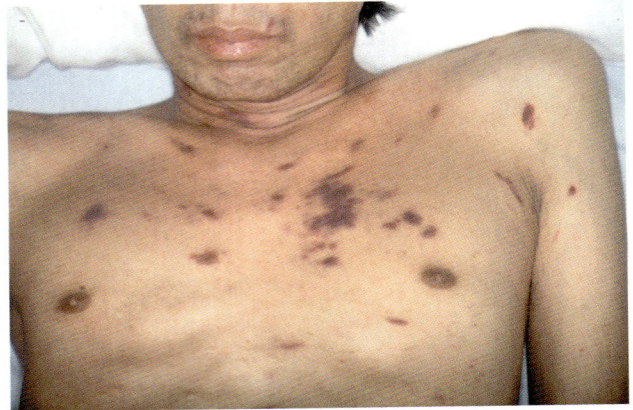

Figure 18–46 □ Kaposi's sarcoma. Nodules coalesce to form firm, hard tumors. Kaposi's sarcoma may precede, develop concurrently with other HIV-related symptoms, or develop late in the course of the disease. Skin lesions may occasionally resolve spontaneously.

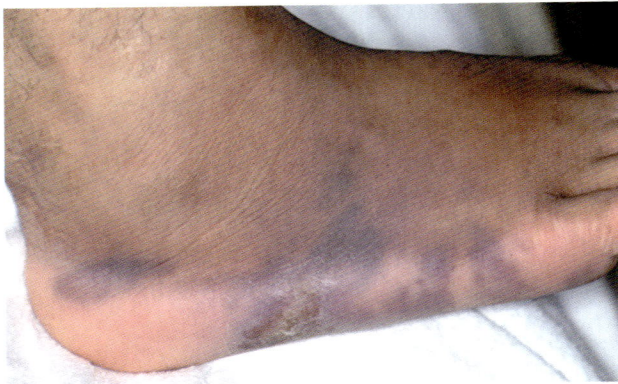

Figure 18–47 □ Kaposi's sarcoma. Lymphedema is especially pronounced on the distal extremities and the face. This may lead to skin ulceration, infection, pain, limit ambulation, and disfigurement. KS-associated herpes virus or HHV8 is the causative agent of Kaposi's sarcoma.

Index

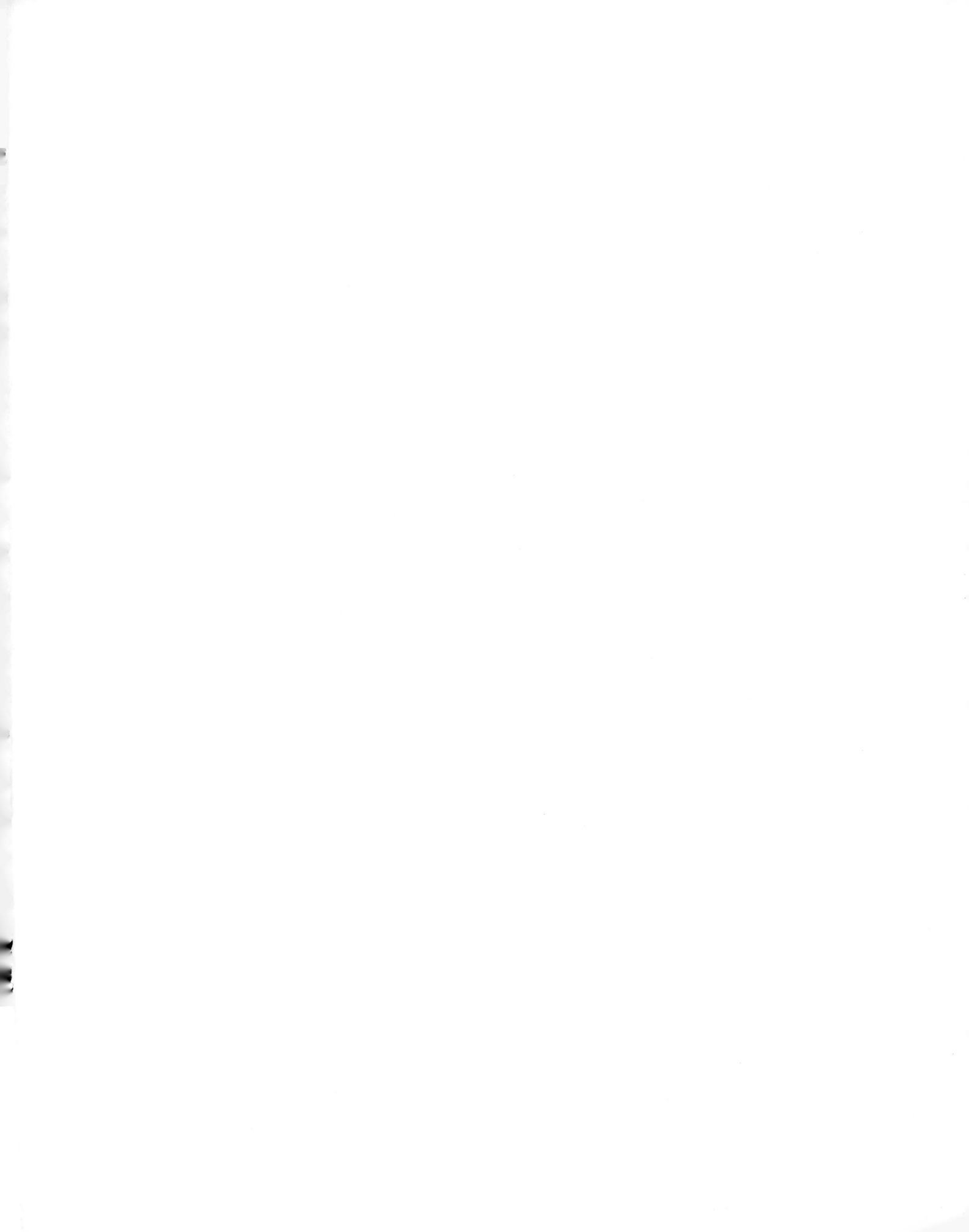

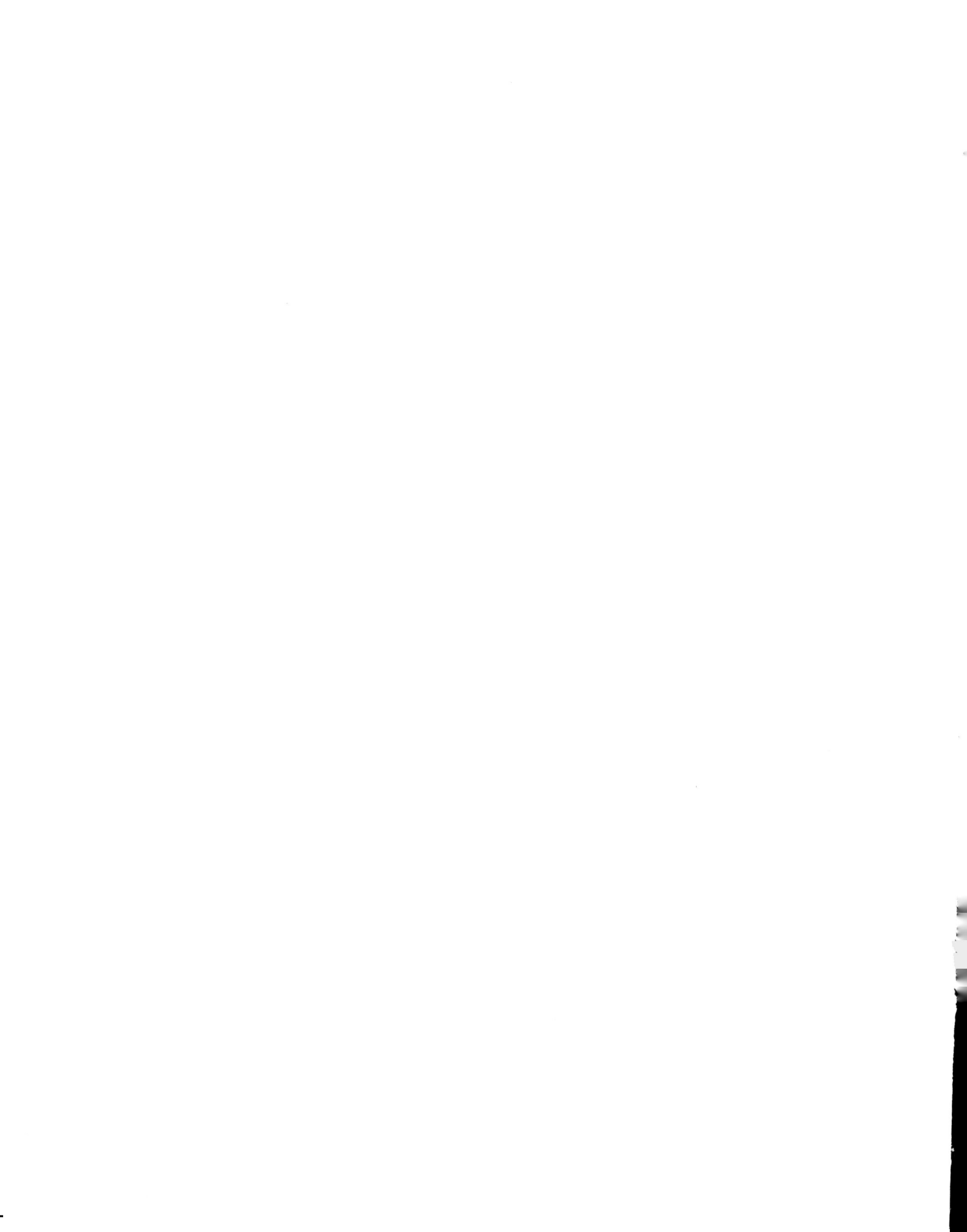